Integrative Assessment of Adult Personality

ERRATA

INTEGRATIVE ASSESSMENT OF ADULT PERSONALITY
Second Edition

Larry E. Beutler and Gary Groth-Marnat

The three equations on page 238 should read as follows:

Fake good = 41.225 + .273Do + .198Em + .538Gi − .255Wb − .168Fx
Fake bad = 86.613 − 1.000Cm − .191Wb + .203Ac − .110Fx
Random = 34.096 + .279Gi + .201Wb + .225Py + .157Fx

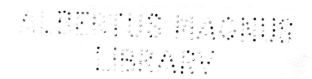

INTEGRATIVE ASSESSMENT OF ADULT PERSONALITY

Second Edition

LARRY E. BEUTLER
GARY GROTH-MARNAT

THE GUILFORD PRESS
New York   London

© 2003 The Guilford Press
A Division of Guilford Publications, Inc.
72 Spring Street, New York, NY 10012

Printed in the United States of America

This book is printed on acid-free paper.

Last digit is print number: 9 8 7 6 5 4 3 2 1

Library of Congress Cataloging-in-Publication Data

Beutler, Larry E.
  Integrative assessment of adult personality / by Larry E. Beutler, Gary Groth-Marnat.—2nd ed.
    p. cm.
  Includes bibliographical references and index.
  ISBN 1-57230-670-X
  1. Personality assessment.   2. Personality tests.   3. Adulthood—Psychological aspects.   I. Groth-Marnat, Gary.   II. Title.
BF698.4.B42 2003
155.2′8—dc21

                                                    2003001946

To Spencer, Parker, Sammi, and baby boy Beutler-Wells.
—LEB

To Dawn Erickson
—GG-M

About the Authors

Larry E. Beutler, PhD, is Distinguished Professor, Chair, and Director of Training at the Pacific Graduate School of Psychology in Palo Alto, California. He is Editor of the *Journal of Clinical Psychology* and former Editor of the *Journal of Consulting and Clinical Psychology.* Dr. Beutler is also a Fellow of the American Psychological Association (APA) and the American Psychological Society. He is a past president of the Society for Clinical Psychology (Division 12 of APA), a past president of the Division of Psychotherapy (APA), and a two-term past president of the international Society for Psychotherapy Research. Dr. Beutler is the author of approximately 300 scientific papers and chapters, and is the author, editor, or coauthor of 15 books on psychotherapy and psychopathology.

Gary Groth-Marnat, PhD, is in private practice in Santa Barbara, California, and is an Adjunct Professor at Pacifica Graduate Institute and the Fielding Institute. He has published more than 100 journal articles and chapters in books and is the author of *Handbook of Psychological Assessment* (2003, Wiley) and *Neuropsychological Assessment in Clinical Practice* (2000, Wiley). Previously, Dr. Groth-Marnat was Senior Lecturer in clinical health psychology at Curtin University in Perth, Australia.

Contributing Authors

Robert P. Archer, PhD, ABPP, is a Frank Harrell Redwood Distinguished Professor and Vice Chair of the Department of Psychiatry and Behavioral Sciences at Eastern Virginia Medical School in Norfolk, Virginia. He is the author of over 100 articles and book chapters related to psychological assessment. Dr. Archer is also the author of *Using the MMPI with Adolescents* (1987) and *MMPI-A: Assessing Adolescent Psychopathology* (1997), and coauthor of the *MMPI-A Casebook* (1994) and *Essentials of MMPI-A Assessment* (2002). He served on the advisory committee to the University of Minnesota Press for the development of the MMPI-A and is a co-author of the MMPI-A manual. In addition, Dr. Archer is the founding and current Editor of the journal *Assessment* and an Executive Board member and Diplomate of the American Board of Assessment Psychology.

Elizabeth J. Austin, DPhil, is Senior Lecturer in Psychology at the University of Edinburgh, Scotland. Her research interests include individual differences, personality, intelligence, and emotional intelligence.

Bruce Bongar, PhD, is the Calvin Professor of Psychology in the doctoral program in clinical psychology at the Pacific Graduate School of Psychology in Palo Alto, California, and Consulting Professor of Psychiatry and the Behavioral Sciences at Stanford University School of Medicine. He is a Diplomate of the American Board of Professional Psychology, a chartered psychologist of the British Psychological Society, and a Fellow of the American Psychological Association and the American Psychological Society. Dr. Bongar has also maintained a small practice for the past 20 years, specializing in psychotherapy, consultation, and supervision in working with the difficult and life-threatening patient.

James N. Butcher, PhD, is Professor of Psychology at the University of Minnesota. He is an internationally recognized scholar on personality assessment and has published widely on the MMPI. Dr. Butcher coordinated the effort to renorm and revise the MMPI, resulting in the creation of the MMPI-2. He is also Consulting Editor for several journals and past Editor of *Psychological Assessment*. He has conducted extensive research on such topics as abnormal psychology, cross-cultural personality, and computer-based personality assessment.

James Choca, PhD, is Professor in the School of Psychology at Roosevelt University in Chicago, Illinois, where he is also Director of the Doctoral Program. A lifelong interest in training and psychological evaluations has led to two books and a number of articles in these areas, particularly dealing with the Millon Clinical Multiaxial Inventory. Dr. Choca is currently involved in the development of a computerized psychological questionnaire, the Emotional Assessment System, designed to measure entities of the DSM-IV.

Martha R. Crowther, PhD, is Assistant Professor and Coordinator of the PhD/MPH program at the University of Alabama in Tuscaloosa. Her primary areas of research include examining the nature, impact, and consequences of custodial grandparenting as well as the relation between spirituality and well-being. Dr. Crowther has published journal articles and book chapters on psychology and aging and diversity in research and clinical training. She is a member of several professional associations including the Gerontological Society of America, the Southern Gerontological Society, and the American Psychological Association.

David A. C. Donnay, PhD, is Divisional Director for Research at CPP, Incorporated (formerly Consulting Psychologists Press), a company that provides assessment-based solutions to meet individual and organizational development needs. He has contributed to recent revisions of the Myers–Briggs Type Indicator and the Strong Interest Inventory instruments, as well as the very recently published Spectrum CPI 260 short form of the California Psychological Inventory. Dr. Donnay's principal research interests are in the areas of personality, career, and executive assessment.

Thomas Dunn, PhD, is Assistant Professor of Psychology at the University of Northern Colorado. His research interests include psychological assessment, malingering, posttraumatic stress disorder, and factors influencing performance of those working in the emergency services.

Timothy R. Elliott, PhD, is Associate Professor and Psychologist in the Department of Physical Medicine and Rehabilitation at the University of Alabama at Birmingham. He is a Fellow of the American Psychological Association and a Diplomate in Rehabilitation Psychology of the American Board of Professional Psychology. Dr. Elliott's principal research and clinical interests are in the areas of health psychology and physical handicaps. He is also coeditor (with Robert G. Frank) of the *Handbook of Rehabilitation Psychology* (2000).

T. Mark Harwood, PhD, is Assistant Professor of Clinical Psychology at Humboldt State University in Arcata, California. His primary research interests include patient–treatment matching, therapist training, substance abuse, and depression. In addition to his teaching and research activities, Dr. Harwood is the Managing Associate Editor for the *Journal of Clinical Psychology*.

R. Sean Hogan, PhD, is a licensed psychologist in private practice in Del Mar, California. He also works as a Psychiatric Liaison for Scripps and Mercy Hospitals, and is an adjunct faculty member of the California School of Professional Psychology in San Diego.

Radhika Krishnamurthy, PsyD, is Associate Professor of Psychology at Florida Institute of Technology, where she teaches assessment courses in the Doctor of Psychology program and serves as Clinical Practicum Supervisor. She is a coauthor (with Robert P. Archer) of the *MMPI-A Casebook* (1994) and *Essentials of MMPI-A Assessment* (2002) and has published several articles on the MMPI-A and Rorschach. Dr. Krishnamurthy serves as Associate Editor of *Assessment*, Consulting Editor for the *Journal of Personality Assessment*, Consulting Editor for *Psychological Assessment*, and Associate Editor of the *SPA Exchange*. She is a Fellow of the Society of Personality Assessment and a member of its Board of Trustees.

Steven Kvaal, PhD, is Associate Professor and Director of Training in the School of Psychology at Roosevelt University in Chicago, Illinois. He also maintains a clinical practice at the Swedish Covenant Pain Center in Chicago. Dr. Kvaal's teaching, research, and clinical work focus on health psychology, particularly the treatment of chronic pain.

Richard W. Lewak, PhD, is a licensed psychologist in private practice in Del Mar, California, and is an adjunct faculty member of the California School of Professional Psychology in San Diego at Alliant International University. Dr. Lewak is a Diplomate of the American Board of Assessment Psychology and has coauthored three books on the MMPI and MMPI-2.

Gerald Matthews, PhD, is Professor of Psychology at the University of Cincinnati. He has a lengthy publication list in the areas of personality, stress, cogntion, and emotional intelligence.

David Mohr, PhD, is Associate Professor in the Departments of Psychiatry and Neurology at the University of California, San Francisco (UCSF), a research psychologist at the San Francisco VA, and Director of the UCSF Behavioral Medicine Research Center. He maintains an active research program on the development and evaluation of psychotherapeutic interventions, as well as testing the efficacy of these interventions in altering pathogenic processes in inflammatory illnesses.

Paul D. Retzlaff, PhD, is Professor of Psychology at the University of Northern Colorado. He has published extensively on the MCMI-I, MCMI-II, and MCMI-III. Dr. Retzlaff's psychometrics and assessment work includes theory, test construction and validation, software development, selection and classification, and multivariate applications in intelligence, neuropsychology, personality, and psychopathology across the aerospace, military, corrections, and pharmaceutical industries.

Rita Rosner, PhD, is a psychologist and lectures currently at the Fridrich-Schiller-University in Jena and the Ludwig-Maximilians-University in Munich, Germany.

Her major area of research is war traumatization in civilians. Dr. Rosner's published papers focus on psychotherapy research and psychological assessment.

Donald H. Saklofske, PhD, is Professor of Educational Psychology and Special Education and Associate Professor in the Department of Psychology at the University of Saskatchewan. He has published extensively on individual differences, personality, intelligence, and psychological measurement and assessment.

Vicki L. Schwean, PhD, is Professor and Head of the Department of Educational Psychology and Special Education at the University of Saskatchewan. She is also Associate Professor in the Department of Psychiatry. Dr. Schwean's research publications focus mainly on behavior disorders, attention-deficit/hyperactivity disorder, and psychological assessment.

Forrest Scogin, PhD, is currently Professor of Psychology and the Director of Graduate Studies at the University of Alabama in Tuscaloosa. His research has been primarily in the areas of psychotherapy, depression, and clinical geropsychology. Dr. Scogin has authored or coauthored over 80 articles, book chapters, and books on these topics. He is a Fellow of APA Divisions 12 (Clinical) and 20 (Adult Development and Aging). He is also chair of the APA's Committee on Aging and chairs the Section II, Division 12 taskforce on evidence-based treatments for older adults.

Ronald A. Stolberg, PhD, is currently a therapist at the Winston School, a private school in San Diego specializing in educating children with learning disabilities. He is also a member of the adjunct faculty in the Department of Psychology at National University. Dr. Stolberg's research interests focus on personality assessment and the sensitivity and specificity of existing personality instruments for the identification of individuals at risk for self-harm and suicide.

Oliver B. Williams, PhD, is currently CEO of Center for Behavioral HealthCare Technologies, Inc., a company that he cofounded with Larry Beutler. He is also a marketing analyst, applications developer, and consultant with numerous corporations in the western United States. Dr. Williams's areas of research and theoretical interest bridge psychopathology, psychophysiology, and treatment. He has written computer programs for clinical patient assessment, data collection, and statistical analysis. He has also written software in several programming languages for respondent/questionnaire applications, graphics and text displays, neuropsychological assessment, and data management.

Moshe Zeidner, PhD, is Professor of Educational Psychology and Dean of Research at the University of Haifa, Israel. He has published numerous research studies with a focus on anxiety, stress and coping, the personality–intelligence interface, psychological testing, and emotional intelligence.

Preface

This book addresses the task of developing integrated adult psychological assessments. As such, we hope it will fill an important need for both established practitioners and students. Most books on assessment provide information on test construction, various tests, and interpretations of patterns of scores. However, they do not provide concepts, strategies, and guidelines on how to combine this information into a coherent interpretation and a problem-oriented psychological report and treatment plan. Instead, concepts and strategies are based on single dimensions or single tests. This single-dimension approach is likely to result in invalid conclusions and incorrect predictions. The conclusions will be invalid not because of anything inherently faulty in the source of information or in the accuracy of the observations, but because a single source or type of information is limited in how accurately it reflects real-world experience.

The above situation is similar to the well-known metaphor about the blind men who were trying to determine the nature of an elephant by touching a part of it. The blind man who touched the long trunk concluded that the elephant was one thing; the blind man touching the leathery and wide leg of the elephant concluded that it must be something else again. Each of the blind men might have been quite accurate in describing what he had touched. None, however, was correct in drawing a generalization about the creature based on what he had touched. They were not correct because they had obtained useful but insufficient (unintegrated) data. The data we collect during the process of personality assessment are useful to the extent we can translate the "snapshots" derived from each instrument into an accurate "moving picture" of the patient or client.

Personality assessment, as a general rule of thumb, is not based on a single issue or observation. An individual's assessment should not be based solely on his or her responses to an MMPI or an MCMI. Similarly, although a clinical interview is extremely important, it may not yield an accurate picture of a patient, unless it is supplemented by objective, normative data. In undertaking a comprehensive assessment of a patient, it is important to collect and utilize a variety of sources and types of information, including psychological testing data, observations, interviews, and collateral reports. It is just as important (or even more so) to integrate that information.

Like the authors of many other textbooks, we began this book because of our belief that there was something missing in the array of textbooks available to our students. Because of the decision of previous authors and editors to focus on one test, a variety of formal tests, or clinical interviewing and observational methods, most of the textbooks currently available are not well suited to constructing the "moving picture" of a complex personality. Few focus on the integration of various observations and the use of the assessment in treatment planning. This narrow view has obscured the fact that personality assessment is not merely a matter of psychological testing or clinical interviewing.

But this book is not designed only for graduate students. The need for integration and systematic observation is at least equally present among practicing professionals. Thus, in undertaking this volume we attempted to step beyond the classroom and address clinicians' needs for information on treatment planning. Clinicians have suffered the constraints of managed care for a decade and, with it, have been discouraged from using formal psychological measurement methods. We believe that this text provides viable options to the common practice of relying solely on an unstructured interview, which current practice encourages. By targeting the assessment process to the questions asked of practitioners and providing more integrative and respectful ways of gathering data, we believe that more focused, efficient, and effective assessments can be conducted.

Our recognition of the weaknesses in available textbooks has always been clearest when we have taught classes and practica in psychological assessment. However, the weaknesses of traditional assessment practices are also apparent in clinical practice. In trying to address these weaknesses, we have each drawn from our efforts to teach assessment practica and to conduct clinical assessments in an integrated manner. In our work, we have always attempted to lead students and professionals to the recognition that personality assessment is partly art and partly science. It is with our students and colleagues in mind, together with a focus on teaching the scientific and artistic aspects of assessment in an integrative manner, that we have organized this book. As we view it, personality assessment is a process that includes the administration, scoring, and interpretation of psychological tests; clinical interviewing, observation, and the gathering of historical and collateral information; and, finally, the integration of those unique pieces of information, so that the final product can be used to predict the patient's functioning reliably and validly and to develop plans that address the clinical needs for treatment.

The integration of assessment information can be understood on a number of different levels. One level requires a conceptual translation of discrete findings into a meaningful description of the client. This level, which was the primary focus of the first edition of this volume, was derived from the observation that many psychological reports do not provide an integrated picture of the patient or client. Instead, they remain at the level of unintegrated summaries of test findings. Signs of such a psychological report are the use of phrases such as "test scores indicate . . . ," "an elevation on scale 5 suggests . . . ," "other persons with similar profiles have been described as . . . ." Poorly integrated reports might also be produced when "clinicians" cut and paste information from computer-generated interpretations. Referral sources do not want to know about "test scores" or "persons with similar profiles" —they want to know about *their particular* client. Just because other people with similar scores had certain characteristics does not then mean that their client also has those characteristics. The philosophy and strategies outlined in this book teach, and encourage, clinicians to combine all sources of data so that their conclusions reflect a combined (integrated) approach rather than a reiteration of single test or subtest findings. The reports are thus person-centered rather than test-centered, and they will help *solve problems* rather than merely *describe client populations.*

A second level of integration involves integrating the data and the assessment process with a *sensitivity to the demands of different referral contexts and populations.* Addressing this level of integration is an addition to this second edition. It acknowledges that a report written for a medical setting will be quite different from that written for a forensic setting. Each context has its own language, expectations, and audience. Comprehensive integration also requires a consideration of the challenges involved in assessing diverse populations. Assessing older patients entails different considerations from assessing younger persons. Special considerations also need to be made when assessing various ethnic groups. We have therefore included a chapter on assessing special populations as well as another chapter on assessing clients in different contexts (i.e., medical, forensic, school, etc.).

Finally, this second edition emphasizes the integration of assessment with the treatment process itself. We have accomplished this goal by expanding on the systematic approach to evaluating clients for treatment that was introduced in the first edition. This approach is embedded throughout the entire book. Our hope is that this will enable readers/practitioners to focus on those variables of assessment that are most relevant for providing treatment recommendations that will optimize outcome. This new focus represents a movement away from merely describing a client to providing information in a manner that facilitates treatment planning. Integrating assessment and treatment also involves providing feedback to the client. Such feedback should be done in a way that conveys a collaborative approach with the client and uses language that is most likely to facilitate client growth. We have thus included a chapter on how this feedback can best be offered. We believe that our efforts, as represented by these different levels of integration, enhance practitioners' skills. These skills will enable the creation of reports that are relevant and useful, and will facilitate interactions that will more effectively reduce clients' pain.

The chapters of this book are arranged to reflect a method of assessment and integration that proceeds from defining the referral question to providing client feedback and writing the psychological report. Chapters 1 and 2 provide basic information on test development, validation, clarifying the referral questions, clinical judgment, and test selection. The information and strategies contained in these chapters describe the initial steps clinicians enact during the early phases of assessment. Chapter 3 outlines those empirically supported variables that are most relevant to treatment planning. This approach ("Systematic Treatment Selection") is not only detailed in this chapter but is also integrated throughout the rest of the book. Chapters 4–9 focus on specific assessment procedures and domains: the clinical interview (Chapter 4), assessing intelligence and personality (Chapter 5), the Minnesota Multiphasic Personality Inventory–2 (MMPI-2; Chapter 6), the Millon Clinical Multiaxial Inventory–III (MCMI-III; Chapter 7), the California Psychological Inventory (CPI; Chapter 8), and the Rorschach (Chapter 9). Although these procedures are useful in obtaining important data regarding a client, these data still need to be related to the larger context of the patient or client. Thus Chapters 10 and 11 discuss the relation between assessment and special settings (i.e., forensic, medical) and special populations (i.e., ethnic groups). Finally, assessment information needs to be effectively communicated to the client and the referral source. Chapter 12 therefore discusses methods of providing feedback to the client, consulting with the referral source, and guidelines for making decisions regarding clients. Since data also need to be formally written into a psychological report, Chapter 13 provides general guidelines, a specific structure, and samples of how to write a psychological report.

This book is the result of many years of work, on both our parts, assessing clients, teaching students, and carefully considering how the assessment might best be accomplished. It would not have been possible without the willing efforts and struggles on the part of students and clients. We have learned from all of you, and we thus extend to you our heartfelt thanks. Of course, writing this book has also been a rich process of learning to work with each other as well. We have enjoyed this process and have found our views to be surprisingly compatible and our interaction highly rewarding.

Many others deserve our additional thanks. Each of the authors who contributed chapters did excellent work. We especially wish to thank them for the efforts they made in sharing our vision of what was involved in "integrative assessment." We know that some of you struggled with this approach. In the end, we are proud of each and every chapter. Our editor at The Guilford Press, Jim Nageotte, provided us with much encouragement and support (as well as patience for yet one more request for an extension of the deadline). Working with him was a pleasure. Our thanks to each of you for making this project possible.

LARRY E. BEUTLER
GARY GROTH-MARNAT

Contents

1

Introduction to Integrative Assessment of Adult Personality

Larry E. Beutler,
Gary Groth-Marnat,
and Rita Rosner

The clinician's skills in integrating sources of information, contemplating the meanings of discrepant cues, formulating opinions, and persuading others to listen constitute the focus of this book. This process involves four steps: (1) identifying the problem, (2) selecting measurement instruments, (3) integrating sources of information about the problem, and (4) deriving and reporting conclusions, opinions, and recommendations.

In this volume, we are concerned with problems that relate to personality. Thus the four steps revolve around issues related to enduring aspects of a person's behavior and applying corrective experiences to those behaviors that are problematic. That is, this book is designed to help clinicians assess a patient's or client's personality in a way that makes a difference in how he or she is subsequently treated in a clinic, hospital, other mental health agency, or even in everyday contact.

Personality is a social construct that refers to behaviors that are socially relevant, enduring, and that are assumed to reflect certain motivational properties. Within a description of an individual's "personality" are dimensions and clusters of related dimensions that describe his or her pre-dilections to behave, feel, and interact. All of these dimensions reflect, directly or indirectly, an aspect of social behavior. People are distinguished from one another, not so much by whether certain traits, such as anxiety, are present, but by the pattern of these traits. Most people have some level of most personality traits. Distinctions among people replete both the amount or intensity of the traits and the patterns with one another. *Personality* designations describe the relative strengths of different traits when compared to other people as well as to other traits. The pattern of behavioral traits—the relative strengths and weaknesses of the traits—forms a social profile that is used by others to describe, and distinguish among, people.

Clearly, not all traits fall within the domain that we call *personality.* Personality traits are assumed to evolve, at least partially, through a process of development, social learning, and choice. A person may have a trait of "baldness"; this is a distinctive quality that transcends situations, but it is devoid of the social behavior and choice aspects that characterize a personality trait.

Because they imply choice, the traits of personality are assumed to reflect aspects of an individual's motivations and aspirations. However, these traits vary in the degree to which, and the directness with which, they signify the presence of both motives and emotions. Some traits directly identify an assumed emotional quality. Thus a person may be said to be a "happy," "anxious," or "moody" person when a particular temperament or pattern of temperaments is frequently present and manifest in a variety of situations. Other traits are described in less affective ways that more directly reflect social interactions. Thus a person may be said to be "gregarious," "extroverted," "introverted," "ascendent," "motivated," "intelligent," "outgoing," "reclusive," or "passive," reflecting different qualities of his or her social behavior, and by inference, social motives or aspirations.

Thus critical to a quality being identified as a "personality trait" are both its reference to socially significant behavior and the assumption that the trait transcends any particular social environment. Simply put, traits are enduring qualities of behavior, distinguished from transitory and situation-specific states of being or feeling. The "behavior" to which these traits refer may involve an external act or an internal motivating process. When a person is described in the terms of personality, a picture is painted of his or her distinctive and volitional predispositions to act. To illustrate the differences among states and traits, on one hand, and personality and nonpersonality traits, on the other, try a thought game.

How would we describe the personalities of George H. W. Bush, Bill Clinton, and Ronald Reagan? In certain ways, these individuals are distinguished from other people. They are all male, and they all are past presidents of the United States. These are attributes and roles that endure, but neither being male nor being a past president can be defined as a personality characteristic. Being male is an attribute that is independent of learned behavior, and being a past president reflects a consequence of social behavior but is not a specific social behavior in itself. Neither term, therefore, reflects identifiable social, volitional, or emotional qualities that are attributable to learning and development.

What personality qualities distinguish these three men? What are the enduring aspects of their social behavior, their dispositions to respond in certain patterned ways? How do these patterned behaviors distinguish one person from another? There are many differences among these three men, but which ones are relevant enough to select as "distinctive," and which are volitional and enduring enough to be called "personality"? To which one would we be most likely to apply the descriptors "nice," "honest," "bright," "sneaky," "dominant," "strong," "tender," or "resourceful"? These are terms that reflect social behaviors, motives, and durability and are often used to describe personality.

In deciding that some of these terms describe our ex-presidents' personalities, we make some important, implicit assumptions. We assume that honesty, sneakiness, niceness, and the like, are qualities that these men carry with them from one situation to another. They are honest in all or most situations; they are sneaky under many conditions; they are nice in most things they do; and so on. That is, these behaviors are not situational; they are recognizable behaviors and behavioral dispositions that will be seen in many situations. We also assume that the behaviors referenced by these terms are meaningful and relevant, and that they relate to other characteristics, the totality of which represents the individual's personality. For what roles and tasks are these traits relevant? For what roles and tasks are they irrelevant? Which of these characteristics are associated with one another? Which are likely to change when the person is not in the role of president?

Psychological assessment is designed to answer such questions, as well as other questions, that have implications for clinical decisions. If an individual's personality describes a relatively unique pattern of interrelated response tendencies that cut across a large number of situations, there must be some way of describing these tendencies that is more specific than simply applying a categorical label, such as "weak," "honest," "extroverted," and the like. Psychological "assessment" or "measurement" is the application of a system of classification or numbering to these qualities, in order to describe the patterns that exist among the qualities and the individual differences that exist among people.

The objectives of psychological assessment in clinical settings involve answering questions that pertain to six clinically relevant domains of behavior: (1) the individual's diagnosis or disorder; (2) the etiology or causes of the disordered behavior; (3) the prognosis or anticipated course of this problem; (4) the nature of the treatments that may ameliorate or alter that course or prognosis; (5) the degree of functional impairment in both routine and specialized life functions; and (6) the person's pattern of strengths and adaptive capacities.

To answer questions relevant to these domains, we must be able to differentiate between behaviors that are a product of single situations (i.e., states) and those that are more general products of personalities (i.e., traits). We also must be able to distinguish between normal or usual behavior and abnormal or pathological behavior. Only by knowing what constitutes "usual" behaviors and "normal" responses to life's situations will a clinician be able to identify the nature and severity of behavioral disturbance and to assess the relevance of the measured behaviors for the questions asked.

WHAT IS THE VALUE AND NATURE OF PSYCHOLOGICAL ASSESSMENT?

All kinds of people seek, or are referred for, psychological assessment. A troubled person may seek information about him- or herself in order to help him or her solve a problem or change his or her feelings; a physician may seek information about a patient in order to identify what is causing a symptom; an adult child may seek information about a parent in order to understand a difficult behavior. Psychological assessment is the process of discovering the social patterns in another person's behavior by (1) distinguishing situational from enduring behaviors, (2) predicting how the person will respond to different situations, and (3) finding an environmental event or treatment that will help or allow a person to change a troubling self-related aspect.

Unfortunately, the already complex process of constructing a helpful picture of a complex person is made all the more difficult by several common practices that are associated with psychological assessment. One of these practices is derived from the custom of Western societies to view various professionals as "experts." This Westernized view of health and mental health professionals tends to perpetuate a fractionated view of patients and contradictory recommendations.

People who want to discover something about themselves or someone else have different ways of formulating the questions that they want answered. The way that they express a question is heavily determined by how the society in which they live has come to think about people who need help and those who are designated to serve them. Thus the questions raised about a person who is having difficulty are embedded within a cultural network that makes certain assumptions about people and about the nature of human behavior. Sometimes these cultural formulations are misleading, as can be seen in the way that psychological assessment is often used in medical or mental health settings by different professionals. The culture of modern, Westernized health care contains many different professions. These professions all claim to have some expertise about a portion of an individual's behavior. Thus, when a healthcare provider seeks to know something, he or she must decide which mental health professional has expertise in that particular area. Often this decision is tendered in such a way that it results in a fragmented view of people. It is not unlikely that a referring professional, who wants a broadly based picture of a person, will send a patient to a psychiatrist to get a "mental status examination"; to a psychologist to get a "personality," "mood," or "intellectual" evaluation; to a social worker to get a "social history"; and to a family practitioner to get a "medical history."

The terms used when professionals or others request consultation and assistance reflect the ways that people subdivide and categorize human experiences and functioning. The labels that we use to describe the domain(s) of behavior we want assessed (1) reveal those aspects of behavior we consider to be relevant, and (2) imply that this domain is different and distinct from other aspects of psychological performance. Such distinctions among different domains of assessment are usually quite arbitrary, however.

We believe that the implication that intelligence, mental state, and personality (among other constructs) are independent of one another creates an inaccurate, fractionated picture of a person. In the course of human functioning, "cognitive" and "intellectual" skills are not independent of "personality"; "mental status" is neither different nor legitimately dissociated from "emotional" or "behavioral" status; and so on. Nevertheless, because the different terms that have been used to describe assessment have been associated with different professional groups, by historical accident, it is not unusual for a client or patient to be referred to three or more different types of mental health professionals in order to obtain essentially the same service. By their unquestioned acceptance of such referrals, referents or consultants implicitly endorse the view that social history can really be considered independently of personality; that mental state can really be considered separately from emotional life; and that personality can exist independently of intelligence or thought. It is therefore not surprising that the recommendations and opinions of one professional may contradict that of other professionals. Indeed, such disparity among consultants is inevitable when members of each discipline frame their opinions in methods, language (jargon), and theories to which the other professionals are neither privy nor considered to hold expertise. In reading different reports from different professionals, it is often not apparent that they are describing the same person. This variability of results perpetuates the myth that different domains of functioning are really being assessed by these different methods.

Kopta, Newman, McGovern, and Sandrock (1986) have demonstrated the profound differences that various theoretical frameworks and procedures can make in the nature and cost of recommended treatment. We need not invoke the story of the blind men and the elephant (see the preface) to see the problems in this picture. Reducing the fragmented and contradictory nature of our descriptions of people promises to lead us to improved efficiency and accuracy when we plan and implement treatments.

A fragmented picture of the client also frequently emerges because of the way in which psychologists choose to report their findings—typically by reporting the conclusions from one psychological test or one type of procedure after another, as if each were of equal value and provided an equally comprehensive and valid view of the person. When reports are written in this "test-oriented" manner, the inevitable contradictions in the findings of different tests are either presented and ignored, omitted, or hastily excused in a summary paragraph. The failure to integrate and explain discrepancies in terms of *person* functions, rather than *test* functions, leaves the reader with a confused picture of the patient.

This book is written with the specific goal of eliminating, or at least reducing, this fragmented view of patients who undergo evaluation for behavioral and emotional problems. It is designed to help clinicians integrate information from different domains of patient experience and to make sense of the discrepant findings that exist among the sources of available information. We have undertaken three tasks in this book:

1. Provide an integrated model of personality and functional concepts that can be used to describe adult functioning efficiently and effectively within the context of responding to a wide variety of referral questions.
2. Outline a general method for resolving conflicts among data sources, while integrating and summarizing clinical information.
3. Provide representative and specific guidelines for extracting and integrating information from a few of the most frequently used and empirically defensible clinical assessment procedures.

The method presented for organizing and integrating sources of information is sufficiently general and flexible as to be applicable to many types of referral questions and assessment methods. Concomitantly, the specific procedures illustrated have been selected not only because of their frequency of use among clinicians, but because they can be adapted to address many of the questions that referents are likely to have in mind when they request "cognitive" assessment, "personality" assessment, "mental status" evaluation, and "diagnostic" testing.

SYSTEMATIC TREATMENT SELECTION:
A MODEL OF FUNCTIONAL ELEMENTS

As clinicians who attempt to respond to a request for psychological assessment, we are faced with the dilemma of deciding which implicit or explicit theoretical perspective we will use when defining qualities of the person and transmitting conclusions. We might ask ourselves a number of questions:

Should I conceptualize and communicate my opinions using the language of unconscious processes or speak only descriptively, of interpersonal ones?
Can or should I speak in a theory-free language?
Should I implicate biological correlates of personality as possible etiological factors in symptom development or stick with situational and environmental ones?

The professionals who refer patients come from many different theoretical perspectives. As consultants, we must be able to transmit findings that will make sense to them, within their own theoretical perspective. However, we often do not know what their perspective is, and even if we do, we may not share their belief in it. Resolving the dilemma of how to conceptualize and transmit our opinions is not as hard as it may initially appear if we make a simple decision to keep our observations (1) as close as possible to the actual, observable data; (2) largely descriptive rather than inferential; and (3) based on concepts whose relationship to the questions being addressed are supported by contemporary research findings.

Beutler and Clarkin (1990) originally developed a cross-theory model for assessing patient behavior that was specifically aimed at addressing the major questions typically encountered by psychological consultants and providing answers unfettered by theoretical jargon and concepts. They identified a set of descriptive patient variables that are implicated in subsequent decisions about treatment, course, prognosis, and the like. This system has become known as "Systematic Treatment Selection" (STS) because of its focus on treatment-related questions as a central perspective that binds together all of the usual referral questions. The STS conceptual system has been updated, refined, and empirically tested (Beutler, Clarkin, & Bongar, 2000; Beutler, Goodrich, Fisher, & Williams, 1999), a process that has resulted in the identification of a relatively small number of constructs and patient variables that can be assessed reliably and used in treatment decision making. The STS has spawned an assessment procedure, based on clinician ratings (Clinician Rating Form, CRF; Fisher, Beutler, & Williams, 1999a), that has been adapted to administration through a computer-interactive platform (Beutler, 2001; Beutler & Williams, 1999). This assessment system (STS-CRF) is described Chapter 3. However, it is imperative that the reader become acquainted with the STS conceptual system at this point, because it is used throughout this volume as the foundational structure for interpreting psychological assessment procedures.

Levels of Decision Making

The process of making decisions in psychological assessment can be conceptualized as proceeding from very general to very specific decisions. At each level, different types of information about the patient are used to make decisions, to respond to referral questions, and to construct treatment plans and recommendations. In formulating the STS model, Beutler and Clarkin (1990) identified four basic levels of information that are implicated in these decisions: (1) patient predisposing factors, (2) treatment-related contextual factors, (3) therapy procedures and therapist relationship qualities, and (4) fit of patient and therapy. Table 1.1 presents a brief outline of these four levels and the informational variables that are considered at each level.

TABLE 1.1. Levels of Systematic Treatment Selection

Patient predisposing factors

Problem characteristics: symptoms, functional impairment, complexity/chronicity
Personality traits: coping style, defensive traits, subjective distress, self-esteem, assets and strengths
Environment: social support, social history, breadth of positive functioning

Treatment contexts (level of care)

Setting: restrictiveness of care
Intensity: frequency and length of treatment
Mode: pharmacological, psychosocial, or both
Format: medication or psychosocial treatment class (i.e., individual, group, family, couple therapy)

Therapy procedures and therapist relationship qualities

Match of therapist and patient demographics and beliefs
Therapeutic actions: directiveness, insight versus skill and symptom focus, cathartic versus supportive, therapist skill and experience
Therapeutic alliance quality: collaboration and relationship strength

Fit of patient and therapy

Fit of functional impairment and complexity with setting, modality, format, and treatment intensity
Fit of coping style with insight orientation versus symptom/task focus of treatment
Fit of trait-like resistance to therapist directiveness
Fit of subjective distress with therapist support versus cathartic evocation

---

These different levels of information interact with one another as increasingly fine-tuned and complex decisions are addressed. Information from each of the four levels is useful only in relation to certain questions. It is the cascading influence of early levels on subsequent levels that allows us to address highly specific referral questions and refine specific treatment decisions (Beutler et al., 2000). For example, in order to address referral questions pertaining to patient diagnosis, level of functioning, or probable prognosis (level 1 questions), only information from the first level of information is needed. The therapist will need to know something about the patient's current and premorbid level of functioning: level of current and past social support, the chronicity and recurrence of the problem, preferred way of coping or interacting with others, how and under what conditions he or she resists the influence of others, and the nature of current symptoms, abilities, and strengths, including level of current distress and history of resilience after crises. This information can be used to respond to many different questions as well as to predict the course of symptom development and resolution.

The second level addresses questions about the optimal level of care (intensity, setting, mode of treatment, etc.) needed by the patient. To respond to such questions, clinicians must make decisions about whether the patient's predisposing qualities fit the available treatment environments. Questions about the desirable length and frequency of treatment, the degree of protective control needed, the advantages of medication and multiple-person treatments, and the selection of the treatment setting, for example, can only be answered by knowing which qualities of the patient serve as indicators for these decisions, what resources and assets are available, and the particular patient's standing on these various factors.

Questions pertaining to the third level of the STS model include such areas as how the patient is likely to interact with health care providers, how to enhance patient cooperation, what treatment model is the best fit for this patient, and how best to develop a good working treatment relationship. Responding to these questions about which particular therapist to use, what model of therapy to apply, or how to alter the patient's prognosis requires information from prior levels as well as knowledge of available treatment options. Information about therapist skill and training, methods that facilitate motivation, the use of relationship enhancement procedures, and the like, is used at this level of decision making.

Finally, the formulation of fine-tuned recommendations about which specific procedures best fit this patient requires an understanding of the patient's predisposing qualities (level 1), the context of the treatment received (level 2), the nature of the available therapist's training and experience in using different treatments (level 3), and the way in which different patient qualities moderate the influence of therapeutic procedures (level 4). At this latter level, questions about differential treatment effects can be addressed by describing the nature of specific applications of procedure to fit patient variables.

PATIENT PREDISPOSING CHARACTERISTICS

Beutler, Clarkin, and Bongar (2000) found that most of the questions posed to consulting psychologists can be addressed by beginning with the assessment of six general but fundamental qualities of patients, then adding to this information all knowledge about environmental demands and the nature of different treatment settings, treatment models, and treatment modes and formats. The clinician can construct responses to referral questions by reference to how these qualities fit certain treatment demands, availabilities, and functions.

Assessment of one's standing on six cross-theory qualities of patients serve as a beginning point for assessment. These to-be-assessed qualities include aspects both of the person and their social environment: (1) the areas of greatest impairment and strength; (2) levels of current and past social support; (3) the chronicity and complexity of the presenting problems; (4) typical and usual ways of coping with stress or resolving problems; (5) the degree of trust and compliance invested in interpersonal, helping relationships; and (6) the level of stress and discomfort currently experienced.

Functional Impairment and Areas of Social Support and Achievement

Assessment of a patient's level of functional impairment must include a determination of both deficits and areas of strength. The principle areas requiring assessment include levels of available support from others, access to social resources, the sense of attachment versus alienation from others, availability of social groups, proximity of family and friends, availability of role models, and the ability to maintain intimacy in relationship with others. These qualities are best assessed as objective qualities, or external perspectives, of behavior, rather than by an assessment of the person's subjective states (Strupp, Horowitz, & Lambert, 1997).

Assessing the positive presence of social attachments and personal resources, rather than just deficits and lack of attachments, is also important in this process. Thus level of social support is usually assessed in the course of assessing areas of impairment and strength. Lacking social support is very different from being actively abandoned or abused. Likewise, merely being in proximity to a friend or family member is significantly different from being actively engaged with other people, and having distal access to nonliquid financial resources is different from actually having money in hand.

The absence of social and financial resources, along with a sense of social isolation or alienation, are poor prognostic signs and suggest the need for enhancing the availability of these resources before other aspects of treatment can be expected to carry much weight. The presence of an intimate relationship, on the other hand, provides a degree of protection from the negative influences of the environment. All of these types of information are important in assessing a patient's level of social functioning.

Problem Complexity/Chronicity

The recurrence and comorbidity of problems are critical in understanding and predicting the course of treatment and a given patient's prognosis (Beutler et al., 2000). The elements that comprise an assessment of this dimensions include (1) information about the recency and length of time during which the patient has had difficulties, (2) the degree of social disruption or stability in his or her life (e.g., maintenance of work and school roles) because of these problems, and (3) the variety of life roles affected by these difficulties.

Stated more simply, assessing the degree of problem complexity requires an understanding of the duration, relapse history, and comorbidity of the patient's presenting problem(s). These factors allow the clinician to estimate the degree to which the patient's problems impair multiple life roles (family, love, work, leisure). Notably, there are indices of positive patterns that tend to protect us from developing chronic and complex problems. An investment in leisure activities, the presence of at least one intimate tie, along with extended periods in which the patient has not manifested social and behavioral problems are positive factors that delimit the patient's problem complexity and improve his or her prognosis for recovery and maintenance.

Coping Style

When interacting with others, and especially when confronted with decisions, problems, and obstructions to their needs or goals, people engage in relatively consistent patterns of behavior that are designed to restore order and reduce discomfort. These characteristic styles of behaving are enduring, trait-like, social, and imply different objectives and motives. Thus they reflect aspects of personality. Efforts to cope with or resolve the problems that arise in daily life, including efforts to escape from stress, can be described as "coping styles" (Beutler, 1983). Simplistically stated, coping styles can be represented by two broad patterns: (1) attempting to resolve problems and escape pain by turning inwardly and thinking, or intentionally not thinking, about the problem, and (2) acting outwardly and directly, on or against the problem. Of course, most people do some of each. They think and they act. It is the relative balance of these two types of behaviors and the order of their use that defines a person's coping style as either "internalizing" (a dominance of thinking and feeling) or "externalizing" (a dominance of acting).

People with an internalizing coping style may reason through a problem, question their own adequacy, insulate and remove themselves from the situation emotionally, divert their attention and thoughts to less threatening objects, or build defenses around their emotions to prevent their acknowledgment or expression. Any or all of these behaviors identify a process of looking inwardly for the solution to problems. Characteristically, internalizing includes, on the negative end of the continuum, self-blame, depression, emotional restriction, avoidance of others, social withdrawal, and exaggerated or restricted emotions; and on the more positive end, a search for internal resources. An externalizing coping style is associated with the relative reliance on behavior, rather than thoughts, reasoning, and feelings, to solve problems. Such people are typically described as "impulsive." An externalizing individual views the source of the problem as external; it is caused, controlled, and resolved by factors outside of the self. These individuals may place blame on others or the environment and feel victimized by fate or insidious intention. In response to these feelings, they may attack the source of frustration, become active in resolving the problem, get involved in an alternative activity, translate the problem explanation into some deficit of physical functioning, or impulsively flee the distressing environment (the "geographical cure").

These externalizing coping strategies are sometimes seen in people who have high needs for stimulation, those who do not carefully think through their decisions before acting, and those who have had problems with the law and authorities at school or work. These individuals are prone to (1) taking drugs to either escape or to keep themselves stimulated, (2) attacking and blaming other people for their problems, or (3) running away. On the positive side, they also tend to take an active role in solving their problems and are not prone to fearful immobilization.

Interpersonal Compliance and Resistance

One way to achieve what is needed to feel safe and solve problems is to rely on those who seem to have more power and authority than we have. Compliance with a treatment recommendation or even entering treatment at all requires (1) some degree of interpersonal trust, (2) the ability to set aside "ego" issues, and (3) a willingness to comply with what the expert advises. At the other end of the spectrum of resistance, a person may (1) rebel against the influence of others, (2) act as if he or she can do everything unaided, and (3) even become oppositional when dealing with those who have either authority or control over him or her. Since such patterns tend to be repeated across situations, "resistance" level reflects a quality of personality. However, most people are likely to resist when their behavioral options are eliminated. Thus situational demands also exert a significant influence in defining a person's level of resistance. *Resistance is both a state and a personality trait.*

Since most of the problems that cause people either to seek or be sent for help involve other people, it is very important to know the degree to which patients or clients are prone or likely to comply and cooperate with those who make suggestions or otherwise attempt to limit their choices. Individuals who are highly prone and vulnerable to being resistant tend to see others as unfriendly, controlling, and demanding. Compliant individuals, in contrast, may perceive the same people as being interested, friendly, and thoughtful. An assessment of these enduring perceptual dispositions can do much to help us predict how and if a person will be receptive to treatment or to the advice tendered by the psychological consultant.

Level of Subjective Distress

Level of dysphoria or unhappiness is a rough indicator of the degree to which an individual perceives the presence of a problem. Discomfort often serves as a motivator for initiating treatment or some other action, and treatment itself may seek to (1) increase motivation by making a patient anxiously aware of his or her difficulty, or (2) reduce the distress to manageable levels. Thus subjective distress is an important aspect of patient functioning, and it is implicated in diagnostic, prognostic, functioning, and treatment decisions. Unlike level of functional impairment, however, this dimension must be assessed by accessing the patient's subjective state. Many patients may function quite well in their social world but still experience a good deal of anxiety about their performance, adequacy, and future. Tapping both objective (functional impairment and resources) and subjective (dysphoria, euthymia, and felt support) dimensions of the individual's functional level is necessary for effective planning and decision making.

Applying Principles of Treatment Planning to Psychological Assessment

Obtaining multilevel sources of information has implications for how clinicians respond to the range of referral questions identified in this chapter. Beutler and colleagues (2000) have illustrated the nature of these dimensions by using them to formulate a set of cross-cutting principles that guide treatment decisions. These authors differentiate between basic and optimizing change principles—a distinction that reflects the specificity of the question being addressed in relation to the particular characteristics of one or more interpersonal relationships, especially the treatment relationship. Thus the basic principles can be used to guide assessment that addresses questions within the first two levels of information. Optimizing principles, on the other hand, guide recommendations about specific treatment relationships, the application of specific treatment models, and the fit of specific treatments to specific patients (differential treatment questions).

We identify specific principles that relate to treatment as we discuss various aspects of predicting patient responses to treatment, and we return to, and refine, these principles throughout this volume as we address various referral questions within the context of particular assessment procedures. Suffice it to point out that assessment methods vary in the type of information that they can usefully and validly assess. Thus the consulting psychologist often must select the methods used to emphasize these different levels of information and ensure that the information derived can be applied to the question(s) being asked. To know how to accomplish this task, the nature of psychological measurement must be clearly understood.

PSYCHOLOGICAL ASSESSMENT AND THE NATURE OF MEASUREMENT

Situational versus Trait-Like Responses

In clinical psychology and psychiatry, the basic task of measurement is translating the qualities that a patient brings to the clinician into a form that answers the questions posed by a referent. Psychological tests are measurement devices and methods that are designed to accomplish this task. The use of modern psychological tests to provide answers to clinical questions and problems is a contemporary representation of a process that is as long as the history of humankind—the effort to identify the nature of individual differences and to account for both the similarities and uniquenesses of each human's experience. These efforts were, and are, imbedded in the perennial attempts of peoples worldwide to predict and control their lives.

Throughout time, the speed at which people gained the abilities to predict and control events around them was governed by how well they overcame two major problems: (1) identifying those particular characteristics that are useful in describing the unique and similar qualities among people, and (2) distinguishing between the situational and personal contributors to (causes of) behavior. The first of these tasks underwrote the development of theories of personality and psychopathology, whereas the second underwrote the development of psychological tests.

The previous section of this chapter described the very basic list of concepts that our understanding of extant research suggests is minimally necessary in order to address the referral questions that are posed to psychological consultants. Now we face the task of identifying how we can move from making observations of a person's behavior to drawing a conclusion that this behavior represents certain distinguishing characteristics of the person rather than the situation in which he or she finds him- or herself.

In order to distinguish among situational and characterological (state vs. trait) aspects of behavior, it is helpful to maintain a constant test environment; doing so essentially eliminates, or at least holds constant, the influence of situational states. That is, across tasks, in a constant environment, clinicians may have some confidence that the resulting variations of behavior among participants or occasions are the result of participants' enduring, trait-like qualities. One of the major advantages of formal psychological measures over informal ones is the presence of standardized administration procedures. These procedures impose certain limitations and structures on a person's response, both by virtue of the explicit instructions used and by the implied expectations and consequences of the response. Such procedures are called "demand characteristics" of the testing environment. The responses to this structured and controlled assessment environment are compared to normative information based on a standardized sample. These "norms" tell us how people usually respond to these demand characteristics. Thus, by comparing a given person's response to these normative values, we can identify the degree to which the respondent's answers deviate from normal or average respondents. By inspecting the nature of the person's response, moreover, and comparing it to the nature of the demand characteristics of the instructions, we also can make some estimate of the degree to which this particular individual is sensitive to, and compliant with, the demands made by the environment. Departures from the expected response depict the ways in which characteristics of the respondent's beliefs and perceptions—qualities that are independent of the task itself—may alter the response to the demand characteristics of the task.

One way to view a response that departs from the established norms of a testing environment is to consider the variance as representing the insertion or modification of "attributed demand" to the demand characteristics. That is, the individual is responding not only to the environmentally imposed demands but also to some idiosyncratic, personal interpretation of these demands. Extreme departures from the conventional suggest the presence of attributed demands that are unconventional. We can see how attributed demands may interfere with the environmental demand characteristics by viewing the two presentations that are illustrated in Figure 1.1. This figure shows two different ways that a respondent might react to the demand characteristics of the Bender Visual Motor Gestalt Test (BVMGT; Bender, 1938).

The instructions and physical properties of the BVMGT impose a demand characteristic that emphasizes accuracy and a distinct consideration of nine geometric figures. Each of the figures is presented on a small card,

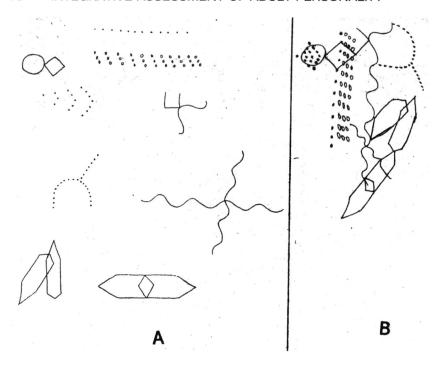

A   **B**

FIGURE 1.1. The Bender Visual Motor Gestalt Test under two demand sets.

and the participant is instructed to "Draw each of the figures the best you can." There are no time constraints on the respondent's performance. The typical or normative response takes about 4 minutes and consists of systematically copying each of the nine figures, beginning in the upper left-hand side of the page and either proceeding down the left side of the page or across the top, separately constructing each figure. Thus the normative response is to reproduce the designs, one at a time, in an orderly sequence. Adherence to this normative response is seen in the first production (set A) shown in Figure 1.1.

The person who drew the second set of designs (set B) was responding to a different set of demand characteristics, demonstrated by this production's departure from the normative expectation. If the BVMGT was administered using the usual instructions—that is, if it imposed the usual demand for accuracy and separation—then we must assume that the respondent inserted some attributed demands into the process. The job of the clinician is to learn something about these attributed demands, and thereby about the respondent, by noting the degree to which the response departs from the norm as well as the nature of that departure. A clinician viewing this second production might conclude that the patient's response is unconventional and poorly organized. It does not reveal a realistic appraisal of, or responsiveness to, the explicit demand characteristics contained in the instructions. In particular, the response shows little sensitivity to the demand of maintaining the boundaries among the separate stimuli. A clinician might conclude that the person who completed set B approached the task with an attitudinal response set that modified the explicit demands by adding attributed demands or expectations to the instructions. These attributed demands were constructed from the respondent's beliefs and attitudes. In other words, this person did not realistically appraise the demands established by the examiner's request because of interference from internal expectations or trait-like qualities. It is these trait-like qualities that are revealed in the production, assuming that the explicit instructions remain constant. A person who changes the demand characteristics of the environment by some internal process of imposing new rules and assumptions may be resistant, schizophrenic—or exceptionally creative.

It is noteworthy that the responses in set B are not disorganized; they are simply organized according to a different set of principles. Indeed, the respondent organized the figures into a design. Perhaps the patient attributed a relational demand to the task that competed with, and overshadowed, the stimulus demand of separateness. Clearly, unless we know the explicit and stimulus-determined demand characteristics of the assessment environment, we cannot interpret the responses that come from psychological measures.

Classifying Behavior through Measurement

The results of psychological measurement, whether formal tests or informal clinical observations, are expressed as either a "categorical" or a "dimensional" classification. An example of a categorical classification is the application of a psychiatric diagnosis. A person is assigned to a diagnostic class or type on the basis of a simple dichotomy of "fit" or "no fit" with certain criteria. Dimensional assessment, on the other hand, assumes that certain qualities are best described as existing in some varying amount in most or all people. It is assumed, therefore, that qualities of this type are only roughly and inaccurately described by a categorical classification. Dimensional assessment is exemplified in quantitative estimates of the magnitude of such attributes as anger, depression, maladjustment, anxiety, neuroticism, extroversion, fear, and so forth.

Interpreting these scores forces us to grapple with the problem of translating them into concepts that have clinical meaning to others. Tests are administered and scored according to established rules and conventions. Such attributes as "problem-solving ability," "anxiety," "conflict," and "personality," however, are inferred, not observed directly. That is, they are hypothetical constructs whose existence can only be estimated from observed behaviors or reported experience. Their value is measured not only by how well they describe or predict behavior, but by how much consensual agreement exists in their meaning among those with whom clinicians communicate. This is why it is valuable to use terms that can be translated easily across various theories. The concepts we presented earlier are a beginning point for the transmission of cross-cutting knowledge. It is valuable to use these concepts and terms to communicate results in common language in order to maximize the value of the communication process itself.

The tasks of integrating, ordering, and transmitting information from both informal and formal measurement procedures are considerably less systematic and technical than those of administering and scoring psychological tests. In this volume, we prefer to use the term *psychological assessment* rather than *psychological testing* to capture this broader clinical function. Psychological assessment includes the use of clinical skills beyond the mechanical administration of tests and computation of scores. Use of this term is a recognition that the measurement instrument of greatest value, in the final analysis, is the clinician, not the test. The clinician who conducts a psychological assessment is a consultant, not a technician who merely administers a test; a consultant delivers opinions, not a summary of procedures.

The Process of Psychological Assessment

The requirements of psychological assessment can be illustrated by addressing the four steps of the assessment process identified at the beginning of this chapter. These steps require (1) an understanding of the social systems through which patients enter or seek assessment; (2) an understanding of the nature of measurement and familiarity with the measurement devices available; (3) knowledge of methods of interpreting these observations; and (4) familiarity with the process of communicating the findings and opinions to others. The four steps, again, are as follows:

1. Identifying the problem to be addressed
2. Selecting and implementing methods for extracting the information needed
3. Integrating sources of information around the problem
4. Deriving and reporting conclusions, opinions, and recommendations

The first of these steps is basic to the psychologist's role in many contexts; the second is the technical function of test selection, administration, and scoring. We assume that the advanced graduate students and professionals for whom this text is intended are familiar with basic psychometric principles and with the technical skills of responding to a referral request, selecting instruments, administering these tests, and scoring them. In this chapter we review only the basic principles associated with the first two steps. Chapter 2 considers the selection of specific tests. The rest of the book is devoted to the third and fourth steps, the advanced principles of formulating, integrating, and communicating opinions—the activities of the consulting psychologist.

Identifying the Problem

We have said that psychological testing is the application of measurement to the description of individual differences. However, in practice, the nature of psychological assessment is more complex than this simple statement suggests. Good clinical assessment begins with translating requests for consultation into questions that can be meaningfully answered by clinical methods. Patients are referred to psychologists for many different reasons, not all of which are stated by the persons making the referrals. Moreover, not all of the ways in which people differ from one another are either likely to be of interest to a clinician or amenable to clinical assessment methods.

For example, let us return to the questions asked at the beginning of this chapter. To a political analyst, the most important distinctions among George H. W. Bush, Ronald Reagan, and Bill Clinton may be their political affiliations. Reagan and Bush were Republicans and Clinton was a Democrat. Although classifying these men by political affiliation represents a method of categorical measurement and scoring, the resultant classification provides little help in deriving an answer to clinical questions. A mental health clinician may find that questions such as "Does any of these men have a clinical disorder?," "Are they depressed?," and "Does any of them pose a danger to himself or others?" are more relevant. That former President Reagan was diagnosed as having "dementia of the Alzheimer's type," that Bush's honesty was called into question regarding the activities of the CIA while he was in office, not to mention the concerns with the honesty of former President Clinton preceding and during his impeachment hearings— all make these questions salient even for former presidents of the United States.

There are many responses to Mr. Reagan's Alzheimer's, Mr. Bush's honesty (or lack thereof), and Mr. Clinton's sexual indiscretions. Some of the questions raised, however, may have little relevance to whether or not they could discharge the functions of the office of President of the United States. A clinician who is asked to assess an individual's personality must begin by distinguishing between questions whose answers will shed light on his or her abilities to carry out responsibilities, tasks, and duties, and those whose answers will serve merely as distractions or matters of interest to others. To assess relevance, clinicians must first determine what question or questions are being asked by whomever is referring the "patient" to the psychological expert. In addition, clinicians also must gauge the consequences of various answers in relation to the person's level of functioning in various life and social roles. Only when clinicians know the likely implications of various answers can they judge (1) whether the questions themselves are relevant, and (2) if so, whether psychological assessment would be a useful method for deriving answers to these questions. Central concerns include (1) estimating whether the questions asked can be answered within the time allotted, (2) using methods that are available, and (3) ascertaining if the findings will be used in a way that is advantageous to the patient. Clinicians must always be aware of who is requesting the information, and the purpose to which the information will be put.

Clinically relevant referral questions seek six general types of information:

1. Descriptions or formulations of the pattern of current behaviors
2. Causes of the behaviors observed
3. Changes that can be anticipated in these behaviors over time
4. Ways in which these patterns may be modified
5. Patterns and areas of deficit
6. Resources and strengths of the person

In other words, the questions address the objectives of determining diagnosis, etiology, prognosis, differential treatment, degree of functional impairment, and assets, respectively, as outlined at the beginning of this chapter.

Diagnostic questions may be phrased as requests to rule in or rule out certain diagnoses, or they may ask how certain symptoms and behaviors are related to one another. Questions of etiology may take the form of inquiring about whether or not traumatic brain damage is present or whether a patient's disturbed interpersonal relationships could be attributed to a recent loss or trauma. Both diagnostic and etiological questions seek to clarify the nature (e.g., interrelationship, severity, etc.) of problematic behaviors.

Questions about whether a given condition is likely to dissipate with time, or whether a given person is at risk for a future problem, are seeking prognostic data to facilitate the prediction of the normal course of change and development in various behaviors and symptoms. Questions of the fourth type, which solicit information to facilitate differential treatment planning, are related to prognostic issues and ask clinicians to anticipate what will happen with the patient's symptoms under certain imposed conditions (e.g., "Is this patient a good candidate for psychotherapy?"; "Should antidepressant or antipsychotic medication be used?"). In addition, some treatment questions are designed to prevent future problems (e.g., "Will education prevent this at-risk person from developing alcoholism?").

Questions about functional impairment may include inquiries regarding the patient's premorbid level of performance (e.g., "How much of this person's impairment predated the trauma?"), and those attempting to estimate some future level of performance (e.g., "What is this patient's employment potential?"; "What level of achievement can we expect of this individual?"). Questions of these types seek to determine (1) expectations others may reasonably hold for patients after their acute symptoms have dissipated, or (2) the cost factors associated with a disability.

Finally, some questions combine information about the patient, his or her environment and the likely course of the patient's problems. Answering many of these questions may require clinicians to integrate information about the patient's assets and strengths. Thus the professional making the referral may ask the clinician for information on probable risk and protective factors, assets, and strengths on which to build an effective treatment program. No diagnostic, prognostic, or etiological picture of a patient is complete without an indication of strengths and assets.

When health care professionals seek consultation from other professionals, they frequently use shorthand communication methods, often without realizing that those with whom they are consulting must be familiar with these abbreviated communications in order to respond to them adequately. Hence a responding clinician must learn to distinguish the stated reasons for referring a patient from the unstated ones. Stated requests are often too general or too specific to allow the responding clinician to address adequately the covert or unstated needs.

For example, the most frequent requests from referring psychiatrists are couched in very broad terms such as "diagnostic testing" or "personality assessment," which are too general to be easily addressed. Such requests do not allow a psychologist to select an efficient way of responding. The request for nothing more specific than "diagnostic testing" could result in an 8-hour neuropsychological evaluation, the administration of 30 different projective tests, 15 hours of interviews and paper-and-pencil tests, and a two-night sleep and penile plethysmographic study—if all diagnoses described by the *Diagnostic and Statistical Manual of Mental Disorders*— Fourth Edition (DSM-IV; American Psychiatric Association, 1994) were to be considered systematically. These procedures not only are very expensive but constitute an inefficient use of time, because the referrant usually has a narrower view of the most likely diagnostic options that he or she wishes to have considered.

On the other hand, some explicit requests are so specific that they do not allow the psychologist enough latitude to develop a reasoned response. A request for the "MMPI" or "projective testing" usually indicates a request for assistance in making a differential diagnosis. However, such specificity prevents the responding psychologist from selecting the most useful measures for addressing this issue and precludes consideration of the concomitant influence of characteristics that may be obtained more reliably and validly from other methods. For example, restricting an assessment either to the MMPI-2 or to a projective method such as the Rorschach would be inadequate if the underlying goal is to find out how the patient functions in his or her family. These tests do not directly consider the family context. Moreover, even under the best of circumstances, a request for a specific test or type of test will be insufficient if test results are not considered in light of the patient's living circumstances and intellectual abilities, both of which must be ascertained through the use of other assessment methods. A given profile on the MMPI-2 will warrant very different interpretations if the patient has borderline intellectual abilities and is living in a group home than if the patient has superior intellectual resources and is living independently.

Reframing or translating the explicit request into a question that reflects the actual problem facing the referrant simplifies the tasks of the consulting psychologist. Reframing a request either for "diagnostic testing" or for the "MMPI," for example, will probably result in an answerable question such as the following: "Is this person's depression of the unipolar or bipolar type?" Similarly, restating the request for "personality evaluation" or "projective testing" as an answerable question will probably result in something like this: "Is this patient able to cope with the stress of job loss without becoming psychotic?"

The first task of the clinician upon receiving a request for evaluation, therefore, is to contact the referrant and discuss the request in sufficient detail that an answerable question emerges or can be developed. An answerable question is one that elicits concepts and issues that are within the domain of psychological experience and that can be measured. Good referral questions often pose hypothetical consequences for various potential answers. The answers obtained must possess the qualities of *sensitivity* (i.e., rightly identifying when the respondent is different from the norm) and *specificity* (i.e., rightly specifying when the respondent is similar to the norm). In order to translate explicit requests into questions that possess these qualities, the clinician usually needs to obtain information concerning the patient's background, current and anticipated treatments, and the time frame in which the answers are needed. For example, the clinician might ask the referrant to (1) elaborate on the patient's current problem, (2) explain why he or she (the referrant) thinks psychological assessment will help, (3) specify what the clinician needs to find out, (4) describe how the information obtained will be used, and (5) indicate what decisions are pending, given the results. Background knowledge in normal development, abnormal psychology, developmental psychopathology, comparative treatments, and differential treatment efficacy will help the clinician frame questions to define the nature of the referral.

Selecting and Implementing the Assessment Tools

Fundamentally, psychological assessment boils down to the task of measuring and classifying observations. The processes of selecting and administering psychological tests are formalized extensions of what we all do in daily life. We meet a person at a cocktail party (identify the situational demands on behavior); observe the person as he or she interacts with us (observe samples of behavior); compare the person's response to that of others or to our prior experiences in similar situations (measure and compare); and conclude that the person is likely to be friendly or unfriendly, likable or unlikable (generalize to unobserved or future situations). We have observed, measured, and classified (diagnosed) the person; queried about his or her history (explored etiology); developed expectations of future responses (determined prognosis); predicted how the person would respond to certain information about us (assessed a differential response to treatment); and drawn conclusions about the person's strengths and weaknesses (identified resources as well as functional impairments). In daily life, our safety and existence often depend on our ability to observe, measure, and classify accurately. If we perform these tasks poorly, we may be socially insensitive (inaccurate measurement), mistakenly assume that others will not hurt us (inaccurate prediction), or find ourselves becoming anxious when others' behavior changes abruptly (inaccurate generalization).

The distinctions between these day-to-day assessments and professional psychological assessment lie primarily in the degree of measurement precision used by clinicians and the theoretical origin of the constructs used to lend understanding, prediction, and control to the realm of behavioral events. A psychologist uses concepts founded on formal psychological theories rather than those contained only within privately derived theories. But, like the cocktail party observer, the clinician looks beyond each subject's responses to the nature of the situation in which the response occurs. Behaviors are judged within their context. All psychological assessment assumes that both the test environment and the associated behaviors constitute representative samples of external environments and of concomitant behaviors in these environments. Hence it is assumed that the relationship between relevant test demands and resultant "scores" will be recapitulated on a magnified scale in an external environment. In other words, clinicians assume that the important elements of the testing environment correspond with similar elements of the real world, and that the symbolized meaning of test scores will be associated with a predictable set of behaviors within these real-world environments.

Because of the various ways they are structured, some tests are better suited than others to assess the domain of cognition; others are best suited to assess the domain of overt behavior; and still others are best suited to tap the domain of emotion. For example, the WAIS-III is a good instrument for assessing cognitive activities, but is not well suited to determining the nature of the testee's emotional experience; the MMPI-2 is well adapted to deriving information about behavioral traits, but is less suited to understanding transitory, situational responses; mood scales are well constructed to evaluate various emotions but poorly suited to assess intellectual and cognitive abilities. Although domains of cognitive, affective, behavioral, and social experiences are not independent of one another, they have some unique qualities and vary in their salience from one environment to another. A psychologist must know both the domain of behavior that is best assessed by a given test and the nature of the environment to which that response domain is best generalized.

As noted earlier in this chapter, test environments are designed to place certain explicit and implicit demands and constraints on the patient's responses. These demand characteristics vary along at least three dimensions that parallel aspects of various external or real-world environments. Observing how patients respond to tests that embody the characteristics of different points along each of these dimensions has value for predicting the nature of behavior. Specifically, these test environments are designed to vary in the degree to which they (1) are structured or ambiguous, (2) attend to internal or external experience, and (3) place stress on the respondent.

Depending on the nature of the referral question, various aspects of these dimensions should be emphasized in the selection of tests. Ambiguity in an environment provides information about the respondent's ability to organize and interpret experience. Tests that vary in ambiguity may suggest something about the patient's ability to use cognitive resources, such as abstract and logical thought, to integrate experience. Likewise, observing how the patient responds to methods that focus variously on internal and external experience may provide information about his or her coping styles, level of impulsivity, vulnerability to threat, and one's accessibility to experience. This information may be important in addressing questions about intellectual abilities, personality disorders, the diagnosis of mood disorders, and suitability for insight-oriented versus behavior-oriented psychotherapies.

Finally, observing whether the patient responds with compliance, defiance, resistance, or decompensation to various levels of stress imposed in the testing environment may provide information about his or her stress tolerance, adequacy of protective defenses, resistance potential, and impulse control. Of course, in most instances, the questions asked are complex, and the patient's response requires the clinician to generalize to environments that vary in several or all of these qualities. Hence instruments are usually selected to permit the systematic observation of response variations at several points along each of these dimensions.

Methods of psychological assessment also differ in the sensitivity and accuracy with which they measure and predict behavior. The clinician's task is thus to select systematic methods for sampling the aspects of situations to which he or she wants to generalize, and to ensure that the behaviors observed in these situations are measured reliably and validly. In order to accomplish this latter task, the clinician must be familiar with good measurement procedures, including (1) the scaling methods used, (2) measurement sensitivity, (3) measurement specificity, (4) availability of normative data, (5) reliability of observations, and (6) validity of the observations. Each of these six areas deserves brief review.

Scaling Methods. Whether the goal is to assess the nature of the clinical question being asked, define the type of situation to which generalizations must occur, or measure an attribute such as intelligence or anxiety, the first and most fundamental quality of measurement is "identity." Simply put, the measurement instrument—be it a clinician's judgment or test score—must translate samples of observed behaviors into a form that fairly represents distinctive qualities of individuals. The failure to identify or classify observations prevents accurate inferences from being made about past, present, or future behavior.

Measurement applies numbers to individuals or attributes as a means of establishing identity among observations. In increasing order of sophistication, there are four methods of preserving identity: nominal, ordinal, interval, and ratio. These four methods are often described as scaling methods because they order and classify observations. Nominal scaling assigns individuals or behaviors to categories. The remaining methods of assigning identity reflect variations of dimensional measurement.

The best example of *nominal scaling*, as applied to people, are diagnostic categories. A DSM diagnosis of major depression identifies a cluster of related symptoms, differentiates those who have the condition from those who do not, and suggests a particular course of development and treatment. Diagnostic labels define discrete categories or "types" of people, and have general application to a wide range of individuals who seek assistance from mental health practitioners. Diagnostic labels are limited in their value, however, because they fail to make some important discriminations among those who meet the criteria for the diagnosis (i.e., those with major depression differ from one another in important, treatment-relevant ways), and they do not provide any information about the large number of individuals who fail to meet the criteria for a diagnosis but who still seek, and can benefit from, mental health services.

That is, nominal scaling methods, such as diagnosis, identify who has a condition but do not allow us to compare individuals either within or across groups. Using a nominal, diagnostic scale, for example, we could not say that depression is "more than schizophrenia" any more than we could say that apples are "more than oranges"—they are entirely different classes.

Ordinal scaling, on the other hand, is a measurement method that identifies the relative *ranking* of observations. We can say that depression is "more prevalent" than schizophrenia, that one person has "more depressive symptoms" than another, or that there are "more apples than oranges in Washington state." This ordinal or ranking method preserves the hierarchy that exists among the observations as well as the identity of each. Thus, while it allows the definition of a dimension, it does not tell us how *much* more frequently depression is observed than schizophrenia, how *much* more depressed one person is than another, or how *many* more apples than oranges are grown in Washington state. Doing any of the latter tasks requires either interval or ratio measurement. These latter scaling methods allow identity, ranking, and comparison.

In clinical assessment it is often important to determine both the category or diagnosis (nominal scale) and how many of the component symptoms are present or how severe they are (one of the three dimensional scales–ordinal, interval, or ratio) in absolute rather than relative terms. To do so, we must construct instruments that apply continuous ratings, in the form of numbers, to our observations. If we can assume that the differences between numbers are the same all along the continuum (the principle of equal intervals), then we can compare one score against another and conclude something about both the presence and the magnitude of observed differences.

Again, both interval scaling and ratio scaling methods allow this latter type of magnitude comparison. Ratio measures can be applied only to characteristics that exist in a continuous quantity *and* do not exist at all (i.e., the scale has an absolute zero). Most psychological qualities do not possess both of these aspects. It is difficult to envision zero levels of anxiety or depression, for example. Unlike physical distance measures, where "0" means that two measurements are identical, it is not possible to measure most psychological properties by a ratio scale. Psychological characteristics are more similar to temperature than to physical distance; in the measurement of psychological qualities, as in that of temperature, a score of "0" is only one point along a scale in which lower scores are always possible. It is conceivable for someone to become even less depressed than a person who scores "0" on a test, much as temperatures can be measured below 0.

Sensitivity, Specificity, and Normative Value. Although necessary, identity as a property of a measurement scale is not sufficient for adequate assessment. If we reflect back on the question of how to describe the three presidents, we can see that the categorical (nominal) identification of political alliance is of little help in assessing clinical referral questions, because it is not sufficiently sensitive to individual variations and is a poor predictor of the degree to which emotions and behaviors may depart from normal expectations. Both Democrats and Republicans can be emotionally healthy, disordered, or dangerous; not all Democrats are like Bill Clinton, and not all Republicans are like George H. W. Bush.

Using the example of the former presidents, we can illustrate three other important concepts in measurement: sensitivity, specificity, and normative value. In a way, we have already discussed the concept of sensitivity. A measurement possesses *sensitivity*—if it can classify a person's uniqueness. That is, a sensitive measure is one that correctly identifies an individual as having a given characteristic or as being a member of a given group. Sensitivity is best understood when applied to categorical measurement and, in this case, is the percentage of "true positives"—that is, the percentage of time the measure identifies a quality as being present when, in fact, it is. The reliability of a measurement is an estimate of the degree to which it is able to identify a condition as present, when it is, in fact, present.

To illustrate the concept of sensitivity, let us first imagine that we have constructed a self-report test consisting of a single question: "Have you ever been President of the United States?" If this test is then administered to Reagan, George H. W. Bush, and Clinton, we may expect that all three will answer affirmatively. By checking their responses against public records, we can then determine that we have successfully identified all three of these individuals accurately. They are "true positives" in that they not only have responded positively to the question, but they actually belong to the class of people defined by our historical criterion. Hence we can conclude that our test has high (even perfect) sensitivity.

The more politically minded, however, may point out that although all three men were indeed elected to the office of president, each can claim unique accomplishments. With a series of subsidiary questions, cross-referenced against historical records, we could develop three subscales for our test. Bush, but neither Reagan nor Clinton, can be identified with a subscale that asks whether he "directed the invasion of Panama"; Reagan, but neither Bush nor Clinton, can be identified with a subscale that asks whether he "negotiated an arms reduction agreement with the USSR"; Clinton, but neither Bush nor Reagan, can be identified with a subscale that asks whether he "proposed an educational indenture program for college students." Thus a measurement system made up of these categories will still possess 100% sensitivity, in that all three former presidents can be accurately classified and distinguished from one another.

Now in terms of mental disorders or personality traits, the case is more difficult than it is with our former presidents. Whereas it is possible to check the presidents' answers against public records, we can check a patient's answers only against defined criteria, such as DSM-IV criteria. But the criteria themselves are only definitions and therefore dependent on cultural and historical norms. Examples of the relativity of definitions are labels such as "homosexuality," which was included as a descriptor of people in DSM-II, or "posttraumatic stress disorder," which was introduced in

DSM-III after observation and acknowledgment of the psychological effects of participating in the Vietnam war. Although this caveat has only limited influence for the actual assessment procedure, it serves to underscore the fact that the certainty of constructs varies, and that caution regarding diagnostic labels is warranted, especially if the empirical support for the diagnostic construct is weak.

Although our presidential designation system possesses impeccable sensitivity, in that it accurately assigns each of the presidents to a categorical class of which he is the only member, psychological assessment requires that the measurement used also be capable of identifying those who do *not* belong to the targeted group. The ability to identify accurately those who do not have a certain quality or group membership is referred to as the scale's *specificity*. Making a determination of our test's specificity is impossible at this point, however, because we have not yet tried it out on people who have not been President of the United States, have not waged war, have not negotiated arms reduction agreements, and have not publicly advanced indenture programs for higher education.

If we asked a large group of randomly selected people the four questions posed to the three presidents, we would find that all (or most) would say "no" to all of the questions. In checking the public records (our criteria), we would probably find that, in fact, none has actually been President of the United States, none has directed troops to invade Panama, none negotiated an arms reduction treaty with the USSR, and none has proposed an educational indenture program to Congress. Hence we could conclude that our test possesses the quality of specificity—it has successfully identified those in our sample who have not been President of the United States—as well as sensitivity.

Once we administer our test to such a large group, it gains some *normative value*. If we assume that the million people we have asked are representative of those in the United States, we can infer that most people would answer "no" to the questions, and that those who say "yes" will be unusual. But because there is so little variability in responses to our scale (1,000,000 people say "no" and only three people say "yes" to our questions), our scale does not allow us to say much of anything about the large number of people who has not been president. As this example illustrates, there must be both *response variability* and a normative value in order for the meaning of responses to be assessed.

To illustrate the importance of these concepts in a different way, consider the following: Say we hold up a pen and ask a classroom full of graduate students to identify what it is (a categorical rating). The characteristics of a pen are so constant and well known that there will be little variation among students' answers. Because all or most of the responses will be the same, we would be able to conclude little about these students beyond the probability that they are sensitive to their environments and familiar with pens. However, suppose one student says, "That is a prince who has been enchanted by a wicked witch." It is the departure of this student's response from the usual or normative response that would allow us to draw conclusions about how realistic his or her perceptions are. If the student comes from an unusual cultural background, in which witches and demons are believed to inhabit all objects, then his or her response may be seen as normal or usual within that particular culture, and our ability to interpret its unique meaning is lost. This illustration underlines the need to consider the meanings of responses in terms of the respondent's social norms and history. Perhaps it is an unfortunate characteristic of psychological assessment that deviation from the "norm" is more informative than compliance with the usual.

If we could rule out the possibility that this student's response is usual or normal within the cultural or religious environment in which he or she lives, by assessing a large number of people who are from the same culture, we could then conclude that the student's response represents some unusual characteristic of him or her. The more unusual the response, compared to the norm that represents the culture with whom the student identifies and in which he or she lives, the more clearly we can conclude that a variant response indicates some form of clinical abnormality. For example, suppose that our student looks frightened, jumps up, and runs out of the room when we hold up the pen. We may infer, with some degree of confidence, that the student is fearful of, and has negative attitudes toward, wicked witches, above and beyond his or her beliefs about pens. If he or she shares with the majority culture a primitive, animistic religion and background, then the unusual nature of this response may be assumed to reflect a deficit in the ability to objectively analyze, interpret, and respond to routine events. However, we can see that it is the deviation or variation of the response that gives us this ability, since we still can say little about the large number of students who has given the expected response, "pen." Even with perfect sensitivity and specificity, in other words, our "Pen Test" may have very limited value, because it only tells us something about those who *deviate* from the norm.

Since no one can be expected to be "average" in everything, we usually construct tests on which there are many ways to deviate from the average or norm. For example, in our illustration of the "President's Test," the large group of randomly selected individuals represents a normative sample because the characteristics of the sampled individuals are likely to be similar to those of the larger population. As in the case of the students in the "Pen Test" example, however, their responses do not distinguish them from one another. In response to the question about having been elected President of the United States, almost all of them have said "no." To be able to draw conclusions about individuals within this group, we must find ways in which their individuality is manifest. If we add an item to our test that asks, "How many people have financially benefited from your decisions during the past year?", we would obtain a number (i.e., a score) from each of them that would manifest response variability. The arithmetic mean of these responses would provide a normative value against which we could compare our three former presidents and all others in the group, even without knowing the accuracy of their estimates. Moreover, the scores (i.e., the number of people who have benefited) among our sample of, say, 1,000,003 people would probably fall within a bell-shaped or normal distribution curve. Some people, like our presidents, will identify a large number of people as having benefited from their actions, whereas others will indicate that few or none has so benefited. Because our sample is both large and randomly selected from the entire population, the distribution of scores is likely to be representative of the general population. That is, the mean and distribution of the sample is likely to be a close approximation of what we would find if we were to ask this question of everyone in the United States.

After first computing the "standard deviation" of our sample, which is an estimate of how the responses are distributed (assuming that the scale measures a normally distributed characteristic), we can describe each individual within our sample by computing an "effect-size" score. This score simply describes, in decimal form, the number of standard deviations separating the individual from the mean of the sample. Because of their visibility and positions of power, it is likely that all three of the presidents in our example will be at wide variance with most of the rest of our sample. They will have highly positive effect-size scores (i.e., they will be several standard deviations above the mean) in the number of people who have financially benefited from their decisions. By inspecting these scores, we can compare the self-rated influence of any of the three presidents and that of any other person in our group.

Comparing individuals to normative standards based upon large numbers of randomly selected (i.e., representative) individuals, however, does not help us understand either what caused any particular observed deviation or the accuracy of the scores given. The questions we still face include a determination of whether or not scores obtained in this way are likely to be accurate or clinically meaningful. Alternatively, do these scores vary as a function of some still unknown quality of the environment? To what degree is their accuracy influenced by momentary distraction? Do these scores indicate a stable aspect of respondents' personalities or intelligence? Are they likely to be influenced by current distress levels or impediments such as a recent bad night's sleep? In reference to our presidents, for example, are their estimates of the numbers of people affected by their decisions a product of their need to feel important, or do these estimates give an accurate indication of their influence? In other words, the measurement must be both reliable and valid.

Reliability and Validity. A measurement provides identity and sensitivity if it reflects the unique features of the patient's experience; it possesses specificity and normative value if it identifies the degree of similarity between an individual and others. The central purpose of psychological assessment, however, is to gather information that allows us to generalize to situations that we cannot observe directly or that have not yet occurred.

We know that behavior does not occur in a vacuum; it arises in response to an environmental quality as well as to the individual qualities and characteristics of the person. Hence, if we are able to provide a constant (i.e., identical) environment for every person who completes our test, the resulting differences in behavior are likely to reflect individual qualities of personality, intellect, and expectations. Psychological tests attempt to provide such a constant environment for individuals, in order to permit testers to (1) observe the variations among their responses, and (2) infer the nature of each of their unique characteristics. We formalize the procedures of observation; study and standardize the environments in which a patient's behavior is sampled; and work to ensure that our instruments for observing and measuring are sensitive, specific, and have normative value. Our observations thereby can be judged to represent samples of how individuals differ in their responses to environments.

The next task that faces us as clinicians is to distinguish between transient and enduring characteristics of people's behavior—states and traits. To the degree that a behavioral characteristic changes from moment-to-moment or occasion-to-occasion, it is said to reflect a *state* and is judged to be an attribute that is influenced by the environment. To the degree that a characteristic remains constant over time and across situations, it is said to be a *trait* and is judged to be a personality quality that is minimally reactive to the environment. Situational anxiety is a state; eye color is a trait; and in between lies a host of qualities that have both state and trait properties—each changes at various rates in response to environments.

Without knowing whether the behaviors we observe are likely to be enduring or situational, we do not know the degree to which our observations or the meanings of test scores can be generalized. The methods of classifying and measuring, in other words, must also possess the ability to be replicated; this is the quality of *reliability*. Reliability is an index of consistency or purity of measurement; it is usually expressed in the form of a correlation. However, because personal qualities vary in how much they are influenced and changed by the nature of the situation, different types of consistency or reliability are relevant for different measures. "Test–retest reliability" is indicated by high correspondence or similarity of responses on two different occasions. If our students say "pen" every time they are asked, we can infer that their familiarity with the object derives from enduring knowledge—a base of knowledge that supersedes changes occurring in the environment. Conversely, if their responses are strikingly different in two different situations or at two different times, we can conclude that whatever their responses are measuring is a temporary or passing state in their experience.

A measurement device with response variability allows us to estimate the likelihood that a given response will recur if the test is administered repeatedly on several different occasions. This estimate is based on the "standard error of measurement," which is derived from a knowledge of the reliability of the test responses. The higher the correlation between scores on the test on two separate occasions, the higher the reliability, and the smaller the error of measurement—that is, there are fewer unintended influences affecting the scores. The standard error of measurement is expressed as a standard deviation that is estimated to be likely to characterize the scores of a single individual if he or she took the test on many different occasions. It is used to estimate the possibility that the variation we observe in each of this individual's responses is an accidental occurrence. We can see in this example how test–retest reliability, as applied to dimensional measurement, is similar to the concept of sensitivity, as applied to categorical measurement. It is an estimate of how sensitive the test is to variations in the condition being assessed.

Another form of reliability is applied to a test when we want to assure ourselves that an entire test or subtest is measuring the same factor. For this purpose, we compute the test's "internal consistency," which is an estimate of the degree to which each item or subpart of the test measures the same factor as the rest of the test items or subparts. Internal consistency is usually expressed as a correlation between the items and the total score. With tests that are designed to measure several different attributes by way of subtests, internal consistency is estimated by the relationship of the items to the subtest scores rather than to a total score. It is expected that these part–whole correlations will be higher than the correlations between items and total scores on subtests, which are designed to measure an attribute differing from one to be measured by an individual item.

"Equivalent-forms reliability" is a method of assessing consistency that combines some of the principles of test–retest and internal-consistency reliabilities. In this method, we may construct two forms of the test and compute the degree to which they measure the same factor, either when administered at the same time or when administered on two separate occasions. This form of reliability is used when there is some reason to believe that the act of responding to the test on one occasion will determine how a person responds on the second occasion. This concern arises when the response is affected either by memory or by corrective knowledge that is gained while the person is taking the test. For example, a subtest from the Wechsler Memory Scale—Revised (Wechsler, 1987) presents paired words and then asks the subject or client to recall the second word of each pair when the first is repeated to him or her. This paired learning task is repeated three times in each administration, and it is likely that the learning that takes place will be carried over to another occasion. Therefore, a different but comparable list of words (an alternate form of the test) is used when the test is repeated, in order to avoid this problem.

Sometimes the test scores are subjective, as in the case where a clinician must make ratings of clients' drawings or the meaning of behaviors. We want to assure ourselves that different raters make similar ratings (i.e., see similar meanings). Thus we may ask the raters to judge the amount of similarity and then compare the judges' ratings for agreement, to be sure that the same factor is being measured by each judge's rating. In such instances, the type of reliability that is desired is called "interrater reliability."

Although high reliability estimates tell us that a similar quality is being measured, and although comparisons of different types of reliability indicate whether the quality measured is a stable quality of the person, the test, the situation, or the rater, they do not tell us what it is that we are measuring. The accuracy with which a test measures the factor or quality we want it to measure is called "validity." *Validity* is the most basic and yet the most difficult criterion to meet in test construction. Because the concept or attribute we are addressing is usually abstract and subjective, there are generally no direct measures of the essence of what we are assessing. Therefore, it is almost impossible to completely establish a test's validity. But by first identifying the particular type of validity that is of principal concern, and then applying some established procedures to the task of measuring this type of validity, we can obtain an estimate of a test's validity that is sufficient for our purposes. The nature of validity, like that of reliability, varies because of the different purposes to which we want our test to apply. The main types are called *content, construct, criterion,* and *incremental* validity.

In clinical appraisal, our desire to identify and distinguish between those behaviors that are situationally governed and those that are constant across situations is often made more difficult by the various meanings of the words and labels we use to define characteristics to different people. In order to be useful, the terms we employ must have the same meaning across situations and cultures. The behaviors and acts that are called *aggression* or *sexual* in one culture must also be identifiable as such in another, even though both the normative levels and the acceptability of these behaviors may differ with the cultural values and norms. The political designations that define the presidents in our earlier example do not have these qualities; they are culture-specific and historically determined, and whatever attributes can be legitimately associated with them do not translate across cultures. The political platforms of the "Christian Democrats" in Italy, for example, may carry little similarity to the collective beliefs of a U.S. Democrat who is also a Christian.

The task of establishing the meaningfulness of the content is central to the derivation of an assessment device's *content validity.* This form of validity deals with the subject of the test and is an effort to define the relevant aspects of the characteristic or construct that is being measured. To the degree that the items appear to the common observer to be related to the quality that is targeted for measurement, we may say that the test has "face validity." However, not all content validity relies on its apparent similarity to the targeted construct or quality. Sometimes the quality that we are measuring cannot be measured by obvious items alone. In order to keep the definition of various words constant and to ensure that the content is accurate in relation to our needs, we often define the meanings that we want for different terms by referring to a formal psychological theory.

Once the terms used in our test items are defined through either their face validity or theoretical content, their meaning must be "operationalized." That is, their meaning must be identified in terms of some behavior that is observable to others. Since these terms are often derived from formal theories in the field, their translation into observable behaviors typically is derived from the ratings of experts who are familiar with the theory from which the definitions and terms are being extracted. The importance of this point can be illustrated by our "President's Test." Let us assume that one of our items asks the former presidents to rate their "success." The meaning of this term to the three men may be judged very differently if the term is extracted from economic theory and judged by economists; if it is drawn from a particular political party's platform and judged by the presidents themselves; or if it is borrowed from communication theory and judged by news correspondents. Therefore, the theoretical as well as the practical meanings of terms must be considered in assessing content validity.

Another form of validity that bears even more directly on the theoretical meaning of the qualities being assessed is *construct validity,* which refers to the degree to which the measurement device accurately identifies the presence of a quality or construct. Since constructs are theoretical rather than observable entities, however, construct validity is usually established by demonstrating that the measured trait or state bears the expected relationships to members of a network of other constructs within our chosen theory. The nature of these relationships is defined by the theory from which the construct has been defined. If our theory defines a president's success by how closely he or she follows a conservative agenda, for example, then one measure of the construct validity of our test is how well it correlates with a measure of political conservatism. As is often true in the establishment of construct validity, scores on an established test are often used as a criterion in order to determine whether the same abstract constructs are also present in the new test. Sometimes this attribute is referred to as *convergent validity,* in that it is a demonstration that two tests converge or measure similar properties.

More than convergent validity is needed, however, in order to establish that a test has construct validity. In addition to demonstrating that the new test correlates with other tests that measure the same theoretically derived construct, a demonstration of construct validity also requires evidence that the new test does *not* correlate highly with tests that are designed to measure different constructs. This demonstration is called *discriminant validity.* A person may score high on our test, for example, because he or she desires to appear conservative in an environment that is politically conservative. In that case, a portion of the test score may reflect the desire to fit in with others, or social desirability, rather than either "success" or "conservatism." If we demonstrate that our test does *not* correlate with a measure of social desirability, however, we have demonstrated its discriminant validity and provided more support for its construct validity.

To illustrate with a clinical example, scores on a test of depression should correlate highly with scores on other tests of depression, but they should not correlate with a test of a supposedly different quality, such as anxiety. Unfortunately, this is a poor but important example of discriminant validity, because although depression and anxiety are theoretically distinctive concepts, few types of psychological measurement (including the ratings of clinical judges) can distinguish them. This fact illustrates an important "Catch-22" problem in demonstrating the validity of measurement: All of these validation estimates assume that it is already possible to measure the construct or concept under investigation. If we can already measure it, why develop the test in the first place? If we cannot measure it now, the new test cannot be shown to be valid.

This problem has led some theorists to suggest that only conceptual or face validity is necessary under most conditions (Reckase, 1996). That is, the test is valid if it appears to be valid and if it is reliable. Alternatively, this problem points to the need for still another type of validity based upon some external criterion. *Criterion validity* is usually subdivided into two types, *concurrent validity* and *predictive validity,* depending on whether the test is expected to relate to external criteria that are present at the time the test is administered, or to those that are expected to occur at some time in the future. If our test of "success," founded upon a conservative political theory, correlates with party affiliation, it may be said to have concurrent validity. If, on the other hand, it correlates with who wins the next presidential election, it may be said to have predictive validity.

The concepts of specificity and sensitivity are related to criterion validity. If a test of diagnosis is sensitive, it accurately identifies those who have the qualities that define the diagnosis—an external criterion. If it possesses specificity, it accurately identifies those who do *not* have the qualities that define the diagnosis—also an external criterion. Both of these examples of criterion validity are also examples of concurrent validity. A test that is able to predict the likelihood that a person will develop a set of symptoms meeting diagnostic criteria at some time in the future has predictive validity. More specifically, if a test of recurrent depression successfully predicts future depression, it may be said to have predictive validity. In clinical practice, the assessment of the course or differential treatment response of a patient relies on predictive validity. Indeed predictive validity may be the most important, but perhaps the most difficult, type of validity to demonstrate.

Finally, *incremental validity* is the demonstration that the test provides more substantial knowledge of, greater ability to predict the behavior of, or more accurate identification of individuals than is possible by using more easily obtained information. Whereas most forms of validity are expressed as correlations or accuracy ratings, incremental validity is usually expressed as a partial correlation—a correlation expressing the relationship between the test and a criterion, while the influence of other variables, or of prior knowledge, is held constant statistically.

SUMMARY

In this chapter, we have briefly reviewed the nature of psychological tests, presented basic descriptive concepts from the Systematic Treatment Selection approach (Beutler et al., 2000), and addressed two of the four tasks required of those who conduct psychological assessment: defining the referral question and selecting the measurement device. This latter issue has been addressed only in terms of the qualities that are needed in order to measure accurately what we seek to measure. We have pointed out the difficulty of translating the shorthand requests for consultation that are frequently received into meaningful questions. We have also pointed out that psychological tests and measures must possess the qualities of scaling identity, sensitivity, specificity, normative value, reliability, and validity. Each of these concepts has been described and illustrated.

Although we have pointed out some of the considerations that are necessary in the selection of test procedures for answering referral questions, we have said little about the usefulness of specific tests, because their usefulness depends on the questions being asked. Specifically, we have pointed to the need to select tests that represent, in some significant and meaningful way, the environment to which generalizations are to be made and that evoke behaviors that are also representative of the behaviors likely to occur in these environments. The remainder of this book addresses the use and usefulness of several specific measures, the interpretative integration of these measures, and the communication of findings. Early chapters provide a conceptual description of the dimensions of the environment that must be considered in the selection of specific tests, and a system for organizing observations in preparation for rendering an integrated summary of findings from different sources and methods. Subsequent chapters describe several specific measures and their integrative interpretation. We wish to alert the reader to the fact that interpretations must be selected to address the referral questions asked. Because these questions are so varied, the thoughtful clinician must use discretion and judgment in extracting and using the information on specific tests for the purposes of responding to any given consultation request.

2

Approaching the Patient
REFERRAL CONTEXTS, TEST SELECTION, AND CLINICAL JUDGMENT

Larry E. Beutler
and Gary Groth-Marnat

While conducting the sequence of activities that comprise psychological assessment, the consulting clinician's role shifts at several critical points. Making these shifts smoothly and effectively requires clear communication, informed intuition, and educated clinical judgment at each point. The clinician begins the process of psychological assessment by defining the nature of the question being asked. For this task, the clinician's role is one of consultant. Once the question has been defined and framed in an answerable fashion, however, the clinician's role shifts into that of measurement expert. In this latter role, the clinician's job is to extract samples of the respondent's behaviors within environments that parallel or mirror those in which problems have occurred. The clinician's task is to match as closely as possible, the demand requirements of the measurement procedure with those of the problematic environment. Then the clinician observes a sample of the patient's behaviors within this contrived, assessment environment, repeating this process until an answer to the referral question becomes apparent.

When applying the measures and scoring them, the role of the clinician becomes (at least, momentarily) that of a psychological technician, whose behavior is controlled by external standardization, performance guidelines, and rules. Once the clinician has completed these technical tasks, however, the role adopted reverts to that of measurement expert. Clinical judgment, experience, intuition, and formal training all have a place in the performance of this role, as the clinician makes sense of and organizes a formal response to the referral question(s). Responses are interpreted, and dissonant findings are resolved. The observations and their assigned meanings are integrated; in this process, the clinician relies heavily upon knowledge of the psychometric qualities of the measurement procedures. Finally, the clinician returns to the role of consultant, as he or she communicates the findings to the referring clinician.

The previous chapter stressed the importance of clarifying the referral questions as well as evaluating the appropriateness of using tests. Later chapters illustrate the application to these questions by referring to a patient whose description is contained in Appendix A. We follow this patient throughout this book.

The current chapter elaborates on the themes developed in Chapter 1. In particular, the clinician must understand not only the importance of clarifying the referral question but also be able to understand the specific issues that arise in various contexts or settings. For example, a medical setting referent might be interested in the relation between psychosocial factors and seemingly organic symptom complaints. In contrast, a referent from a forensic context would be more interested in information that might assist in sentencing or deciding on the magnitude of compensation in a personal injury case. One of the major skills of the psychological consultant is to understand each of these contexts in a way that enables him or her to communicate competently with the referral source. This chapter introduces the demands of context/setting, a consideration that is amplified in Chapter 10. The current chapter also provides more detailed information on the types of tests that are relevant for various domains of patient functioning.

CONTEXTS OF ASSESSMENT

Each setting or context in which a clinician is asked to provide services implicitly contains its own way of approaching the client, which will be reflected in the typical types of referral questions asked (see Table 2.1). In addition, each context has its own (1) language, (2) role expectations for the professionals within these contexts, (3) sets of issues that must be addressed in confronting the client, and (4) theoretical beliefs. These variables require psychologists to be familiar with each context or setting in which they work, so that they can tailor their reports accordingly. The context influences such specific report-writing strategies and characteristics as the length

TABLE 2.1. Typical Referral Questions According to Different Contexts

Context	Typical referral question
Psychiatric	Is this patient a danger to self or others? To what extent might this patient be suffering from cerebral impairment? What challenges are likely to occur with this patient in psychotherapy? What is this patient's prognosis?
General medical	Does this patient have an undiagnosed psychological disorder? What are some appropriate psychosocial treatments for this patient, who has a known medical condition? Given a patient's psychological condition, might he or she have particular difficulties with surgery?
Legal	Is this witness's testimony credible? Is this client competent to stand trial? What is the extent and nature of this client's injury? What is the optimal custody arrangement for this child? Is this client likely to benefit from treatment? What are the strengths and weaknesses of this professional's report?
Vocational	What is the degree of match between this client's personality and various vocations in which he or she is interested? Can this person with a disability return to work? If so, what would be most suitable for him or her? Which of these candidates would be most suitable for the position?
Psychological	Is there clinically relevant information that I, as the treating clinician, am missing? What type of intervention would this client respond to best? How is this client progressing compared to other similar cases? What are the medical and legal aspects of this case, for which I might need to seek consultation?

of the report, the types of language and phrases used, and the extent to which technical test information is included.

The most important and frequently encountered contexts in adult personality assessment are those from psychiatric, general medical, legal, vocational, and psychological settings (Groth-Marnat, 1999b). Chapter 10 reviews these and other settings that call for special skills, materials, and knowledge on the part of psychologists. This latter chapter offers suggestions that may allow psychologists to select procedures and approach problems in a manner that is relatively specific to the setting in which they work. Here we provide a few short examples of the kinds of demands that arise in different contexts.

The Psychiatric Setting

Psychiatric settings constitute the most time-honored arena for the use of formal psychological testing. Indeed, the birth of clinical psychology can be considered to have occurred largely because of psychiatrists' need for formal testing information about their patients. In the early years of clinical psychology, psychiatrists were assigned the roles of administrator, therapist, and consultant. The early roles of clinical psychologists were as technicians who provided what would be analogous to "lab tests" based on their test data. The roles of all mental health professionals have changed greatly since these early years. Psychologists, nurses, social workers, and counselors now frequently play administrative and consultative roles. Nurses and psychologists are asked to provide consultation on medication management and to plan and conduct psychotherapy.

In the domain of psychological assessment, the level of expertise, types of information, and responsibilities assumed by psychologists have expanded considerably since these early days. However, psychologists should realize that sometimes nonpsychologist mental health professionals may still consider psychological testing in a relatively narrow "lab test" manner that keeps it disembodied from the contexts that influence interpretations and conclusions. For example, this perception may be observed when a psychiatrist requests information from a specific test ("I would like a WAIS-III done on this patient"). As emphasized in Chapter 1, the psychologist's optimal response would be to translate such a request to one that focuses on the domains that need to be measured (i.e., What is the patient's level of cognitive functioning?) rather than the specific method of doing so. The psychologist should then establish what decisions need to be made regarding the patient (i.e., Can this patient function independently?). Then the psychologist can inform the referrant about what method and procedure would best answer the desired questions, serving both an educative and consultative function. This process can be greatly enhanced by understanding the issues and roles typically faced by those who seek psychological consultation.

In each setting, the psychologist's report should reflect the specific questions raised and the values of the system. Many psychiatric settings, particularly those that embody a traditional, psychoanalytic perspective, value elaborate formulations of patient personality and relationships. These reports require more interpretation of the dynamics that are at play than do those required in other settings. For example, more biologically oriented psychiatric settings tend to be quite pragmatic and less tolerant of reports that provide an interpretation of a patient's personality or "dynamics."

These settings may best be served with short, descriptive reports that concentrate on the question(s) being asked. By attending to these differences among the contexts in which assessments are initiated, psychologists can act as effective consultants (rather than technicians), in that they will fulfill a broad role that provides optimally useful information for the clients they assess.

The Medical Setting

Among the many contexts in which a psychologist may consult, medical settings are perhaps the ones that most challenge the consultant's need to understand the demand characteristics represented. The extensive technical knowledge necessary to appreciate medical treatments, the complexity of many health conditions themselves, the sheer number of allied health professionals working in these settings, and the manner in which the patient is likely to be referred through the system make understanding the context essential. In order to be maximally useful, psychologists should not only develop a clear, focused approach to assessment, but also take the time to become familiar with the patient's medical conditions and their treatment.

In medical and health care settings, psychologists are frequently asked to make determinations regarding patients' emotional status, prognosis, the etiology of their condition, their strengths and resources, possible appropriate treatments, and their probable psychiatric diagnosis. In other words, the referral questions presented in these settings cover the entire range of those addressed in this book. Indeed, the essence of personality assessment conducted in medical and health settings is not very much different from that done in more traditional mental health settings. The core difference lies in access to the patient, the nature of the normative comparisons used, the frequent availability of a multidisciplinary treatment team in these settings, and the rules and regulations that pertain to the tasks and objectives of the specific setting.

Long narrative reports are typically not useful in a medical context since the subculture expects far briefer, focused reports than would be tolerated in most other settings. Reports should run from two to three pages, be highly specific, use bullets to highlight the major points, and have a strong focus on symptoms, diagnosis, and treatment.

The Legal Setting

Psychologists are consulted for many different purposes within legal settings: assessing a defendant's competency to stand trial, determining insanity, contributing to child custody decisions, evaluating the significance of personal injury, and assessing the presence of malingering, deceit, and exaggeration (Ackerman, 1999; Blau, 1998). In recent years, the definitions and requirements of "expert testimony" that are applied by the court to psychological testimony have shifted. The *Daubert* criterion, which is becoming the most accepted standard by which to define psychological experts, requires that the testimony be consistent with established scientific findings. This criterion, compared to its predecessors, places relatively less emphasis on the mere fact of an expert's experience and training.

At the core of psychological practice in a forensic or legal setting is the requirement that the professional psychologist be able to translate relevant technical psychological knowledge into clear, everyday terms that are understandable by individuals who vary widely in education, training, and experience. For example, a frequent complaint of attorneys is that many reports by psychologists use language that is highly specific to psychology and very technical. To reduce this problem, it is particularly desirable for legal reports to avoid referring to such items as test scales, scores, and profiles and to instead focus on what the results mean for this particular person within their specific situation. One must be aware that within legal contexts, words carry very distinct, legal meanings that are often different from the way the same terms are used in psychological circles. Psychologists who consult in these settings must be aware of distinctions between such phrases as "preponderance of evidence" and "beyond reasonable doubt." A psychologist must also become familiar with the legal meanings of such terms as "insanity," "reasonable certainty," and "incompetent." It is these definitions and the manner in which the psychologist comes to his or her conclusions, that will be given scrutiny in court. Accordingly, these matters are discussed at greater length in Chapter 10.

In comparison to those written for medical settings, legal reports are often quite lengthy because careful detail needs to be given to (1) explaining the nature of the support for various opinions, as well as (2) anticipating and responding to potential challenges. It is not unusual for legal reports to include responses to previous reports that have been made by other professionals. As a result, reports can sometimes be up to 20 pages, although 6 to 10 pages is a more typical range. Legal reports must be particularly clear in identifying the specific referral question being addressed, and the report must be addressed specifically to these questions. Usually this specificity can be accomplished by numbering the referral questions at the beginning of the report and then providing a similarly listed set of responses at the end of the report.

Other Contexts

There are a variety of additional settings in which psychologists work, such as schools, industry, and the military. Each setting is somewhat different, and all call for specific clinical knowledge and skills. It is important to understand that in addition to the general guidelines and expectations for different kinds of settings (e.g., psychiatric, medical, forensic), there are also specific expectations and standards that arise from the composition of the staff at each particular facility. Thus it is imperative for psychologists to become familiar with the general nature of the setting in which they work as well as with the specific ethos that governs that specific setting.

Summary

The foregoing discussion of referral settings has highlighted several key themes in working within various referral contexts. Psychologists should be clinical consultants rather than merely technicians who administer tests. This means they need to learn the roles, language, values, and types of disorders that are most likely to be seen in these contexts. For example, in forensic contexts psychologists are likely to encounter a high proportion of persons with personality disorders, whereas in general medical settings a high proportion of physically ill and somatizing patients is the rule. Furthermore, there are context-specific expectations regarding the length and nature of psychological reports, and each setting has its own preferred and defined technical terms. Psychologists should be aware of, and knowledgeable about, the expectations that characterize the setting(s) in which they work.

In all cases, psychologists usually are faced with unclear referral questions that, first and foremost, must be clarified. One of the most important strategies is to remember that most referral sources will need to make a variety of decisions regarding the client and, as such, psychologists can often clarify the referral question by focusing on which decisions and actions are being considered. Another important theme is to view the client and his or her presenting problem in a wider environmental and psychosocial context. This perspective is sometimes difficult to achieve, particularly given that psychological testing lends itself toward formulating the client's difficulties in narrow, individual terms rather than with reference to the larger system in which the person is living.

TEST SELECTION

Selecting the optimal instrument for assessment involves a number of interacting factors. As discussed previously, one of the most important considerations is ensuring that the instruments used can elicit the type of information required by the referral question. It is thus necessary to clarify the referral question and to fully understand the setting in which the referral is made. Matters of test reliability and validity, other aspects of psychometrics, how the test will be used, and for whom it is appropriate must also be considered. Additional and related considerations include understanding

(1) the dimensions of psychological tests, (2) the advantage of a fixed or "core battery" (one that is given to everyone) in relation to a flexible battery, (3) how to best become familiar with the instruments within the field (based on patterns of test use), and (4) how best to become acquainted with the different domains of functioning assessed by each instrument.

Dimensions of Psychological Tests

Psychological tests are essentially exercises that are performed according to instructions in situations that are constructed to bear some similarity to problematic environments, and in which a person is requested to respond to a set of stimuli that is presented in a standardized manner. It is assumed that the testing situation is analogous to the everyday environment in which the person lives and that the responses given can be generalized to how the patient will act in everyday life. It is this assumption that makes psychological tests useful. If the client's responses were so specific to the testing environment itself that they could not be generalized to real life, then it would be impossible to make meaningful statements related to the various referral questions. Much of the most relevant research on psychological tests relates to the ability to make statements about the client's everyday life. The ability to generalize is referred to as the "everyday" or "ecological" validity of the test. It also should be noted, however, that no single, contrived environment or test procedure can represent fully the varied aspects of any real-world environment in which a patient lives. Given that tests are, to a greater or lesser extent, analogous to the environments of actual interest (as noted, sometimes called "analogue environments"), they nevertheless vary in the extent to which they (1) measure changeable versus more permanent aspects of the person (i.e., states vs. traits), and (2) favor the disclosure of different types of information (demand characteristics). Demand characteristics vary in terms of (1) the degree to which the instruments are structured versus unstructured, (2) the focus on internal versus external experience, (3) the degree to which they are experienced by the client as stressful, and (4) whether they yield qualitative versus quantitative data.

States versus Traits

As we discussed in Chapter 1, *traits* refer to our enduring qualities or response tendencies; they are recognizable across situations and transcend varying situational demands. States, on the other hand, are temporary and situationally induced reactions. Although our state reactions may be affected by our traits, state reactions are less stable and more susceptible to change in response to changing environments. In reality, this distinction is not particularly clear since most qualities that are identified as describing human experience have both state- and trait-like aspects. Terms such as *personality* and *intelligence* are used to describe attributes that are primarily trait-like, whereas terms such as *acute, distress,* and *resistance* are used to describe attributes that are primarily state-like. When clinicians discuss differences between baseline and current functioning, they are usually talking about the relative elevation of various state responses. Likewise, when clinicians discuss differences among a patient's level of performance, coping style, and normative values, they are usually discussing trait tendencies.

In addition, different tests or subscales of multiscale inventories often emphasize the extent to which the variable has trait- or state-like qualities. For example, the State–Trait Anxiety Inventory (Spielberger, Gorsuch, Lushene, Vagg, & Jacobs, 1983a) makes this distinction particularly clearly. Some of the scales on the MMPI-2 (Butcher, Dahlstrom, Graham, Tellegen, & Kaemmer, 1989) are also considered to reflect highly stable trait-like qualities (e.g., hysteria, introversion/extroversion), whereas others reflect more changeable and state-like aspects (e.g., depression).

One task of the behavioral scientist is to determine which qualities of a patient are trait-like and which are state-like. Another task is to determine how to define both states and traits in operational (i.e., observable and replicable) ways, so that the definitions will be useful for answering the questions related to diagnosis, etiology, prognosis, treatment, functional impairment, and client strengths that comprise the task of psychological assessment. Often, appropriate test selection can facilitate this process.

Demand Characteristics

To respond most effectively to a referral question, a clinician selects a variety of analogue environments to present to the patient. The instructions and format of presentation that establish the nature of each of these selected environments are designed to limit the patient's response in various ways. As noted, these limits are referred to as the "demand characteristics" of the test. In other words, the implicit and explicit rules that govern what the respondent can and must do constitute a test's demand characteristics. Because the clinician systematically manipulates these analogue environments by altering the instructional qualities and the nature of the test material, the demand characteristics of a test are conceptually similar to the manipulation of an independent variable in an experiment.

Concomitantly, the various constructed demand characteristics of an analogue environment are designed to evoke different classes of response. Some demand characteristics are best described by how the instrument is formatted (e.g., structured or unstructured), whereas others are best described by identifying the particular type of response domain assessed by the instrument. An example of the latter representation is found in the difference between instruments that require an individual to think, thereby eliciting information about thought processes, and those that require the individual simply to identify the presence of symptoms, thereby eliciting information about emotional and interpersonal behaviors. The forms that these behaviors take in response to the demands of an instrument are referred to as the "response characteristics" of the eliciting environment. An individual's response characteristics indicate something about the domain or area of experience that is targeted for observation by the demand characteristics of the assessment environment. Although the domains of functioning that distinguish different responses must be identifiable when different demand characteristics are encountered, it is variations in the client's responses within each response domain, and to each analogue environment, that are observed and interpreted. Hence, the observations and measurement of the patient's behavior and experience serve the same functions as the dependent variable in an experiment.

Two cardinal assumptions are made by the clinician in order to formulate generalizations based on the observations within the analogue environments of the consulting room regarding the environments of interest in the external world: (1) The variations that exist in the demand characteristics of the test environments are similar to critical aspects of the everyday environments of patients; and (2) the response characteristics that are observed are diminutive or symbolic representations of behaviors likely to be exhibited in real-world environments. Stated another way, in order to make accurate interpretations, the clinician counts on the ability to predict accurately the parameters of both stimulus generalization and response generalization.

Stimulus generalization is the basis for predicting the likelihood (i.e., probability or frequency) that a response that has been observed in a test environment will also be exhibited in a real-world environment. In contrast, *response generalization* is the basis for predicting the nature and form that a real-world behavior will take. Whereas stimulus generalization is a function of the similarity that exists between the demand characteristics of the analogue and the real-world environments, response generalization is a function of the similarity of the responses that occur in these two types of environments.

The value of clinical assessment is contingent on the ability of the clinician to (1) identify relevant similarities between the real-world and analogue environments, and (2) construct a testing environment that evokes generalizable and relevant behaviors. It is therefore important to give some consideration to the *demand characteristics* that clinicians alter by selecting and using different instruments in order to construct a generalizable testing environment, and to the domains of *human experience and performance* to which test responses are generalized.

Structured versus Ambiguous Environments. Assessment procedures vary in the degree of structure imposed on the respondent. High levels of structure are maintained by test instructions that either limit the number of responses available to the patient or identify responses as either "correct" or "incorrect." The true–false format of the Minnesota Multiphasic Personality Inventory (MMPI-2) and the open-ended format of the Wechsler Adult Intelligence Scale—Revised (WAIS-III; Wechsler, 1997) are examples of the two ways in which high levels of structure are provided.

Varying the degree of structure places a demand on the respondent to impose various levels of order on his or her response. High levels of structure relieve the individual of the need to impose order and organization on, or to attribute meaning to, the stimulus material or task. There is little ambiguity in what the clinician wants. The structured subtests of the WAIS-III are reliable and valid measures of knowledge; they tap cognitive content and assess observational accuracy. The true–false format of the MMPI-2 provides reliable and valid measures based on self-observations, attributions, and decisiveness.

In contrast, ambiguous tasks require construction and selection of responses in the relative absence of information. The methods used for inducing ambiguity in an assessment environment include reducing cues that indicate the number or nature of acceptable responses, and introducing instructions that lack specificity. One of the crucial behaviors that arises from a certain set of demand characteristics in an analogue environment is the set of features we refer to as "projection." This is because the person "projects" aspects of themselves into their responses.

Projection, in this context, is a hypothetical process, not one that is directly measured. Projection is inferred to have occurred whenever meaning is attributed to an ambiguous event. The meaning ascribed is assumed to reflect the internal qualities of the respondent rather than a quality of the external world. Projective theory maintains that when structure is removed, the respondent attributes his or her own private meanings or aspects of his or her own internal experiences to the ambiguous stimuli. In interpreting the Rorschach, for example, it is common to view a large number of small-detail responses as indicative of a person who focuses, similarly, on small details in other aspects of life. It is the instructional ambiguity that evokes organizational and projective responses. From the response characteristics and content (i.e., number of small details), the clinician infers the presence of such defining traits as conventionality, order, and a selective bias toward making external or internal causal attributions. The imposition of order on the stimuli serves as an index of the patient's ability to organize disparate elements in problem tasks; the degree of conventionality (assessed by normative criteria) serves as an index of social compliance; and the failure to discard unusual percepts serves as an indication of low sensitivity to social conventions.

Obviously, the assumption that projection is elicited by ambiguous stimuli is central to some interpretations of a person's responses to ambiguous environments. However, responses also can be seen more parsimoniously as representative of the person's efforts to solve ambiguous problems. In this latter case, a clinician can explore "empirical relationships" between various response characteristics and both concomitant and future behaviors, or the clinician can observe aspects of the patient's general problem-solving skills and assume that these observations reflect qualities of the patient's response to situations in which answers and implications are not clear. Thus the response characteristics of speed, accuracy, and problem-solving efficiency remain relevant, even when the validity of the projective hypothesis is suspect. Clinicians can select different types of assessment procedures, depending on the importance of ambiguity for the evaluation. If ambiguity is important, then assessment procedures, such as the Rorschach or open-ended interviewing would be recommended. If ambiguity is less important, then using more structured procedures, such as the MMPI-2 and structured clinical interviews, would be appropriate.

Internal versus External Experience. Another variation in the demand characteristics of instruments is the domain of experience that the patient is encouraged to explore or reveal. That is, test environments vary in the nature of the experience on which respondents are asked to focus and reveal. A clinician may select assessment procedures that request a patient to disclose (or behave in such a way as to disclose) internal experience, or the clinician may directly observe external events. Different tests vary in the extent to which they elicit subjective versus objective behavioral samples. Overt behaviors that can be directly observed constitute objective experience, whereas internal behaviors that can only be inferred from what a respondent says or does are classes of subjective responses. Direct observations of behavior are the most usual methods of sampling objective behavior. Rating the behavior or the environment is another method of sampling objective experience, although such ratings are positioned more toward the subjective end of the continuum than are direct observations. In contrast are measures that assess more internal aspects of experience, such as the Rorschach, or even behavioral responses to the WAIS-III (e.g., a client stating "I'm no good at these types of tasks," which suggests low self-efficacy). Much of the assessment of subjective behavior must rely on self-reports of some kind or on observations of behaviors that are considered to be symbolic expressions of internal experience.

Most procedures that purport to assess "personality" elicit responses that reflect several points along the dimension of subjective–objective experience. This range is employed because "personality traits" are thought to be operative not only in a variety of environments but also in the process of enacting subjective experiences in the form of objective behaviors. The

MMPI-2, for example, includes questions that require self-observations and revelation of overt behavior (e.g., "I have used alcohol excessively," "I have very few quarrels with members of my family"), and others that require awareness of internal states (e.g., "Parts of my body often have feelings like burning, tingling, crawling, or like 'going to sleep,' " "I am worried about sex"). Likewise, clinical interviews ask respondents to report on both subjective experience (e.g., "How often do you feel depressed?") and observable behaviors (e.g., "How many times have you been in trouble with the law?").

Comparing the results of procedures that variously sample subjective and objective experiences may be especially helpful in addressing questions of differential diagnosis and treatment. Comparisons of a patient's sensitivity to, and ability to report on, subjective and objective experience, for example, may reflect the degree to which the patient's personality or coping style is expressed primarily through internal processes and behaviors that are only indirectly observed externally, or through external behaviors directly. Reports of subjective anxiety in the absence of observed or reported behavioral disturbances suggest that a given individual internalizes experience; reports of drinking, hostile interactions, and legal difficulties, without concomitant reports or observed indications of internal distress, suggest that an individual acts out (i.e., externalizes) conflicts. If both external behavioral disruption and internal distress are present, it may indicate that an individual uses both types of coping strategies.

Information about the relative use of internalizing and externalizing coping styles also has been found to be predictive of an individual's response to different treatments. The identification of an internalizing coping style may serve as an indicator for the use of insight-oriented therapies, while an externalizing coping style may serve as an indicator for the use of behavior-focused, skill-building, and cognitive therapies (Beutler & Clarkin, 1990; Beutler, Clarkin, & Bongar, 2000). These points are discussed at greater length in Chapter 3.

Level of Stress. A third demand characteristic of the instrument is the level of stress that it imposes on the patient. Note that *stress* is a characteristic of the environment and should be distinguished from *distress,* which is a quality of discomfort in the individual; stress may precipitate distress. The demand imposed by varying levels of stress requires the respondent to cope in some manner, whereby he or she reveals an aspect of his or her coping style. By altering characteristics of the assessment, the examiner "draws out" information about how the individual responds to different levels of stress.

Stress levels in the assessment environment can be controlled by varying the degree of administrator directiveness, the nature of the interpersonal environment, and by the use of instructions that present conflict.

A frequent means of manipulating the degree of stress is altering the degree of *directiveness*. High levels of control and direction may be used to increase the level of stress in the administration of materials. In contrast, relatively noncontrolling procedures include unstructured interviews and requests for free associations; in these, the nature of the respondent's alternatives is not greatly limited, and little stress may be induced. Procedures such as individually administered IQ tests (e.g., the WAIS-III) have a high degree of directiveness, on the other hand, and the requirement of "right answers" may ensure that stress is transmitted. Clinicians can increase directiveness further by introducing frequent reminders to attend to accuracy or quality—"Remember, do the best you can"; "Try a little more to get it right."

A different type of stress can be introduced by imposing a requirement for speed. This type of clinician control is usually imposed and increased by varying the frequency of the time reminder ("Do it as fast as you can") and by varying the extent of making an obvious show of tracking performance time (holding a stopwatch in a visible position).

Still another type of stress can be imposed on the patient by selecting assessment procedures that vary the nature of the *interpersonal environment*. The goal of placing stress on the respondent by varying the interpersonal context is to elicit behaviors that reflect interpersonal sensitivity, the ability to engage with others, and thresholds of compliance and defiance. Procedures that have written instructions and can be completed in a room alone are likely to induce less acute distress than ones that are individually administered. Sentence completion tasks, personality questionnaires, group forms of intellectual tests, and the like, impose little interpersonal stress. Individual intelligence tests, most individually administered projective tests, and interviews all include a component of interpersonal stress.

A third method for introducing stress into an analogue assessment environment is to present an *irreconcilable conflict*. The demand quality of contradiction calls on the respondent to make choices. The instructions are typically contradictory and require that a person modulate between impulses and constraints. The responses observed under these conditions are interpreted as reflecting the propensity of the respondent's cognitive organizational skills to decline. Environments that embody this type of stress are of particular help in determining whether an individual can utilize cognitive strengths to override frustration without any negative effect on the quality or organization of problem-solving output. For example, in pitting instructional demands for precision against those for speed, a clinician may require a patient to be maximally accurate and to utilize maximal speed in reproducing a series of designs (i.e., "Do it as well and as fast as you can"). Under the joint pressures of interpersonal stress and high levels of directive demand, the clinician can observe the respondent's ability to find a compromise between tendencies to over- and undercontrol behaviors.

Here the clinician is interested in making a generalized interpretation about how well a respondent is able to maintain baseline levels of performance during high stress conditions. A qualitative decline in the number of conventional responses; an increase in the number of regressive, unusual, or immature responses; the emergence of impulsive responses; and a relative increase in the number of affect-laden responses all suggest that the respondent has difficulty maintaining perspective in the face of strong emotions. Low tolerance for external control may be manifested through various forms of defiance and rebellion. In contrast, high levels of tolerance may be manifested through consistent efforts to please the clinician. The clinician can assess the strength of the patient's propensity to respond in a defiant or compliant fashion by systematically increasing the strength of the directives offered and observing the consequences.

An additional area of functioning that may be sampled by introducing environmental stress, and one that particularly arises in environments that vary clinician control, is the ability of the respondent to comply with the demands of treatments. All treatments require at least some sacrifice of personal freedom, along with a willingness to accept the validity of external authorities. Although treatments may vary in these qualities, the patient's willingness to sacrifice control to the clinician during assessment may indicate the patient's ability to subjugate him- or herself to treatment in the interest of experiencing long-term gains.

Quantitative versus Qualitative Data

"Empirical" tests are based upon the demonstration that the scores (numbers) elicited are different among patients with different, known characteristics (i.e., normative and criteria-group comparisons). These empirical demonstrations are at the very foundation of quantitative assessment, and, of necessity, rely on the demonstration of *group* differences in numerical scores. However, some professionals in the field have become disillusioned with quantitative methods and have criticized academic psychology and measurement theorists for the failure to attend to individual idiosyncrasies (Headland, Pike, & Harris, 1990; Rutter, 1994). These individuals attach far less importance to subgroup norms as the basis for assessing the value of clinical methods. They maintain that comparing a given individual to a standard based upon small criteria groups, as a means of determining the meaning of that individual's behavior, obscures clinically relevant uniqueness. They favor, instead, an "ipsative" description of the person, in which each individual serves as his or her own reference point for describing relative strengths and weaknesses.

Not surprisingly, practitioners who work daily with people are often less persuaded by demonstrations that an individual's test scores are either different from or similar to those of various reference groups than are academic psychologists, who are more familiar and comfortable with numerical concepts. Hence, although academic psychologists frequently criticize and even eschew tests such as the Rorschach, clinicians continue to use such tests as a basis for developing clinical impressions. The complex and multidimensional relationships described in clinical formulations of personality functioning are difficult to distill into numbers. Some approaches, such as Exner's scoring system for the Rorschach (Exner, 1993), have attempted to translate narrative descriptions into numerical formulations (see Chapter 9). Even if such procedures were used and found to have some validity, many clinicians would remain concerned that these numbers fail to preserve the character of the phenomena being observed. They ask such questions as these: Do ratios and combinations of numbers adequately capture the essence of love? Do they adequately distinguish among different kinds of nonobservable experiences (e.g., love, anger, lust, etc.)? Do numbers adequately allow us to compare the amount that people love their wives or husbands with the amount that they love their mothers? Can numbers capture the variations in love-driven behaviors that occur when a child's life is threatened or when a spouse or lover is unfaithful?

Advocates of the methods of "narrative assessment" and "hermeneutics" represent increasingly persuasive forces within contemporary measurement theory. These qualitative methods, which attend to the wholistic structure and content of natural language, have a particular affinity for clinicians for whom quantitative methods do not appear to be adaptable to describing the complexities and colors of individual differences.

We believe qualitative methods offer an additional perspective in the measurement of human experience. However, we also believe quantitative and qualitative methods are not inherently in opposition to each other; in fact, they are potentially synergistic (i.e., they can complement each other). Qualitative methods of interpretation emphasize idiographic (i.e., idiosyncratic) patterns, whereas quantitative methods are distinguished by their nomothetic (i.e., normative) basis of deriving meanings from patient productions. The former methods rely on an ipsative comparison, in which various qualities of the patient serve as a standard of relative comparison; the latter methods emphasize a normative or group comparison, in which the patient is compared to an outside norm reflective of others' responses. Narrative descriptions can enliven and deepen an understanding of test scores, while test scores can be used to ensure the objectivity of narratives and allow a normative interpretation.

Test selection often reflects both the type of information the clinician wants to elicit from the patient (i.e., demand characteristics) and the extent to which the clinician values qualitative versus quantitative information. For example, tests such as the Rorschach and the Thematic Apperception Test lend themselves to a more qualitative interpretation. The degree to which a clinician emphasizes such factors as behavioral observations and history also might reflect the value placed on qualitative information. Even quantitatively oriented tests such as the MMPI-2 and WAIS-III can be embellished with qualitative information. For example, a clinician might list several critical items from the MMPI-2 as a means of representing the types of item content that elicit client response. This addition may serve to add some richness to themes that emerge from quantitative interpretations. Most interpretive procedures for the Wechsler intelligence scales also add a qualitative dimension. For example, a clinician might include the excessive detail from a word definition to exemplify the thought processes of a compulsive client. We encourage practitioners to develop a balance between such quantitative and qualitative types of information.

Even though we encourage such a balance, we also encourage the awareness that qualitative interpretations of test materials are subject to several sources of error. The interpretations may not be accurate; they may not be replicable or constant; they may reflect a client's mood or diet rather than actual internal characteristics; and they may have no heuristic value for predicting and planning treatment. Even qualitative interpretive methods must come to grips with issues of reliability and validity. In order to be useful, non-numerical concepts (such as the complex verbal ones that characterize narrative descriptions) must be capable of reliable classification, and each category must be distinguishable from others. That is, a clinician must be able to assert that a conflict with a mother is manifestly different from a conflict with a wife; that two ego states are different; that aggressive impulses are different from sexual ones; or that two dynamic intrapsychic patterns differ from each other.

Fixed versus Flexible Battery Approaches

Ever since the work of Rapaport, Gill, and Schafer (1946), most clinical treatment programs have advocated and employed a standard set of assessment devices as part of the intake procedure. Although the same instruments are administered to all incoming patients, with little or no modification, the interpretation itself is usually modified according to patients' ethnic background, sex, and referral problems. This "standard" or "core" battery approach to assessment is designed to provide a broad base of similar and reliable information from which to compare patients, make diagnoses, evaluate areas of patients' strength and weakness, determine prognoses, and plan treatment.

Approaching assessment through the use of a core battery of devices has several advantages over more flexible, individualized assessment procedures. For example, through the consistent and repeated use of the instruments from a core battery, a clinician may develop a set of explicit expectations about the characteristics of those patients who seek services at a given clinical institution. By referencing a client's performance against a set of specific norms, and by observing the patient characteristics that are associated with a good response to the treatment in a particular setting, the clinician develops the ability to extract very individualized interpretations from the test materials. A core battery thereby may allow highly individualized interpretations because of the increased expertise resulting from an in-depth familiarity with the instruments used.

In addition, a core battery permits the accumulation of a database that allows a clinician to review the changes, over time, in patients applying for service at a given site (and, where applicable, the changes within individuals from one admission to another). Even the overall efficacy of various treatment programs in a facility can be determined if postdischarge follow-up evaluations are included in the standard battery. In contrast, if each entering patient receives a different set of tests based upon his or her particular presentation, it is difficult to compare patients entering the facility at different times or to estimate the efficacy of the treatment programs established.

On the other hand, there are drawbacks to using a core battery that is applied to everyone. The primary drawback is the lack of flexibility for addressing the unique needs of individual patients. That is, there are questions that a single, all-purpose test battery is simply unable to answer. As a result, some authors (Clarkin & Hurt, 1988; Sweeney, Clarkin, & Fitzgibbon, 1987) argue for a more focused or problem-specific form of evaluation as an alternative to the use of a core battery. This type of assessment battery comprises instruments that are focused on the issues most salient to the patient's diagnosis and treatment; such assessments may be very different for different individuals, depending upon the nature of the questions asked by referring professionals. The advantages of this "individualized" approach lie in its ability to respond specifically to presenting issues and referral questions. Problem-focused assessment allows a more in-depth analysis of a given patient's problems than the usual core battery, because it acknowledges that some tests are better suited to addressing certain problems than are others.

The professional debate about the virtues of using a core/standard versus flexible/problem-focused assessment procedure is, in reality, overly polarized. More typically, clinicians use a small group of standard tests combined with additional tests tailored to the specifics of the client's presenting problem. For example, a clinician may use several different batteries flexibly in a given setting, each tailored to particular problems typically presented by patients who come to that setting. Many clinics have specialized treatment programs for anxiety disorders, depression, and eating disorders. Depending on a patient's initial complaints, as assessed by the first telephone contact or interview, one of several core batteries may be administered to address these complaints separately and flexibly. Flexibility also can be introduced by supplementing these batteries with individualized tests that reflect the needs of specific patients. For a person with initial complaints of depression, for example, a standard battery (an omnibus personality test, a symptom checklist, an assessment of social background, and a test of interpersonal relationships) could be augmented with tests that are sensitive to mood and affect, memory, and suicidality. Such supplemental tests allow desirable individualization in assessing those functional areas that are presented in the referral question, whereas the core tests allow comparisons to be made across patients and time.

Patterns of Test Usage

The kind of test most frequently selected in the modal standard battery is an omnibus personality test of trait-like qualities. One or two instruments of this type are often included in an assessment battery in order to obtain behavioral samples from both subjective and objective experience domains. The next most frequently selected instrument type consists of intellectual and cognitive tests designed to determine level of abstract reasoning, problem-solving efficiency, and the nature of cognitive organization. We believe it is important to assess these functions in order to accurately interpret personality and symptom presentations.

Symptom and other state measures, though high on the list of preferred measures, are less frequently selected in the standard battery than tests of either global personality or general cognitive functioning (Camara, Nathan, & Puente, 2000). When symptom measures are included, however, tests that evaluate several different problem domains and provide both an estimate of the objective level of social dysfunction and an indication of patient subjective distress are favored.

In terms of specific instruments, the Wechsler intelligence scales (WAIS-III and WISC-III) consistently have been found to be the most frequently used cognitive measures in clinical practice (Camara et al., 2000). These instruments are closely followed, in frequency of use, by the MMPI-2 and Rorschach. Other frequently used instruments include the Bender Visual Motor Gestalt Test (BVMGT), Thematic Apperception Test, Wide Range Achievement Test–III (WRAT-III), projective drawing procedures (i.e., house–tree–person), Wechsler Memory Scale–III (WMS-III), and the Millon Clinical Multiaxial Inventory–III (MCMI-III). However, there is a trend toward an overall decrease in the amount of time professional psychologists spend doing assessment (Piotrowski, 1999). This decrease is considered to be largely the result of reduced reimbursement from managed care organizations. There also seems to be greater emphasis on brief, targeted instruments that have direct relevance to treatment planning and outcome assessment (Maruish, 1999, Piotrowski, 1999). Such instruments include the Symptom Checklist 90—Revised, Beck Depression Inventory–II, and the State–Trait Anxiety Inventory. This emphasis on brief, targeted in-

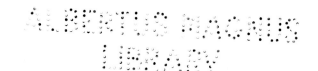

struments is most likely a response to greater cost-containment efforts by managed care (Groth-Marnat, 1999a). Associated with this new emphasis is the more recent development of instruments specifically designed for treatment planning, patient tracking, and outcome assessment, such as the Systematic Treatment Selection Clinician Rating Form (Fisher, Beutler, & Williams, 1999a), Butcher Treatment Planning Inventory (Butcher, 1998), and the Outcome Questionnaire (Lambert et al., 1996). As might be expected, forensic and educational settings, which are minimally impacted by managed care programs, have patterns of test usage similar to the patterns found prior to the impact of managed care (Piotrowski, 1999).

A final pattern that should be noted in test usage is that projective assessment seems to be losing favor among psychologists and is decreasing in frequency of use. Again, this is most likely due to the lack of reimbursement from managed care companies and the perception that they are overly labor intensive and do not yield sufficient information relevant for treatment planning and outcome assessment.

Selecting Instruments Based on Domains of Client Functioning

Imbedded in the various referral questions is information related to different areas or domains of a client's functioning. For example, a referral from a general medical setting might request information related to whether a patient is translating psychosocial stress into physiological symptoms. In order to answer this question, the clinician will need to investigate the pattern and severity of symptoms as well as develop a diagnosis. The most central domains for most referral questions are (1) historical background, (2) cognitive functioning, (3) emotional functioning, (4) interpersonal–intrapersonal functioning, (5) diagnostic status, (6) prognosis and treatment response, and (7) client strengths and resources. The typical report is organized around these domains (see Chapter 13). In order to choose which test or group of tests to administer, the first step is to clarify which of the domains need to be addressed. The clinician can then choose various instruments that assess these domains. Each instrument may be more adept and reliable for assessing some areas of functioning than others.

Clarkin and Hurt (1988) identified a number of areas in which reliable and sensitive instruments exist for specific purposes. Their suggestions are adapted in Table 2.2, which identifies the instruments whose focus and content are most useful for each of the seven response domains listed above. Two points should be noted in reference to Table 2.2. First, the list of tests is only representative, not comprehensive; it does little justice to the very large number of available measures that may be used to assess each area. Indeed, there are instruments that may be better suited for specific purposes than those presented here. In particular, the many neuropsycholo-

TABLE 2.2. Recommended Instruments for Various Response Domains

Domain/instrument(s)	Rater
1. Historical background	
Life Experiences Survey	Patient
Social Support Questionnaire (SSQ)	Patient
2. Cognitive functioning	
General functioning	
Mini-Mental State Examination (MMSE)	Clinician
Intellectual functioning	
Wechsler Adult Intelligence Scale–III (WAIS-III)	Patient
Shipley Institute of Living Scale	Patient
Memory functions	
Wechsler Memory Scale–III (WMS-III)	Patient
Cognitive process/content	
Rorschach	Clinician
Perceptual–motor functioning	
Bender Visual Motor Gestalt Test (BVMGT)	Clinician
3. Emotional functioning	
General severity and pattern	
Symptom Checklist 90—Revised (SCL-90-R)	Patient
Brief Symptom Inventory (BSI)	Patient
Client Emotional Configuration Scale	Clinician
Depression	
Hamilton Rating Scale for Depression (HRSD)	Clinician
Beck Depression Inventory–II (BDI-II)	Patient
Anxiety	
State–Trait Anxiety Inventory (STAI)	Patient
Anger/hostility	
State–Trait Anger Expression Inventory (STAXI)	Patient
4. Interpersonal–intrapersonal functioning	
Coping style	
Minnesota Multiphasic Personality Inventory–2 (MMPI-2)	Patient
Inventory of Interpersonal Problems	Patient
Structural Analysis of Social Behavior	Clinician
Sexual disturbance	
Derogatis Sexual Functioning Inventory	Patient
Child Abuse Potential Inventory	Patient

(continued)

TABLE 2.2. (continued)

Domain/instrument(s)	Rater
Marital/family disturbance	
Dyadic Adjustment Scale	Patient
Family Environment Scale	Patient
Marital Satisfaction Inventory	Patient
Social adjustment	
Social Adjustment Scale—Self-Report	Patient
Michigan Alcoholism Screening Test	Patient
5. Diagnosis	
Structured Clinical Interview for DSM-IV (SCID)	Clinician
Structured Interview for DSM-III Personality (SIDP)	Clinician
Anxiety Disorders Interview Schedule (ADIS)	Clinician
Millon Clinical Multiaxial Inventory–III (MCMI-III)	Patient
6. Prognosis and risk	
Suicide potential	
Scale of Suicide Ideation	Clinician
Beck Hopelessness Scale (BHS)	Patient
Alcohol abuse potential	
Alcohol Use Inventory	Patient
Schizophrenia prognosis	
Camberwell Family Interview	Clinician
7. Client strengths and resources	
Bar-On Emotional Intelligence Inventory	Patient
California Psychological Inventory	Patient

gical instruments are not included (see Groth-Marnat, 2000; Lezak, 1995). This list of instruments represents an effort to balance the adequacy of the information obtained with the time–cost of using each instrument.

Second, the table does not account for the fact that omnibus, trait-oriented instruments (e.g., the Millon Clinical Multiaxial Inventory–III [MCMI-III], the MMPI-2, and the Rorschach) also include special scales and procedures that can be extracted and used for more specific purposes, such as assessing risk for depression, severity of alcohol abuse, and anger control. The reader will find more information about some of these special scales and their uses in the chapters of this book devoted to these tests. As indicated above, a number of the most frequently used instruments (i.e., MMPI-2, MCMI-III, CPI, Rorschach) are discussed in more depth in test-oriented chapters later in the book.

It should be noted that many of the instruments listed in Table 2.2 are not discussed in *Integrative Assessment of Adult Personality*. Further information on these instruments (as well as the ones that are discussed later in the book) can be found by consulting various textbooks and abstracting resources on psychological testing (e.g., Buros, 1978). It is also essential to read through the test manuals carefully to check their reliability, validity, and normative base. The tests listed in Table 2.2 can be ordered from various publishers. We have included a listing of publishers and the tests they publish in Appendix B. Note that these publishers have many more tests than are listed in Appendix B; we have only included those instruments that are included in *Integrative Assessment of Adult Personality*.

A brief description of the various domains of the psychological report is included below to introduce the tests listed under each of these domains as well as preface how these domains can be organized in a psychological report.

Historical Background

Details about a patient's history can best be obtained with the interview procedures discussed in Chapter 4. It is not sufficient simply to know *what* has happened to an individual, however; a clinician also needs to have an understanding of the impact of these events and the resources that are available to support change.

Objectively measuring life changes and their impacts is a very complex task. In order to accomplish such a task in the most complete fashion, a very extensive, multidimensional assessment procedure is required (Monroe, 1982; Schulz & Tompkins, 1990; Zimmerman, 1983). A less intensive approach to this problem may focus on two related dimensions: life changes and social support systems. The information provided in assessments of these two dimensions will ordinarily be supplemented by the historical information, available from diagnostic interviews and procedures (discussed later in this chapter).

Cognitive Functioning

Cognitive functioning is a multidimensional domain. The aspects of functioning that are most salient for most patients include problem-solving level, abstract reasoning abilities, attention, memory, perceptual content and accuracy, and perceptual–motor integration. Cognitive functioning (including these several subareas) is given the greatest attention in the assessment of organic and intellectual impairment. The numerous neuropsychological procedures that are used for very specific purposes are not reviewed here. Instead a few instruments that, together, provide a range of information within and across the various subareas of cognitive functioning are surveyed. Chapter 5 elaborates on the relation between cognitive functioning and personality.

Emotional Functioning

The domain of emotional functioning includes (1) the assessment of both mood and affect; (2) estimates of the chronicity of dysphoria, when present; (3) evaluation of emotional stability; and (4) a determination of the level of emotional control that the patient exhibits. The instruments listed in Table 2.2 are designed to facilitate the assessment of general emotional qualities, symptoms of emotional dysphoria and disturbances, and specific aspects of behavior that are related to depression, anxiety, and anger. These latter areas of disturbance are the most likely ones in which mood and affect will be noted.

Interpersonal–Intrapersonal Functioning

Chapter 3 outlines some of the dimensions of symptomatic and interpersonal functioning that have been proposed as being among the most relevant for making treatment decisions (see also Beutler et al., 2000). Of particular concern to the present discussion are (1) patient conflict areas, (2) coping styles, and (3)potential for resisting the influence of others. It is often important to distinguish between trait-like and state-like qualities. The trait-like aspects are typically described as aspects of personality, whereas the state-like aspects often reflect levels of distress and reactivity to stress. Thus, to some degree, these latter concepts overlap with the more general concepts considered in connection with emotional functioning. The instruments presented here include both state and trait components.

Diagnosis and Prognosis

With the advent of recent versions of the *Diagnostic and Statistical Manual of Mental Disorders* (DSM) of the American Psychiatric Association, a concerted effort has been made to base patient diagnosis on objective and observable qualities of their experience. The use of behavioral descriptors have replaced elaborate analyses of internal processes as central to the task of diagnosis. Likewise, theoretically based speculations about treatment course have been replaced by empirically derived information about relapse and recurrence in the diagnostic system.

While these changes have improved the reliability with which diagnoses can be assigned from the DSM, simply agreeing on observable diagnostic criteria has not been sufficient to assure that the diagnostic process is accurate and helpful in treatment planning. Structured questionnaires and interviews have been required, many of which entail extensive study and practice to apply effectively. Virtually all research protocols and, increasingly, clinical treatment protocols require the use of structured assessment before diagnosis is recorded and treatment is planned. Table 2.2 gives some examples of these instruments, most of which rely on clinician judgment and observation. The use of these structured assessment materials improves the replicability of assigning diagnoses, but weaknesses in the diagnostic system itself precludes these diagnoses from being highly effective in selecting effective treatment procedures or predicting response to selected treatment.

To accomplish the latter purposes, separate instruments are often used to estimate a patient's prognosis in relation to a certain class of risk behaviors. For example, Table 2.2 lists instruments to assess the risk of drinking relapse, suicidal behavior, and thought disorder, among the most important risks facing psychiatric patients. These prognostic instruments can be used along with diagnosis to provide a more comprehensive picture of patient status and probable treatment response.

Client Strengths and Resources

Although understanding a client's presenting problem is certainly crucial, it is equally important to identify and understand a client's strengths and resources. In the past, clinical psychology has rightly been criticized for focusing on pathology to the exclusion of clients' positive levels of functioning. These concerns have been expressed by professionals within the field as well as by clients. Imagine, for example, how it would feel for clients to read through reports that focus almost exclusively on their deficits. Given increased client rights to freedom of information, this is a salient issue. Thus it is highly likely that clients will see the reports that have been written about them. From a treatment perspective, it is crucial to identify any available skills and resources that can be used to assist patients in overcoming whatever difficulties are contained within their presenting problem. These skills and resources may be found in social support available to the patient, level of insight, resilience, community resources, and level of emotional intelligence. Often treatment can be most productively accomplished by focusing and expanding on these strengths and resources. Thus, clinicians should strive to identify these strengths and resources and ensure that there is a balance between the positive and the pathological descriptors used in psychological reports

MAXIMIZING CLINICAL JUDGMENTS

Psychological assessment involves integrating various sources of information to form judgments about such areas as personality, diagnosis, treatment recommendations, dangerousness, or vocational selection. The ultimate test of this process is the degree of accuracy of these judgments. It is thus crucial for clinicians to be aware of the research on clinical judgment and be able to apply these research findings to increase the accuracy of their judgments.

Research on judgment accuracy for personality assessment indicates that judgments by psychologists vary according to the domain being assessed. The reliability of ratings for symptoms has been found to be quite accurate (Garb, 1998; Groth-Marnat, 1999b). In contrast, there has been considerable variation in rating accuracy for personality traits, and ratings of defense mechanisms have been found to be quite unreliable (Garb, 1998). Accuracy of diagnosis has been found to be variable but usually within acceptable limits when clinicians clearly follow DSM-IV criteria. The diagnostic accuracy of reports can be increased further by obtaining and integrating information related to the nature, course, etiology, and treatment of the disorder (Rorer & Widiger, 1983). It has also been found that, in cases where a diagnosis was unclear, psychological testing can help to clarify the diagnosis (e.g., Walters, White, & Greene, 1988). Unfortunately, many clinicians do not adhere closely to DSM-IV criteria when applying a diagnosis, which thus results in inaccuracy. A further difficulty is that when clients are given a primary diagnosis, a secondary diagnosis, such as substance abuse, is frequently overlooked (so-called "overshadowing," see Garb, 1998). For example, Mollinare, Aames, and Essa (1994) found that if patients were given an Axis I disorder, an underlying personality disorder was likely to be overlooked. Substance abuse and dissociative symptoms were also likely to be particularly underdiagnosed in psychiatric settings. Although underdiagnosis might occur in psychiatric contexts, in many other contexts, psychologists are likely to overemphasize pathology and overlook positive aspects of clients' functioning (see review by Wills, 1978). This overemphasis is particularly likely to occur if the clinician is using projective tests (Soskin, 1959) or tests that emphasize psychopathology, such as the MMPI-2 or MCMI-III.

A humbling finding has been that clinicians are generally overconfident regarding the accuracy of their judgments (Kleinmuntz, 1990; Smith & Dumont, 1997). This dismaying conclusion is further compounded by the counterintuitive finding that clinicians with less experience and knowledge tend to be more confident (but no more accurate) than those with greater experience and knowledge (Garb, 1998). The exception to this finding is that extremely knowledgeable clinicians tend to have moderate levels of confidence regarding their judgments. Part of the reason for the above finding is that clinicians, particularly during the early stages of practice, do not usually receive feedback regarding the accuracy of their judgments. Over a period of time, they gradually receive feedback that results in a more accurate assessment of their own accuracy.

Developing accurate treatment decisions is a crucial aspect of clinical practice. Unfortunately, the accuracy of decision making in this area has been disappointing. For example, Bickman, Karver, and Schut (1997) found that agreement among clinicians regarding the level of care for patients was low to undetectable. Somewhat similarly, agreement among behavior therapists regarding which behaviors to change has been quite low (Felton & Nelson, 1984; Persons, Mooney, & Padesky, 1995). Treatment decisions for clinicians having similar theoretical formulations have been good to adequate (Witteman & Koele, 1999). In contrast, there has been little agreement for treatment decisions for clinicians with divergent theoretical orientations. Potential biases in treatment decisions have been found to be related to race, age, socioeconomic status, private (vs. public) treating facility, and gender (see Garb, 1998, and Chapter 12). Given the frequently disappointing literature related to treatment decisions, throughout this book we emphasize a systematic, empirically supported method that is likely to produce a high level of clinician agreement as well as to optimize treatment outcome (see Chapter 3).

Our intention in providing this very general overview of a quite extensive literature is to extract practical guidelines that can enhance clinical judgment. Accordingly, the following points summarize some of these guidelines:

- Diagnosis should be made using clear, consistent criteria.
- Clinicians should be cautious in assessing some areas (e.g., defense mechanisms) whereas other areas (client symptoms, some aspects of personality) can be assessed with more confidence.
- Clinicians should avoid letting one diagnosis overshadow the possibility of additional relevant complaints (e.g., personality disorders, substance abuse).
- Clinicians should describe client strengths.
- Clinicians should avoid overconfidence regarding their clinical judgments.
- Clinicians should learn as much as possible about the theoretical and empirical literature related to each client's type of problem.
- In order to increase accuracy, clinicians should seek not only evidence that confirms tentative conclusions, but also challenge these conclusions with arguments or information that might disconfirm the conclusions.
- Clinicians should seek feedback whenever possible (i.e., request referral sources to rate the accuracy and usefulness of psychological reports).

SUMMARY

This chapter has summarized three dimensions that play a crucial role when clinicians approach clients. The first is to develop an understanding of the setting from which the referral comes. Practitioners from each of these settings are likely to ask different questions. In addition, they have different terminology, ways of conceptualizing the client, and even different expectations regarding the length of the report. Effectively working with the client and communicating the results of an assessment requires knowledge of the issues and concepts existing in these settings.

A large number of issues is relevant to the optimal selection of test instruments. Clearly the referral question and psychometrics of the tests are crucial. Sometimes it might be useful to consider a relatively stressful type of test (and test environment) to determine how clients function in these situations. Do they give up easily or persevere? The relative ambiguity of a test might provide relevant types of information. Having clients answer true–false questions/statements will clearly provide little information related to how well they can initiate, organize, and articulate their responses. If such initiating/organizing information is required, then the examiner might wish to create ambiguity.

The selection of tests, as well as how they are interpreted, also may vary in terms of the amount of qualitative versus quantitative information that is required. Furthermore, the selection of tests will vary in the extent to which clinicians use a core/fixed versus a flexible battery. We recommend the use of several core tests, with which a clinician is quite familiar, combined with additional instruments that can be introduced flexibly, based on the referral questions and the characteristics of the client. The core tests are likely to be those that are most frequently used in the profession. Clinicians also will choose tests based on the various domains in which they are interested. To assist in this process, we have listed some of the more frequently used tests of the various domains.

Finally, clinicians should be aware of the different factors that might enhance or compromise their clinical judgment. Accuracy can be enhanced by following various rules of practice, such as using clear diagnostic criteria, knowing which domains of personality can be most accurately judged, not letting one diagnosis overshadow other relevant areas, describing client strengths, resisting feeling overconfident, keeping informed about relevant literature, and seeking feedback on the accuracy and usefulness of assessment findings.

3

Identifying Treatment-Relevant Assessment
SYSTEMATIC TREATMENT SELECTION

T. Mark Harwood and Oliver B. Williams

Systematic Treatment Selection (STS; Beutler & Clarkin, 1990; Beutler, Clarkin, & Bongar, 2000; Gaw & Beutler, 1995) is a procedure for planning treatments that are compatible for individual patients. It is both a formulation for identifying effective treatments and a system of assessment that is specifically designed to address the concepts and dimensions presented in Chapter 1. The material presented in this chapter provides background for this assessment procedure and describes the application of the STS to R.W., the patient followed throughout this volume.

The foundation of STS, both as a method of treatment planning and as an assessment system, is a set of 18 research-informed principles that suggest the conditions under which various families of interventions, modalities of treatment, and formats are likely to be associated with change. Prescriptive Therapy (PT; Beutler & Harwood, 2000), an application of 10 of the 18 STS principles to the specific case of individual therapy (see Table 1.2), is an individualized, psychosocial treatment designed to provide targeted and highly effective interventions that fit the problems and personality styles of the particular patient. It is unique in the fact that it is derived from the use of intervention principles, rather than from a particular model or theory of treatment or a prescriptive set of techniques. The principles were defined initially by an extensive review of empirical literature and then subjected to independent cross-validation (Beutler et al., 2000). Thus, PT is an empirically supported method for matching treatment-relevant predisposing characteristics of patients with specific types of therapeutic interventions. Although PT may be delivered in a variety of treatment formats that vary in length and intensity to fit a variety of problems, for most applications, it is a relatively brief (i.e., 20 or fewer sessions) therapy. This empirically derived patient–treatment matching model has been demonstrated to increase the efficacy of therapy in an efficient and systematic fashion, improving treatment outcome and patient productivity while reducing the time in, and the subsequent costs of, treatment for both the patient and the health care system (Beutler et al., 2000; Beutler, Moleiro, Malik, & Harwood, 2002; Beutler, Moleiro, Malik, Harwood, et al., 2002).

The guidelines and strategies of the STS system that are presented in this chapter were developed primarily from an inspection of depressive spectrum disorders; however, these matching guidelines and strategies have been cross-validated and applied to a wide variety of problems in which dysphoria, chemical abuse, and anxiety were present as either primary or secondary features (Beutler et al., 2000; Beutler & Harwood, 2000; Beutler, Moleiro, Malik, Harwood, et al., in press). Depression is the most widely occurring comorbid condition, and its major symptoms, especially dysphoria, signal the possible presence of most types of psychological difficulties. Because depression is a general indicator of distress, does not appear to have a specific pathogen or course, and does not have a specific, identifiable treatment (see Beutler et al., 2000; Beutler & Malik, 2002a), we believe that it is unfortunate and even misleading for treatments of depression to be applied as if the condition were an isolated and independent mental health condition. In reality, depression typically arises in response to the convergence of a complicated cluster of problems. It usually co-occurs with other diagnoses, often serving as a marker for the presence of general disturbance and distress arising from almost any condition.

Substance abuse and personality disorders (operating as initiating and/or maintaining elements in the course/etiology of depression) are among the most difficult comorbid conditions in the treatment of depressive spectrum disorders. Patterns of recurrence, chronicity of mental disorders or problems, comorbidity, and generalized disturbances in interpersonal relationships have all been identified as indicators of disorder complexity (Beutler et al., 2000). Among therapies for complex disorders, it is especially important that the treatment be flexible and multifaceted in order to address noncompliance, preemptive treatment termination, and the comorbidity that typically characterizes these problems.

PRESCRIPTIVE THERAPY

There is no universal personality type, living environment, or lifestyle that characterizes all or even most people who present for mental health treatment, and research findings indicate that no particular treatment works for everyone. Research also indicates that (1) important variations predispose people to be differentially receptive to various interventions, and (2) this pattern of reaction appears to be similar across a wide variety of problems. PT addresses the predisposing variations that exist among patients by extracting strategies and techniques from several different theoretical models to provide the best, most efficacious fit for individual patients.

The 18 principles comprising the STS treatment planning model identify six patient dimensions that are used to assign various levels of care, contexts of treatment, and specific interventions. These six dimensions, described in Table 3.1, reiterate those presented in earlier chapters of this volume. Collectively, these dimensions have been used to (1) assign varying levels of treatment intensity, (2) predict the likelihood of responding to pharmacotherapy and psychotherapy, (3) enhance the roles and power of therapeutic relationships, and (4) explain differential responses to therapist interpersonal styles and techniques (Beutler et al., 2000).

PT concentrates on four of these dimensions (impairment level, coping style, resistance level, and distress level) and 10 of the 18 STS principles and applies them to the specific case of individual psychotherapy. These four patient dimensions serve as prognostic indicators for determining likely treatment response as well as specific indicators and contraindicators for employing different families of treatments. The four dimensions have been validated in a variety of research studies, and three of them (impairment level, coping style, resistance level) have been recognized, by a special task force (convened by the Division of Psychotherapy of the American Psychological Association) as effective for assisting psychotherapy treatment planning (Norcross, 2002). This task force has identified qualities that contribute to effective therapeutic relationships. Moreover, our own research has confirmed the predictive validities of all four of these dimensions when used to select compatible families of interventions

---

TABLE 3.1. Treatment Matching Patient Dimensions

1. Level of functional impairment in social and intimate activities and relationships.
2. Level of social support, an indirect and inverse correlate of impairment level.
3. Problem complexity, an index of comorbidity and chronicity.
4. Characteristic ways of coping with, and adapting to, changing environments.
5. Levels of trait-like resistance to external demands.

(Beutler, Harwood, Alimohamed, & Malik, 2002; Beutler, Moleiro, & Talebi, 2002). It is on the strength of these observations that these dimensions were chosen to serve as binding threads for the many assessment devices and procedures described throughout this volume.

Guiding Objectives of Systematic Treatment Selection/Prescriptive Therapy

STS (and its individual extrapolation, PT) attempts to establish the scientific bases of the assumptions that are inherent in psychotherapeutic practice. It provides a model for selecting interventions differentially to accommodate a variety of patient qualities and characteristics. In this process, it advocates using multicomponent methods of intervention that are systematically derived from a variety of psychotherapeutic approaches. Like all available prescriptive treatment models, the STS model eschews the so-called comprehensive clinical theories of either psychopathology or psychotherapy as guides to intervention. Instead it focuses on specific and individual patient dimensions that indicate the likely efficacy of equally specific treatment strategies. The application of a truly prescriptive and differential psychotherapy requires (1) the identification of the patient cues that reliably indicate the presence of treatment-relevant traits and states, (2) an assessment of the levels at which these qualities occur, and (3) a selection of the appropriate therapeutic interventions to fit these qualities and levels.

For example, one of the 18 guiding principles of STS asserts that "therapeutic change is greatest when a patient is stimulated to emotional arousal in a safe environment, until problematic responses diminish or are extinguished." This statement identifies *exposure* and *extinction* as cardinal qualities underlying treatment efficacy. Such principles as this identify classes of intervention, rather than specific techniques, as central to effective psychotherapy. Thus, rather than recommending the use of specific procedures (e.g., response prevention or imaginal exposure) as the favored means of treatment, this principle of PT requires therapists to identify and select procedures, from within their own repertoire of skills and knowledge, that can promote exposure to feared events and can be maintained long enough to produce extinction of avoidant responses. From an identification of avoided interpersonal situations, one therapist may use the technique of *in vivo* exposure, another may use imaginal desensitization, and still another may use role-playing exercises. By operating from principles of change, rather than from a particular theory or a menu of techniques, therapists gain a flexibility that allows them to extend their work beyond the mere treatment of, say, phobia to a host of behaviors that arise from emotional avoidance. This shift in perspective ensures the exercise of maximal flexibility and creativity on the part of therapists.

A Process of Clinical Decision Making

The STS model of treatment planning is constructed around four levels of decision making:

- Assessment/quantification of the six patient predisposing dimensions (listed in Table 3.1).
- Assignment of the level of care and context of treatment.
- Development of the therapeutic relationship and selection of families of interventions.
- Fitting families of interventions to the particular needs of the patient.

Each of these four decision-making levels entail more refined levels or sublevels, which together move from gross, general decisions to specific and highly refined decisions.

The first level of decision making in the application of the STS system involves the selection of means to measure the six *patient predisposing dimensions* (listed in Table 3.1), and associated variables, which are then used to answer referral questions and plan treatment. At this level, clinicians may decide (1) which of the six variables are relevant to the referral question, (2) the instruments to use, and (3) how to present the assessment environment and demands to the patient. Decisions about prognosis, strengths, and treatment are premature at this beginning stage. This is a preliminary level, requiring knowledge of assessment and measurement processes.

The patient dimensions targeted for assessment at this level will affect the decisions made at the subsequent three levels. These dimensions measured must allow the clinician to respond to the referral questions and, ultimately, to develop an understanding of the patient's treatment planning needs. The range of measurement targets at this level includes (1) aspects of normal adjustment (coping style, interpersonal attitudes, etc.), (2) aspects of the patient's environment (social support, role demands, expectations, etc.), and (3) attributes of the presenting problem itself (symptoms, severity, impairment level, distress level, chronicity, etc.). These dimensions are implicated in several of the reasons for referral, ranging from predictions of prognosis to assessment of strengths and level of functioning. The use of these dimensional variables for determining the etiology of a set of problems, however, is the least effective role played by the STS system. Conversely, assistance in treatment planning is the strength of the STS system.

The second level of decision making is devoted to assigning *level of care* and *context of treatment* for individual patients. Within this level are three subareas or sublevels of decision making. The first of these latter levels of prediction applies selected patient dimensions (e.g., social support, complexity, and subjective distress) to estimating patient prognosis (i.e., likelihood of recovery). This prediction serves as a baseline estimate against which the clinician can then determine the added benefit that can be attributed to specific treatments. Accordingly, the second level of prediction is based on patient dimensions (e.g., complexity, impairment level, social support) that are used in assigning the level and context of care (intensity, setting, mode, and format). More specifically, the level and context of care are determined by decisions about the applications of pharmacotherapy, psychotherapy, family therapy, probable treatment duration, relapse probability, dangerousness, and treatment format.

Context decisions include those related to the intensity of treatment required (beginning with the decision of whether to treat at all), the setting in which treatment would be offered (e.g., inpatient or outpatient), the modality (medical vs. nonmedical), and the format (individual vs. family, group, etc.) of treatment. The available literature suggests that although patient diagnosis is often claimed as a factor in these decisions, more often, clinicians use patient functioning, previous episodes, chronicity, flexibility, cooperation, and other indicators of severity as determiners of treatment context (Beutler & Harwood, 2000; Beutler et al., 2000). Indeed, empirical evidence is generally supportive of these contentions and indicates that a patient's prior history of similar problems, along with levels of impairment, may be particularly important in choosing the appropriate form of treatment and context in which to administer that treatment.

At the third level of prediction, the clinician uses knowledge of patient predisposing dimensions to inform the development of the treatment *relationship* and the selection of specific classes of *therapeutic procedures*. Here the clinician focuses on the nature of the specific treatment that will best fit a given patient. Patient qualities (e.g., coping style, resistance level, distress level, and expectations) are used to guide the clinician in establishing and maintaining a relationship and applying a set of interventions that are most likely to resolve the presenting problem/disorder. These qualities also suggest the focus of treatment (symptom-related, skill building, conflict resolution), the level of therapist strategies (i.e., directive vs. evocative), and approaches to managing the patient's emotions. This optimal level of refinement in the treatment planning process is used to guide individual interactions between patient and therapists.

Decisions at the third level are always made with due regard for previous decisions about the level and context of treatment. For example, research (see Barber et al., 2001; Beutler et al., 2000; Castonguay, Goldfried, Wiser, Raue, & Hayes, 1996) has found that the nature of an effective treatment relationship varies as a function of the setting in which it occurs and the nature of the specific interventions used. Therefore, effective treatment planning must take into account how well the assigned therapist or clinician adapts to the patient and to the context in which treatment is offered, and how well the therapist provides procedures that are effective and useful within that particular environment.

The STS model calls for relationship and procedural decisions to take place at several different points. For example, certain decisions are made when a therapist is selected or assigned, in order to ensure that this therapist's views and expectations are compatible with those of the patient. Other decisions occur when procedures are selected, in order to ensure that these procedures enhance the patient's expectations and facilitate the development of a productive treatment alliance. A third type of decision ensures the availability of skills and professional experiences that can be suited to the level of patient need. The particular therapist, his or her therapeutic skills and experience, and the procedures and techniques employed all interact with the predisposing patient dimensions.

The fourth level of decision making in the STS model, *treatment fitting*, provides the most refined level of treatment planning. Here the clinician fits particular classes of intervention to the varying needs of the patient. Only after taking into account the requirements and "demands" of the therapeutic process, and the nature of the therapeutic relationship (which will provide both motivation and support) can the clinician confidently and competently select the particular treatment techniques and strategies that fit the particular and specific needs of each patient. For example, treatment is most likely to be effective under the following conditions:

- The therapist adjusts the level of directiveness and guidance to the patient's ability to tolerate external control (*resistance level*).
- The use of symptom-removal and/or insight-related interventions corresponds to how the patient acquires and adapts to new information (*coping style*).
- The use of abreactive and affect reduction procedures are consistent with the patient's level of motivation (level of emotional arousal and *subjective distress*).
- The intensity of treatment is modified in relation to the level of *functional impairment* experienced by the patient.

In sum, PT is intended to fit the setting as well as the patient and to match the dispositions of the clinician to the predilections of the patient.

MATCHING PATIENT AND TREATMENT DIMENSIONS: CROSS-THEORETICAL APPLICATIONS

A major disadvantage of most manualized therapies, as used in contemporary clinical trial studies, is that they often are insufficiently flexible to address a given patient's needs (Anderson & Strupp, 1996; Henry, Schacht, Strupp, Butler, & Binder, 1993). Single-theory formulations are likely to proscribe the use of interventions that are inconsistent with their theory, even if those interventions have been found to be effective in empirical re-search. Unfortunately, the limited range of the interventions contained in most conventional manuals does not accurately reflect the pragmatic, cross-theory "eclecticism" that characterizes most psychotherapists' styles (Garfield, & Kurtz, 1977; Norcross & Prochaska, 1988) or that is repre-sented in the many "empirically supported treatments" (e.g., Chambless & Ollendick, 2001). As a multifaceted intervention, PT (Beutler & Harwood, 2000) promises more flexibility of application as well as access to a wider range of effective interventions than single-theory models.

The central six patient dimensions that carry the preponderance of the burden for making decisions at the four levels of decision making (level of functional impairment, level of social support, problem complexity/chronicity, patient coping style [particularly level of externalization and impulsivity], level of patient resistance, and level of patient distress) repre-sent continuous dimensions of patient functioning and collectively include both state and trait qualities. For each of these patient dimensions (one through six), one or more corresponding classes or families of treatment in-tervention or treatment type have been found to contribute to, or enhance, outcome. These corresponding treatment classes/families include:

1. High versus low treatment intensity
2. Treatment modality
3. Treatment format
4. Skill building and symptom-focused versus insight- and awareness-focused interventions
5. High versus low therapist directiveness
6. Relative level of emotional experiencing and enhancement (manipu-lating emotional arousal) employed in the treatment of the patient.

The bidirectional quality of most of these treatment dimensions is aligned with the mediating role played by the corresponding patient dimen-sions, and identifies the range of strategies that therapists must have at their disposal in order to work with patients who display different levels of a particular dimension. For example, among patients who are experiencing high or low levels of functional impairment, the planned intensity of treat-ment should be correspondingly high or low. One way of increasing treat-ment intensity is to increase the number of sessions per week offered (up to three or four sessions); another way may be to add phone calls or addi-tional therapies (e.g., group, couple). As a patient's functioning improves, the number or frequency of treatments might be allowed to decrease (e.g., to two or one session per week).

Likewise, among patients with externalizing coping styles, symptom-focused behaviorally oriented treatments are indicated internalizing pa-tients can benefit from the use of a set of procedures focused on conflict resolution and self-exploration that follow the initial use of symptom-focused interventions. For patients with high levels of resistance, therapists would employ nondirective and patient-driven therapies; however, for those with low levels of resistance, directive treatments and interventions appear to outperform less-directive treatments.

Arousal levels are thought to be inversely related to the application of arousal-inducing strategies and techniques (Beutler & Harwood, 2000). That is, therapists should attempt, in general, to maintain a moderate level of arousal in patients. This level is optimal because it helps to keep the patient alert, engaged, and motivated without overwhelming him or her with excessive levels of anxiety. Patients with low levels of arousal, for example, need to experience arousal-inducing interventions in the therapy session until moderate levels of arousal are achieved, and then these levels should be maintained. Conversely, patients experiencing high levels of arousal require the application of arousal-reducing interventions to bring anxiety down to manageable (moderate) levels; from there, the therapist endeavors to maintain this level of arousal.

Functional impairment is related to problem complexity/chronicity and degree of available social support. Complex/chronic problems and functional impairment typically covary, and complex/chronic problems tend to respond best to longer-term and more intensive treatments that focus on interpersonal relationships. Additionally, patients with high problem complexity/chronicity tend to benefit most from broadband treatments that include both psychosocial and interpersonal components. Although modern research has failed to find evidence that combining psychosocial and pharmacological interventions produces a reliable increase of benefit over either alone (Antonuccio, Danton, & DeNelsky, 1995; Barlow, Gorman, Shear, & Woods, 2000), there do appear to be some specific indications of when to prescribe antidepressant and antianxiety agents. Pharmacotherapy achieves its greatest efficacy among individuals with high levels of problem complexity/chronicity, especially in relation to depressive symptoms (Beutler et al., 2000). The patient's location along the complexity/chronicity dimension is derived from an evaluation of the longevity of the problems, the depth and breadth of problems, and the presence of nuclear/original family issues.

Complexity/chronicity is also reflected in the patient's level of social impairment—a dimension that is the inverse of the patient's level of social support. A patient's social support systems and resources include *inhibitors* (problematic aspects of the patient's unique social support system) and *facilitators* (resources that are positive) of change. An evaluation of the quality and quantity of social resources provides (1) an indication of the likelihood that the patient will seek and use information or advice from others, and (2) information regarding the individual's available resources for coping. Low levels of social support typically indicate a need for longer-term treatments, whereas higher levels of social support provide a general marker for briefer treatments. As can be gathered from the foregoing, the quantification and qualification of a patient's level of complexity/ chronicity, social support, and functional impairment help guide the determination of the treatment context that includes intensity of treatment, psychosocial and/or pharmacological modes of treatment, and format of treatment (e.g., individual, couple, or group treatment).

It is beyond the scope of this chapter to provide detailed information on the various assessments and patient cues that can be used to identify a patient's "location" on the predisposing dimensions. Additionally, a thorough discussion of the myriad interventions (indicated by principles of use) that are effective for the management of treatment in relation to each guiding dimension is beyond this chapter's parameters; however, a few illustrative examples are provided. The interested reader is directed to Beutler and colleagues (2000) and to Beutler and Harwood (2000) for detailed outlines and examples of applicable interventions for each of the patient–therapy guiding dimensions.

In its simplest form, functional impairment is managed either by increasing or decreasing the number or frequency of sessions (i.e., the intensity) of treatment. High impairment may be indicated by (1) low (< 60) Global Assessment of Functioning (GAF) scores (American Psychiatric Association, 2000), (2) signs of disturbed family/household functioning (e.g., patient was "kicked out" of the home), (3) signs of social isolation (e.g., seeks to be alone an excessive amount of the time), and (4) lack of social support (e.g., patient has no family members in which he or she can confide). Low impairment is suggested by the absence of the foregoing indicators.

Coping style is typically assessed *objectively*, using a combination of MMPI-2 scores formulated to produce an internalization ratio (IR); and *clinically*, using a variety of patient-provided cues. An IR score reflects the degree to which externalizing scales (Hy, Pd, Pa, Ma) dominate over internalizing (Hs, D, Pt, Si) ones. Scores of less than 1 indicate that the patient utilizes an internalizing coping style; externalization is indicated by scores greater than 1. Observable patient cues that are suggestive of internalization include timidity, introversion, and a greater likelihood of feeling hurt instead of angry. The range of clinical cues that one can expect to observe from those who are "externalizers" includes gregarious sociability, impulsivity, and high needs for stimulation (i.e., easily bored). Externalizers tend to exhibit behaviors that are characterized by active avoidance of blame or responsibility, impulsivity, denial, and aggression.

Symptom-focused strategies that employ interventions to address these externally observed symptoms or to facilitate the acquisition of new skills are suggested for externalizers (e.g., skill building, confrontation with the feared consequences that result in avoidance behaviors, behavioral contracts). In contrast, "internalizing" patients typically benefit the most from interventions that facilitate awareness of thematic patterns and an understanding of the genesis of their behaviors, and that enhance self-esteem (e.g., by reducing self-criticism). Internalizers typically exhibit behaviors that emphasize self-reflection and self-criticism, social withdrawal, and emotional isolation/internal control. Among patients with an internalizing coping style, therapists can increase the likelihood and magnitude of change by adopting a primary therapeutic stance that involves a focus on insight. This style of therapy employs any strategy that increases the patient's awareness of how specific behaviors or interpretations of events operate to affect him or her. Insight-focused strategies include reflection, interpretation, and emotive/expressive (i.e., experiential) treatment procedures. (For interested readers, Daldrup, Beutler, Engle, & Greenberg, 1988, is an excellent example of an empirically supported experiential treatment manual.)

Resistance level can be measured with the Dowd Therapeutic Reactance Scale (DOWD-TRS) or the TRT (negative treatment indicators), Pd$_2$ (authority problems), TPA2 (competitive drive), or Do (dominance) MMPI-2 subscales that are indicative of interpersonal defensiveness (relative to the scale median or mean). Low resistance is also suggested by patient history and in-session cues that indicate a willingness to follow the advice of those in authority, avoidance of confrontation, and related tendencies. High resistance is suggested by behaviors and cues that include frequent resentment of others, enjoyment of competition, and attempts to "get even" when provoked. Generally speaking, directive and guiding therapies are most helpful among those patients who are nonresistant. Directive interventions include closed-ended questions, interpretations, activity scheduling, and confrontation. Resistant patients respond best to the use of nondirective interventions, including open-ended questions, self-directed therapy work or self-monitored homework, paradoxical interventions, and reflection.

As we indicated previously, managing the patient's level of acute distress and arousal is an important aspect of therapy. State and trait levels of arousal should be assessed (e.g., using the State–Trait Anxiety Inventory [STAI]; Spielberger, Gorsuch, Lushene, Vagg, & Jacobs, 1983b). Because arousal encompasses a state-like and highly mercurial dimension, the therapist should be mindful of in-session cues that suggest counterproductive changes in arousal levels. Patients who are experiencing high levels of acute (state) distress (as might be indicated by a score above the normative patient 75th percentile) are typically unable to process or function in a planful manner and fail to benefit from procedures that emphasize emotional awareness or emotional processing (e.g., Litz, Gray, Bryant, & Adler, 2002). Patients with very low levels of arousal lack motivation and energy to work through problems. High levels of arousal frequently follow some traumatic or unexpected experience and are indexed by patient cues of restlessness, inability to focus, distractibility, flashbacks, feelings of derealization, irritability, agitation and anxiety, unfocused kinesthetic behaviors (e.g., inappropriate smiling, lack or reduction of spontaneous facial expressions, and limb and trunk movements), and changes in vocalization (tense, jerky, reduced speech fluency, etc.). Low levels of arousal are indexed by patient cues suggesting apathy, lack of energy, malaise, and the absence of the foregoing signs.

A patient's arousal may be increased to a moderate level and then directly alleviated through exposure strategies. Debilitating levels of arousal can be reduced by providing structure (e.g., role and homework assignments, structured relaxation procedures, free expressive methods, automatic thought work) and implementing supportive interventions (e.g., direct suggestions of relaxation, self-instruction).

INTRODUCTION TO THE THERAPEUTIC PRINCIPLES OF TRAINING IN SYSTEMATIC TREATMENT SELECTION

STS treatment planning and PT adhere to the assumption that the selection of strategies and techniques of effective treatment will best be derived from an understanding of basic principles of therapeutic change, rather than by adhering to constrictive theories or menus of techniques. The guidelines presented in the STS model, including the PT model of individual treatment, are based on sound, research-derived principles of behavior change. These principles are designed to enable the clinician to construct strategies for implementing change, which are then transmitted through the use of procedures and techniques. Each level of implementation provides more opportunity for flexibility and creativity; however, flexibility and creativity must operate within the context of the guiding principles that have an impact on relationship development among patients, treatment considerations, and selection of intervention families. This progression from firm principle to creative application of technique stands in contrast to the usual method of constructing treatment guidelines that increasingly restrict treatment options in the application of technical procedures.

Here we present the 18 guiding principles that are used in Systematic Treatment Selection to promote change. Within these principles are 8 specific ones that are used in PT to induce differential rates of response (listed as items 5, 12, 13, 14, 15, 16, 17, and 18). For a more thorough treatment of the guiding principles, strategies, and techniques and their relationship to patient predisposing variables, the interested reader is directed to Beutler and Harwood (2000) or Beutler and colleagues (2000). These principles of therapeutic change represent the broadest conceptualization of treatment. Attention to these principles in the selection of appropriate strategies and techniques increases the likelihood and magnitude of positive change. These principles are reviewed in Table 3.2.

Of the principles listed in Table 3.2, the first 10 are categorized as "reasonable and basic principles" (Beutler et al., 2000) because they are general and can be implemented without observing the psychotherapy process in various sessions. The subsequent eight principles are identified as "optimal principles" because they are designed to be applied selectively and differentially, and because they function best through direct feedback based on observations of the treatment process.

These principles, when restated to identify the nature of treatment for a specific patient, constitute treatment strategies. *Strategies* are families of interventions or techniques that share a common objective. They operate within and originate from the principles of therapeutic change, but do so in a manner that is specific to a given patient. For example, principle 18 emphasizes that patient stress should be moderate. Applied to a particular patient, however, this principle may mean that the patient's level of distress should be lowered and that procedures should be employed to reduce it from high to moderate levels. For this patient, the indicated strategy would be to reduce affective arousal; reflections, closed-ended questions, stress-management procedures, and providing structure are techniques that may be implemented to comply with this objective strategy.

At a minimal level, effective strategies for implementing the foregoing principles will accomplish the following:

- Provide a safe and respectful environment.
- Expose the patient to the external precipitators of the symptom or to the internal experiences that are avoided (e.g., via *in vivo* exposure, repeated interpretation of a consistent dynamic theme, adopting a here-and-now focus on daily problems and relationship change).
- Adapt the level of treatment to the level of patient impairment (e.g., adjusting frequency and length of sessions, assigning group and/or individual treatment).
- Select interventions that build skills and alter symptoms (for externalizers and internalizers) or that evoke insight and awareness (for internalizers almost exclusively) and apply them differentially to reflect differences in patient coping styles.
- Adopt either a directive or nondirective role with the patient to lead him or her toward action and change (e.g., alter level of directiveness, utilize paradoxical interventions, make behavioral contracts, and/or establish support [*note:* internalizers typically respond best to structure]).
- Provide either support or confrontation and exposure to fit the patient's level of emotional distress (i.e., provide structure and support if emotional arousal is high, and confrontative, experiential, and open-ended/unstructured procedures if arousal is low).

TABLE 3.2. Principles of Systematic Treatment Selection

Reasonable and basic principles

Prognosis

1. The likelihood of improvement (i.e., prognosis) is a positive function of social support level and a negative function of functional impairment.

2. Prognosis is attenuated by problem complexity/chronicity, and by an absence of patient distress. Facilitating social support enhances the likelihood of good outcome among patients with complex/chronic problems.

Level and intensity of care

3. Psychoactive medication exerts its best effects on those patients with high functional impairment and high problem complexity/chronicity.

4. Likelihood and magnitude of improvement are increased in patients with complex/chronic problems by the application of multiple-person therapy.

5. Benefits correspond to treatment intensity in functionally impaired patients.

Risk reduction

6. Risk is reduced by careful assessment of risk situations in the course of establishing a diagnosis and history.

7. Risk is reduced and patient compliance is increased when the treatment includes family interventions.

8. Risk and noncompliance are minimized if the patient is realistically informed about the probable length and effectiveness of the treatment and the roles and activities that are expected of him or her during the course of the treatment.

9. Risk is reduced if the clinician routinely questions patients about suicidal feelings, intent, and plans.

10. Ethical and legal principles suggest that documentation and consultation are advisable.

Optimal principles

Relationship principles

11. Therapeutic change is greatest when the therapist is skillful and provides trust, acceptance, acknowledgment, collaboration, and respect for the patient, within an environment that both supports risk and provides maximal safety.

12. Therapeutic change is most likely when the therapeutic procedures do not elicit patient resistance.

Principle of exposure and extinction

13. Therapeutic change is most likely when the patient is exposed to objects or targets of behavioral and emotional avoidance.

14. Therapeutic change is greatest when a patient is stimulated to moderate emotional arousal in a safe environment, until problematic responses diminish or disappear.

Principle of treatment sequencing

15. Therapeutic change is most likely if the initial focus of change efforts is to build new skills and alter disruptive symptoms.

(continued)

TABLE 3.2. *(continued)*

Differential treatment principles

16. Therapeutic change is greatest when the relative balance of interventions favors the use of skill-building and symptom-removal procedures with patients who externalize, or the use of insight and relationship-focused procedures with patients who internalize.

17. Therapeutic change is greatest when the directiveness of the intervention is either inversely correspondent with the patient's current level of resistance or authoritatively prescribes a continuation of the symptomatic behavior.

18. The likelihood of therapeutic change is greatest when the patient's level of emotional stress is moderate (i.e., not excessively high or excessively low).

AN INTERNET-DISTRIBUTED APPLICATION FOR IMPLEMENTING SYSTEMATIC TREATMENT SELECTION

The model of treatment planning outlined by the STS model has been applied to a computer-driven procedure for assessing patients and constructing interventions. Fisher, Beutler, and Williams (1999b) developed an instrument for measuring, within a single framework, the six STS patient dimensions (described earlier in Table 3.1). This instrument (the Systematic Treatment Selection—Clinician Rating Form, STS-CRF) has been adapted to a computerized version (Beutler, 2001) that administers, scores, and interprets the results. An online system to help clinicians develop and plan treatments is now available; this system capitalizes on the extensive STS research findings to produce more effective treatment protocols for a variety of patients (*www.systematictreatmentselection.com*). This Web-enabled program has incorporated patient demographic characteristics, diagnostic information, therapist performance data, and patient change profiles into a user-friendly ("users" may be therapists, patients, or case managers) interface that can expedite treatment and improve the efficacy of psychotherapy. The STS system, codeveloped by Beutler and Williams, has undergone a 9-year evolution to its current form as an Internet-distributed application that incorporates a Web browser interface, multiple SQL data servers, and a telephone (interactive voice response [IVR]) intake–update system.

The STS system consists of a clinician response and a patient self-report version, both of which are available in English or Spanish. The patient response-prompted system employs voice renditions (IVR) that efficiently guide patients through a telephone intake process and provides treatment-relevant information. Both response-prompted systems provide the same types of highly graphic and visually rich outputs for the clinician (or case manager) and reduces reliance on written language. Although a clinician can quantify the six treatment-relevant patient dimensions without the help of a computer, the Web-based STS system provides information that is accessible only from the system. For example, the STS system matches therapists to patients (as well as treatments to patients), and it provides treatment trajectories for actual treatment progress as well as a prognosis trajectory based on a population of patients with similar treatment relevant qualities.

The remainder of this chapter is devoted to illustrating the principles of STS as they relate to a case example. For more information on the computer-driven administration of the Web-based STS system, the interested reader is referred to Appendix C and the URL provided in this section.

CASE EXAMPLE

R.W. is a 22-year-old, Mexican American woman. She has a history of panic attacks, associated with apparent agoraphobia, social phobias, and significant paranoid ideation. She carries a provisional diagnosis of undifferentiated schizophrenia (295.9) and social phobia (300.23). Her history (presented in Appendix A) suggests a good deal of social distrust and isolation, largely deriving from her initiation of a long-term but illicit relationship with a high school teacher while she was yet underage.

The clinician employing the STS model typically would gather background information on R.W. and administer several assessment tools (e.g., MMPI-2, STAI, DOWD-TRS, and/or STS-CRF) to elicit the information in the foregoing paragraph and to quantify the patient's status on the six treatment-relevant dimensions. The STS-CRF (introduced previously) is a clinician-administered semistructured interview that may be used to supplement or replace the foregoing measures. The STS-CRF is designed to tap the six STS patient dimensions and provide profile information when entered into the STS computer system. Diagnostic and profile information may be gathered from more conventional measures (e.g., MMPI-2) or from the STS-CRF. Regardless of the method used to gather the information, the clinician would establish the patient's symptom profile, paying particular attention to areas that reveal significant elevations (over $T = 50$). In the case of R.W., symptoms in the domains of thought disturbance and hypomania are most elevated.

R.W.'s assessment results reveal a tendency toward externalizing over internalizing qualities (indicated by the IR and STS-CRF), providing information for the STS treatment planning dimensions. Thus she may be expected to have many external fears, to anticipate being harmed, and to be hypersensitive to other's opinions and criticisms. She also has a high level of trait-like resistance (also called "reactance" and indicated by the TRS, STS-CRF, and various MMPI-2 scales), suggesting that she invests a good deal of energy in asserting her autonomy and may have problems with authorities and with any perceived loss of interpersonal control. Elevations also suggest that her problem is complex/chronic, that she experiences a moderate level of subjective distress, and that she has adequate social support.

Based on assessment results in the context of the STS model, the clinician would suggest long-term treatment, including the use of psychoactive medications designed to affect thought processes, and efforts to structure the patient's environment to reduce the degree of instability and variability of response. The externalizing patterns suggest the need to focus on discrete symptoms and to utilize a concrete and structured approach that trains the patient in more effective thought and emotion management, effective interpersonal skills, and helps her to test out suspicions of other's motives and behaviors. The high levels of resistance lead to the suggestion that self-directed treatments should supplement therapist activities to reduce the degree of confrontation. Self-help manuals focusing on impulse control, anxiety management, and cognitive skill building are recommended.

SUMMARY

STS represents a theoretical therapeutic perspective, an empirically supported method of treatment, and a state-of-the-art system of delivering high-quality mental health care that capitalizes on an extensive database of continually updated empirical findings. The technical eclectic method that STS employs is one that utilizes the most useful strategies and interventions available, without the constraints imposed by single-theory formulations of patient care. That is, STS therapists should be opportunistic (flexible) in their adherence to strategies, willing and able to select the best from among the myriad interventions that are consistent with any specific principle and strategic plan. It is not enough to simply do what sometimes appears to work; STS therapists are guided to identify and do what *consistently works best*.

STS is based on rigorous research that began in the 1980s. A succession of large-scale randomized clinical trials has provided the empirical support for the STS model, and each investigation has resulted in an expansion and refinement of the model. As new treatment-relevant dimensions are identified, they are incorporated into an updated STS treatment package—the ultimate goal of each iteration is to produce an incremental increase in the efficacy and effectiveness of mental health treatment.

When therapists incorporate the information provided by the research on patient dimensions (i.e., by utilizing the STS model or system), they are able to provide a highly focused and targeted treatment. In other words, patient management, symptom reduction, and change are optimized because the STS program is based on research findings that have been incorporated into a system that both maximizes the likelihood of positive outcome and increases the magnitude of change.

4

—

The Integrative
Clinical Interview

David Mohr and Larry E. Beutler

The interview is the evaluation procedure used most frequently in clinical practice, and it has many uses, such as obtaining historical and current status information from the patient and informing decisions about suitability for initiating psychotherapy or psychopharmacological treatment. It is also used to monitor the progress of treatment and alter treatment when progress is slow. Although it is frequently used as a "stand-alone" procedure for responding to specific referrals, it is also used as part of formal psychological and neuropsychological evaluations (Lezak, 1995).

OVERVIEW OF INTERVIEW FORMATS

Interviews vary along a continuum from unstructured to very highly structured. Unstructured formats are those that vary from clinician to clinician, patient to patient, and occasion to occasion. There is no standardized format, and the responses obtained are not compared to any external norms; interpretation relies solely on the initiating clinician. The questions asked, the topics discussed, and the decisions made are a product of the clinician's individual judgment. In other words, the unstructured clinical interview is characterized by maximal flexibility. It follows a sequence of topics that is developed and modified by the individual clinician to fit any circumstance that arises. It is tailored to the patient's presenting problem, requires no special materials, and capitalizes upon the clinician's personal creativity and skill. However, precisely because it is so wedded to individual clinicians and because skill and competence vary widely among clinicians, the unstructured clinical interview is also among the least reliable and, therefore, potentially the least valid measures used in psychological assessment. The information rated by clinicians frequently is disparate from the responses of patients on self-report measures. Agreement between patient and therapist is difficult to obtain, even regarding very fundamental personal qualities of the patient. For example, even categorical identifications of a patient's ethnicity may be inaccurate, when based on information from unstructured formats (Root, 1992). Variability in rated ethnic assignment varies nearly 50% of the time among raters (Good, 1992a).

One of the reasons behind such variability is the high level of inference that is usually applied to data obtained in an unstructured fashion. To overcome some of these problems, major changes were initiated in the *Diagnostic and Statistical Manual of Mental Disorders* (DSM), beginning in the early 1970s (American Psychiatric Association, 1994). The resulting structure of the modern DSM reduced the role of inference and, thereby—at least, as applied to diagnostic decision making—has imposed a degree of structure on the interview procedure. The demands of diagnosis require the clinician to focus on specific symptoms and signs that characterize each diagnostic condition. This indirect structure has been translated to more obvious and direct applications in the form of structured interview formats for assigning diagnostic labels. The most noted of these are the Diagnostic Interview Schedule (DIS; Kessler & Eaton, 1985; Robins, Helzer, Croughan, & Ratcliff, 1981), the Structured Clinical Interview for DSM-IV (SCID; First, Spitzer, Gibbon, & Williams, 1995; Spitzer, Williams, Gibbon, & First, 1992), and the Schedule for Clinical Assessment in Neuropsychiatry (SCAN; Eaton, Neufeld, Chen, & Cai, 2000).

Structured interview formats require the clinician to (1) follow a specific regimen in asking questions, (2) cover specified topics, and (3) address a finite list of identifiable symptoms and signs associated with various disorders. Although this structure has improved the reliability of assigning diagnoses and identifying problem areas (e.g., Spitzer et al., 1992), clinicians frequently find structured interviews to be very constraining and time consuming. Furthermore, such interviews are still too reliant on patient self-report to overcome the problems of validity, so validity is still suspect when complex disorders and conditions are involved. Eaton and colleagues (2000) conclude, "It is unlikely that the highly structured self-report modality will ever be satisfactory for disorders such as schizophrenia or bipolar disorder, in which lack of insight precludes relying heavily on subject's judgment as to the presence or absence of a symptom, or the impairment it may generate" (p. 222).

There is a place, however, for interviews whose content is specified and whose results can be corroborated by standardized procedures that are amenable to identification by a skilled and experienced clinician (Summerfeldt & Antony, 2002). "Semistructured" interview formats are designed to combine the flexibility of the traditional clinical interview with the validity and reliability of structured assessment methods. Because such interviews invariably suffer from either low or unspecified reliability and validity levels, however, they cannot be expected to function as stand-alone procedures. Nevertheless, they may supplement evidence from other sources and capitalize on the clinician's training and experience. Self-report instruments can augment the clinical judgment that is applied to open-ended interview responses and clinician inference, providing information that is different from that obtained in structured formats. Moreover, research in the domain of job interviews suggests that procedures that provide feedback to the interviewer and that explore the consequences, to the clinician, of the decisions made, may produce more valid and reliable interview results than when these steps are not taken (Brtek, & Motowidlo, 2002; Huffcutt, & Arthur, 1994; McDaniel, Whetzel, Schmidt, & Maurer, 1994). It is possible that procedures that increase the continuity between the clinician's behaviors and the outcome of the evaluation can facilitate the development of both methods as well as motivate clinicians to improve the validity and reliability of clinical procedures.

Structured interviews and self-report devices rely on different procedures for establishing normative data, different scaling methods, and different validity criteria (Eaton et al., 2000). Some of the more useful instruments to use as adjuncts to the interview were reviewed in Chapter 2, and the most frequently used ones are explored more thoroughly in Chapters 6, 7, and 8.

Clinicians should be careful in interpreting some of the differences between the results of interviews and the results of standardized tests, however. At one level, interview and self-report data all derive from the same source, the patient. Both types of self-report rely on the patient's own set of experiences to define problems and severity, and this common factor may result in over- or underreporting of the significance of problems. For example, a high-functioning patient who has had little experience with psychological difficulties may rate symptoms as very severe, whereas another patient who has experienced considerable difficulties might rate the same symptom as mild. The results of self-report measures also can be influenced by extraneous variables that may distract the respondent and reduce the value of the report. More specifically, for example, reports of having difficulty meeting job/career obligations (a common item on depression self-report measures) can be strongly influenced by a variety of external factors, such as a transitory disruption in the work environment, more enduring economic conditions that interfere with transportation, or even patient characteristics such as medical illness, disposition and coping style, or psychological dysfunction/disorders such as depression (Mohr et al., 1997). Although self-report measures often confound the effects of external and internal factors, structured interviews help clinicians make an objective and hopefully less confounded determination of symptoms and symptom severity. Because the structured interview provides objective criteria and norms, the resulting information may be more meaningful for communication with other health care professionals and more useful in monitoring the progress of treatment.

This chapter presents a model of the semistructured clinical interview that combines elements of both structured and unstructured formats. First, we summarize some of the strengths and components of both unstructured and structured interviews that can be integrated into a systematic treatment plan, and then we describe the use of the Systematic Treatment Selection—Clinician Rating Form (STS-CRF; Fisher, Beutler, & Williams, 1999a; see Chapter 3)—the hard-copy version of the STS described in the previous chapter.

STRENGTHS OF INTERVIEW FORMATS

The Unstructured Interview

Although some psychotherapists have begun to supplement their therapeutic procedures with objective assessment measures, informal assessment and what are called "clinical impressions," derived from an unstructured interview, remain the most common methods of establishing diagnoses, evaluating patients for treatment, and monitoring treatment efficacy over time. The unstructured interview offers four major advantages over a highly specified and structured interview procedure. First, the unstructured interview is better suited than structured interviews to facilitate rapport between clinician and patient, which is important to the success of treatment. Second, the unstructured interview allows the clinician maximal flexibility. That is, the clinician can adapt the interview to fit the emergence of unusual and unexpected material and can pursue certain problems or symptoms in depth, while limiting focus on areas of functioning deemed to be unproblematic. Third, the interview may be modified at the clinician's discretion to create particular demand characteristics that correspond with those that exist in the environments in which the problems occur. Fourth, the unstructured interview is not limited by unavailability of specific assessment tools or norms.

However, there are also limitations and weaknesses to this method. First, since every clinician's interview is different, it is impossible to know either the reliability or the validity of any one clinician's use of these methods. Moreover, it is generally conceded that unstructured interviews are lacking in reliability and are highly susceptible to clinician biases (Garb, 1998). One of the authors recalls an experience during a predoctoral internship, when the clinical psychology interns made individual and highly accurate predictions about each new patient's diagnosis, based solely on which psychiatrist was on intake duty. It was commonly known that the chief of service would diagnose every patient as paranoid schizophrenic, whereas one of the younger psychiatrists had a disposition to see every patient as having a bipolar disorder. Extant evidence confirms that the way patients are perceived, diagnosed, and treated is more dependent on the clinicians who treat them, the type of setting in which they are evaluated (i.e., outpatient vs. inpatient), and the culture from which the patients come than on individual symptomatic presentations (Garb, 1998; Gillis, Lipkin, & Moran, 1981; Gillis & Moran, 1981). Given that the results of the clinical interview are central in communication among health care providers and treatment planning, it is clear that a procedure is needed that combines the flexibility of the unstructured interview with the ability to estimate accurately the reliability and validity of the interview, as is available in structured methods.

Structured Interviews

Structured interviews, such as the DIS, SCID, and SCAN, consist of a predetermined set of questions that is presented in a defined order. This standardized administration enhances the reliability of the presentation among interviewers and allows the development of normative values to aid in interpretation. The SCID for Axis I disorders, for example, typically earns reliabilities in the range of .70 to .96 for different disorders (Skre, Onstad, Torgersen, & Kringlen, 1991), which are substantially higher than those interviews that use less structured formats (e.g., Eaton et al., 2000; Summerfeldt & Antony, 2002).

Typically there are two types of structured interviews, based on their objectives and the nature of the format used. The aims of structured interviews, which are commonly used in clinical settings, vary along two dimensions: the nature of the problem that is targeted for assessment and the scope or breadth of problems assessed. The targeted problem, for example, may be depression, anxiety, marital, or some combination of symptoms and behaviors. The breadth of an assessment procedure may be increased by either increasing the number of areas of life activities assessed or by assessing a greater variety of symptoms. For example, the targeted problem of a structured interview is usually framed as either a diagnostic condition (broadly focused) or a particular symptom (narrowly focused). Structured interviews for diagnosis, such as the DIS or SCID, often take two or more hours to complete, and frequently are best suited for research settings rather than for clinical settings, because they do not have a strong relationship to defining a specific treatment. Symptom-focused methods for assessing anxiety-related symptoms, such as those described by Antony, Orsillo, and Roemer (2001), are much more useful than diagnostic assessments in clinical practice, because they identify symptoms that are susceptible to direct correction via relatively specific and focused psychotherapy procedures. It should be underscored that the narrower and more specific the assessment of problems, the stronger the relationship between this assessment and the assignment of a particular treatment. The more general the assessment, the less its value for predicting the value of a specific treatment.

Because the scope of structured interviews can be either broad or narrow, depending on the number of areas explored, these interviews can be adapted to particular needs. For example, useful structured interviews are available to assess a wide variety of nonsymptomatic and nondiagnostic areas, such as level of social support (Barrera, 1983) and psychosocial stress (Leserman et al., 1997). These are more general concepts than symptoms but less general than Axis I diagnosis. Moreover, these specific (if broad) areas have specific implications for treatment: They identify problem areas in need of correction, areas that may slow progress in treatment or that may be used for monitoring change and progress.

Broad Focus

Broadly focused structured diagnostic interviews are usually designed as freestanding, comprehensive assessment procedures. Indeed, if the interview is to be the only assessment method used, then a broadly based structured interview provides the most valid and reliable diagnostic information available. The Structured Clinical Interview for the DSM-IV (SCID; First et al., 1995) is the gold standard for obtaining a thorough diagnostic profile of the patient. The SCID directs the clinician through a sequence of choice points—a "decision tree." The patient is systematically queried about critical symptoms associated with the syndromes represented in DSM-IV (American Psychiatric Association, 1994). The clinician relies on the content of the responses as well as on his or her observations of the patient to rate the presence and severity of specific symptoms. The result of this approach is a list of formal DSM-based diagnoses, for which the patient is likely to qualify. The SCID can be used to establish a diagnosis for both Axis I and Axis II disorders. Among the alternatives to the SCID are the Diagnostic Interview Schedule (Kessler & Eaton, 1985), which is more structured than the SCID, and the Composite International Diagnostic Interview (Robins et al., 1988), which can be applied to the International Classification of Diseases (ICD).

The SCID interview is divided into modules (self-contained interview questions), each representing a particular set of related diagnoses (e.g., depression, drug abuse, anxiety, thought disorder). The time required to administer a fully structured diagnostic interview varies in relation to the number and severity of symptoms and syndromes presented. Patients with many psychiatric symptoms will trigger numerous diagnostic modules, the administration of which results in an interview lasting several hours. Furthermore, it is recommended that clinicians undergo an initial training period to learn how to administer it reliably. Such training can take 20 or more hours. Although some good reliabilities have been reported (e.g., Skre et al., 1991), success in achieving these levels has been inconsistent. For example, even after extensive clinician training, reliability and criterion validity indices have been found, in some studies, to vary widely as a function of the particular diagnostic groups studied and the levels of clinician experience (Eysenck, 1986; Frances et al., 1991; Kendler, 1990; Sandler, Hulgus, & Agich, 1994; Widiger & Spitzer, 1991). The variability across studies suggests that the diagnostic reliabilities and accuracies of the diagnostic interview schedules are (1) marginal for establishing general groupings of diagnostic classes, and (2) highly dependent on extraneous factors. Moreover, periodic retraining is necessary to prevent decay or drift in clinician reliability, but this retraining is not a procedure that is endorsed, encouraged, or even possible in many clinical settings. Finally, because of its weak relationship to treatment planning and selection, many clinicians do not find that the information generated from broadly focused diagnostic interviews is worth the time required for training and administration.

Narrow Focus

The length and complexity of broadly focused structured interviews have motivated investigators to develop short diagnostic interviews that require little training. By definition, such interviews are not as comprehensive as broadly based ones. One example of this format is the Prime MD (Spitzer et al., 1994). Initially developed for physicians, this structured interview takes an average of 8 minutes to administer and covers the most common psychiatric problems, including mood, anxiety, alcohol, eating, and somatoform disorders. It is very simple to use, requiring virtually no training for psychologists. The Prime MD also can be used as a screening tool in clinics. With some training, it can be reliably administered by clinic staff with medical (e.g., nurses) or mental health (e.g., social workers) backgrounds.

Alternatively, for the assessment of specific disorders, the individual modules of the SCID, DIS, or CIDI can be administered separately. These instruments can be particularly useful when the patient's symptoms are uncertain, changeable, or obscure, or when the diagnosis is uncommon and infrequently encountered by the therapist.

Structured Symptom Interviews

Broad Focus

The structured symptom interview is usually not formulated in a decision-tree format, nor is it centered on any particular, formal diagnostic criteria. The broadly focused structured symptom interview evaluates a wide array of psychiatric symptoms that suggests areas of potential pathology or problems. The Present State Examination (PSE; Wing, Nixon, Mann, & Leff, 1977) is an example of a comprehensive, broadly focused structured symptom interview. The PSE has both a long form, consisting of 140 ratings of psychiatric symptoms, and a short form, consisting of 40 items. Although items can be combined into symptom clusters or syndromes, the PSE is not designed as a diagnostic tool. Due to its length and its focus on rating symptoms to the exclusion of other information of potential clinical utility, the value to clinicians of using or personally administering the PSE may be limited. However, the PSE can be reliably administered by people without specific mental health training (Rodgers & Mann, 1986) and therefore may be a useful screening tool in medical or group practice settings where paraprofessional or support staff are available.

The Mental Status Exam (MSE; Amchin, 1991) is a relatively brief and widely used structured interview that focuses on a broad range of potential symptoms. The MSE provides information on the severity of impairment within a wide array of functional areas comprising the overall integration of cognitive, affective, mood, and personality functioning. It is left to the clinician's judgment, however, to translate the assessed symptoms into diagnostic impressions or treatment recommendations, or determine if any of the areas requires more careful and detailed evaluation.

Narrow Focus

Narrowly focused structured symptom interviews target a particular area of functioning or set of related symptoms. These measures focus on the severity of symptoms with far more sensitivity than diagnostic tools, but they do not indicate the degree to which a patient's symptom pattern is consistent with specific diagnostic criteria or syndromes. Such tools are useful in monitoring treatment progress, reporting symptom severity to referents, and justifying treatment or treatment progress to third-party payers. The most commonly used structured interviews target depression, anxiety, or cognitive functioning. The most widely used interview for depression is the Hamilton Rating Scale for Depression (HRSD; Hamilton, 1960). The HRSD has been in use for more than 40 years and has been revised so many times that it is impossible to claim that there is just one HRSD (Grundy, Lunnen, Lambert, Ashton, & Tovey, 1994). Initial revisions shortened the HRSD to 17 items. Other revisions, seeking to improve reliability, added structure to the HRSD by including sample questions, and added specificity to the way that the scales are anchored (Whisman et al., 1989).

The Hamilton Anxiety Rating Scale (HARS; Hamilton, 1959) is very similar to the HRSD in format. Compared to the HRSD, few alterations to the HARS have been published. Hence, the scales used for ratings remain unanchored and may pose problems for reliability in the absence of rigorous training. More widely used is the Anxiety Disorders Interview Schedule (ADIS; DiNardo, Brown, & Barlow, 1994). This semistructured interview covers a variety of relevant demographic data, background, medical history, the presenting problem, and associated symptoms. It yields considerable detail about specific anxiety symptoms and indicates an individual's conformity to various diagnostic criteria in the domain of anxiety disorders. Two versions of the ADIS are available: One version provides information about current status, and the other assesses symptomatology over the person's lifetime.

Cognitive functioning is perhaps the most important area to assess using a structured interview procedure. With improved medical care for acute conditions and an aging population, ever greater numbers of people have chronic medical conditions. It is estimated that more than 45% of the American population has at least one chronic medical condition (Hoffman, Rice, & Sung, 1996). Many of these conditions, including coronary problems and pulmonary disease, diabetes, autoimmune conditions, AIDS, and many other diseases, can potentially involve some cognitive impairment. Thus it can be anticipated that a high percentage of patients in the average psychotherapist's caseload will have some cognitive problems. Yet the vast majority of such problems go undetected (Derogatis & Lynn, 1999).

Unlike most other areas of psychological assessment, objective assessment is the only valid alternative for identifying the presence of cognitive impairment. Self-report can be very unreliable (Schwartz, Kozora, & Zeng, 1996). A variety of brief screening tools has been developed to assess cognitive status. The Mini-Mental State Exam (MMSE; Folstein, Folstein, & McHugh, 1975) is the most widely used. The High Sensitivity Cognitive Screen (Faust & Fogel, 1989) was developed to detect milder impairments than the MMSE. The Cognitive Capacity Screening Test (Jacobs, Merhard, Delgado, & Strain, 1977) was developed to evaluate organic mental syndromes in medical patients, although some testing with psychiatric and normal patients was also conducted. These evaluations typically require 10–20 minutes to administer. Although they can be administered by trained assistants, in our experience administration of interviews by the clinician elicits more information and can increase confidence in the therapist, particularly among patients with medical illnesses.

THE INTEGRATED, SEMISTRUCTURED INTERVIEW

Rather than arguing the merits of unstructured versus structured interviews, this chapter emphasizes ways in which clinicians can organize and develop their own preferred interview methods in order to gather relevant assessment data. We believe that an integrated, semistructured approach offers a compromise that includes (1) the flexibility and rapport of the unstructured interview, (2) the structure that ensures a comprehensive evaluation, and (3) the flexibility of adding structured assessments to facilitate treatment decisions, monitor treatment outcome, and aid in communication with other health care providers or payers. We believe that this approach complies closely with what clinicians are likely to find most useful. It has several advantages:

• In an integrated, semistructured approach, the clinician may choose to alter the level of structure or stress employed to assess the patient's likely response to external demands and his or her ability to collaborate with treatment. In doing so, the clinician can selectively draw attention to type of experience (i.e., sensitivity to internal or external events) in order to generate hypotheses about the patient's response to these domains of experience.

• Another strength of the integrated, semistructured clinical interview is its use as a direct measure of the content of recalled experience. It is very helpful for identifying the external experiences and events associated with the patient's living contexts, and for taking a personal history. Although formal tests and computer-interactive software often have been used to gather social and developmental information that will help construct the patient's history, the semistructured interview allows a degree of follow-up that can provide a fuller description of the unique experiences and events affecting a given individual's behavior.

• The integrated, semistructured clinical interview allows the clinician to observe the development of an interpersonal relationship at first hand, and to adapt his or her responses to the changing nature of the patient–clinician interactions. In this way, the semistructured interview elicits behaviors that are similar to those that are likely to occur in the treatment relationship itself. Thus the responses observed may form the foundation for hypotheses about a patient's ability to establish rapport and to cooperate with treatment demands.

• While the integrated, semistructured interview capitalizes on the flexibility of unstructured interviews, it also incorporates standardization through the organization of the interview and the potential introduction of standardized assessment tools. This standardization enhances the validity and reliability of the assessment, facilitates the organization of assessment information, and ensures a comprehensive evaluation.

Next we review three basic components of this interview method: the *context* in which the interview is conducted, the *format* of administration, and the *content* of the interview itself.

Interview Context

The "interview context" refers to the environmental structure in which the interview is conducted. The degree of control a clinician has over the context can vary greatly. Certainly clinicians have considerable control over the context within their own offices, but many institutional settings, such as hospitals, medical clinics, jails, and prisons, may not afford the same flexibility. The clinician's primary concern in establishing the interview context is to ensure that the patient achieves the desired expectations and mind set. Ideally, the patient should be interviewed in a quiet, protected environment, designed to provide reassurance that the information obtained will be treated responsibly and confidentially. Moreover, the environment should convey a sense of order and management, so that the patient can feel assured that the clinician is able to protect the safety of the material or information. Disorder in the contextual arrangements of the interview may create the expectation that the clinician may become overwhelmed by the stress of the patient's problems or be unable to maintain confidentiality in protecting the patient's disclosures.

In addition to any explanations that might be offered by telephone at the time the patient schedules a visit, it is good practice to follow the initial phone call by mailing some written materials to the patient. These materials may include the following:

Directions for finding the office
A map of parking facilities, if necessary
A description of all the services available through the clinician's practice or clinic
The specific services to be provided on this occasion
Materials that address the limits of confidentiality and potential risks and benefits of the service
An outline of the fee structures
Billing and cancellation policies
Confirmation of the appointment time
Emergency contact information (even if it is only referral to 911)
A contact person, should the patient have any further questions.

Although some clinicians prefer to give these materials to the patient in the office, mailing this information prior to the visit is increasingly recommended for both ethical and legal reasons.

Efforts to enhance the patient's sense of safety and comfort should be continued and enhanced by the atmosphere provided by the staff and setting when the patient arrives for the session. A good deal of research has been devoted to discovering the nature of environments that promote disclosure, facilitate a sense of safety, and lead to the development of confidence in the clinician (see Norcross, 2002; Wohlwill & Carson, 1972). By and large, this literature suggests the importance of open spaces, light, and friendly reception personnel in order to enhance the sense of personal freedom and comfort in the waiting area.

Ordinarily there are a few registration and insurance forms to be completed by the patient upon arrival. Some clinics have somewhat more extensive intake procedures. For example, clinics in medical settings often conduct some screening evaluations prior to the initial visit or interview with the clinician. Sometimes this involves paper and pencil assessments, and sometimes it may involve more objective, structured assessment. In such cases, if possible, the clinician should meet briefly with the patient to explain the clinic's procedures and their rationale, answer any preliminary questions, reassure the patient of confidentiality, clarify the patient's right to refuse the evaluation, and reassure the patient that they will meet shortly.

To facilitate the development of a relationship that encourages disclosure, the arrangement of seats should be such as to allow, but not to force, eye contact with the interviewer. Soft lighting and comfortable furniture convey safety and relaxation. However, these characteristics may not be desirable for extended formal assessment in which firm seating, a table, and bright lights for reading are required. The variability required of the interview and testing environments requires either an office that is flexible and easily adaptable, or the availability of different rooms used for testing and therapy. The clinician must ensure smoothly conducted but relatively few transitions among these settings, however, in order to maintain the sense of orderliness.

Interview Format

When initiating the interview itself, the clinician should be on time and ready to attend to the patient's presentation. The clinician should greet the patient in the waiting room, introduce him- or herself, if they have not met earlier, and escort the patient to the examining room or office. If the subsequent administration of the tests is to be carried out by an assistant or someone other than the interviewer, it is helpful if the assistant is introduced before the procedures are begun and remains with the patient and clinician throughout the initial interview.

The interview is usually the first assessment procedure administered because (1) it is the method in which most clinicians place the most faith (usually without justification), (2) (more realistically) it is the easiest method of facilitating the patient's cooperation, and (3) it is readily adapted to providing a context in which the other instruments can be selected and interpreted. As noted above, when the patient is invited into the office, he or she should be given a choice of seating accommodations, varying both in distance from the clinician and in comfort level of the chairs. Facilitating patient choice among such options not only because it provides the clinician with an opportunity to construct hypotheses about personality functioning and interpersonal relatedness, it also reinforces the patient's sense of control and self-governance.

The actual interview usually begins by reiterating major points presented in the standard pre-appointment preparation materials, including the purpose of the evaluation, what questions are being addressed, what information the clinician already has received and from whom, and the anticipated consequences of the findings. At this point, it is useful for the clinician to ask about the patient's impression and to provide his or her own impression of how the results may be used. This latter information is especially important to discuss with the patient whenever the referral questions involve social consequences in the form of employability, insurance coverage, prescription of medication, recommendations for hospitalization, and/or some form of social stigma (e.g., loss of child custody, denial of parole). Assurance of the right to refuse evaluation and treatment is particularly important when the evaluation may result in the loss of freedom or in a major life change. Forensic evaluations dealing with questions of guilt, insanity, competence, disability, and sentencing are examples of such situations, as are custody evaluations and assessments of dangerousness.

Before ending these preliminary comments, the clinician should invite the patient to ask questions about what has been presented. Moreover, the patient is reminded about the time limits of the evaluation, and the procedures to be used are briefly described.

All of the foregoing information is designed to provide reassurance to the patient and to emphasize the freedom that he or she has in the situation. This reassurance is of the same consequence in self-referred evaluations as it is in forensic examinations (when the patient is under court order) and in mental health examinations (when the patient may be incoherent), though in these latter circumstances it is often more difficult to provide such assurance. As a practical matter, the clinician should err in the direction of providing more information than the patient can adequately understand. It is wise not to take the risk of failing to provide information that is later deemed to have been important to the patient's ability to grant informed consent to the procedure.

From this point on, the format of the interview is organized around the desired content, but the clinician attempts to adjust the order of the content of material discussed in order to maintain a smooth flow from topic to topic. That is, the clinician should avoid moving mechanically from question to question and topic to topic. The approach should be conversational in tone, with each new topic introduced as smoothly as possible, flowing naturally from what the patient has just reported.

This smooth conversational flow is usually enhanced by proceeding from general topics to topics associated with problem areas. Both rapport and the amount of information obtained will be enhanced if the clinician begins topics with open-ended and general questions, and subsequently progresses to more specific, closed-ended questions. It is easier to proceed from these general questions to specific ones than vice versa. By proceeding in this manner, the clinician gathers the information within a smoothly flowing and topical conversation, seeking additional information, as it is needed, without losing the focus or appearing overly rehearsed.

Note that a clinician who begins with closed-ended questions is likely to obtain relatively flat and unrevealing answers, as in this example:

THERAPIST: What did your father do?

PATIENT: He was a carpenter.

THERAPIST: How did you get along with him?

PATIENT: Oh, pretty well, most of the time.

THERAPIST: And what did your mother do?

Contrast this exchange with the responses generated by more open-ended questions:

THERAPIST: Tell me about your parents.

PATIENT: Well, they were poor people; my father was a carpenter and my mother was a housewife.

THERAPIST: What was it like living with them?

PATIENT: Oh, it was OK most of the time, but my father was very strict, and my mother often felt like she had to protect us kids from him.

THERAPIST: Tell me more about how that happened.

PATIENT: My father just had a very, very clear idea about how he wanted us kids to be. And when we did anything he didn't like, he would really fly off the handle.

THERAPIST: Is there an example of this that stands out in your mind?

Note that the use of closed-ended questions has the effect of focusing the patient's attention on the clinician's questions. Most patients will try to accommodate the clinician by answering, often dutifully. Open-ended questions invite the patient to explore, thereby permitting the emergence of a broader spectrum of material, which the clinician can then focus on with more specific questions.

All material elicited must be received with a matter-of-fact attitude. Indeed, in asking about sensitive subjects, it is a good idea to phrase the questions positively, so that it is assumed that everyone has done everything. Thus, for example, "How old were you when you began masturbating?" is generally preferable to "Have you ever masturbated?"

When it is necessary to change topics, it is worthwhile to keep the difference between interrogative/mechanistic and conversational styles in mind. A clinician using the mechanistic interviewing style may go from one topic to another, as follows:

THERAPIST: And was there anything else about your brothers and sisters?

PATIENT: No.

THERAPIST: How has your health been?

A clinician using a more conversational style may proceed thus:

THERAPIST: What else can you tell me about the relationship between you and your brothers and sisters?

PATIENT: Well, there's really not much to tell. They . . . (*concludes the thought*).

THERAPIST: What kind of health problems did they have?

PATIENT: Oh, they were all healthy, but my mother . . . (*continues*).

THERAPIST: What similar kinds of problems have you had?

Note that the lead-in question in the second example is more open-ended than the one in the first example, and that the clinician introduces the patient's health as a topic within the context of a discussion about the family. In this way, the change in topic flows smoothly from a discussion of the siblings, avoiding an abrupt transition from talking about the brothers and sisters to again talking about the patient. There may be times that such smooth transitions are not possible, either due to contextual constraints, such as limited time, or patient characteristics, such as perseveration or excessive talkativeness. In such cases, it is best to let the patient know that you are about to change subject by saying something like "I'd like to shift gears now, and find out. . . . "

The clinician may find it useful to incorporate more formal assessment tools into the interview. Such instruments can be introduced effectively by providing a brief explanation. For example:

THERAPIST: You mentioned that you've been having some problems with your thinking and memory. The kinds of problems you describe are not uncommon in people with HIV, but they also can result from the emotional distress you've been having. Would it be OK with you if we evaluated these problems a little more carefully to try to understand where they might be coming from?

At the conclusion of the interview, the clinician is advised to invite comments and additional information that the patient might think are important:

THERAPIST: What have I missed that you think might be important for me to know?

PATIENT: Well, I don't know. Did I tell you that my uncle committed suicide?

After processing new information that is highlighted in this way, and before employing other assessment procedures, the clinician should again invite questions and comments. Moreover, before terminating the session at the end of the testing period, the clinician typically provides some limited feedback to the patient. If the patient has been with an assistant for the test administration, the clinician and the assistant provide this feedback together, after a brief private meeting to share and organize their thoughts. After feedback, another appointment is scheduled (1) to complete the assessment procedures, if necessary, (2) for more detailed feedback following the scoring and analysis of results, or (3) for the beginning of treatment. Even if the end-of-session feedback seems satisfactory, it is wise to plan for at least one additional feedback session to be conducted after all materials are analyzed and before the final report has been sent to the referring clinician. This session allows the clinician to incorporate, in the final report, any relevant new material that the feedback session itself elicits.

In this feedback session, it is wise to reiterate the purpose of the evaluation and to summarize the findings and recommendations. If the patient was evaluated as part of an intake for psychotherapy, a clear description of the proposed treatment and the roles of the patient and clinician should be presented. In the case of general or specific evaluations, the patient may usefully be invited to read a penultimate draft of the report and to comment on its content. Even if the findings and recommendations are not likely to please the patient, this summary should take place frankly and openly, so that nothing provided by the referring clinician to the patient, following receipt of the report, will come as a surprise. Since these records are available to the patient, allowing input may alleviate some of the potential negative effects of the patient's being confronted with some of the critical or controversial material. Certainly, under these conditions, the language and description should minimize the potential for harming the patient.

Interview Content

The interview provides information about all six STS dimensions (functional impairment, degree of social support, chronicity/complexity of problem, coping style, resistance level, and distress level), that can then be cross-validated against other instruments. In addition, the interview offers a unique opportunity to explore areas that extend beyond these dimensions. Thus details about the person's history, information about the development and course of the problem, and details about interpersonal relationships are assessed more directly through the clinical interview than in any other medium. Information on all of these topics is interwoven in the responses to the structured or semistructured interview.

The content of the interview includes both verbal and nonverbal elements. Whereas the verbal content is adapted to the referral questions being addressed, behavioral observations that arise in response to the context and format of the interview are blended with the verbal content to provide the basis for making inferences and drawing conclusions about the areas of functioning that are later described in the written report. The areas of functioning to be addressed in the report include, but are not limited to, the dimensions and concepts presented in Chapter 1, and all are weighted in importance during the interview by the nature of the referral question and the confidence that the clinician can legitimately place in his or her observations. As we discuss the nature and content of the clinical interview, we integrate these concepts with other information that is (relatively) uniquely amenable to the interview format.

In addition to its usefulness as an after-the-fact tool for integrating clinical impressions, the STS-CRF form (see Chapter 3) can be used by the clinician to direct and guide the semistructured interview. It cannot replace other procedures or even replace the interview itself, but the computer-based application, perhaps supplemented by the self-report format, can help ensure that relevant topics are covered while flexibility in administration and focus is maintained. The computerized form includes subroutines that circumvent questions that do not generate positive responses on critical items. It also allows the insertion of standardized test scores from the MMPI-2, MCMI, SCL-90-R, BDI-II (Beck, Steer, and Brown, 1996), and other instruments, in lieu of separate assessment of state- and trait-like variables. These modifications shorten the procedure and increase its clinical usefulness.

In integrating verbal and nonverbal observations, the clinician pays

close attention to any discrepancies that may exist between observed behaviors and the verbal content of the patient's responses. A patient who is
animated and excited but who describes him- or herself as "depressed" is a
very different individual from one who is sluggish and unresponsive as well
as subjectively "depressed." Such discrepancies are used to infer qualities of
involvement or investment and motivation for undergoing the evaluation
or subsequent treatment, and provide the basis for making inferences about
aspects of prognosis as well as cognitive, emotional, interpersonal, and
intrapersonal functioning. In addition, the clinician attempts to extract information that will bear on diagnostic decisions, and observes patterns of
interaction that will bear on treatment prognostications. In so doing, it is
conventional to explore different areas of patient functioning. Thus, as a
way of extracting information about the dimensions that are pertinent to
the referral questions, the interviewer considers aspects of the problem and
then the way it has developed and manifested in different social contexts.

Since some of the particular strengths of the interview procedure are in
its adaptability for use with very different and varied problems, this aspect
of the interview bears particular consideration. Table 4.1 provides an outline of the content areas and contexts that are usually explored in the clinical interview. It should be noted that the order in which the information
obtained may be, and usually is, somewhat different from the order in
which it is reported, although usually the interview roughly follows the
outline that will be used for the written description.

Identifying Information

It is important to establish certain information about the patient at the out-
set of the interview. The clinician should inquire about the name that the
patient prefers, as well as his or her formal name, age, self-defined ethnicity, and the name and relationship to the patient of the referring professional. This information should be presented in the written intake report.
Discrepancies between the patient's report and the clinician's impressions
regarding age, ethnicity, and the like, are surprisingly common (Beutler,
Brown, Crothers, Booker, & Seabrook, 1996) and should be noted in the
written intake report as a means of alerting the reader to the demographic
qualities and preferences that may help determine the patient's culture, cultural roles, beliefs, and value systems.

Presenting Complaint/Problem

The next task is to define the nature of the problem that brings the patient
in for assessment. This task is accomplished by asking the patient to describe the major problem or difficulty for which he or she is seeking help. In

TABLE 4.1. Systematic Treatment Selection, Clinician Rating Form

INTAKE OUTLINE

I. Identifying Information

   A. This section includes preferred name, legal name, ethnicity, and gender of patient.

II. Presenting Complaint/Problem

   A. This section is comprised of the patient's description.

III. History of Problem

   A. Course and history, level of social and functional impairment, and efforts to alleviate problems and symptoms are covered here.

   B. Also report the history of prior treatment, including how successful or unsuccessful.

IV. Social and Family History

   A. This section presents the client's developmental social history, including historical and present levels of social support. It provides a baseline from which to estimate complexity/chronicity and impairment level. It describes the structure of the early family, the nature of early environmental factors, and how important family relationships have changed over time. Experiences of early abuse or deprivation should be elicited.

   B. This section also should include information about friendships, including ability to relate to peers in school, problems with the law or with authorities, educational achievements, work history, and the demonstrated ability to develop close relationships. It should include an assessment of how disruptions to social relationships have been handled and a comparison of current and past attachment levels.

   C. Sexual history also should be covered here, including any history of sexual abuse, marriages, pattern of sexual difficulties, etc.

V. Medical History

   A. This section includes a review of medical problems experienced, the formal and informal treatments sought, the effects of these treatments, and the prescribed and nonprescribed drugs that have been, and currently are being, taken.

   B. This section also should include a description of any current illicit drug use as well as patterns of alcohol use.

VI. Mental Status, Coping Patterns, and Response Dispositions

   A. This section covers current status in the following areas:
      1. Appearance
      2. Cognitive functioning
      3. Affect and mood
      4. Coping styles
      5. Resistance potential

(continued)

TABLE 4.1. *(continued)*

VII. Integrated Formulation and Treatment Plan

   A. This section should identify the problems that will be addressed in treatment and indicate the level of danger to self or other that is present.

   B. The section should identify plans for treatment, referral, and additional consultation. It should refer to problems that are likely to arise, and alternatives that would be considered in that event.

   C. Considerations regarding the need for special treatment settings, special consultations, and other special arrangements for treatment should be considered here.

   D. The section concludes with a statement of the client's prognosis.

the intake note, this description of the problem is usually noted succinctly in the patient's own words, along with notations of any relevant nonverbal indicators of distress. The clinician attempts to distill the patient's verbal response into one or two sentences that best describe how the patient identifies the purpose of the referral and evaluation. This verbatim patient description provides important information on its own as well as when compared to the assessing clinician's and the referring clinician's impressions of the problem and the purpose of the evaluation. Along with the patient's manner as he or she presents a description of the problem, any discrepancies observed between verbal reports and behaviors provide initial indications of the patient's investment in and willingness to change. Moreover, by succinctly paraphrasing the problem in a way that is acceptable to the patient, the treating clinician can periodically refer to this description when assessing the significance and relevance of changes that are observed later in the treatment process.

As previously described, it is at this early point of describing the patient's problem that the clinician can easily explore misunderstandings that may exist about the evaluation process and explain how the results of the evaluation will be used. At this juncture the interviewer should be concerned with the discrepancies that may exist among the informed opinions of interested others (significant others, the referring clinician, the interviewing clinician, etc.) as well as with obtaining the patient's informed consent to undertake the procedures. Obtaining informed consent is imperative not only from an ethical and legal perspective but also from a practical one. A patient who feels informed and autonomous is likely to be more cooperative than one who feels controlled and coerced. Therefore, before going into depth about the nature of the problem itself, the clinician must be assured that the patient has a clear understanding of the purpose and use of the procedures.

History of Problem

After learning how the patient conceptualizes the problem, the clinician begins to elicit information about symptom onset, pattern, and treatment. It is here that the clinician begins to uncover information on various treatment-planning dimensions and begins to formulate a response to the referral question. Once again, the clinician is interested in the verbal content of the patient's impressions as well as in the more subtle indicators of stress and coping provided by accompanying nonverbal behaviors. Although overall assessment is not always concerned with the consensual accuracy of the patient's verbal report, cross-validating evidence is often sought to support the reliability of the interview content and to observe discrepancies that may exist among three interrelated aspects of the verbal presentation of history.

In exploring the history of the problem as well as the patient's interpersonal and social history, the six STS dimensions on which treatments are planned form a framework around which information can be sought within each content area of the interview. The interview, however, is organized around content reflecting different areas of manifestation and development. The content extracted in these areas is not uniform in the degree to which it yields information on the treatment planning dimensions. Thus, while obtaining information about the patient's problem, the level of severity, chronicity, problem complexity, and level of impairment will easily emerge, whereas information on the closely related concept of social support will more easily emerge when the patient's family and social history is reviewed. The skilled clinician will integrate the information obtained from all of these content areas when formulating the problem, responding to the referral, and developing the treatment plan.

In the following paragraphs, we present the interview structure based on the topical contents discussed, highlighting how and when certain information that is specific to the treatment planning dimensions is likely to emerge, such as: (1) the level of functional impairment, (2) the chronicity and course of the condition, and (3) the patient's efforts to alleviate or prevent the problem (coping style).

Level of Functional Impairment. The first aspect of symptom or problem evaluation in the STS treatment planning procedure is a determination of the severity of the symptom or problem. Level of functional impairment, in our usage, is an estimate of the degree to which the patient's functioning is impaired in such activities as work, family life, intimacy, and social contacts. Evidence for functional impairment must include actual behaviors that disrupt one or more of these areas of daily functioning. Functional impairment is only poorly correlated with level of felt, or subjective severity of, distress (Fisher et al., 1999a), since the latter requires no external estimate of performance. However, together, functional impairment and subjective distress may provide some motivation for seeking treatment. Noting changes in severity of functional impairment is frequently a critical component in both patient and third-party judgments of treatment effectiveness. Functional impairment can be evaluated in the interview with the patient, but for more specific information that is not colored by level of distress, the clinician may need to interview collateral contacts, such as spouses, parents, or adult children.

For many of the most common symptom clusters, such as depression or anxiety, well-established structured and semistructured interviews are available (see the earlier discussion of the HRSD and HRSA) that provide an estimate of impairment in life activities. The use of an objective instrument can give the clinician a concrete measure of severity. This marker can be used to monitor the progress and effectiveness of treatment, and it can also be useful to share with patients, periodically. In successful cases, objective evidence of progress in specific symptoms and progress can be validating. When difficulties arise, this information can be used to initiate a discussion of problems in treatment and a search for new treatment strategies.

Functional impairment also should be assessed through a semistructured clinical interview that typically focuses on the impact that problems and symptoms have had on such activities as work, school, and interpersonal relationships. Multiple perspectives are often helpful, since symptom presentation and severity are typically influenced by level of distress and patient coping styles, which produce either exaggerated or minimized reports. Hence, to the degree possible, it is a good idea to cross-validate the historical information presented by the patient with sources of information that are external to the patient, including significant others, treatment records, and the referrer. The interviewer should be aware that the impact of symptoms and problems on life routines is affected by physical well-being, social support, and general interpersonal functioning. Cross-validation of indicators can help the clinician tease apart the relative contributions of the presenting complaint, symptoms, health, distress level, coping style, and interpersonal function on the patient's life routines.

There are many clinical instances in which discrepancies between the patient's and external observers' assessments of impairment serve as differential diagnostic or etiological indicators. For example, patients with dementia of the Alzheimer's type are often distinguished from those with dementia associated with depression by the latter group's tendencies to overestimate the degree of actual impairment of functions as well as by their excessive concern with loss of memory or verbal fluency. Similarly, patients with externalizing coping styles or delusional disorders are characterized by the tendency to attribute the problem to others rather than to self. However, the criteria for "exaggeration" are frequently elusive, and reviewing the observations of those who have viewed the patient in real-world settings may help clarify the matter.

Of course, when comparing the patient's reports, the reports of significant others, and the interviewer's own observations, the interviewer must keep in mind that family members and friends may have vested interests that lead them to minimize or exaggerate the significance of the problems being addressed. When discrepancies are significant and the likely consequences are severe, objective evaluation via standardized assessment tools, indirect and direct observations of the patient, collateral information on grades or work performance, and interviews with disinterested parties can be employed to derive reliable hypotheses about the roles of denial, minimization, and exaggeration among the parties involved. For example, work records, school reports, and sometimes even bank or spending records may be requested as supplements to the clinician's other assessments of performance, in order to determine what patterns and changes are occurring.

Chronicity and Course of the Condition. Obtaining information on symptom course requires a detailed consideration of (1) the events that were present when the symptom patterns or presenting problems were first noticed, (2) how long and with what frequency the patterns have occurred, (3) how they have changed over time, and (4) how the patterns or problems came to the patient's attention. This effort at discovery is extended into an exploration of the pattern of problem recurrence and change that has been noticed by the patient. This information may be compared with the reports that are available or that can be conveniently obtained from significant others, prior treatment records, and the referring professional. Specifically, in the interview the patient is asked to report on (1) the circumstances under which he or she (or someone else) first noticed the problems; (2) how he or she and significant others initially explained the problems; (3) the frequency and nature of the circumstances in which the problems have recurred; and (4) the changes that have been noted, over time, in both the problems and the circumstances.

A historical review of social and family functioning establishes the level of chronicity and complexity of the patient's problem and the level of social support for change. *Problem chronicity* is indicated by the time over which the problem has developed. *Complexity,* which is highly correlated with chronicity, reflects the multiplicity and recurrence of problems and their pattern of change over time. The patient's unique history of problem development, remission and recurrence, and resolution must be considered in juxtaposition with a general history of current and developmental social conditioning experiences. A long period of low normative functioning, dating to early development, as well as a history of recurring problems are poor prognostic indicators for change. Recently developed and single-

episode problems have a better prognosis, but in either case, only by knowing the developmental course and early functioning of the patient can the
clinician determine the level of impairment or change and the chronicity of
the difficulties. Direct questioning during the interview may provide the
most direct access to the baseline that allows determination of chronicity/
complexity and impairment levels, since correspondent sources of data are
frequently unavailable among adult patients.

Efforts to Cope with and Alleviate Problems. The third aspect of the
symptom history consists of (1) the patient's descriptions of how he or she
has coped with and attempted to alleviate, the symptoms, (2) how effective
these efforts have been, and (3) what resources have been used in the process. Although information about these efforts will provide clues to the patient's coping style and general personality, the main focus here is determining how successful the patient has been in obtaining relief through his or
her own, or others', efforts. In other words, the effectiveness of coping efforts, rather than the particular nature of them, is the point. The clinician
particularly wants to determine (1) whether the patient or others in his or
her environment can predict the recurrence and exacerbation of the symptoms or problems, (2) the level of self-efficacy or hope for success, (3) what
prior efforts have been made to initiate treatment, and (4) the success levels
of such treatments. In pursuing these aims, the clinician elicits the patient's
description of what cognitive resources and patterns are used to help explain and adapt to the problem, and how helpful these are in managing the
difficulty. The clinician also seeks to elicit what types of behavior have been
used in the service of self-protection, and what roles others play in altering
the problem manifestation and severity of impairment. Thus a review of the
person's formal efforts to seek treatment, the nature of these resources, and
patterns of interactions with informal sources of help (e.g., family, friends,
books, self-help groups, etc.) are necessary.

The clinician can increase the reliability of inferences made about interpersonal functioning by knowing the roles that others play in the patient's problem. The roles performed by others can be judged on the basis
of the patient's report and whatever ancillary information is available regarding how these others support the patient, impede problem resolution,
or contribute to problem development and maintenance. Notably, from information about (1) the level of the person's functional impairment, especially as it pertains to how, and under what circumstances, others in the patient's environment become involved in the problem; (2) what the patient
thinks when under duress; and (3) how the patient seeks to alleviate distress, much will be learned about how the patient copes more generally.
Thus, as this information about the patient is gathered, the clinician uses it
to infer the presence of certain patterns in the patient's manner of coping
with interpersonal closeness and aggression. We return to this point later in

this chapter, when we focus more specifically on the patient's general coping style.

Efforts to gain information from what the patient or significant others report are indirect ways of estimating how effectively the patient has tried to redress the problem. Direct evidence of how appropriately and effectively the patient has sought relief is also available though observations of behavior that occurs during the evaluation process itself. Patients who have given up and are hopeless often exhibit negative responses to assessment tasks, asserting that they cannot do the task or making self-recriminating complaints that they have performed inadequately. Such hopeless patients either seek additional assistance or withdraw and give up as they experience a devastating loss of self-efficacy in dealing with their problems. These patterns also may reflect their general styles of adapting to the world, but such an assumption cannot be made without evidence of a preexisting and long-enduring pattern.

Social and Family History

Of course, level of impairment can be judged only from a baseline of long-term functioning that preceded the patient's entry into treatment. The most important feature of the information obtained on family history relates to the availability of, and felt support from, family members. It is also important to gain information about how family members deal with each other and what they inadvertently or directly communicated to the patient about handling such important issues as sexual feelings, anger, fear, and love. Then, as the clinician reviews the patient's social and interpersonal history, he or she can determine if the interpersonal themes and patterns observed to occur in family interactions have been reenacted in other relationships.

Social Support. Interpersonal attachment and relationships are critical to patients' adjustment. Indeed the level of social support is strongly and consistently (inversely) related to the level of functional impairment (Beutler, Harwood, Alimohamed, & Malik, 2002). Even the availability of a single person in whom the patient can confide comfortably may significantly reduce rates of relapse and improve his or her ability to cope with problems.

Many aspects of social support may be useful, but perhaps the most important is the degree to which the patient finds comfort and reassurance in a family environment. Inquiries about the nature of the family unit during the patient's early developmental years as well as currently are helpful to determine whether this environment fostered such assets as independence, personal achievement, interpersonal cohesion, opportunity for play, and use of leisure time. Moos (1974) has suggested that good family relations accomplish three cardinal tasks: They foster supportive relationships, allow and encourage personal development and growth, and maintain order and organization.

Not only does a review of family development help establish a baseline to which the clinician can compare current behavior, it also facilitates the determination of whether there are social systems available to the patient to support change. Toward this end, the clinician must elicit information from the patient about the following factors:

Structure of the family
The patient's roles within that structure
Level of felt support and frequency of contact
Significant formative events
Patterns of reinforcement and punishment to which the patient was subjected
Progress in reaching key developmental milestones
Changes that have occurred in important family relationships over time.

The effort here is to determine the nature of both past and present roles and allegiances within the family structure so that the clinician can see what changes have occurred and estimate the level of decline from, or maintenance of, lifelong patterns. The following questions may initiate leads that can be followed fruitfully:

"As you were growing up, who in your family were you the most like?"
"To whom were you the closest? . . . Are you still close?"
"How did you find out when there were problems between your father and mother?"
"What did other members of your family do when there were problems? . . . What do they do now?"
"What were your most and least favorite family traditions? . . . Do you still participate in those?"

The interview is virtually unique in its ability to identify and explore sensitive issues that might play a formative role in the patient's current presentation. Special care should be taken to elicit any experiences of early abuse, emotional withdrawal, or emotional/physical deprivation, as well as any instances of drug, alcohol, or sexual difficulties that may have been experienced by the patient or by other family members. Examples of family attitudes toward aggression, sexual expression, and achievement should be requested. The following questions may be helpful in initiating these topics:

"How did members of your family feel [or react] when you got angry?"
"How was discipline managed in your family?"
"What was the worst experience you had growing up in your family?"

"What did members of your family do when you discovered sex?"

"How did members of your family teach you about sex?"

"How did the various members of your family show it when they were angry? Sad? Hurt? Happy?"

"Who in your family got into the most trouble because of drinking or drug use?"

"What attitudes did your parents have about sex? How did they convey these to you?"

"What role did religion play in your family?"

This information about the patient's functioning and support within the nuclear family should be supplemented by the patient's description of early and changing friendships and social interactions. The concern here is to evaluate levels of support, symptomatic changes (including relapses and recurrences), and acuteness of impairments to the patient's capacity for intimacy, attachment, and autonomy. For most content areas, the subjectivity of these data is as relevant as their factuality. Indeed, the patient's subjective responses to early friendships, love relationships, and sexual attachments are specifically sought. In eliciting such information, the clinician is seeking to determine not only past and present patterns in the way the patient deals with others, but also to form an impression about his or her capacity for forming a therapeutic treatment alliance. Patients who report having had few friendships or who do not recall having lasting friendships and love relationships are at greater risk for failure to develop the therapeutic attachment that is often necessary for supporting change.

Other aspects of social support concern persons outside of the family. For example, the clinician can obtain a simple count of the number of people the patient perceives as being available to provide support and encouragement during times of trouble, and then ask the patient to rate the degree to which he or she is satisfied with that level of support. For narrative detail, the clinician can ask the patient to describe the nature of these relationships. The Social Support Questionnaire (SSQ; Sarason, Levine, Basham, & Sarason, 1983) can be used to supplement these interview impressions.

When undertaking such an assessment, it is helpful to begin with a conceptual structure. Barber, Luborsky, Crits-Christoph, and Diguer (1995), for example, employ an interview procedure to develop an understanding of the themes around which patients organize their interpersonal lives. They use a three-step method of exploring interpersonal relationships, the Core Conflictual Relationship Theme (CCRT) method, which identifies key people in the patient's life, beginning with parents, siblings, and other family members, and proceeding to peers, early and later love attachments, employers, teachers, and other authorities. The patient is asked to describe each of these relationships, with special attention given to identifying (1) the wishes and wants that the patient sought in these relationships, (2) the actions of these other people when the patient tried to achieve these desires, and (3) the consequential acts of the patient him- or herself when the wishes were, or were not, realized.

Strupp and Binder (1984) offer a conceptual system that is similar to the CCRT method, with the addition of a separate step regarding patient expectation of the relationship. They propose that the persistence of maladaptive patterns can be assessed by determining patients' (1) wishes, fears, or desires in initiating a relationship; (2) what response they expected from the other person; (3) what behavior they initiated in order to achieve or avoid the expected response; and (4) consequences following this behavior, especially within the relationship in question.

Luborsky and Crits-Christoph (1990) have suggested that the clinician should not be guided by social structure while gathering information about interpersonal patterns. That is, it is not important only to evaluate a sibling, a lover, a work colleague, or whatever other figure exists in the social structure of the person's life. Rather, the clinician should also focus on the function these people play or have played in the patient's life:

To whom can the patient talk about emotional problems?
To whom can the patient turn for help with concrete problems, such as moving to a new dwelling or completing basic chores when illness strikes?
To whom does the person turn for physical affection?
How much of a need does the patient have in these areas?
What are the patient's expectations in each of these areas?
How much social contact does the person have in these areas?
How satisfied is the person with the social contact in each of these areas?

To the degree that similar needs, expectations, and levels of dissatisfaction are found across different relationships, periods of time, and types of relationships, the clinician can infer that the pattern observed is pervasive, chronic/complex, rigid, and ritualistic. That is, the patient's relationships are more dominated by his or her fixed needs than by the nature of the person to whom the patient is relating or the emergence of any particular crisis. Alternatively, if different needs and expectations are found to be expressed in different relationships, it may be inferred that the patient has the ability to be discriminating, flexible, and realistic in social interactions.

These thematic patterns have been found to be consistent across different relationships (Crits-Christoph et al., 1988; Shefler & Tishby, 1998). The degree of pervasiveness also can be used to indicate a focus for treatment interventions and to identify aspects of interpersonal functioning that can be changed to improve the person's ability to adapt and grow. From a review of the patient's report about these relationships, the clinician can begin to develop an understanding of the patient's patterns in relating to others. Do they tend to develop close attachments? Lasting friendships? Love relationships? Do they receive assistance and care from family members?

People who feel alienated from others frequently reveal this information spontaneously, as they discuss how relationships with key people in their lives have changed over time. Thus asking about early relationships with parents and siblings, and then asking about current and recent relationships with these people, can reveal important patterns that indicate alienation or closeness. Pressing the inquiries further to determine what the patient wishes for, wants, and expects in these family relationships can help the clinician evaluate how realistic the person's images of, and aspirations about, attachment might be.

Inferences about the chronicity and complexity of problems also can be based on the factual information reported about the prevalence and longevity of adolescent group behavior, legal difficulties, postadolescent love relationships, sexual experiences, and relationships to school and work authorities. Special attention is frequently given to key points in time, during which the patient went through social changes. The following questions may provide leads for further exploration:

"What happened to the best friends you had as a child and adolescent?"
"On whom can you rely for help and support in your life now?"
"What is the worst trouble you got into as a young person? . . . How is that trouble similar to the problems you have now?"
"What was your first sexual experience like?"
"What kind of homosexual experiences have you had?"
"What was the worst trouble you got into with teachers at school?"
"What kind of trouble have you had with the law?"
"How frequently have these problems recurred?"
"To whom have you turned for help or support?"

These questions often concern sensitive topics. Again, it is important to treat the responses in a matter-of-fact way and to phrase the questions in a way that assumes that every behavior is "normal" or expected.

Patient descriptions of sexual history are particularly important to establish the genesis of problems and general adaptability, although it is not often possible to cross-validate these descriptions. These reports should encompass the areas of sexual or physical abuse, patterns of sexual difficulty and dysfunction, marital disruptions, and both extramarital and premarital sexual problems. The patient's social and sexual evolution should be explored sufficiently to provide the clinician with an informed opinion of how disruptions to social relationships have been handled in current and past attachments.

Medical History

Obtaining a description of the patient's significant medical history is nearly as important as developmental background to estimating patient level of functional impairment and chronicity/complexity. As noted above, a third or more of the populations of the developed nations have some form of chronic illness due to aging and our success at treating life-threatening illnesses. Many of these illnesses and/or their treatments can produce emotional or cognitive problems. Thus exploration of their course may reveal information about the chronicity/complexity of the current problem(s).

In obtaining medical information, factual rather than subjective information is at a premium, and cross-validation of the patient's reports should be actively sought. Available sources of information about objective data (e.g., medications, medical complaints, doctors' visits, surgeries, hospitalizations, etc.) should be reviewed to determine the nature of past and current medical problems, associated treatments, and lists of treatments (including prescription and nonprescription drugs) that have been, and are currently being, taken. Because increasing numbers of Americans are using complementary and alternative treatments, the clinician also should ask about the use of nonprescription or herbal remedies as well as nontraditional treatments (e.g., acupuncture, homeopathy). This section also should include a description of any illicit drug and alcohol use, along with perceived benefits, drawbacks, and side effects. Questions that open up these areas in the interview may include the following:

"For what conditions/reasons have you been hospitalized in your life?"
"For what illnesses have you consulted a doctor?"
"What health problems do you currently have?"
"Have you talked about these problems/symptoms with your doctor?"
"What medication are you taking currently? . . . How long have you taken this medication?"
"What nonprescription medications, herbs, or naturalistic remedies are you taking?"
"What nontraditional methods have you used or are you using?"
"What street drugs do you use or have you used?"
"What alcoholic beverages do you prefer?"
"Has anyone ever said that alcohol was a problem for you?"
"How often have you gotten into trouble because of your use of drugs or alcohol?"

When information is elicited about prior medical problems and symptoms, as well as their treatment, some pointed inquiry is often helpful in order to determine the degree to which emotional problems might have been implicated in the problem for which the patient was being treated. Questions about symptoms, nature of treatments, the treatment site, and the specialty of the caregiver are areas for exploration. Particular attention should be given to previous experiences in psychotherapy. These experiences may help the clinician anticipate methods of working with the patient that might be helpful, or problems to be avoided in the conducting of psychotherapy.

Eliciting the types of medications and their dosages will also often unobtrusively reveal the treating physician's possible concern about the role of emotional factors in prior conditions and complaints. Disclosure of having used medication for "nerves," "tension," "stress," or "depression," for example, is suggestive of prior emotional disturbances that may not have been recognized, as such, by the patient. The clinician cannot assume that the patient either knows or is willing to disclose the purpose of various medications, however. Furthermore, patients often keep old medications around for later use. It is helpful to ask what medications (both prescriptive and nonprescriptive) the patient keeps at home, and even to request that he or she bring in the medication bottles for inspection.

Not only is a knowledge of medication usage helpful for determining the chronicity of problems and the degree to which treatment has been focused on emotional difficulties or symptoms; it is imperative that the clinician explore possible misuse of prescriptive medications and their potentially iatrogenic effects before reporting information to the referrer that may result in additional prescriptions being offered.

Mental Status, Coping Patterns, and Response Dispositions

To this point, we have addressed the role of the interview in identifying the nature of the patient's problems, levels of functional impairment, social support systems, and chronicity/complexity of the problem. We have specifically pointed to some of the unique types of data that can be obtained from interviewing the patient and collateral contacts (i.e., significant others). The interview, for example, has no equal in establishing baseline data by which to assess change, chronicity, and impairment levels. Other aspects of functioning that are important to systematic treatment selection are gleaned from a comparison of these historical descriptions to current estimates of personality and mental functioning. These comparisons (1) further establish and affirm level of patient impairment and problem chronicity, (2) allow us to assess more specifically the complexity of the presenting problem(s), (3) facilitate an assessment of the patient's coping style as well as (4) likely level of resistance to the assigned treatment, and (5) level of motivational distress. These treatment planning variables can be obtained through formal self-report instruments, but they can also be reliably assessed through the clinical interview.

Mental Status. Mental status evaluation usually addresses current behaviors within the domains of appearance, cognitive functioning, affect, mood, and personality style and integration. The STS qualities of coping style and resistance level are important components of assessing personality style and integration. Mental status evaluation is best used to establish the level of functional impairment and determine the complexity of the patient's condition. It provides estimates, which can be cross-validated with other procedures, of the patient's distress (mood and affect), coping style, and resistance level. Complexity, a correlate of chronicity (Beutler, Clarkin, & Bongar, 2000) and a reflection of multiple or recurrent problems, is indicated by disturbance in several aspects of mental functioning. This disturbance level can be identified by using the mental status examination.

The assessment of mental status is best performed using a structured interview. In this chapter, we have mentioned a few such interview procedures that can be used; however, this list is not exhaustive, by any means. The astute clinician will not rely solely on the quantitative data but will give careful attention to the patient's behavior throughout the interview. To assist in the distillation of the several sources of information derived from the interview, the clinician should note observations within the following areas of functioning.

Appearance. Appearance provides one estimate of current level of functioning. The clinician should make note of how appropriately the patient is dressed and how well he or she is groomed, as well as any evidence of inadequate self-help skills. Deficiencies in appearance may indicate deterioration of coping ability, inadequate or inefficient cognitive resources when planning and anticipating the consequences of behavior, inadequate fiscal resources, the absence of caring social support systems, or lack of social judgment. Declines in appearance may indicate increasing depression, schizophreniform intrusions, or emerging manic behaviors.

Cognitive Functioning. Cognitive functioning performance provides another estimate of functional impairment, especially when it is compared to records of school performance and historical indices of chronicity of deficits in intellectual development. Intellectual level, memory, perception, verbal fluency, and visual–motor organization are most reliably evaluated by standardized assessment procedures, some of which have been listed above. However, this information can be augmented by clinical interview, which establishes a historical baseline by which to estimate the chronicity of the problem.

The degree of verbal fluency and coherence observed during the interview is a supplemental avenue into assessing the nature of some cognitive processes. For example, the clinician should note the degree to which verbal output is impeded (sluggish) or exaggerated (pressured) as a potential diagnostic indicator of level of cognitive efficiency, mood, and problem severity. The abilities to retain a topical focus and associate logically when moving from topic to topic are especially important to note as diagnostic indicators. Thought intrusions are indicated by spontaneous and usually momentary changes of verbal content, especially if these interruptions contain unusual or unconventional ideas. Thought content impairments and lowered cognitive efficiency are reflected in this pattern.

Circumstantial logic and tangential associations are other indicators of a current thought process disturbance. In the former case, details and extraneous topics provide momentary distractions from topical focus, but the patient retains a general and contextually logical framework. Frequently, the patient reports information in excruciating detail and develops expanded but loosely related side stories while attempting to make and emphasize a point. In contrast, tangential associations are revealed in the inability to stay on the same topic and within a single framework of logic. Often, however, the distinction between circumstantial and tangential associations lies only in how conventional the association is between the main and the adjunctive topics. Tangential logic is characterized by very loosely associated topics and unusual patterns of logic. The patient is unable to complete a story in even fractured detail because of the apparent competition of other, unrelated, and frequently unusual or morbid story lines.

Thought content disturbances are noted whenever the patient inserts topics at inappropriate times and in inappropriate amounts. A tendency to insert contents and words associated with sexuality, aggression, potential victimization, or religious activities and figures into discourse are the most usual and indicative patterns. Fixed beliefs, delusions, and obsessions may be revealed in these preoccupations. In their extreme, the presence of unusual thought content is apparent; however, in less extreme forms, the nature of thought content disturbances may be difficult to delineate without special sensitivity to their subtle indicators. There is no substitute for prior experience with people who present serious cognitive disturbances, or for the comparisons possible through the use of standard and criteria-related norms.

Affect and Mood. The patient's affect and mood offer clues from which the clinician can estimate quality and level of distress as well as level of impairment in social functioning. *Mood* refers to the type and severity of subjective feelings of distress, whereas *affect* refers to the degree of integration and consistency in the expression of various feelings in social discourse. Under ideal circumstances, a person's recall of emotionally trying events is a balanced mixture of appropriateness, empathic resonance, and congruence between affect and mood. That is, the feeling the person recalls having is one that would be expected to characterize most people's response in similar circumstances: He or she is sad at loss, happy when desired events occur, and angry when frustrated in his or her goals. Likewise, when the person recalls the emotional event, some of the same feelings are reactivated in the present moment. This process of "empathic resonance" may be reflected in the recall of the person's own experience or activated by another person's experience. Finally, there is general congruence between the feeling that is experienced or reported and the one conveyed through facial, verbal, and postural expressions.

There are three types of incongruence between mood and affect. First, the failure to show emotion when discussing a topic that would usually evoke sadness, anger, or pleasure may suggest that the range of emotions is constricted and that excessive control is being exerted to keep emotions in check. Second, exaggerated displays of the emotions being discussed suggest the inability to step back from experience in order to gain objectivity. Third, a display of emotions that is at variance with those that normally would be evoked by the topic may indicate either an ineffective effort to reject and distance the self from the emotional experience or a lack of capacity for empathic resonance.

As a final distillation of these observations, the clinician estimates the strength of distressed feelings by noting the degree to which the patient is able to keep feelings and emotions in check without restricting or overcontrolling affect. From observations of the variations in the range of available affect and associated nonverbal behavior, the clinician attempts to determine whether the patient can identify and reexperience the feelings that were present at a previous time without becoming impaired by their recurrence.

Coping Patterns and Response Dispositions. The clinical interview permits an assessment of patient coping styles and response dispositions. Reported and observed information from the interview, as well as from formal assessment, can reveal a pattern of behaviors that identifies the nature of the patient's interpersonal and intrapersonal conflicts and his or her coping style. For example, during the interview, those patients who rely on internalizing coping strategies will often make self-deprecating comments, whereas those who rely on externalizing behaviors to reduce stress are more likely to become angry, blame the test, or resist the test administrator.

Coping styles are loosely grouped into two categories: internalizing and externalizing. Patients who tend to locate the cause of their problems, even more than the resolution of these problems, within themselves are generally "internalizers." Patients who habitually internalize their problems often experience or report higher levels of distress, but they may also have a greater capacity for insight. To elicit coping styles, the therapist should inquire about how the patient conceptualizes the problems he or she encounters and to whom/what he or she attributes responsibility for their cause. This determination entails explorations of how the patient explains the problem to others and how others have accepted or altered this interpretation. Patients who tend to locate problems outside themselves may report lower levels of distress, with the exception of frustration or anger. For these patients insight may be a more difficult goal to achieve.

In making judgments of the relative dominance of internalizing or externalizing behaviors, the clinician relies on historical descriptions and direct observations of the patient's response to the interview itself. As always, discrepancies among these sources of information are interpreted in terms of (1) the relative reliabilities and validities of the assessment procedures, and (2) the nature of the demand characteristics represented. The reader is reminded and cautioned that the clinician's confidence in interview-based observations is almost always excessive. While dispositional coping styles may affect the likelihood that an individual will use one coping strategy or another, the clinician should bear in mind that coping behaviors are highly situation-specific. In other words, under some circumstances an unabashed externalizer will likely accept responsibility or blame him- or herself for a given difficulty.

The clinician should also determine how the individual acts around others when unexpected problems arise. Obtaining descriptions of behaviors and actions in response to particular events, both routine and troubling, is helpful. Questions about how the patient gets along with neighbors, friends, parental figures, legal officials, and authorities tend to reveal information about coping styles. Those who enjoy social gatherings, loud and active parties and other recreational activities, and stimulating events (i.e., parties, racing, dangerous activities, etc.) tend to rely on externalizing styles of behavior. Those who enjoy solitary activities (e.g., reading, hiking alone, listening to music, working at the computer, etc.), seek solace by reducing stimulation (e.g., withdrawal), and participate in relaxing events (e.g., watching TV, napping, etc.) tend to rely on internalizing patterns.

When assessing coping styles, special but not exclusive attention should be given to unexpected or crisis situations. These situations tend to exaggerate—but may also misrepresent—general coping style, especially among people whose coping style reflects strong or nearly equivalent dispositions toward both active and passive coping activities.

Resistance Potential. Resistance potential is indicated by patients' receptivity to directives, suggestions, and loss of control. It is also reflected in how patients attribute responsibility for the resolution of problems (as opposed to their cause). If patients perceive the therapist as an important source of help, they may be more prone to cooperate than if they believe that they should be able to correct problems on their own.

Careful evaluation of previous treatment experiences may also help the clinician predict treatment-specific resistance to interventions. If previous treatment has included group, individual, or family psychotherapy, the clinician should attempt to discover who the therapist was, what was discussed and not discussed, the patient's overall response, and a description of those interventions that were both helpful and not helpful in the process. In this way, the clinician can begin to narrow down potential treatment recommendations and formulate suggestions for treatment that will capitalize on the patient's prior responses. If time permits, the clinician should request a release-of-information form and subsequently seek to obtain treatment summaries from prior treatment sources to supplement the patient's reports.

Finally, in assessing patient receptivity the clinician observes the patient's pattern of response to the clinician him- or herself. Under the best of circumstances, the requirement of revealing oneself to a stranger is difficult. It is made even more difficult by the frequent fear that the clinician has special powers and can see things that even the patient does not know are there. Hence the interview is an ideal opportunity to observe interpersonal patterns of defense and expression; these observations further supplements the more indirect but standardized assessments of personality.

In order to capitalize on the opportunity available, the interviewer notes the efforts the patient makes to establish a relationship with the clinician. These include efforts to solicit reassurance about accuracy, normality, or acceptability, as well as any verbal and behavioral rejections of the assessment procedures. These observations are noted as representing the patient's effort to balance needs for acceptance with needs for autonomy. Special tendencies either to comply with, or to reject and abandon the effort, are noted. These directly observed patterns are considered along with the factual data and descriptions reported by the patient and others, in order to derive hypotheses about coping style, patterns or levels of resistance, social judgment, and level of distress.

Strengths and Special Behaviors or Needs. Other observations made directly by the clinician include the adaptive capacities of the patient, the presence of particular skills, and past accomplishments. Strengths are not restricted to attributes of the patient him- or herself. Strengths also reside in the presence of family members, reference organization, past achievement, and future hopes. These are the resources that provide positive motivation for making changes and overcoming problems. These positive attributes serve as points at which growth may be encouraged and comprise the person's capacity to defend the self against stressors.

The clinician should also note other special behaviors or needs of the patient that will have a bearing on the need for special treatment settings, extra consultations, and other unusual arrangements for treatment. These special behaviors or needs include physical limitations and challenges, language differences, unavailability of support systems, and current medical or educational needs. Depending on the patient, treatment settings may need to include wheelchair accessibility; a reference or support group of a given ethnic background or age range; staff members who can speak and understand the patient's primary language; or materials for teaching learning-disabled, deaf, or blind patients.

Integrating Information from the Semistructured Interview

The integrated, semistructured interview provides a vast amount of information that may be used for a variety of purposes, including responding to referral questions and providing justification for treatment to third-party payers. These purposes often provide an intrinsic organizational framework that facilitates integration of the information. However, the most common use for such an interview—intake into psychotherapy—does not necessarily provide a method of organizing information in a manner that informs treatment decision making. Although clinicians commonly learn or develop some methods of distilling information, few, if any, of these methods have any empirically supported relationship to treatment planning and determining the differential prognoses of various treatment strategies.

The STS computer-assisted system provides an empirically supported framework for integrating information from several sources in the service of selecting psychotherapeutic interventions or methods that are most likely to succeed. These conclusions are based on patient characteristics as assessed by the research-informed model of Systematic Treatment Selection (Beutler & Clarkin, 1990; Beutler et al., 2000). As noted, the treatment planning dimensions used in the STS model include level of impairment, level of social support, chronicity and complexity of the problem, level of subjective distress, coping style (externalization vs. internalization), and resistance potential. Although this system cannot replace the diagnostic interview or other methods of gleaning clinical data, it can be used to help organize findings around treatment recommendations.

The computer-based administration of the STS Clinician Rating Form (STS-CRF) also can be used to prompt the clinician to explore different areas of functioning and problem profile during the interview, thereby helping to ensure that the relevant topics are covered in a way that facilitates patient understanding and treatment development. Chapter 3 includes examples of questions from the STS-CRF. Following the STS-CRF procedure assures that adequate attention is given to (1) patient demographics (Section IA), (2) major symptoms (Section IB), (3) areas of family and social functioning (Section IC and II), and (4) several problem and patient attributes that help define the nature of optimal psychotherapeutic interventions (Sections III, IV, V).

The STS-CRF includes 29 items that evaluate subjective distress, 21 items for externalization, 12 items for internalization, and 24 items for resistance potential. Embedded in these items are measures of specific symptoms, severity, chronicity, and social support. Initial trials have shown this rating form to be reliable and moderately correlated with patient self-report measures assessing similar constructs (Fisher et al., 1999a). We can illustrate the use of the STS-CRF as an assessment system by the example of R.W., whose background information was presented in Chapter 3.

CASE EXAMPLE

We know certain facts about R.W. from the presentation given in Appendix A, most of which were obtained through the interview. For example, we know that R.W. is a female, 22 years old, was referred by Dr. Renny, and identifies herself as Mexican American. We also know that she was referred because Dr. Renny wanted help establishing the diagnosis. We can assume that the clinician attempted to clarify the referral question by asking Dr. Renny which diagnostic alternatives were being considered, which ones had been rejected, and why. The patient has reported to Dr. Renny that she has a history of panic attacks and social anxiety. These symptoms led her to seek therapy about a year ago. We know that, at that time, she was unable to go outside because of panic attacks. This, and the history that is contained in the referral itself, sounds like a fairly typical description of an individual with mixed anxiety symptoms, including agoraphobia with panic. But this easy-to-make diagnosis may be misleading, given that Dr. Renny has now referred the patient due to questions about diagnosis, and in view of the patient's report of a chaotic family history of physical abuse, sexual intimidation, and deprivation. This reported history has apparently led Dr. Renny to wonder if the anxiety symptoms are associated with a more complex and chronic problem of identify diffusion or dissociation.

Our interview with the client will ask her to describe the problems that are most salient at the present time. We will pay particular attention to the symptoms of anxiety and the history of trauma and crisis. If possible, we will seek external validation of some of these emotionally charged events. We will also obtain historical information about her symptoms, their previous and current treatment, and her family. We will attempt to place in a historical perspective her first and subsequent experiences with abuse, panic attacks, feelings of derealization, and internal voices. Her description of the relationship with her current male friend, which was initiated when she was still a minor, as well as the descriptions of sexual intimidation and emotional abuse by her stepfather, will immediately raise legal and ethical questions about the need to report and how to maintain confidentiality. These issues can be addressed adequately only in the clinical interview and require talking to the patient about the legal and ethical requirements as well as about the impact of these relationships on her feelings of power, self-regard, and ability to attach to others.

We will seek information about her reactions to the rejection she received from others when they discovered that she was dating a married man, including the reactions of her parents and friends. Her history suggests a relatively acute reaction to this latter social rejection, but this is, or may be, superimposed on a more chronic history of physical and emotional abuse and deprivation. The highly charged nature of the patient's response, however, may compromise the accuracy of her report and should not be trusted without some confirming evidence of traumatic events. It can be observed, however, that the patient's coping adequacy may be relatively low, exacerbated by a described pattern of withdrawal during these times. This pattern might lead us to suspect a dominantly internalizing coping style, but this conclusion must be tempered by what motives may have led her to develop this relationship in the first place as well as by the descriptions of associated periods of impulsivity and poor judgment.

All of this information would probably lead us to think of this problem as chronic/complex, highly distressing to the patient, and involving high levels of functional impairment. The history presented (Appendix A and Chapter 3) also will suggest to us that she has few social supports, a mixture of internalizing and externalizing coping patterns, and is likely to be quite resistant to treatment. The complexity of the problem remains more uncertain. It is clear that many symptoms are currently present (panic attacks, agoraphobia, dissociation, social phobia, highs and lows, etc.), but it is less clear as to whether these symptoms are a manifestation of the relatively recent problems associated with her illicit relationship, or whether there are many different and somewhat separate problems evolving from earlier abuse and neglect. The relationship among proximal (relationship) and distal (family rejection and abuse) events, dissociative symptoms, internal critical and accusing voices, social anxiety, and depression will only be untangled by a careful detailing of the chronology of each of these symptoms. This history will give us a clearer clue as to whether the problems are all reflective of a common anxiety or whether there are, as she presents, several problems that have evolved over time.

In the course of exploring the patient's medical, family, and social history, we will also inquire about her mood and the cycling of high and low feelings that she describes. We especially would like to know about her vegetative symptoms; to assess these reliably, we may supplement our observations by administering the Hamilton Rating Scale for Depression and possibly the Hamilton Rating Scale for Anxiety. Her descriptions of "emotional changeability," including "highs and lows," will lead us to look for manic symptoms that might suggest cyclothymic patterns. We need to know when each set of symptoms started, how often each occurs, and how quickly each dissipates. The descriptions presented in Appendix A, however, do not

strongly suggest a cyclothymic pattern, although they do suggest the perme-
ation of depression as a coexisting and probably secondary response to her
anxiety.

The mixture of internalizing patterns such as withdrawal and seclu-
sion, along with externalizing pattens (sexual promiscuity, drinking, etc.),
should be investigated through contacts with collateral associates. The immediate description suggests a dominant internalizing coping style with
some episodic externalizations and excessively high levels of distress, which
may account for the derealization and fragmentation that she reports. Although she identifies various "persona," we would be disinclined to interpret these as alternative personalities. The level of her awareness of them
and their emergence to crisis suggest that they are more likely to be metaphorical expressions of her conflicts and confusion. This confusion, along
with a history of parental abuse and deprivation, if confirmed, may lead us
to expect a high level of resistance to an authoritative treatment approach.

SUMMARY

This chapter has presented an integrated, semistructured approach to psychological evaluation that is designed to achieve a reasonable balance between interview flexibility and comprehensiveness by combining the unstructured and structured approaches. The strengths of the unstructured
procedure include its flexibility and its unique adaptability to the quest for
factual and historical information. However, it is not wise to use such an
interview as a stand-alone assessment device, for its weaknesses include uncertain reliability and validity and the tendency of clinicians to place more
confidence in its results than may be warranted. Structured approaches
have demonstrated reliability and validity, but they are inflexible, very formal, and sometimes require considerable time investment for training, administration, and maintenance of reliability.

The clinical interview often establishes the context and mind-set for
conducting the rest of the assessment. That is, a clinician can emphasize
and capitalize on the qualitative strengths of the interview by using it as an
entrée to the assessment process, and by structuring it in such a way as to
encourage cooperative and realistic expectations on the part of the patient.
Moreover, providing adequate pre-assessment information within a safe
and comfortable setting can enhance the patient's cooperation and disclosure in the interview as well as in the other structured assessment procedures.

The interview is especially useful for extracting factual information
from the patient. However, the clinician's qualitative observations—particularly in regard to discrepancies between (1) the factual content provided
by patients and that provided by others, (2) verbal content and nonverbal

indicators of affect, and (3) judged affect and mood—can be helpful sources of information when constructing hypotheses about functioning to supplement the information obtained in more structured and standardized ways. Moreover, direct observations of the methods used by the patient to establish and maintain the interviewer–interviewee relationship can form the basis for inferences about the nature of habitual coping strategies and self-presentation efforts. Although interview-derived observations are no more important and sometimes less valid than observations made through less direct psychological assessment devices, they add a valuable dimension to the overall effort to distill the meanings of current behaviors and to predict future ones.

An integrated, semistructured interview format combines the strengths of unstructured and structured approaches. This approach provides validity and reliability where it is required, while preserving flexibility and a format that is conducive the development of rapport.

5

Integrating Intelligence and Personality

Donald H. Saklofske, Elizabeth J. Austin,
Gerald Matthews, Moshe Zeidner,
Vicki L. Schwean, and Gary Groth-Marnat

A key focus in classical assessment is a patient's intellectual functioning. Assessing intelligence provides essential information about individuals in relation to the types of vocations they might enter, the extent to which they can understand and work with many types of psychotherapeutic information, and the level to which their emotional functioning might be interfering with their cognitive abilities. In this chapter, we focus on how intelligence and personality are interrelated and on how clinicians should interpret intellectual assessments in the context of an overall clinical evaluation and treatment plan. Personality cannot be fully understood without taking into account how it is related to, and affected by, intelligence. This point is underscored by Wechsler who stated that "general intelligence cannot be equated with intellectual ability, however broadly defined, but must be regarded as a manifestation of the personality as a whole" (quoted in Matarazzo, 1972, p. 79). Intelligence cannot be adequately assessed or even conceptualized as distinct from nonintellectual aspects of functioning, such as need for achievement, motivation, persistence, or curiosity. Despite this acknowledgment by psychologists over the previous decades, there has been little attempt to integrate the assessment and descriptions of intelligence and personality until relatively recently.

A number of typical clinical scenarios illustrate the importance of integrating personality and intelligence. For example, a referral source might feel it is quite important to know whether a client's level of anxiety is likely to disrupt intellectual functioning, such as attention and memory (high functional impairment). A vocational assessment might find that a job applicant has high intelligence, as measured by a standardized IQ test, but the applicant still may not be appropriate for a job if he or she has difficulty applying this intelligence toward solving interpersonal conflicts. Yet another person may have average intellectual ability, but further assessment may find that he or she is not open to a wide range of experiences and new situations. This lack of openness may constrict her intellectual ability to a fairly narrow range of areas. Clinicians are frequently in the position of providing feedback to clients (and referral sources) regarding the meaning of traditional intelligence test scores. It is often important to point out that many abilities that are frequently considered signs of "intelligence" are not represented by an IQ score, including practical intelligence (common sense), emotional intelligence, sense of humor, ability to resolve conflict, and level of self-awareness. A complete assessment of a client often involves evaluating some of these personality and conative characteristics in addition to determining his or her cognitive and intellectual ability(ies).

A fairly wide range of intelligence/personality perspectives has emerged (see Collis & Messick, 2001; Saklofske & Zeidner, 1995). In part, this range is due to calls for a "unified psychology" (Sternberg & Grigorenko, 2001); in addition, a greater realization that traditional conceptions of intelligence often do not provide sufficient information about how well someone will adapt and perform in educational, social, or vocational settings, has stimulated research and theory building. Personality is often perceived as the crucial link in answering these questions. The most important clinical contributions in an extensive literature that attempts to integrate research on intelligence and personality explore (1) correlations between major personality traits and intelligence, (2) the relation between intelligence and mental health, and (3) various conceptualizations of emotional intelligence.

CORRELATIONS BETWEEN INTELLIGENCE AND PERSONALITY TRAITS

Intelligence and Major Personality Traits

In earlier work, Eysenck (1971) contended that personality and intelligence were not correlated, although both the psychoticism and the lie scale of his personality measures tended to show small negative correlations with intelligence. In contrast, Robinson (1985, 1986) reported that introverts earned higher scores on the Wechsler verbal subtests compared to extroverts, who tended to score higher on tests tapping perceptual organization abilities. However, the magnitude of the correlations and mean score differences between groups (extroverts, amibiverts, and introverts), when found, tended to be small (Saklofske & Kostura, 1990).

The personality factors most often described in current clinical research reflect the five-factor model (Costa & McCrae, 1992; Digman, 1990; Goldberg, 1990) that includes neuroticism (N), extroversion (E), openness (O), agreeableness (A), and conscientiousness (C). These five factors that are clearly correlated with intelligence are summarized in Table 5.1. The correlations are typically of small-effect size, except for openness to experience, where the effect size is moderate. This larger correlation makes conceptual sense in that openness has been described as a variable on the boundary between personality and cognition (McCrae, 2000). However, the links between intelligence and openness are not straightforward, in the main, and include associations with (1) typical intellectual engagement, (2) the amount of intellectual effort that an individual applies to everyday life situations (Goff & Ackerman, 1992), and (3) intellectual curiosity and need for cognitive stimulation (McCrae, 2000; McCrae & Costa, 1997).

Correlations between intelligence and other measures in the personality domain, such as anger, locus of control, and hostility, have also been examined. These measures can be thought of as "downstream" from personality, in the sense that they are more directly related to specific behaviors than are broad traits such as extroversion and neuroticism. An idea that can be used to provide a framework for examining correlations between these traits and intelligence is that intelligence aids adjustment to the environment, including the facilitation of personal and social adjustment, as well as resiliency. A general prediction, based on this viewpoint, is that intelligence is positively correlated with traits that can be regarded in broad terms as socially and/or personally adaptive, and negatively correlated with those that can be regarded as maladaptive.

TABLE 5.1. Summary of Associations
between Intelligence and Major Personality Traits

Sign of correlation		Typical correlation magnitude
N	−	0.1
E	+	0.1
O	+	0.3
P	−	0.1

Note. N, neuroticism; E, extroversion; O, openness; P, psychoticism.

A recent study investigating this idea used four large data sets (originally gathered for other purposes) that included scores on intelligence tests and on a range of personality traits (Austin et al., 2002). For each of the datasets, a general ability factor (g) was extracted from the ability test scores, and correlations between g and traits of interest were examined. A number of the correlations were significant, showing that there are associations between these traits and g (see Table 5.2). These correlations were significant, even when neuroticism was partialed out (indicating that the correlations are independent of neuroticism). Effect sizes were similar to those for major personality traits (correlations around .1–.2). In the remainder of this section, the results shown in Table 5.2, together with findings from other studies, are used to provide a framework for the discussion of intelligence and adaptivity associations.

Traits Related to Negative Affectivity

It would stand to reason that persons with higher intelligence would be more able to adapt to, and solve, problems related to personal, interpersonal, and work relationships. This reality is reflected in several of the characteristics listed in Table 5.2, including the negative correlation between intelligence and negative affect or neuroticism (Watson & Pennebaker, 1989), anxiety (Zeidner, 1995), depression (Endler & Summerfeldt, 1995), and somatic symptom reporting (Vassend, Watten, Myhrer, & Syvertsen, 1994). Each of these characteristics is related to maladaptive personal adjustment.

In terms of proposing a mechanism that might link negative affect and intelligence level, it is possible that higher intelligence enhances the effectiveness of the cognitive appraisal of and response to stress, leading to a lesser tendency to depression and negative emotions. However, in the case of clinical depression, it is not clear whether cognitive deficits should be regarded as an antecedent or an outcome of the condition. If lower intelligence were an antecedent to depression, then the depressive schemata and cognitive distortions that usually precede depression would be somehow related to lower intelligence (Larsen, 1992: Saklofske, Kelly, & Janzen,

TABLE 5.2. Associations between General Ability and Traits Related to Personal and/or Social Adjustment

Positive associations with g	Negative associations with g
Anger control, type A, hard driving, internal locus of control	Depression, public self-awareness, social anxiety, hostility, (negative) emotionality, unassertiveness, somatic symptom reporting

Note. Data from Austin et al. (2002).

1995). In contrast, it may be that depressive symptoms themselves (e.g., slowed thinking, sleep disturbances, low energy level) actually lower cognitive functioning. Those tasks most sensitive to depression are those requiring effortful and controlled processing, in contrast to automatic processing (Zeidner, Matthews, & Saklofske, 1998). Thus the WAIS-III subtests of Matrix Reasoning, Digit Symbol-Coding, Block Design, and Similarities are more sensitive to depression. The above findings suggest that a potentially relevant assessment agenda is to determine the extent to which depression may be lowering cognitive functioning, as well as to determine the possible existence of cognitive schemata/distortions that may have existed prior to the onset of depressive symptoms and increased the risk of depression.

Anger, Aggression, Hostility, and Related Traits and Behaviors

The negative correlation with hostility and positive correlation with anger control and intelligence shown in Table 5.2 are consistent with literature showing negative associations between intelligence and aggression (Huesmann, Eron, & Yarmel, 1987). Conduct disorders in children and juvenile and adult criminality have been found to be associated with below-average intelligence (e.g., Goodman, 1995; Herrnstein & Murray, 1994; Moffit, Gabrielli, Mednick, & Schulsinger, 1981). A possible mechanism underlying these findings is that the cognitive processes that moderate the expression of anger and aggression might be facilitated by higher intelligence levels (Zeidner, 1995).

Matthews, Saklofske, Costa, Deary, and Zeidner (1998) have suggested some possible explanations for the inverse relation between IQ scores and aggression, anger, and delinquency. Although these findings are correlational, the clinician may wish to consider whether a client's aggression is related to lower ability to (1) manage stress and frustration, (2) inhibit or control impulses, or (3) delay gratification. As well, less intelligent persons may have greater difficulty acquiring insight into cause-and-effect relationships. Alternatively, anger and aggression may disrupt both intelligence and the learning of intellectual skills, and this disruption may limit the acquisition and appropriate use of socially desirable traits.

Locus of Control and Type A

The positive correlation between intelligence and internal locus of control is consistent with the perception of having control over one's environment. This sense of control may help to provide a sense of well-being, resilience, and enhanced adaptive functioning (DeNeve & Cooper, 1998; Diener, 1984). High locus-of-control individuals display an above-average ability to deal with extremely negative life events and circumstances, such as childhood maltreatment (Heller, Larrieu, D'Imperio, & Boris, 1999). Resilience is also associated with higher measured intelligence (Fergusson & Lynskey, 1996).

The mechanism explaining the relation between intelligence and locus of control, self-agency, self-efficacy, perceived control, and causal attributions has yet to be determined. One possibility is that self-efficacious individuals view intelligence as more of a skill that is developed by active efforts to gain knowledge and competencies. In turn, personal goal setting may be influenced by self-appraisal of abilities, including intelligence. For persons with high self-efficacy, errors are interpreted (and expected) as part of the process of mastery rather than being seen as sources of distress or threat. In contrast, persons with low self-efficacy will interpret tasks (e.g., tests) as threats and contend that they lack the resources to successfully manage task demands (i.e., "I am so stupid in math"). This negative self-talk may not only increase anxiety level (test anxiety) but further reduce the person's sense of control related to changing or controlling the situation. The positive correlation between ability and type A trait (in Table 5.2) is somewhat harder to interpret theoretically, but it fits with the finding that high type A scores are associated with enhanced subjective quality of life and a heightened sense of instrumentality (Bryant & Yarnold, 1990).

POSSIBLE MECHANISMS FOR INTELLIGENCE–PERSONALITY CORRELATIONS

Unfortunately, much of the research on intelligence and personality has not demonstrated directional or causal relationships between the two variables. In the previous sections, possible mechanisms by which intelligence and adaptive personality traits are linked were briefly discussed. Regression analysis and structural equation modeling can be used to further explore intelligence–personality relationships. For example Figure 5.1 shows three possible relationships between general ability, neuroticism, and anger control. In the first model, general ability and neuroticism act as independent predictors. In the other two models, either g or N take mediating roles. Comparing models of this type for goodness of fit indicates that a model in which neuroticism mediates the effect of g on anger control is the best fit (Austin et al., 2002). This model also indicates a contribution from agreeableness (A) (see Figure 5.2).

Cross-sectional data cannot provide information on the underlying causes of intelligence–personality associations. In order to obtain information of this type, intelligence and personality development from childhood to adulthood must be studied. Data are sparse; however, Huesmann and colleagues (1987) reported aggression and intelligence scores for a group of participants at age 8, and later at age 30. Early IQ did not predict changes

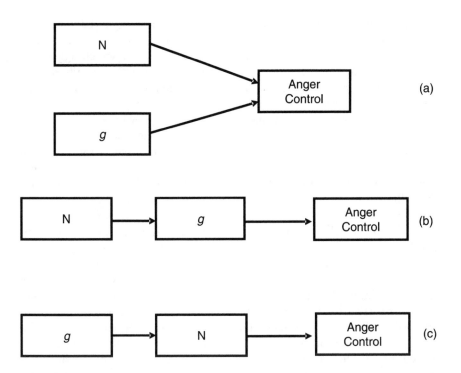

FIGURE 5.1. Possible models for the relationship between general ability (g), neuroticism (N), and anger control: (a) regression model with independent contributions from g and N; (b) g as a mediator; (c) N as a mediator.

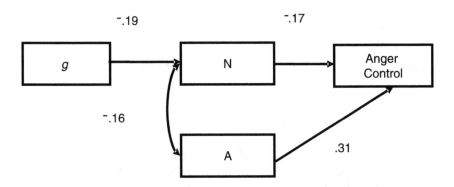

FIGURE 5.2. Best-fitting model for anger control. N, neuroticism; g = general ability; A, agreeableness.

in aggression after age 8, but differences between early IQ and adult intelligence were predictable from early aggression scores. These findings suggest a mechanism (at least, in children age 8 and above) by which aggression impedes learning opportunities (e.g., aggressive children's typically disruptive classroom behavior). The study data provide no information on development of the aggression–intelligence association in younger children. However, the authors suggest that children with higher intelligence may be able to learn nonaggressive problem-solving strategies more easily.

An evolutionary framework for understanding associations between intelligence and traits related to social adjustment could be helpful. For example, the underlying idea of the comparative psychology concept of "Machiavellian" or "social" intelligence is that the evolution of primate and human intelligence was driven, at least in part, by the complexity of the social environment as well as by problems presented by the physical environment (see Byrne & Whiten, 1997). If this thesis were correct, some linkage between intelligence levels and socially adaptive personality traits might be expected. As a case in point, it may be simplistic to characterize aggressive coping as simply a cognitive deficit. However, Bjorkqvist and Oesterman (2000) reported that high social intelligence is positively correlated with all types of conflict behavior, including aggression, thereby implicating social intelligence as a factor that promotes participation in conflict. They also reported that the correlation between social intelligence and the use of different strategies increased with the safety of the behavior (i.e., .22 for physical aggression, .55 for indirect aggression, .80 for peaceful conflict resolution). Empathy, which in general acts to mitigate aggressive impulses, was strongly correlated with intelligence; however, empathy and aggression differed in their relationship with intelligence. Controlling for social intelligence, empathy was negatively correlated with all forms of aggression but positively related to conflict resolution. This finding led to the formulation: "Social intelligence – empathy = aggression." It would appear that the socially intelligent but nonempathic person may use aggression as a coping mechanism—but intelligently, using violence sparingly.

Ability Level and Response to Test Items

An important consideration is that respondents with varying ability levels interact with items on personality measures in different ways. For example, more intelligent persons may understand the items better because of their higher vocabulary and education. As a result, they respond more consistently, resulting in higher reliabilities. Differential responding to test items also may result in differences in the factor structure of the scales or the degree to which the scales accurately measures personality across various intelligence levels.

An outline of possible causal mechanisms is provided in Table 5.3. The first proposed effect in Table 5.3 hypothesizes that high-ability respondents find the scale more meaningful for describing themselves; therefore, the personality scale is *more* reliable for more intelligent individuals. Again, persons with greater intelligence also might understand the items better, resulting in more consistent (reliable) responses (Goldberg & Kilkowski, 1985; McFarland & Sparks, 1985). The second proposed effect hypothesizes that less able respondents perceive a scale as being a measure of a single trait (unidimensional). In contrast, the more able make more subtle distinctions between items and perceive the same scale as having two or more dimensions (e.g., the more able might be more inclined to perceive distinctions between the diligence and orderliness items of a conscientiousness scale). The consequence would be an opposite outcome to the first possibility: lower-ability individuals would respond more consistently than their higher-ability counterparts. This outcome would lead to *lower* scale reliability among persons with higher ability. Alternative explanations for both findings are also shown in Table 5.3.

TABLE 5.3. Proposals on the Variation of Personality Structure with Ability

Effect of ability level on personality factors	Expected empirical findings	Alternative interpretations
Scales are a better match to self-description for the more able and are perceived more coherently by them.	Higher proportion of extreme scores in high-ability groups; larger score standard deviation and increased scale reliability.	Item content more meaningful to the more able; items understood better; more able to perceive underlying construct and respond more consistently; ability-related differences in self-presentation strategy or its success.
Scales perceived as unidimensional by the less able, multidimensional by the more able.	An extreme form of this effect would lead to more factors being extracted in high-ability groups. A more likely outcome is that the number of factors is unchanged but scale standard deviations and reliabilities decrease with increasing ability. Correlations between factors larger in low-ability groups.	Ability-related differences in self-presentational strategy or its success.

Evidence for either of the effects described above is sparse, in part, because very few studies have measured both intelligence and personality in groups covering a sufficiently wide ability range. However, a number of studies has found a rise in personality scale reliability with ability level for such constructs as neuroticism and openness to experience (Austin, Deary, & Gibson, 1997; Brand, Egan, & Deary, 1994; Myers & McCaulley, 1985; Shure & Rogers, 1963). In contrast, Austin, Hofer, Deary, and Eber (2000) report evidence from the Cattell psychopathology scales that intelligent respondents made more subtle distinctions among items related to distress. These more subtle distinctions actually resulted in lower scale reliabilities. They also noted that higher-ability persons made clearer distinctions between the psychoticism and neuroticism scales. This outcome resulted in more valid assessments of these constructs for the higher-ability, as opposed to the lower-ability, group.

Socially Desirable Responding

It is possible that the intelligence–adaptivity associations discussed above could arise from socially desirable responding; that is, people who seek social desirability may exert more effort to produce adaptive behaviors. For example, a person attempting to create an unrealistically good impression might fake answers in the direction of low hostility, low depression, high anger control, and so on. There is certainly evidence that personality scores can be faked under instruction (e.g., "Answer these questions the way a depressed, worried, or easygoing-sociable person might") and in job application contexts (see Paulhus, Bruce, & Trapnell, 1995; Scandell & Wlazelek, 1996; Topping & O'Gorman, 1997), and it seems likely that more intelligent respondents would be better at doing so, which might induce, or at least make a contribution to, the intelligence–personality correlations discussed above. The relationship between overt faking and scale reliability is harder to predict (Austin et al., 2000).

That socially desirable responding does *not* account for personality–intelligence correlations is suggested by evidence that social desirability and lie scale scores are negatively correlated with intelligence (Austin et al., 2002; Egan, 1989; Ones, Viswesvaran, & Reiss, 1996; Saklofske & Kostura, 1990). These findings suggest that more intelligent people actually have less tendency to fake their responses to personality items. In instances of malingering, of course, it is possible that an effort could be made to produce lower-ability scores. It is not really possible to fake "higher" scores on an intelligence test, but lower scores could certainly be created. Thus a client who may gain financially from demonstrating lower-intelligence test scores that presumably have resulted from a head injury sustained in a traffic accident could deliberately fail on particular items assessing memory, visual spatial reasoning ability, and so on. Thus the relationship between personality and intelligence for individuals prone to malingering could be a contrived one that serves a particular purpose. Fortunately, psychologists have various test taking and other observations available to them to assist in detecting malingering.

Implications and Conclusions

This brief review of research highlights a number of modest but consistent relations between intelligence and personality. Higher ability is associated with persons who are more open to experience, can more effectively control their anger, and have a high internal locus of control. They are also more likely to be hard driving and have more type A characteristics. In contrast, lower ability is associated with persons who are more depressed, unassertive, socially anxious, hostile, experience more negative emotions, and are more likely to express somatic complaints. Understanding why these relationships occur is more difficult. One possibility that has some support is that the traits of neuroticism and agreeableness mediate the link between intelligence and the extent to which a person will express his or her anger. Thus it is the combination of intelligence, neuroticism, and agreeableness that determines whether or not a person will express his or her anger. Self-efficacy and higher locus of control might be the products of more instances in which more intelligent persons successfully solved a problem situation.

Similarly, a person's level of empathy interacts with intelligence to determine whether or not an intelligent person will express aggression (i.e., a person with high intelligence but low empathy would be more likely to act aggressively). Finally, links between intelligence and personality may, in part, be an artifact resulting from more consistent and meaningful responses to personality scale items by more intelligent persons. In order to better understand these causal relationships, future research should employ more longitudinal methods and extend beyond self-report measures by using such strategies as simulations.

MENTAL HEALTH AND INTELLIGENCE

A logical question that follows from the above discussion is whether there is a relationship between intelligence and various psychological disorders. For example, an examiner might find evidence of cognitive slowing associated with depression (e.g., Endler & Summerfeldt, 1995) or lower scores on processing speed among children with attention-deficit/hyperactivity disorder (ADHD) (e.g., Schwean & Saklofske, 1998). It is often essential to determine the extent to which such cognitive functions are affected by the disorder. The above examples illustrate how certain disorders may actually cause cognitive disturbances. However, more recent research has also investigated the extent to which various levels and patterns of abilities precede, and can even serve as risk factors for, some types of disorders.

At a theoretical level, there are several rationales for expecting that low intelligence might act as a risk factor for subsequent disorders. Biological models of intellectual function suggest that high intelligence may be associated with brain qualities that confer resistance to disease. The most straightforward example derives from research on brain injury associated with dementia conditions such as Alzheimer's disease. Satz (1993) proposes that ability tests index a "brain reserve capacity" that controls the threshold at which neural damage becomes sufficient to cause functional impairment. From the different perspective of cognitive, self-regulative models of disorder, reciprocal relations between intelligence and mental health are expected (Zeidner & Matthews, 2000; Zeidner et al., 1998). Lack of self-knowledge and insight may contribute to "disorders of self-regulation," as described by cognitive "schema" models of depression and anxiety. Conversely, more effective routines for self-regulation, such as functional coping skills, may foster the development of "emotional intelligence."

Several issues need to be addressed to achieve a satisfactory synthesis of research findings that has viable implications for clinical practice. The first is the reliability of the empirical findings. In the case of schizophrenia, for example, controversy continues regarding the question of whether or not all the intellectual decline seen in patients reflects premorbid impairment (David, 1998; Gold, 1998; Russell, Munro, Jones, Helmsley, & Murray, 1997). In the case of adolescent delinquency, an inverse relationship with IQ is well-established, but arguments for intelligence as a risk factor (Lynam, Moffitt, & Stouthamer-Loeber, 1993) have been challenged on both conceptual and analytical grounds (Block, 1995). There are uncertainties too over whether deficits should be attributed to loss of general intelligence or to more specific abilities.

A second issue is the status of intelligence as a causal factor. As Satz (1993) points out, some of the literature supporting the cerebral reserve hypothesis shows effects of education level as a protective factor, and discriminating effects of intelligence from confounding variables such as education and socioeconomic status (SES) is a generally acknowledged difficulty. A third source of difficulty is the diverse theoretical basis of the mental health field, within which biological, cognitive, and psychodynamic approaches coexist, sometimes synergistically, at other times, in opposition.

Certainly, then, there is evidence that intelligence is an important and practically significant predictor of various mental disorders, including depression, suicide, schizophrenia, personality disorders, and dementias related to age and HIV infection (Zeidner et al., 1998). However, these relationships may reflect a variety of competing models that should be considered by practitioners engaged in diagnosis and prognosis as well as in decision making regarding primary, secondary, and tertiary prevention programs.

Explanations of Intelligence as a Risk Factor for Psychological Disorders

In modeling associations between intelligence and psychological disorders, it is important to distinguish between latent and manifest attributes of both constructs. First, it is essential to distinguish between a person's score on some test of general intelligence, which can be loosely termed "IQ," and the hypothetical underlying g construct, identified as a latent trait within a structural covariance model. The g factor represents an intellectual competence, whereas the test score assesses performance on a specific occasion and may be sensitive to situational influences such as attention and motivation (especially in clinical patients). Psychological disorders may influence both competence and the additional factors contributing to performance. In treating g as a possible causal entity, we are conceptualizing it as an index of a molar package of neural functions (e.g., brain size and neural interconnectiveness) and/or cognitive functions (e.g., working memory, executive processing). These functions can act causally on other aspects of brain and mental function. Second, illness assessed at the symptom level (e.g., via a DSM-IV diagnosis) must be distinguished from the underlying pathology of neural or cognitive function. For example, the cerebral reserve hypothesis (Satz, 1993) implies that neural pathology is not necessarily expressed in functional impairment (i.e., in high-reserve individuals). Conversely, lack of insight or use of counterproductive coping strategies may accentuate the functional consequences of maladaptive cognitions (Wells & Matthews, 1994).

A number of causal factors may explain the relation between intelligence and the later development of psychopathology. For example, intelligence may be predictive of future mental health because it directly indexes health-promoting processes or because it buffers against disease processes. Intelligence also may function as an indirect indicator, in that premorbid test scores may be reduced because of attentional impairments, for example, that are causally linked to future pathology. In addition, associations between intelligence and future health may be essentially artifactual if, for example, both are a product of education or SES. Such processes might be based in a person's biology, psychology, or the interaction between the two. With these distinctions in mind, four causal models linking measured intelligence ("IQ") to pathology have been proposed.

1. *The etiological model—g as a direct causal factor.* One possibility is that neural or cognitive processes associated with intelligence directly cause subsequent health or illness (see Figure 5.3a). An example is provided by

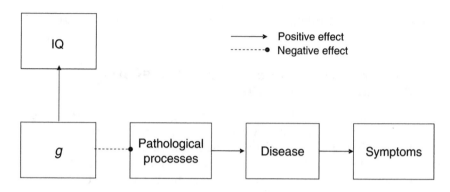

FIGURE 5.3a. Intelligence as a direct causal factor in mental illness.

the hypothesis that positive symptoms of schizophrenia (e.g., hallucinations and delusions) are a consequence of deficient inhibitory processes in selective attention, which leads to the inability to distinguish relevant from irrelevant information (Beech & Williams, 1997). If intelligence influences the efficiency of inhibitory processes (Dempster & Corkill, 1999), then it functions as a direct etiological factor in schizophrenia. In this picture, one source of vulnerability to the illness is the ineffective screening of irrelevant stimuli and thoughts conferred by low intelligence. To establish the model empirically, it is necessary to show that intelligence influences a neural or cognitive process that, in turn, influences subsequent pathology.

2. *The compensatory model.* An alternative possibility is shown in Figure 5.3b. Rather than affecting underlying pathology, intelligence affects the extent to which that pathology disrupts adaptive functioning and generates symptoms. For example, a patient with insight into his or her condition may be better able to cope with the illness. To establish this mechanism, it is necessary to demonstrate that intelligence is correlated with the putative buffer (e.g., degree of insight) and that the buffer acts as a predictor of severity of symptoms, when severity of pathology is controlled.

3. *The performance deficit model.* A third possibility, depicted in Figure 5.3c, is that intelligence test performance is sensitive to factors linked to developing pathology that are not themselves part of intellectual competence. For example, conditions such as depression and chronic fatigue syndrome are associated with deficits in motivation and energy. Individuals predisposed to depression may show cognitive and motivational deficits prior to the development of clinical pathology. These deficits may signal emerging problems in maintaining attention and task-directed effort that have an impact on IQ test performance but are unrelated to underlying intellectual competence. Distinguishing this mechanism from the etiological one requires investigation of the deficit's contextual sensitivity in a pre-

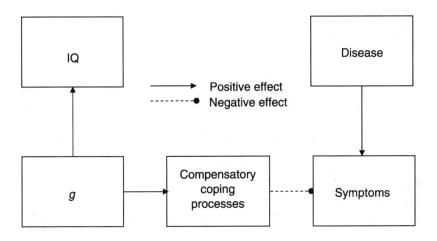

FIGURE 5.3b. Intelligence as a contributor to compensatory processes for coping with symptoms.

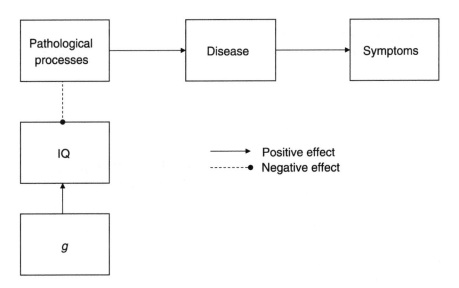

FIGURE 5.3c. The disease and the observed performance deficit are independently influenced by the same processes.

morbid test score. For example, performance deficits of test-anxious individuals may be eliminated by the provision of reassuring instructions (see Zeidner, 1998), demonstrating that the deficit is one in performance rather than competence. If the performance deficit model applies, then test scores obtained in conditions that eliminate the deficit should not be predictive of pathology. As a contrary example, Macklin and colleagues (1998) reported that in combat veterans, premorbid IQ predicted the likelihood of posttraumatic stress disorder (PTSD), suggesting an effect of g on the pathological processes that produce PTSD. The correlation between PTSD and concurrent IQ was reduced to nonsignificance when premorbid IQ was controlled, indicating that the maladaptive cognitions associated with PTSD do not seem to impair IQ test performance.

  4. *The common cause model.* Figure 5.3d presents a final possibility. Here, the model suggests that a common developmental cause underlies both ability level and psychopathology. Examples include genetic or environmental factors capable of influencing both intelligence and psychopathology. If the common cause model applies, controlling for the confound will eliminate the intelligence–psychopathology relationship.

  There is an expanding literature investigating the relationship between intelligence and a number of psychological disorders. This knowledge can provide potentially useful information relevant to assessing the risk, man-

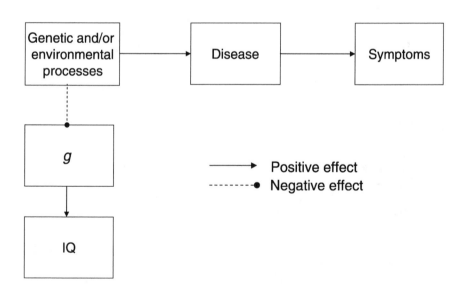

FIGURE 5.3d. Common genetic and/or environmental factors independently influence the development of both the disease and intelligence.

ner of expressing, and prognosis for a number of disorders. Two of the most important and well-researched areas are the links between intelligence and schizophrenia, and those between intelligence and depression.

Intelligence and Schizophrenia

Despite noteworthy exceptions (e.g., Nobel prize winner John Nash, depicted in the film *A Beautiful Mind*), people with schizophrenia tend to have lower average intelligence than either matched controls or general population samples. Research has consistently found that lower intelligence exists prior to the onset of clinical symptoms, rather than occurring entirely as a consequence of the illness, although there is also evidence for intellectual decline after illness onset (Aylward, Walker, & Betts, 1984). Two recent large-scale studies, using military draft-board psychometric test scores and their relation to later psychiatric hospitalization, found that the IQ distribution of those later diagnosed with schizophrenia had shifted downward by approximately 8 IQ points, compared to noncases (David, 1998; David, Malmberg, Brandt, Allebeck, & Lewis, 1997; Davidson et al., 1999). A logistic regression analysis demonstrated a linear relationship between low IQ and schizophrenia risk in both studies. A reanalysis of Table 2 in David and colleagues' (1997) research gives an odds ratio of around 1.5 for a one standard deviation decrease in IQ. In each study, the diagnosis of schizophrenia occurred a number of years after the IQ measurement, long enough to rule out the possibility that lower IQ is simply an early symptom of the illness. In the David and colleagues study, the risk due to low IQ was found to remain significant after correction for a range of potential confounders, including socioeconomic status.

Schizophrenia is well known to have multiple causes (Zuckerman, 1999), including genetic components, risk factors for prenatal brain damage, and associations with birth complications. Given these risk factors, the intelligence–schizophrenia link may have two possible explanations. One possibility is that low intelligence acts independently of other risk factors to increase the likelihood that schizophrenia will occur (Figure 5.3a). An alternative possibility is that a common cause (genetic or environmental) might be associated with both lower IQ and other risk factors (Figure 5.3d). In addition to the lower IQ scores of patients, a number of other markers of schizophrenia have been found. In particular, brain-imaging studies of first-onset cases reveal structural abnormalities that must have existed prior to the onset of the illness. A history of childhood behavioral abnormalities is also characteristic of people with schizophrenia.

These indicators, taken together, provide strong evidence for schizophrenia as a neurodevelopmental disorder (Davies, Russell, Jones, & Murray, 1998). If this were the case, lowered IQ could be a symptom of the underlying disorder, with developmental brain abnormality acting as the cause of both lowered IQ and schizophrenia. Further evidence for the common cause mechanism comes from studies of the unaffected relatives of people with schizophrenia, wherein relatives have been found to show impaired cognitive performance compared to normal controls (Krabbendam Marcelis, Delespaul, Golles, & van Os, 2001; Laurent et al., 1999; Staal, Hijman, Pol, & Kahn, 2000). Such findings do not necessarily rule out an independent role of intelligence in disease risk and progression. One possible mechanism by which low intelligence might act as a direct risk factor for schizophrenia is by associated deficits in social cognition and information processing, increasing the likelihood of psychotic symptoms such as delusions and hallucinations (David et al., 1997).

The study of insight in people with schizophrenia and other psychoses, and the associations between insight and illness progression, provide additional, if indirect, evidence of the association between schizophrenia and intelligence. Insight was originally conceptualized as the extent to which a patient accepts that he or she is suffering from a mental illness. Recent work has suggested that a multidimensional approach to insight is more helpful, and several instruments to assess insight dimensions have been developed (McGorry & McConville, 1999). In the formulation developed by David (1990), three overlapping dimensions of insight were measured: acceptance of mental illness, compliance with treatment, and ability to relabel psychotic phenomena as abnormal. A number of studies investigating associations between insight measures and intelligence has been performed, with most reporting positive associations (David, 1999). These findings suggest that higher intelligence is associated with a greater awareness of illness and a greater readiness to comply with treatment. Furthermore, positive associations between insight, treatment compliance, and outcome have indeed been reported (McGorry & McConville, 1999). However, there is evidence that insight can have negative as well as positive aspects. Lack of insight into a serious mental illness can be regarded as a defense mechanism or a coping style that may aid the patient in dealing with his or her condition. Conversely, high insight can have negative consequences such as depression and increased risk of suicide (Amador et al., 1996; McGorry & McConville, 1999; Moore, Cassidy, Carr, & O'Callaghan, 1999).

Intelligence and Dementia

Research on normal cognitive aging suggests that age may be "kinder to the initially more able" (Deary, MacLennan, & Starr, 1999, p. 26), most likely because high intelligence (or its covariates) might protect against cognitive decline. Results from longitudinal and cross-sequential studies demonstrate that people of higher education level, higher social class, and higher intelligence do indeed show a smaller decline in ability test scores as they age (Deary et al., 1999).

There is also considerable evidence that the good fortune of the more able extends to a reduced risk of dementia. One particularly well-known result comes from a study of a group of elderly nuns who had written brief autobiographies in early youth. These biographies were scored for linguistic ability. It was found that low early-life linguistic ability was a strong predictor of both cognitive decline and Alzheimer's disease in later life (Snowdon et al., 1996). A series of larger longitudinal studies has shown that the incidence of dementia falls with increasing education level, occupational status, and premorbid IQ (Ott et al., 1995; Schmand, Smit, Geerlings, & Lindeboom, 1997; Stern et al., 1994; Whalley et al., 2000). Somewhat similarly, HIV-infected adults of lower occupational status and low premorbid IQ were more likely to develop neuropsychological deficits related to their HIV status (Pereda et al., 2000; Satz et al., 1993; Stern, Silva, Chaisson, & Evans, 1996).

Since educational level, socioeconomic status, and intelligence are positively intercorrelated, the interpretation of the above findings is not a straightforward task. One explanation is that more intelligent persons have more brain "reserve" (Satz, 1993). In other words, they have a greater amount of backup, so that when they lose neurons, they have additional resources that can compensate for the loss. Brain reserve is considered to be biologically based and, in some sense, a measure of redundant brain capacity. Within this framework, intelligence, educational level, and occupational status act as indirect measures of reserve capacity. It is assumed that the incidence of the degenerative brain changes observed in dementia is actually the same in groups with differing levels of reserve capacity, but that the more redundant brain structure of individuals with high reserve confers a degree of protection on them. One proposed measure of reserve capacity is brain size (known to be positively correlated with psychometric intelligence [Deary, 2000]). In this model, dementia-induced lesions would compromise the function of a greater fraction of the brain in a low-reserve, compared to a high-reserve, individual. The low-reserve person would be more likely to display clinical symptoms of the disease. Brain size as an indicator of reserve is supported by a number of clinical studies. For example, the onset of Alzheimer's disease was found to occur later for persons with larger intracranial volume than for persons with smaller intracranial volume (Schofield, Mosesson, Stern, & Mayeux, 1995).

Although there is considerable evidence to support the reserve hypothesis, there are reported differences in how g relates to this reserve. Some researchers imply that general ability, g, is a direct measure of reserve. In contrast, others state that g and *reserve* have a common cause, such that g is merely a marker for reserve. The latter view corresponds to the model shown in Figure 5.3d. Dementia is clinically defined in terms of a range of impairments in intellectual performance, and diagnostic criteria for dementia are inevitably measures of intellectual ability, meaning that dementia screening test scores are positively correlated with intelligence test scores. In this context, the "g = reserve" idea predicts that, for a given degree of brain degeneration, a less intelligent person is more likely to be diagnosed as demented than is a more intelligent person, because his or her intellectual performance has less far to fall to cross the clinical threshold (see Figure 5.4a; Gold, Deary, MacLeod, & Frier, 1995). This hypothesis may well be correct but does not add anything to the theoretical understanding of dementia risk. The studies of normal cognitive aging (described above) escape this trap by addressing differential rates of intellectual decline. Examples of models with more substantive content are shown in Figures 5.4b and 5.4c. Future research will need to (1) identify those aspects of brain biology that account for differences in susceptibility to dementia, and (2) explain individual differences in dementia susceptibility not accounted for by initial intelligence level.

Other explanations have been proposed for the associations between intelligence, education level, and dementia risk. Katzman (1993) suggests a mechanism in which education increases synaptic density in the neocortical association cortex. Although there is no direct evidence for this process in humans, a number of animal studies (Swaab, 1991) suggest that an enriched environment can promote brain development throughout the lifespan. This leads to the hypotheses that mental activity in later life can

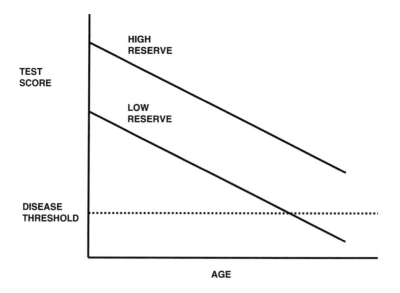

FIGURE 5.4a. An uninformative formulation of the reserve model, in which *reserve* is simply a measure of initial test score. High- and low-reserve groups decline in score at the same rate, so members of the low-reserve group receive an earlier diagnosis.

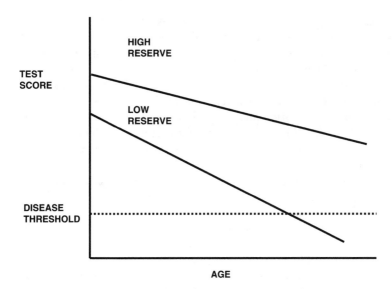

FIGURE 5.4b. A possible explanation for the findings on dementia. Low- and high-reserve groups start at different cognitive levels, but the high-reserve group also experiences a slower decline. This is the finding for normal cognitive aging.

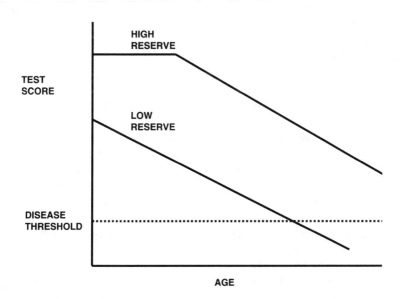

FIGURE 5.4c. Alternative explanation for the findings on dementia: Onset of decline is delayed to a later age in the high-reserve group.

maintain reserve capacity (the "use it or lose it" idea), suggesting that the relationship between intelligence and dementia is best described by the compensatory process model (see Figure 5.3b). There is certainly evidence that social and leisure activity in later life protects against cognitive decline and dementia (Fabrigoule et al., 1995; Kondo, Niino, & Shido, 1994).

Insight into the relative likelihood of competing views regarding the causal status of education and ability in dementia can be obtained by determining which variable acts as a stronger predictor of dementia vulnerability. For example, it was shown that premorbid intelligence predicts dementia incidence better than does educational level (Schmand et al., 1997). This finding provides support for the idea that a reserve factor linked to intelligence is more important than merely engaging in intellectual activities (via education). The same conclusion can be drawn from behavioral–genetic studies that assess the association between scores on a dementia screening instrument (Mini-Mental State Examination) and education level (Carmelli, Swan, & Cardon, 1995; Pedersen, Reynolds, & Gatz, 1996). The education–MMSE correlation was found to be largely accounted for by heritable cognitive ability, thus supporting the existence of a biologically based reserve factor. The alternative models described above, in which brain structure is affected by education and other activities, would require the correlation to be environmentally mediated.

Clearly, further work is needed to uncover a definitive explanation of the associations between intelligence and intelligence-related markers for risk of dementia. However, there does appear to be evidence for a biologically based brain reserve model, but more work is required to confirm this model and to test its explanatory power against competing environmentally based models

EMOTIONAL INTELLIGENCE

The concept of emotional intelligence (EI) received widespread, international attention following Goleman's (1995) popular book on the topic. The general theme underlying EI is not new, as noted in the efforts of Binet, Thorndike, Wechsler, and others to describe and measure a kind of social–emotional, interpersonal–intrapersonal capacity (see Kaufman & Kaufman, 2001). However, the development of a number of scales that purport to tap EI has operationalized the concepts of EI as well as made it possible to assess the constructs underlying EI. Given the growing concerns about the eruption of aggressive acts and violence on school grounds and in the world community, some psychologists and allied professionals view EI as a key factor in describing and understanding these aspects of behavior

EI is at the crossroads of ability and personality; the term refers to competence in understanding and managing emotion and the outcome of emotional encounters supported by skills for emotional awareness, interpersonal sensitivity, and mood regulation. More emotionally intelligent persons should perform better on certain kinds of tasks, such as identifying emotions in pictures and stories, and choosing the appropriate course of action in challenging circumstances. EI also refers to many psychological functions frequently linked to personality, such as self-awareness, sensitivity to others, coping with stress, and positive emotional experiences (McCrae, 2000). Zeidner and Matthews (2000) identify various attributes that appear to link personality and intelligence, including openness, self-efficacy, and ego resiliency, which might be seen as facets of EI.

From an applied perspective, EI is attractive as "an intelligence anyone can have." It is considered more malleable and trainable than general intelligence, and raising EI has even been seen as the answer to the multifold social problems of industrialized nations (Goleman, 1995). Occupational success may depend on EI as much as cognitive intelligence, and education should instill skills for emotional regulation as well as abstract knowledge. Moreover, even psychotherapy may benefit from techniques that help clients "get in touch with" their emotions

At the same time, caution and even skepticism are in order (for critical reviews, see Matthews, Zeidner, & Roberts, 2002; Roberts, Zeidner, & Matthews, 2001). The claims made for the importance of EI, especially in popular accounts, though sometimes extraordinary and inspiring, are often unsupported by acceptable evidence. There are also differences of opinion regarding the assessment of EI, especially the higher-level components of emotional regulation. One question that must be addressed is how to determine the "correct" answer to a test item that asks respondents how they would handle situations such as resolving an argument, comforting a depressed person, or dealing with their own troublesome emotions. Indeed, EI recapitulates the assessment problems posed by the construct of "social intelligence," for which, despite several decades of research, there is still no generally accepted and validated measure of the ability to understand and manage social interactions (see Kihlstrom & Cantor, 2000). Another potentially significant problem is the overlap with existing personality measures. Readers are directed to a comprehensive scientific debate on the conceptual and methodological status of EI, published in the journal *Emotion* (Volume 1, Number 1, 2001).

Theoretical Issues

Since much of the research on EI is atheoretical, two key assumptions are rarely made explicit or tested. The first assumption is that *individual differences in EI are correlated with neural or psychological processes that influence the outcome of real-world emotional encounters.* Construct validation of EI requires a demonstration that individuals differ appropriately at this processing level. Some speculations have been put forward. Goleman (1995) suggests that EI depends on subcortical and cortical "emotion centers" of the brain, working in harmony with, rather than in opposition to, each other. Neuroscience evidence (e.g., Rolls, 1999) supports the role of structures such as the amygdala and prefrontal cortex in the mediation of emotion. However, there is little compelling evidence that individual differences in normal emotional functioning directly correspond to parameters of these brain systems (Matthews et al., 2002). Still another approach is to link EI to individual differences in cognitive functioning, such as coping skills (Salovey et al., 2000), but, again, evidence is lacking.

The central problem for both biological and cognitive models is that although emotional functioning is supported by a multiplicity of different processes, there is no evidence that these processes cohere around some central construct of EI. For example, recognizing facial emotions probably depends on (1) brain systems such as the amygdala, (2) both unconscious and conscious appraisal processes, and (3) the person's use of contextual information such as background knowledge and cultural norms for expression (e.g., a fearful expression is entertaining in a horror film or uncomfortably amusing on the face of a clown). These processes operate at different levels of abstraction and appear to be both biologically and cognitively separate. A particular problem for assessment is the fact that unconscious implicit processes supporting "proceduralized" skills are especially important for real-world social functioning (e.g., Bargh & Chartrand, 1999), but it is unclear whether or not these social skills are validly assessed by the items on both ability- and personality-like tests that require explicit or "declarative" knowledge.

The second theoretical assumption is that *individual differences in processing related to emotion actually control the success or failure of real-world adaptive outcomes.* In other words, even if we assume that tests of EI assess some genuine competencies or skills, the question still remains: Do these skills have any substantial impact in real life? Matthews and Zeidner (2000) argue that it is difficult to rank-order adaptive outcomes on any continuum of success versus failure. Stress outcomes are more often qualitative rather than quantitative and produce a pattern of costs and benefits that changes over time. How these costs and benefits are weighted depends on individual and cultural values. For example, consider a person who works long hours and eventually gains an important promotion. At a personal level, benefits of job satisfaction and achievement are balanced against costs of fatigue, possible health problems, and loss of opportunity to engage in other activities. At a social level, the person might neglect his or her family in the short term but gain financial security for them in the long term. At a cultural level, there might be a conflict between the work ethic and the value of finding fulfillment outside work. In other words, there is no a priori "emotionally intelligent" resolution of such dilemmas and conflicts; different decisions produce qualitatively different outcomes that cannot be evaluated without reference to personal and societal values (Matthews et al., 2002).

Consistent with this analysis, *different styles of coping are not strongly linked to better or worse adaptive outcomes* (Matthews & Zeidner, 2000; Zeidner & Saklofske, 1996). There is a weak tendency for problem-focused strategies, which seek to tackle the issue proactively, to work somewhat better than emotion-focused strategies, which may lead to prolonged reflection rather than direct action. However, sometimes emotion-focused coping, or avoidance coping, is more effective in coming to terms with an event, and, in general, the outcomes of coping styles are highly dependent on the context (Lazarus, 1991a, 1991b). The remarks made so far refer to individual differences in the functioning of "normal" individuals without clinical pathology. Of course, persons with mental disorders show styles of coping that are clearly maladaptive. However, Matthews and colleagues (2002) caution against the identification of mental disorder with low emotional intelligence, since there appear to be multiple, independent sources of pathology in emotional functioning.

The overlap between some operationalizations of EI and established personality constructs raises the further issue of whether traits such as emotional stability (i.e., low neuroticism) and extroversion are truly adaptive. Again, reviews of the evidence (Matthews, 1999; Matthews et al., 2002) suggest that personality traits relate to mixed adaptive outcomes. For example, neuroticism is reliably linked to negative affect. However, lack of emotional stability does not, in general, seem to be a disadvantage in the workplace. Meta-analytic reviews (e.g., Barrick & Mount, 1991b) show that neuroticism predicts less than 1% of the variance in job performance overall. In fact, neuroticism may be a disadvantage in jobs characterized by overt stressors, but it is sometimes advantageous in nonstressful occupations where sensitivity to future threat may drive effort and achievement (Matthews, 1997a, 1997b, 1997c; Mughal, Walsh, & Wilding, 1996). Some personality dispositions may carry more severe potential costs than others, such as the vulnerability to anxiety and mood disorders that is associated with neuroticism (Bagby, Joffe, Parker, Kalemba, & Harkness, 1995; Saklofske et al., 1995). However, to claim that some trait characteristics are more "emotionally intelligent" than others is to grossly oversimplify the sometimes subtle costs and benefits linked to specific traits. Matthews (1999) suggests that traits control adaptations to specific environments. For example, emotional stability predisposes the person to handle stress, whereas neuroticism is an advantage when threats are disguised or delayed. How "emotionally intelligent" the person appears may thus depend on the "fit" between personality and environment.

Assessment of Emotional Intelligence

Differing conceptualizations of EI have resulted in ability versus mixed models that are reflected in different assessment strategies (Mayer, Salovey, & Caruso, 2000b; Mayer, Salovey, Caruso, & Sitarenios, 2001). Ability models seek to operationalize EI through objective tests akin to intelligence tests, and are comprised of items with right or wrong answers. Such tests should be moderately correlated with other mental ability measures and with general intelligence. According to Mayer and colleagues (2000b), the four components or "branches" of EI are (1) identification of emotions, (2) understanding emotions, (3) assimilation of emotions in thought, and (4) regulation of both positive and negative emotions in the self and others. In contrast, mixed models are broader in scope, in that they encompass personality factors that promote adaptive emotional functioning in addition to more specific abilities. For example, Bar-On (1997, 2000) identifies the following five areas of emotional functioning that might have both ability and personality components: intrapersonal skills, interpersonal skills, adaptability, stress management, and general mood.

The Multi-Factor Emotional Intelligence Scale

The most comprehensive and original EI ability-like measure is the Multi-Factor Emotional Intelligence Scale (MEIS; Mayer, Caruso, & Salovey, 2000a). An abbreviated and refined version of the MEIS, the Mayer–Salovey–Caruso Emotional Intelligence Test (MSCEIT), has recently been released. Other seemingly objective tests measure more specific abilities, such as perception of emotion (Davies, Stankov, & Roberts, 1998) and the ability to articulate the feelings appropriate for particular circumstances (Lane, 2000). The MEIS is comprised of 12 subtests that, together, provide scores for the four branches previously described, and an overall EI measure. Although there are concerns about the reliability of some of the subtests, reliability for overall EI is very good, exceeding .90 (Mayer et al., 2000b).

Correlations with ability measures have been reported as .36 with verbal intelligence (Mayer et al., 2000a), .32 with a crystallized intelligence measure derived from the Armed Services Vocational Aptitude Battery (Roberts et al., 2001), and a nonsignificant .05 with fluid intelligence as measured by the Ravens Matrices (Ciarrochi, Chan, & Caputi, 2000). Importantly, test scores appear to be distinct from standard personality measures. Roberts and colleagues (2001) found that the highest correlations between the MEIS and scales for the five-factor model were for high agreeableness (.24) and low neuroticism (–.18). Nevertheless, a recent empirical study and review of data (Matthews et al., 2002; Roberts et al., 2001) identified various areas of concern. Research on mental abilities (e.g., Carroll, 1993) has produced sophisticated multilevel models that establish a hierarchy of factors ranging from relatively narrow primary abilities up to general intelligence, or g, as an overarching top-level factor. Broad abilities, such as fluid and crystallized intelligence, occupy an intermediate tier. The limited research on the MEIS and ability measures does not indicate the "level" of EI within such a hierarchical model. It is unclear, for example, whether EI might be seen as a primary ability that could be subsumed under crystallized intelligence (as a collection of learned skills) or as a higher-order factor of greater scope.

In addition, evidence on the predictive validity of the MEIS is limited. Mayer and colleagues (2000a) found that scores predicted criteria, including empathy, parental warmth, and life satisfaction, but correlation magnitudes were modest, ranging from .11 to .33. Relationships with parental warmth and life satisfaction fell to nonsignificance ($r < .10$) when verbal intelligence and empathy were controlled. Rather oddly, under these circumstances, the MEIS was slightly but significantly negatively correlated with attempted self-improvement and with culture seeking. Thus the discriminant validity of the MEIS requires further investigation.

Perhaps the most fundamental problem is that of scoring the MEIS test items as right or wrong. Mayer and colleagues (2000a) used two alternate scoring methods. Expert scoring is based on a priori judgments of the correct responses to items, made by experts in the field of emotion. However, experts are fallible, and experts from different disciplines may disagree. Consensus scoring is based on the assumption that the pooled response of large normative samples is veridical. This method, in effect, computes the match between the respondent's answers and those of a normative sample, with the degree of congruence indicating the level of EI. One may question whether popular beliefs about emotion are, in fact, true or false, such that this method may assess social conformity rather than an ability (Roberts et al., 2001). For example, a talented but unconventional artist with original perspectives on emotions and their significance might well obtain a low score on the MEIS.

The Emotional Quotient Inventory

The Bar-On Emotional Quotient Inventory, or EQ-i, is comprised of 15 scales grouped together into five composite dimensions: intrapersonal skills, interpersonal skills, adaptation, stress management, and general mood (see description in case description). Bar-On, creator of the instrument, conducted quite extensive development work in demonstrating scale reliability in different cultures, and in showing that the EQ-i predicts relevant criteria such as mental health, coping level, work satisfaction, and personality traits associated with hardiness in stressful circumstances. Indeed, the EQ-i is one of the most extensively researched instruments measuring

EI. Although the EQ-i has predictive validity, it is unclear whether the scale has discriminant validity. Bar-On (1997) himself reports very substantial correlations (exceeding –.80 in some cases) between the EQ-i scales and measures of pathological symptoms. This high correlation may imply, however, that there is little that is novel about the instrument. Dawda and Hart (2000) showed high correlations between the EQ-i and the dimensions of the well-known five-factor model of personality, with the magnitude of the correlation between total "EQ" and neuroticism exceeding –.60 in men and –.70 in women. Another concern is that the EQ-i does not converge well with the MEIS. However, Bar-On (2000) reports a correlation of .46 between the two measures. This modest correlation means that, despite some overlap, they are essentially different constructs. Unlike the MEIS, the EQ-i appears to be independent of general intelligence (Bar-On, 2000). Of interest is that both a short form (Bar-On, 2002) and a youth version have recently been made available (Bar-On & Parker, 2000).

The Emotional Intelligence Scale

The Emotional Intelligence Scale (EIS) questionnaire is similar to the EQ-i. The factor structure suggested by Schutte and colleagues (1998), in their initial article in which this scale was introduced, has not been clearly established in confirmatory factor analysis (Petrides & Furnham, 2000). The most satisfactory empirical solution appears to place a general EI factor superordinate over four lower-level factors of optimism/mood regulation, appraisal of emotions, social skills, and utilization of emotions (Saklofske, Austin, & Minski, in press). Like the EQ-i, the EIS predicts criteria related to well-being but overlaps substantially with existing personality traits. Compared with the EQ-i, the EIS has two points in its favor. First, its correlations with the five-factor model are somewhat smaller though still substantial (the highest correlation was a .51 with extroversion; Petrides & Furnham, 2000). Second, Saklofske and colleagues (in press) showed that the EIS predicted well-being indices, even with the five-factor model dimensions statistically controlled, although the increment in variance explained was very modest for all criteria.

Summary and Conclusions

Much of the excitement surrounding the new idea of emotional intelligence is not well-founded in empirical research. On the positive side, the more rigorous approaches to the topic (e.g., Mayer et al., 2000b) have focused attention on the potential importance of an individual's awareness and regulation of emotion. At this early stage, no final judgment on the value of the concept can be made; future research may solve some of the problems about EI we have identified in its current stage of development. Published scales for EI fail some elementary psychometric tests. Different measures, and even different scoring methods, fail to converge on a common dimension, raising questions about reliability. Although both ability and self-report tests have some predictive validity, the gains offered by assessing EI, in addition to standard personality and ability scales, seem modest, at best. The theory of EI, which might guide better assessment, is in its infancy. The best articulated theory (Mayer et al., 2000a) makes some plausible distinctions between different components of EI but has little to say on some fundamental issues, including possible biological bases and the roles of "implicit" and "explicit" processing. Existing data also suggest that it is hard to link, in any simple way, success of adaptive outcome to information processing, coping, or even personality.

Given these cautions, the practical utility of assessing EI seems somewhat limited. Certainly, current tests of EI should not be used exclusively for making important decisions about individuals. The most fundamental objection is that whether a person appears as more or less emotionally intelligent depends, to a large degree, on the instrument used (or even on how it is scored). Interest in EI has been valuable in stimulating interest in emotional functioning in educational and occupational settings, but there is little evidence that research on EI has added substantially to existing practice (see Matthews et al., 2001, for a review). There is no study in a peer-reviewed journal supporting Goleman's (1995) claim that EI may be more important than IQ in predicting job success following hiring. However, more narrowly defined concepts may be useful in refining current techniques. For example, work on alexithymia has led to the development of methods for treating patients who find it hard to verbalize their inner states (Parker, 2000). At present, it would seem that questionnaire measures and theoretical understanding of EI will not revolutionize assessment of individual differences in emotional functioning, but they may add incrementally to existing knowledge.

INTELLIGENCE–PERSONALITY AND SYSTEMATIC TREATMENT SELECTION

When traditional measures of intelligence are combined with measures of emotional intelligence, it is possible to make inferences regarding several of the STS variables. One frequent concern is whether or not a person's emotional difficulties are sufficient to disrupt his or her level of cognitive functioning. In order to evaluate this area, clinicians should note the degree of functional impairment and distress from other forms of data (e.g., history, behavioral observations, MMPI-2) and then consider whether or not the impairment and distress are sufficiently high to disrupt measures on cognitive tests. In general, those subtests that require the most effort are most likely to be affected. For example, anxiety may lower scores on the WAIS-III subtests of Arithmetic, Digit Span, and Digit Symbol-Coding.

A number of qualitative observations made during individual intelligence testing can be used to infer STS variables. For example, depressed patients who appear confused and show a slow response time may be manifesting reduced cognitive abilities related to high functional impairment. Patients who are high in resistance also will be likely to express this resistance on formal intelligence testing as well. They might make comments such as "These tests seem stupid" or "I think this is a waste of time." Although the behavioral observations described above are not likely to carry the same weight as more formal measures of functional impairment or resistance, such observations can be used to add support to more formal measures. More importantly, these measures provide a further contextual framework that will aid the clinician in addressing questions of both diagnosis and prescription.

Even though measures of intelligence (especially IQ) do not provide direct measures of social support, EQ-i type subtests do assess respondents' level of interpersonal skills and ability to adapt. The underlying assumption is that, if their EQ is high, they should be more able to develop and maintain supportive relationships. As with social support, a person's coping style is not measured directly by the assessment instruments (or concepts) described in this chapter. However, persons who have a high internal locus of control and high self-efficacy are also likely to have higher intelligence as well as an internalizing coping style. In addition, persons with higher EQ-i scores (and higher g) will be more likely to regulate their mood effectively. Level of resistance is not readily assessed by measures of general or emotional intelligence, although malingering may be observed on tests such as the WAIS-III. Clinicians will need to rely on other forms of assessment to evaluate this variable.

As indicated above, level of distress (and functional impairment) may result in reduced performance on tasks requiring a high degree of effort (especially if attention is required). However, this level of assessment does not measure distress directly as much as assess the impact that distress may be having. A somewhat more direct measure of distress might be EQ-i subtests that assess the degree to which a person can manage stress. If these scores are low, the person is more likely to be distressed at the time of assessment. Thus short-term reduction of stress may be an important focus of therapy, with longer-term development of stress management skills.

CASE EXAMPLE

The following case example is used throughout the book to illustrate the contributions that each of the test-oriented chapters can make toward effective assessment of adult personality. As noted previously, the entire case (history, tests administered, interpretation of all test data, etc.) is included as Case 2 in Chapter 13. In addition, all test scores are listed in Appendix A, including the patient's profile on the Wechsler Adult Intelligence Scale–III as well as the Bar-On Emotional Quotient Inventory. The following case discussion focuses on concepts and domains relevant for the interface between intelligence and personality (relevant concepts are italicized).

To reiterate, the client (R.W.) is a 22-year-old, Mexican American female who is currently supported by her 42-year-old boyfriend of 6 years. She reported complaints of panic attacks, social anxiety, and insecurity in her current relationship. Although she has received her GED, the client is not currently employed or in school. She was referred for evaluation in order to clarify her diagnosis and assist in treatment planning.

One of the central concerns of many personality assessments is whether or not the *severity of a patient's emotional difficulties is sufficient to disrupt his or her cognitive functioning*. A review of R.W.'s cognitive functioning indicates an average intelligence, but her emotional quotient (EQ) is below average. Her history and other test results strongly suggest that she is not optimally using her cognitive abilities. In particular, many of the WAIS-III subtests that reflect cognitive efficiency related to working memory and processing speed were among her lowest scores (Digit Symbol-Coding, Arithmetic, Digit Span, Symbol Search, Letter–Number Sequencing). Together with her symptom severity, this is sufficient to disrupt her cognitive functioning. Her thoughts are often disorganized and, under stress, she is likely either to withdraw or act out (sexually or with drugs). In either case, she does not think her way through conflicts by trying to develop new problem-solving strategies (i.e., use problem-focused coping). In addition, her academic achievement is low, in part, because she directs her energy toward resisting persons in authority (teachers) rather than focusing on the academic tasks presented to her. Thus, while she certainly has the potential to perform at a significantly higher cognitive level, her levels of distress, cognitive style, and interpersonal orientation result in a far less than optimal utilization of her general cognitive ability.

R.W. also experiences internal and external events as happening *to* her (high external *locus of control*). In particular, her panic attacks feel beyond her control and seem to occur at random intervals. Interpersonally, she relies heavily on her boyfriend to organize her day-to-day life and to take care of her. Much of her neediness (and resulting difficulties) in the relationship is the result of her feeling that she will be abandoned and may even be suggestive of a dependent personality. Since she is threatened both internally (panic attacks, disorganized thoughts, social anxiety) and externally (fear of abandonment), she works to maintain a narrow range of experiences (low *openness to experience*).

The client has a number of *cognitive distortions* that help to explain her symptoms, and these distortions may also be targeted in psychotherapy. She is extremely sensitive to the real or imagined perceptions of other people ("What will they think of me?"). Many of these concerns revolve around the judgments she imagines people make because she is dating an older man. Thus she "mind reads" that people are rejecting her when she and her boyfriend appear in public (e.g., "People think I'm no good" and "I know they don't like me"). In addition, she has a difficult time distinguishing internal from external reality and misinterprets her internal states. Misintrepreting her internal states is likely to be an important causal factor in the development of her panic attacks.

Her overall *emotional quotient* was in the low average range (EQi = 85). Relative strengths were that, during the interview itself, she was able to describe her symptoms and history clearly, in a relatively articulate and assertive manner. She was also oriented to time and place, responded in an open, direct manner, and appeared to have relatively good insight into her condition. At the same time, however, she reported that under stress, she withdraws and her thoughts become disorganized. She described these experiences as frightening. In addition, she appears to be extremely dependent on her relationship with her boyfriend. He makes most decisions for her and cares for her financially. Thus she does not need to engage actively in problem solving, since he does so for her. Although she adapts to this dependency most of the time (i.e., generally good impulse control), she also occasionally rebels against it by impulsively acting out.

A review of the above points suggests several conclusions relevant to the STS model. First, R.W.'s level of functional impairment is sufficiently high to disrupt her cognitive functioning; the level of impairment also indicates that treatment would need to be of relatively long duration. Her level of social support is quite narrow and highly dependent on a single source (i.e., her boyfriend), which suggest the need to expand her social support network as well as assist her in improving her interpersonal problem-solving style (e.g., greater independence via assertiveness training and social skills development). Given her relatively young age, it is premature to conclude that her difficulties are of a long duration, but they do appear to be complex and include a number of cognitive-related difficulties (cognitive distortions, poor reality testing under stress, etc.). It is difficult to draw conclusions related to coping style and resistance based on intellectual assessment (i.e., WAIS-III, EQ-i), so interpretation on these variables is best deferred to more appropriate assessment instruments. It is clear, however, that she is sufficiently distressed to be highly motivated for treatment (assuming, of course, that her level of resistance is not too high). Indeed, her overall susceptibility to stress seems to be high.

In summary, R.W.'s strengths include (1) good to average level of intelligence, (2) potential to be aware of her emotions, and (3) ability to articulate how she feels when asked direct questions. However, her cognitive ability is reduced by her current symptoms, she keeps her experience within a narrow range, has a number of cognitive distortions, perceives events as occurring beyond her control, and has a low tolerance for stress. Of concern is that when she is under stress, she may withdraw, have a difficult time regulating her emotions, and experience poor reality testing.

SUMMARY

Personality and intelligence are cornerstones in the study and description of individual differences. As psychological science entered the realm of application and practice, there was an increased emphasis on understanding the uniqueness but also the connectedness of personality and intelligence variables in relation to assessment, diagnosis, prescription (for both intervention and prevention), and also process and outcome evaluations of treatments. Explorations of the interface between personality and intelligence have been facilitated by advances in research methodology and statistical techniques (e.g., structural equation modeling); efforts to resolve the schism between theory, research, and application; a general endorsement of the scientist-practitioner model; and an increased appreciation of the relevance of psychology to all aspects of human life (see Collis & Messick, 2001; Saklofske & Zeidner, 1995). Contemporary definitions now reflect personality as the study of the whole person needed to "bring order and consistency to the explanation of an individual's behavior" (Monte, 1995, p. 33).

To reinforce these perspectives, we presented some research evidence linking intelligence to some of the more familiar personality variables of interest to clinicians. It has been established that there are consistent correlations of small effect size between personality traits and intelligence measures (Ackerman & Heggestad, 1997). However, in spite of the massive knowledge generated from psychological research, there continues to be gaps between what is known and needed by practicing psychologists in schools, health settings, industry, and so on, who are regularly presented with the full range of human issues and needs. We encourage practicing psychologists to be informed by empirical findings; this is critical to separating psychology as a scientifically grounded discipline and practice from pseudosciences such as astrology. Furthermore, it discourages practices where "belief trumps evidence"!

We have also described several potential pathways linking intelligence to mental health. Such theoretical models have considerable heuristic value to the practicing psychologist (there is no better tool than a good theory, except of course, facts) as illustrated by brief discussions of both schizophrenia and dementia. Attention is then turned to a critical examination of emotional intelligence as a recent example of a construct linking intelligence, affect, and behavior. There is growing interest in EI from, for example, industry and education, but it must account for variance not captured by other intelligence and personality constructs if it is to have practical utility in a description of individual differences.

The case study illustrates how an empirically grounded psychology (nomethetic framework) may inform practitioners and in turn how they must integrate these often complex and diverse findings into an accurate and contextually sensitive description of the individual client (idiographic framework). For example, while the research literature presents a negative correlation between intelligence and aggression, forensic psychologists are quick to point to such nonconforming examples as Dr. Hannibal Lecter, the fictional brilliant but cruel psychopath, or the Nazi elite who were responsible for some of the most horrific crimes against humanity. There are many ways of earning an IQ of 100 (e.g., VIQ = 112, PIQ = 88 vs. VIQ = 100, PIQ + 101) that are of potential diagnostic relevance. However, the integration of this cognitive information with other client factors such as achievement motivation, self-concept, performance anxiety, and extreme shyness, will contribute significantly to describing and understanding a client's social and vocational issues. The eminent psychologist, Hans Eysenck, once informally commented that there is a considerable difference between bright and less intelligent extraverts just as there is between introverts and extraverts who are similar in measured intelligence.

Diagnostic descriptions are becoming increasingly more refined, as illustrated in DSM-IV, and the effectiveness (empirically validated) of psychological treatments (e.g., cognitive behavior therapy) for conditions ranging from anxiety to depression is quite impressive. Meyer and colleagues (2001) offer compelling support for the validity and efficacy of psychological testing and assessment. They suggest that the focus should now be on psychologists who select, use, and interpret tests that lead to diagnoses and treatments. The psychologist is the architect who is informed by theory and research on personality and intelligence, and uses it in a reciprocal fashion with client "data" for systematic treatment selection. This is exemplary of best practices in psychology.

6

The MMPI-2

James N. Butcher and Larry E. Beutler

Clinical assessment of mental health patients in the 1930s was a difficult and somewhat flawed activity. The difficulties resulted, for the most part, from the lack of a valid, objective means of obtaining information about patients' problems and symptoms. Although personality questionnaires were available, they were not considered to be effective in the clinical assessment of psychiatric patients because they were (1) too closely tied to psychological theories to be useful, (2) developed with college students, or (3) intended to measure variables that were unrelated to psychopathology. A developer of the Minnesota Multiphasic Personality Inventory (MMPI), Starke Hathaway (1965), pointed out that sheer frustration in understanding clinical patients was what led him and psychiatrist C. McKinley to begin the research in 1939 that resulted in the publication of the original MMPI. Initially, the MMPI was developed at the University of Minnesota Hospitals to aid clinicians in the routine tasks of assessing and diagnosing patients with mental disorders; however, it became immediately successful at filling the void in clinical assessment by providing a useful and practical assessment technique for individuals reporting mental health symptoms and problems in a variety of settings.

The MMPI provides information that is useful in predicting individual client's problems and behaviors in a cost-effective manner. More than 60 years after its publication, the MMPI (now the MMPI-2 and MMPI-A) is still the first and most frequent choice for practitioners when it comes to understanding patients' problems (Camara, Norton, & Puente, 2000). What gives the MMPI approach to assessment the utility and tenacity it has enjoyed? Hathaway (1965) pointed out several features of the MMPI, in addition to its validity, that he considered important in accounting for the instrument's popularity as a clinical assessment device: "the provisions for some control over undesirable response patterns, detection of invalid records such as those from nonreaders, the use of simple language, the simplicity of administration and scoring, and, finally, the general clinical familiarity of the profile variables" (p. 463). He further noted that other qualities of the MMPI enhanced its reputation as an objective psychological assessment procedure: It furnishes reliable evaluations across administrations and provides a ready means of evaluating a person's score on each scale within a normative framework. That is, a patient's scores on the scale can be compared with the responses of others, and the clinician directly determine whether a given patient's scores are low or high compared to a normative control group as well as to a clinical patient group.

The extensive normative base and the ease with which its information can be utilized makes the MMPI-2 a particularly useful instrument for identifying clients' strengths, weaknesses, and unique characteristics. Meyer and colleagues (2001), after surveying empirical validation research for psychological and medical procedures, emphasized this latter point, concluding that psychological assessment (including instruments such as the MMPI-2) show strong and compelling evidence of their value as a unique source of information about clients.

BACKGROUND

Development of the Original MMPI

In developing the MMPI, Hathaway and McKinley (1940) chose as their response format the use of statements to which the client could respond either "True" or "False." This straightforward self-administration task enabled individuals with a relatively low reading level to complete the inventory in a short time, usually about 1½ hours. Hathaway and McKinley did not select items for the scales according to their content; they considered the selection of scale items based on face validity to be too subjective. Instead they compiled a large pool of potential items (about 1,000), which were, for the most part, indicative of symptoms of mental disorders. Before the initial norm development, they reduced the item pool to 504 items. (Later, the MMPI item pool was expanded to 550 items by the inclusion of two additional scales, Masculinity–Femininity and Social Introversion.) In constructing scales, Hathaway and McKinley had no preconceived idea as to how items should be grouped. They used empirical contrasts between a sample of normal subjects and groups of well-defined patients to determine the items comprised by a particular scale.

Their concept of "scale" for the MMPI was relatively uncomplicated. Hathaway and McKinley believed that patients who endorsed similar symptoms or items in the MMPI pool were diagnostically more alike than they were different. If an item empirically discriminated a criterion group (say, people with depression) from a normal group, it was considered to have validity and was included on the Depression scale. For example, they believed that individuals endorsing many symptoms related to having a depressed mood were likely to be more similar to other depressed patients than they would be to other clinical diagnostic groups. In order to quantify the relationship between reported psychological symptoms and diagnostic similarity, Hathaway and McKinley developed scales (groups of items) with norms based on particular diagnostic groups by which individuals could be compared on particular qualities. A pattern of response that was more similar to one diagnostic group than another tended to indicate a greater likelihood that a diagnosis represented by this normative group would be viable. Rather than reflecting contemporary diagnostic groupings, however, the current MMPI scales are best viewed as dimensions reflecting particular problems and symptom clusters, such as depression or psychopathic deviation, than particular diagnoses.

In developing norms for the original MMPI, Hathaway and McKinley collected responses from a large group of "normals," defined as men and women who were not presently under a doctor's care. Most of the subjects in the original normative sample were visitors to the University of Minnesota Hospital. These individuals were usually people waiting at the hospital who had time on their hands and were willing to participate in the study. The means of the scale distributions were assigned a value of 50, and the standard deviations of each distribution were assigned a value of 10. The T-score distributions allow for comparison of scale scores across scales. A score of 70, which indicated two standard deviations above the mean, was considered clinically significant.

Almost as soon as the inventory was published (Hathaway & McKinley, 1943a), it began to gain acceptance in clinical assessment settings. The scale construction method produced clinical scales that proved to have high generalizability across diverse settings, and the MMPI became the most widely used and researched objective personality inventory in the United States (Lubin, Larsen, & Matarazzo, 1984; Lubin, Larsen, Matarazzo, & Seever, 1985; Piotrowski & Lubin, 1990) for patients in general medical settings, adolescents in schools, inmates in correctional facilities, individuals in alcohol and drug problem treatment units, military personnel, and eventually applicants for highly responsible or sensitive positions in industrial settings (e.g., airline pilots, police officers, or nuclear power plant operators). The MMPI also became the most widely used measure of psychopathology in psychological, psychiatric, and medical research studies.

International adaptation of the MMPI followed shortly after its publication. During the 1940s translations were completed in Cuba, Germany,

Italy, Japan, and Puerto Rico, and by 1976 there were approximately 150 foreign language translations available in over 40 countries (Butcher, 1985; Butcher & Pancheri, 1976). The MMPI has been viewed by mental health professionals in other countries as a more efficient way of providing effective assessment instruments than constructing entirely new indigenous instruments. Various reviews of cross-national MMPI research (Butcher, 1985; Butcher & Pancheri, 1976; Cheung, 1985) have suggested that the MMPI has demonstrated the same level of acceptance in mental health settings in many other countries as in the United States.

Revisions: The MMPI-2 and MMPI-A

Over time, several problems with the original MMPI became apparent. Many of the items in the inventory were found to be out of date or objectionable (Butcher, 1972; Butcher & Owen, 1978), and it was recommended that the instrument be revised by deleting obsolete items and broadening the item pool to include more contemporary topics. In addition, the use of the original MMPI norms became problematic, because the normative sample on which the original MMPI scales were based was not appropriate for many present-day comparisons (Butcher, 1972). The original MMPI normative sample was comprised of white rural subjects from Minnesota, yet it was being used across the United States with broadly diverse clients. Colligan, Osborne, Swenson, and Offord (1983) and Parkison and Fishburne (1984) conducted studies showing that the original MMPI norms were inappropriate for use with that decade's subjects.

In the early 1980s, the University of Minnesota Press, the copyright holder, decided to sponsor a revision of the MMPI. The revision program, initiated in 1982 by a committee comprised of Grant Dahlstrom, John Graham, Auke Tellegen, and James Butcher, was aimed at maintaining the integrity of many scales of the original MMPI, because of their demonstrated advantages, as well as at expanding the range of clinically relevant measures in the inventory (Butcher, Graham, Williams, & Ben-Porath, 1990). Of primary concern to the committee was the need to maintain the acceptability of the original instrument in its restandardized versions, the MMPI-2 and the MMPI-A.[1] Initially, the MMPI revision committee decided to develop two separate experimental booklets, one for adults and one for adolescents, for use in data collection. Each experimental booklet included all the original MMPI items, some with minor wording improvements (Butcher, Dahlstrom, Graham, Tellegen, & Kaemmer, 1989; Butcher et al.,

---

[1]Because this chapter focuses on assessment of adults, detailed information about the MMPI-A is not included. Readers interested in the assessment of adolescents should consult the manual for the MMPI-A (Butcher et al., 1992) or the interpretive guide by Butcher and Williams (2000).

1992). Items measuring new content (e.g., suicidal behavior, treatment readiness, type A behaviors, problematic substance use) were added to both experimental booklets. In addition, developmentally relevant items were added to the appropriate booklets (e.g., work adjustment items were added to the adult form, and school adjustment items to the adolescent form).

Items that constitute the validity and standard scales, except for the objectionable items, were retained in the MMPI-2. However, new items measuring additional clinical problems and applications were added to the inventory, replacing the out-of-date items from the original booklet. Thus broader content coverage, allowing for new scale development, was accomplished without altering the standard scales. In order to modernize the MMPI, new normative and clinical data were collected on adults (Butcher et al., 1990) and adolescents (Butcher et al., 1992). In the development of the MMPI-2 and MMPI-A, the following goals were pursued:

1. Revise and modernize the MMPI item domain by deleting objectionable, nonworking, or otherwise obsolete items and replacing them with items addressing contemporary clinical problems and applications.
2. Assure the continuity of the original validity, standard, and several supplementary scales by keeping these measures relatively intact.
3. Develop new scales to address problems that were not covered in the original MMPI.
4. Collect new, representative, randomly solicited, and nationally based nonpatient samples of adults and adolescents, in order to develop age-appropriate norms.
5. Develop new normative distributions for the MMPI-2 and MMPI-A scales that would better reflect clinical problems.
6. Collect a broad range of clinical data for evaluating changes in the original scales and for validating the new scales.

Development of New Norms

The MMPI-2 normative sample consisted of 2,600 subjects (1,462 women and 1,138 men, ages 18 through the adult years), sampled from seven states in different geographic regions (California, Minnesota, North Carolina, Ohio, Pennsylvania, Virginia, and Washington). The normative sample was balanced for gender and important demographic characteristics such as ethnic group membership. Normative subjects were randomly selected, initially contacted by letter, and asked to come to a prearranged testing site for completion of the test battery. All subjects were administered the 704-item experimental form of the MMPI, a biographical questionnaire, and a questionnaire assessing significant life events in the past 6 months. In addition to the normative study described in the manual for the MMPI-2, a number of other normative and clinical studies provided additional validation for the MMPI-2 standard scales and new content scales.

The norms for the MMPI-2 were constructed to eliminate two problems with the original MMPI norms. First, as noted above, the norms were based on a large contemporary sample of individuals drawn from across the United States. Second, the norms were expressed as standard scores (T-scores), each with a mean of 50 and a standard deviation of 10. Employing T-scores assured that the meaning of each scale, relative to a normative value, would be uniform for any given level. That is, for a given T-score, the percentile value of the clinical and content scale scores would be equivalent. As a result of the new normative procedures, there are small differences between T-scores generated by the original and new procedures. However, it is important to realize that the relationship between the uniform T-score distribution and the original MMPI distribution is very strong, and that both are based on a linear T-score transformation for the raw scores (Tellegen & Ben-Porath, 1992).

As a result of maintaining the continuity between the original MMPI and the MMPI-2, the validity research on the original scales has been shown to apply equally well to the MMPI-2 (Graham, 1988, 1990). In addition, a number of studies was conducted to provide new validation information for the scales, to ensure that they maintained their validity during the revision process. Several recent studies have provided evidence of the validity of the traditional clinical scales on the MMPI-2 (Ben-Porath & Butcher, 1989a, 1989b; Ben-Porath, Butcher, & Graham, 1991; Butcher et al., 1991; Butcher, Graham, Dahlstrom, & Bowman, 1990; Butcher, Jeffrey, et al., 1990; Egeland, Erickson, Butcher, & Ben-Porath, 1991; Hjemboe & Butcher, 1991; Keller & Butcher, 1991). Several additional scales, often referred to as "supplemental scales," were retained from the original MMPI (the Anxiety, Repression, Ego Strength, MacAndrew Alcoholism, and Overcontrolled Hostility scales). In addition, several new supplementary scales were published in the MMPI-2 to assess specific problems, such as drug and alcohol abuse (the Addiction Potential scale and Addiction Acknowledgment scale) and marital problems (the Marital Distress scale) (Weed, Butcher, Ben-Porath, & McKenna, 1992). A brief description of the MMPI-2 validity scales is provided in Table 6.1, and the clinical and supplemental scales are described in Table 6.2.

Development of the MMPI-2 Content Scales

Interpretation of item content is based on the view that responses to items are communications about an individual's feelings, personality style, and past or current problems. It is assumed that the individual wishes to reveal his or her ideas, attitudes, beliefs, and problems, and then cooperates with

TABLE 6.1. Description of the MMPI-2 Validity Scales

Cannot Say (?) score. The total number of unanswered items. A defensive protocol with possible attenuation of scale scores is suggested if the ? raw score is more than 30.

Lie (L) scale. A measure of unsophisticated or self-consciously "virtuous" test-taking attitude. Elevated scores (T > 65) suggest that the individual is presenting him- or herself in an overly positive light—attempting to create an unrealistically favorable view of his or her adjustment.

Infrequency (F) scale. The items on this scale are answered in the nonkeyed direction by most people. A high score (T > 80) suggests an exaggerated pattern of symptom checking that is inconsistent with accurate self-appraisal and suggests confusion, disorganization, or actual faking of mental illness. Scores above 110 invalidate the profile.

Defensiveness (K) scale. Measures an individual's willingness to disclose personal information and discuss his or her problems. High scores (T > 65) reflect an uncooperative attitude and an unwillingness or reluctance to disclose personal information. Low scores (T < 45) suggest openness and frankness. This scale is positively correlated with intelligence and educational level, which should be taken into account when interpreting the scores.

Back F (FB) scale. This scale was incorporated into the MMPI-2 to detect possible deviant responding to items located toward the end of the item pool. Some subjects, tiring of taking the test, may modify their approach to the items partway through the item pool and answer in a random or unselective manner. Since all of the items on the F scale occur before item 370, the F scale, or F–K, may not detect such changes in response pattern. This 40-item scale was developed in a manner analogous to the development of the original F scale—that is, by including items that had low endorsement percentages in the normal population.

Variable Response Inconsistency (VRIN) scale. The VRIN scale consists of 49 pairs of specially selected items. The members of each VRIN pair have either similar or opposite content; each pair is scored for the occurrence of an inconsistency in responses to the two items. The VRIN score is the total number of item pairs answered inconsistently. A high VRIN score is a warning that a test subject may have been answering the items in the inventory in an indiscriminate manner, and raises the possibility that the protocol may be invalid and that the profile is essentially uninterpretable.

True Response Inconsistency (TRIN) scale. The TRIN scale is comprised of 20 pairs of items that are opposite in content. If a subject responds inconsistently by answering "True" to both items of certain pairs, 1 point is added to the TRIN score; if the subject responds inconsistently by answering "False" to certain item pairs, 1 point is subtracted. A very high TRIN score indicates a tendency to give "True" answers to the items indiscriminately ("acquiescence"); a very low TRIN score indicates a tendency to answer "False" indiscriminately ("nonacquiescence"). (Negative TRIN scores are avoided by adding a constant to the raw score.) A very low or very high TRIN score is a warning that the test subject may have been answering the inventory indiscriminately, so that the profile may be invalid and uninterpretable.

Note. Adapted from J. N. Butcher, MMPI-2 workshops and symposia, University of Minnesota.

TABLE 6.2. Description of the MMPI-2 Clinical and Supplemental Scales

Clinical scales

Scale 1: Hypochondriasis (Hs)

High scores: Excessive bodily concern; somatic symptoms that tend to be vague and undefined; epigastric complaints; fatigue, pain, weakness; lacks manifest anxiety; selfish, self-centered, and narcissistic; pessimistic, defeatist, cynical outlook on life; dissatisfied and unhappy; makes others miserable; whines, complains; demanding and critical of others; expresses hostility indirectly; rarely acts out; dull, unenthusiastic, unambitious; ineffective in oral expression; longstanding health concerns; functions at a reduced level of efficiency without major incapacity; not very responsive to therapy; tends to terminate therapy when therapist is seen as not giving enough attention and support; seeks medical solutions to psychological problems.

Scale 2: Depression (D)

High scores: Depressed, unhappy, and dysphoric; pessimistic; self-deprecating, guilty; sluggish; somatic complaints; weakness, fatigue, and loss of energy; agitated, tense, high strung, irritable, prone to worry; lacks self-confidence; feels useless and unable to function; feels like a failure at school or on the job; introverted, shy, retiring, timid, and reclusive; aloof; maintains psychological distance; avoids interpersonal involvement; cautious and conventional; has difficulty making decisions; nonaggressive; overcontrolled, denies impulses; makes concessions to avoid conflict; likely to be motivated for therapy.

Scale 3: Hysteria (Hy)

High scores: Reacts to stress and avoids responsibility through development of physical symptoms; has headaches, chest pains, weakness, and tachycardia; anxiety attacks; symptoms appear and disappear suddenly; lacks insight about causes of symptoms; lacks insight about own motives and feelings; lacks manifest anxiety, tension, and depression; rarely reports delusions, hallucinations, or suspiciousness; psychologically immature, childish, and infantile; self-centered, narcissistic, and egocentric; expects attention and affection from others; uses indirect and devious means to get attention and affection; does not express hostility and resentment openly; socially involved, friendly, talkative, and enthusiastic; superficial and immature in interpersonal relationships; shows interest in others for selfish reasons; occasionally acts out in a sexual or aggressive manner with little apparent insight; initially enthusiastic about treatment; responds well to direct advice or suggestion; slow to gain insight into causes of own behavior; resistant to psychological interpretations.

Scale 4: Psychopathic Deviate (Pd)

High scores: Antisocial behavior; rebellious toward authority figures; stormy family relationships; blames parents for problems; history of underachievement in school; poor work history; marital problems; impulsive; strives for immediate gratification of impulses; does not plan well; acts without considering consequences of actions; impatient; limited frustration tolerance; poor judgment; takes risks; does not profit from experience; immature, childish, narcissistic, self-centered, and selfish; ostentatious, exhibitionistic; insensitive; interested in others in terms of how they can be used; likable and usually creates a good first impression; shallow, superficial

(continued)

TABLE 6.2. *(continued)*

relationships, unable to form warm attachments; extroverted, outgoing; talkative, active, energetic, and spontaneous; intelligent; asserts self-confidence; has a wide range of interests; lacks definite goals; hostile, aggressive; sarcastic, cynical; resentful, rebellious; acts out; antagonistic; impulsive outbursts, assaultive behavior; little guilt over negative behavior; may feign guilt and remorse when in trouble; is free from disabling anxiety, depression, and psychotic symptoms; likely to have personality disorder diagnosis (antisocial or passive–aggressive); is dissatisfied; shows absence of deep emotional response; feels bored and empty; poor prognosis for change in therapy; blames others for problems; intellectualizes; may agree to treatment to avoid jail or some other unpleasant experience, but is likely to terminate therapy before change is effected.

Scale 5: Masculinity–Femininity (Mf)

Males
   High scores (*T* > 80): Shows conflicts about sexual identity; insecure in masculine role; effeminate; aesthetic and artistic interests; intelligent and capable; values cognitive pursuits; ambitious, competitive, and persevering; clever, clear thinking, organized, logical; shows good judgment and common sense; curious; creative, imaginative, and individualistic in approach to problems; sociable; sensitive to others; tolerant; capable of expressing warm feelings toward others; passive, dependent, and submissive; peace-loving; makes concessions to avoid confrontations; good self-control; rarely acts out. (The interpretation of high scores should be tempered for males with advanced academic degrees.)
   High scores (*T* = 70–79): May be viewed as sensitive; insightful; tolerant; effeminate; showing broad cultural interests; submissive, passive. (In clinical settings, the patient may show sex-role confusion or heterosexual adjustment problems.)
   Low scores (*T* < 35): "Macho" self-image, presents self as extremely masculine; overemphasizes strength and physical prowess; aggressive, thrill seeking, adventurous, and reckless; coarse, crude, and vulgar; harbors doubts about own masculinity; has limited intellectual ability; narrow range of interests; inflexible and unoriginal approach to problems; prefers action to thought; is practical and nontheoretical; easygoing, leisurely, and relaxed; cheerful, jolly, humorous; contented; willing to settle down; unaware of social stimulus value; lacks insight into own motives; unsophisticated.

Females
   High scores (*T* > 70): Rejects traditional female roles and activities; masculine interests in work, sports, hobbies; active, vigorous, and assertive; competitive, aggressive, and dominating; coarse, rough, and tough; outgoing, uninhibited, and self-confident; easygoing, relaxed, balanced; logical, calculated; unemotional and unfriendly.
   Low scores (T < 35). Describes self in terms of stereotyped female role; doubts about own femininity; passive, submissive, and yielding; defers to males in decision making; self-pitying; complaining, faultfinding; constricted; sensitive; modest; idealistic. (This interpretation for low scores does not apply for females with postgraduate degrees.)

(continued)

TABLE 6.2. *(continued)*

Scale 6: Paranoia (Pa)

Extremely high scores (*T* > 80): Frankly psychotic behavior; disturbed thinking; delusions of persecution and/or grandeur; ideas of reference; feels mistreated and picked on; angry and resentful; harbors grudges; uses projection as defense; most frequently diagnosed as schizophrenic or paranoid.

Moderately high scores (*T* = 65–79 for males, 71–79 for females): Paranoid predisposition; sensitive; overly responsive to reactions of others; feels he or she is getting a raw deal from life; rationalizes and blames others; suspicious and guarded; hostile, resentful, and argumentative; moralistic and rigid; overemphasizes rationality; poor prognosis for therapy; does not like to talk about emotional problems; difficulty in establishing rapport with therapist.

Extremely low scores (*T* < 35): Should be interpreted with caution. In a clinical setting, low scores in the context of a defensive response set may suggest frankly psychotic disorder; delusions, suspiciousness, ideas of reference; symptoms less obvious than for high scorers; evasive, defensive, guarded; shy, secretive, withdrawn.

Scale 7: Psychasthenia (Pt)

High scores: Anxious, tense, and agitated; high discomfort; worried and apprehensive; high-strung and jumpy; difficulties in concentrating; introspective, ruminative; obsessive and compulsive; feels insecure and inferior; lacks self-confidence; self-doubting, self-critical, self-conscious, and self-derogatory; rigid and moralistic; maintains high standards for self and others; overly perfectionistic and conscientious; guilty and depressed; neat, orderly, organized, and meticulous; persistent; reliable; lacks ingenuity and originality in problem solving; dull and formal; vacillates; is indecisive; distorts importance of problems, overreacts; shy; does not interact well socially; hard to get to know; worries about popularity and acceptance; sensitive, physical complaints; shows some insight into problems; intellectualizes and rationalizes; resistant to interpretations in therapy; expresses hostility toward therapist; remains in therapy longer than most patients; makes slow but steady progress in therapy.

Scale 8: Schizophrenia (Sc)

Very high scores (*T* = 81–90): Blatantly psychotic behavior; confused, disorganized, and disoriented; unusual thoughts or attitudes; delusions; hallucinations; poor judgment.

High scores (*T* = 65–79): Schizoid lifestyle; does not feel a part of social environment; feels isolated, alienated, and misunderstood; feels unaccepted by peers; withdrawn, seclusive, secretive, and inaccessible; avoids dealing with people and new situations; shy, aloof, and uninvolved; experiences generalized anxiety; resentful, hostile, and aggressive; unable to express feelings; reacts to stress by withdrawing into fantasy and daydreaming; difficulty in separating reality and fantasy; self-doubts; feels inferior, incompetent, and dissatisfied; sexual preoccupation and sex-role confusion; nonconforming, unusual, unconventional, and eccentric; vague, longstanding, physical complaints; stubborn, moody, and opinionated; immature and impulsive; high-strung; imaginative; abstract, vague goals; lacks basic information for problem solving; poor prognosis for therapy; reluctant to relate in meaningful way to therapist; stays in therapy longer than most patients; may eventually learn to trust therapist.

(continued)

TABLE 6.2. *(continued)*

Scale 9: Hypomania (Ma)

High scores ($T > 80$): Periods of excessive activity; accelerated speech; may have hallucinations or delusions of grandeur; energetic and talkative; prefers action to thought; wide range of interest; does not utilize energy wisely; does not see projects through to completion; creative, enterprising, and ingenious; little interest in routine or detail; easily bored and restless; low frustration tolerance; difficulty in inhibiting expression of impulses; episodes of irritability, hostility, and aggressive outbursts; unrealistic, unqualified optimism; grandiose aspirations; exaggerates self-worth and self-importance; unable to see own limitations; outgoing, sociable, and gregarious; likes to be around other people; creates good first impression; friendly, pleasant, and enthusiastic; poised, self-confident; superficial relationships; manipulative, deceptive, unreliable; feelings of dissatisfaction; agitated; may have periodic episodes of depression; difficulties at school or work; resistant to interpretations in therapy; attends therapy irregularly; may terminate therapy prematurely; repeats problems in stereotyped manner; not likely to become dependent on therapist; becomes hostile and aggressive toward therapist.

Moderately elevated scores ($T > 65, \leq 79$): Overactive lifestyle; exaggerated sense of self-worth; energetic and talkative; prefers action to thought; wide range of interest; does not utilize energy wisely; does not see projects through to completion; enterprising and ingenious; lacks interest in routine matters; becomes bored and restless easily; low frustration tolerance; impulsive; episodes of irritability, hostility, and aggressive outbursts; unrealistic, overly optimistic at times; shows some grandiose aspirations; unable to see own limitations; outgoing, sociable, and gregarious; likes to be around other people; creates good first impression; friendly, pleasant, and enthusiastic; poised, self-confident; superficial relationships; manipulative, deceptive, unreliable; feelings of dissatisfaction; agitated; views therapy as unnecessary; resistant to interpretations in therapy; attends therapy irregularly; may terminate therapy prematurely; repeats problems in stereotyped manner; not likely to become dependent on therapist; becomes hostile and aggressive toward therapist.

Low scores ($T < 40$): Low energy level; low activity level; lethargic, listless, apathetic, and phlegmatic; difficult to motivate; reports chronic fatigue, physical exhaustion; depressed, anxious, and tense; reliable, responsible, and dependable; approaches problems in conventional, practical, and reasonable way; lacks self-confidence; sincere, quiet, modest, withdrawn, seclusive; unpopular; overcontrolled; unlikely to express feelings openly.

Scale 0: Social Introversion (Si)

High scores ($T > 65$): Socially introverted; is more comfortable alone or with a few close friends; reserved, shy, and retiring; uncomfortable around members of opposite sex; hard to get to know; sensitive to what others think; troubled by lack of involvement with other people; overcontrolled; not likely to display feelings openly; submissive and compliant; overly accepting of authority; serious, slow personal tempo; reliable, dependable; cautious, conventional, unoriginal in approach to problems; rigid, inflexible in attitudes and opinions; difficulty making even minor decisions; enjoys work; gains pleasure from productive personal achievement; tends to worry; is irritable and anxious; moody, experiences guilt feelings; has episodes of depression or low mood.

(continued)

TABLE 6.2. *(continued)*

Low scores ($T < 45$): Sociable and extroverted; outgoing, gregarious, friendly, and talkative; strong need to be around other people; mixes well; intelligent, expressive, verbally fluent; active, energetic, vigorous; interested in status, power, and recognition; seeks out competitive situations; has problem with impulse control; acts without considering the consequences of actions; immature, self-indulgent; superficial, insincere relationships; manipulative, opportunistic; arouses resentment and hostility in others.

Supplemental scales

Anxiety (A) scale. This scale defines the first, and largest, factor dimension in the MMPI-2. It measures general maladjustment or emotional upset.

Repression (R) scale. This scale assesses emotional overcontrol and reliance on denial and repression. It defines the second main factor in the MMPI-2.

Ego Strength (Es) scale. This scale was developed as a means of predicting successful response to psychotherapy. To develop the scale, "successful" therapy patients were contrasted with another group of patients who had failed to benefit from treatment.

MacAndrew Alcoholism (MAC-R) scale. The MAC-R scale is the revised version of the MAC scale on the original MMPI. It is an empirically derived scale that assesses the potential for developing substance abuse problems.

Dominance (Do) scale. This scale was developed to identify dominant individuals by asking their peers to identify them as one or the other. The Do scale measures comfort in social relationships, self-confidence, strong opinions, persevering at tasks, and ability to concentrate.

Social Responsibility (Re) scale. This scale was developed as a means of predicting an individual's feelings of responsibility to others.

Overcontrolled Hostility (O-H) scale. This scale was developed to identify individuals who have difficulty expressing anger and usually overcontrol their hostile impulses, yet have engaged in assaultive behavior.

Post-Traumatic Stress Disorder (PTSD-PK/PS) scales. The PK scale, developed to assess PTSD in veterans, uses an empirical scale construction strategy to discriminate individuals who are experiencing symptoms of PTSD.

Marital Distress scale (MDS). This scale was developed for MMPI-2 and was designed to identify distress or discord in close relationships.

Addiction Potential scale (APS). This scale was constructed as a measure of personality characteristics and life situations associated with substance abuse.

Addiction Acknowledgment scale (AAS). This scale began with a rational (as opposed to statistical) search through the pool for items with content indicating substance abuse problems, and was refined by statistical methods. The scale assesses the degree to which the individual acknowledges alcohol or drug problems.

Note. Adapted from J. N. Butcher, MMPI-2 workshops and symposia, University of Minnesota.

the testing by truthfully acknowledging them. Most people taking the inventory provide accurate information about themselves.

The content scales for the MMPI-2, described more fully in Table 6.3, were developed to assess the main content dimensions in the revised inventory (Butcher, Graham, Williams, et al., 1990). The new MMPI-2 content scales were developed by a multimethod, multistage scale construction strategy, in which both rational and statistical procedures were employed to ensure content homogeneity and strong statistical properties. The new MMPI-2 content scales assess several important areas of symptomatic behavior (Anxiety, Fears, Obsessiveness, Depression, Health Concerns, and Bizarre Mentation). They also include two personality factor scales (Type A Behavior, Cynicism), two externalizing scales (Anger, Antisocial Practices), a negative self-view scale (Low Self-Esteem), and important clinical problem area scales (Family Problems, Work Interference, Negative Treatment Indicators).

The MMPI-2 content scales have been shown to have strong internal psychometric properties, along with external validity. For example, comparisons between the MMPI-2 content scales and the original MMPI clinical scales using the same behavioral descriptors showed the content scales to possess external validity equal to, or greater than, that of the clinical scales (Ben-Porath et al., 1991; Butcher, Graham, Williams, et al., 1990). Additional studies confirmed the external validity of many of the content scales. The FAM scale was associated with marital and family problems (Hjemboe & Butcher, 1991); the ASP scale has been found to be significantly related to antisocial personality and behavior (DSM-III-R-based; Lilienfeld, 1996); the ASP scale also differentiated mothers who had been identified as at high risk for abusing their children from other women taking the test (Egeland et al., 1991); the HEA scale significantly discriminated chronic pain patients from the MMPI-2 normative sample (Keller & Butcher, 1991); the ANG scale was found to be correlated significantly with other measures of anger (Schill & Wang, 1990); and the LSE scale showed high internal consistency and strong assessment of a global self-esteem assessment (Brems & Lloyd,1995).

Two studies provided empirical verification for MMPI-2 content scales. Faull and Meyer (1993) found that the Depression content scale on the MMPI-2 outperformed the MMPI-2 Depression clinical scale in assessment of subjective depression in a group of primary medical patients. In another study, Clark (1993) reported that patients in a Department of Veterans Affairs chronic pain program who had high scores on the MMPI-2 Anger content scale showed frequent and intense anger, felt unfairly treated by others, felt frustrated, were oversensitive to criticism, were quick-tempered, tended to externalize anger, had tenuous anger control, were impulsive, and had anger control problems. Munley, Busby and Jaynes (1997)

TABLE 6.3. Description of the MMPI-2 Content Scales

1. *Anxiety (ANX; 23 items)*. High scorers on ANX report general symptoms of anxiety, including tension, somatic problems (i.e., heart pounding and shortness of breath), sleep difficulties, worries, and poor concentration. They fear losing their minds, find life a strain, and have difficulties making decisions. They appear to be readily aware of these symptoms and problems, and are willing to admit to them.

2. *Fears (FRS; 23 items)*. A high score on FRS indicates an individual with many specific fears. These specific fears can include blood; high places; money; animals such as snakes, mice, or spiders; leaving home; fire; storms and natural disasters; water; the dark; being indoors; and dirt.

3. *Obsessiveness (OBS; 16 items)*. High scorers on OBS have tremendous difficulties making decisions and are likely to ruminate excessively about issues and problems, causing others to become impatient. Having to make changes distresses them, and they may report some compulsive behaviors, like counting or saving unimportant things. They are excessive worriers who frequently become overwhelmed by their own thoughts.

4. *Depression (DEP; 33 items)*. High scores on this scale characterize individuals with significant depressive thoughts. They report feeling blue, uncertain about their future, and uninterested in their lives. They are likely to brood, be unhappy, cry easily, and feel hopeless and empty. They may report thoughts of suicide or wishes that they were dead. They may believe that they are condemned or have committed unpardonable sins. Other people may not be viewed as a source of support.

5. *Health Concerns (HEA; 36 items)*. Individuals with high scores on HEA report many physical symptoms across several body systems. Included are gastrointestinal symptoms (e.g., constipation, nausea and vomiting, stomach trouble), neurological problems (e.g., convulsions, dizzy and fainting spells, paralysis), sensory problems (e.g., poor hearing or eyesight), cardiovascular symptoms (e.g., heart or chest pains), skin problems, pain (e.g., headaches, neck pains), and respiratory troubles (e.g., coughs, hay fever or asthma). These individuals worry about their health and feel sicker than the average person.

6. *Bizarre Mentation (BIZ; 24 items)*. Psychotic thought processes characterize individuals high on the BIZ scale. They may report auditory, visual, or olfactory hallucinations, and may recognize that their thoughts are strange and peculiar. Paranoid ideation (e.g., the belief that they are being plotted against or that someone is trying to poison them) may be reported as well. These individuals may feel that they have a special mission or power.

7. *Anger (ANG; 16 items)*. High scores on the ANG scale suggest anger control problems. These individuals report being irritable, grouchy, impatient, hotheaded, annoyed, and stubborn. They sometimes feel like swearing or smashing things. They may lose self-control and report having been physically abusive toward people and objects.

8. *Cynicism (CYN; 23 items)*. Misanthropic beliefs characterize high scorers on CYN. They expect hidden, negative motives behind the acts of others—for

(continued)

TABLE 6.3. *(continued)*

example, believing that most people are honest simply for fear of being caught. Other people are to be distrusted, for people use each other and are only friendly for selfish reasons. They likely hold negative attitudes about those close to them, including fellow workers, family, and friends.

9. *Antisocial Practices (ASP; 22 items).* In addition to holding similar misanthropic attitudes as high scorers on the CYN scale, high scorers on the ASP scale report problem behaviors during their school years and other antisocial practices, such as being in trouble with the law, stealing, or shoplifting. They report sometimes enjoying the antics of criminals and believe that it is all right to get around the law, as long as it is not broken.

10. *Type A Behavior (TPA; 19 items).* High scorers on TPA are hard-driving, fast-moving, and work-oriented individuals who frequently become impatient, irritable, and annoyed. They do not like to wait or be interrupted. There is never enough time in a day for them to complete their tasks. They are direct and may be overbearing in their relationships with others.

11. *Low Self-Esteem (LSE; 24 items).* High scores on LSE characterize individuals with low opinions of themselves. They do not believe that they are liked by others or that they are important. They hold many negative attitudes about themselves, including beliefs that they are unattractive, awkward and clumsy, useless, and a burden to others. They certainly lack self-confidence and find it hard to accept compliments from others. They may be overwhelmed by all the faults they see in themselves.

12. *Social Discomfort (SOD; 24 items).* SOD high scorers are very uneasy around others, preferring to be by themselves. When in social situations, they are likely to sit alone rather than joining in the group. They see themselves as shy and dislike parties and other group events.

13. *Family Problems (FAM; 25 items).* Considerable family discord is reported by high scorers on FAM. Their families are described as lacking in love, quarrelsome, and unpleasant. They even may report hating members of their families. Their childhood may be portrayed as abusive, and marriages may be seen as unhappy and lacking in affection.

14. *Work Interference (WRK; 33 items).* A high score on WRK is indicative of behaviors or attitudes likely to contribute to poor work performance. Some of the problems relate to low self-confidence, concentration difficulties, obsessiveness, tension and pressure, and decision-making problems. Others suggest lack of family support for the career choice, personal questioning of career choice, and negative attitudes toward coworkers.

15. *Negative Treatment Indicators (TRT; 26 items).* High scores on TRT indicate individuals with negative attitudes toward doctors and mental health treatment. High scorers do not believe that anyone can understand or help them. They have issues or problems that they are not comfortable discussing with anyone. They may not want to change anything in their lives, nor do they feel that change is possible. They prefer giving up, rather than facing a crisis or difficulty.

Note. From Butcher, Graham, Williams, & Ben-Porath (1990). Copyright 1990 by the Regents of the University of Minnesota. Reprinted by permission.

showed that the BIZ and DEP scales separated depressed inpatients from schizophrenic inpatients more effectively than did the MMPI-2 clinical scales D and Sc.

Two other studies conducted research on the construct validity of the content scales: the DEP scale had higher internal consistency and greater convergence with other depression measures than Scale 2 (D) of the MMPI-2 (Faull & Meyer, 1993). The DEP content scale was found to be significantly related to other measures, including those for depression, hopelessness, low self-esteem, and suicidal ideation (Boone, 1994).

Current Status of MMPI-2 Use

The MMPI-2 has been reported to be the most widely used personality assessment instrument in recent surveys of licensed mental health professionals (Frauenhoffer, Ross, Gfeller, Searight, & Piotrowski, 1998). Other surveys have reported similar conclusions (Borum & Grisso, 1995; Lees-Haley, 1992; Lees-Haley, Smith, Williams, & Dunn, 1996). In fact, 100% of frequent assessors surveyed in one survey used the MMPI or MMPI-2 in personal injury cases (Boccaccini & Brodsky, 1999). They also reported that the MMPI was the only instrument used by the majority of psychologists conducting emotional injury assessments. Piotrowski (1998) reported that the MMPI/MMPI-2 was the most frequently used instrument for assessing pain, with 76% of respondents reporting that they "almost always" use the instrument for pain assessment. The original MMPI was withdrawn from use by the test publisher, the University of Minnesota Press, in 1999 and is no longer available or recommended for use.

Since the publication of the MMPI-2 in 1989, the instrument has been widely adapted into other languages and cultures. There are over 25 available translations in a variety of languages, and the test is widely used as a clinical and research instrument in many other countries at this point (Butcher, 1996; Butcher et al., 1998).

ADMINISTRATION AND SCORING

The MMPI-2 provides a relatively easy administration format compared with many other clinical assessment methods. Most people are accustomed to completing paper-and-pencil surveys, and can, with brief instructions, become readily engaged in the task. Since the MMPI-2 is a structured task, it is important that the person administering the test follow the test instructions closely. It is also important to determine, in advance, whether clients can understand the items and mark their responses in the appropriate place. It takes a fifth- or sixth-grade reading level to understand the MMPI-2 items. The inventory can be administered in several ways: by the traditional paper-and-pencil form, by audiocassette, or by computer. Individuals are instructed to read the items and determine whether each item is true or false, as applied to them. They are asked to mark a T or F in the appropriate place on the answer sheet, or to respond by pressing the appropriate key on the computer keyboard.

The scoring of the MMPI-2 scales is easy and objective. In the case of manual scoring of the test, the practitioner simply places a scoring template over the answer sheet and counts the number of items endorsed in the scored direction on each scale. The raw scores are then placed in the appropriate place on the profile sheet. Once all of the scales are scored, the profile is drawn by connecting the dots that mark the appropriate raw score level on the profile. In the case of five of the clinical scales, a correction factor for test defensiveness (the Defensiveness or K factor) is added to the raw score before plotting the profile.

The objective administration, scoring, and interpretation procedures for the MMPI-2 make it particularly well suited to computer processing. Many practitioners today make use of a computer interpretation program to provide the "raw material" or test-based hypotheses for interpreting the MMPI-2. Later in this chapter, a computer-interpreted MMPI-2 protocol is presented to provide the reader with an illustration of an objective test interpretation.

Developing Hypotheses about Clients

Useful hypotheses about client functioning can be obtained from various sources of information within the MMPI-2. One valuable interpretive strategy involves examining the MMPI-2–based test indices with certain questions in mind, in order to generate interpretive hypotheses about the individual's personality functioning and current behavior:

What is the motivation of the client to participate in the assessment process?
What are the client's cognitive and ideational processes like?
How is the individual functioning in interpersonal contexts?
Is he or she likely to remain stable over time, or is change possible?
What are the likely clinical diagnostic issues?
Is this individual amenable to psychological treatment?

In the discussion that follows, we examine a general strategy for interpreting MMPI-2 profiles and explore the variables in the MMPI-2 that address the questions of interest. Then we present a case illustration, analyzed by a computer-based MMPI-2 system, to show how an objective appraisal of the MMPI-2 indices can provide the practitioner with a substantial amount of information that can be incorporated into a diagnostic evaluation.

The interpretation of MMPI-2 scales and profiles involves a sequential analysis based on several types of information in the test. First, and often considered to be the most important to interpretation, is an assessment of the individual's approach to the test items by appraising the MMPI-2 validity scales. The next step in the interpretation process involves the determination of the likely empirical behavioral correlates that have been established for the clinical and supplementary scales. In the third step, the MMPI-2 item content, as noted above, can be used as a direct source of information about specific concerns that can, in turn, be incorporated into the interpretive process. We demonstrate how these levels of analysis work in the following sections of this chapter, as we consider each in turn.

Assessment of Profile Validity

Understanding the client's motivation and investment in the assessment process is a key factor in the interpretation of self-report instruments (Ben-Porath & Tellegen, 1993). Individuals taking the MMPI-2 under certain conditions may have clear motivations to present themselves in particular ways. For example, litigants in personal injury cases may tend to exaggerate their complaints; men and women being evaluated in family custody cases tend to present themselves in a highly virtuous and unrealistic manner. It is extremely important for a practitioner to assure that a test protocol was produced in a cooperative and open manner, without test-taking response patterns that prevent the practitioner from obtaining valid information.

The MMPI-2 contains a number of measures that address test-taking attitudes and provide the clinician with a means of knowing whether the client has cooperated sufficiently with the evaluation to provide an accurate portrayal of his or her personality characteristics and problems (see Table 6.1). For example, the motivation for respondents to present themselves in a favorable light or to be defensive in the assessment is usually detected by the Lie scale or the Defensiveness scale (Baer, Wetter, & Berry, 1992). On the other hand, individuals who wish to be perceived as having extreme psychological problems tend to exaggerate their symptoms. This exaggerated symptom-checking approach usually produces extreme elevations on the two scales that assess faking: the Infrequency scale and the Back F scale (Berry, Baer, & Harris, 1991; Graham, Watts, & Timbrook, 1991; Rogers, Bagby, & Chakraborty, 1993; Schretlen, 1988; Wetter, Baer, Berry, Robison, & Sumpter, 1993; Wetter, Baer, Berry, Smith, & Larsen, 1992).

In addition to these invalidating conditions, there may be unusual, noncontent-oriented response sets operating in the test performance. These conditions are detected by other measures in the MMPI-2: For example, random responding is detected by the Variable Response Inconsistency scale, and mostly true or mostly false response patterns are detected by the True Response Inconsistency scale (Berry et al., 1992; Tellegen & Ben-Porath, 1992).

Assessment of STS Dimensions of Personality and Behavior

The second step in MMPI-2 analysis involves the translation of scale scores and patterns into meaningful predictions of behavior. This step includes two tasks: (1) the identification of the types of problems characterizing a given patient, and (2) the prediction of how this person will respond to treatment, both generally and specifically.

Identifying Patient Characteristics. This section demonstrates how the MMPI-2 clinical, supplemental, and content measures can be employed to provide information about the client's functioning in several areas related to mental status: (1) cognitive/ideational functions, (2) mood and affect (including emotional stability), (3) specific conflict areas, and (4) diagnostic considerations. Embedded within these areas of functioning is information on the six STS dimensions that relate to predicting prognosis, diagnosis, and treatment planning. This information is frequently incorporated into the psychological report.

1. *Cognitive/ideational functions.* The MMPI-2 clinical scales provide a valid picture of the behavioral problems or symptoms the individual is experiencing, especially as related to the STS dimensions of functional impairment. Generally (there are a few exceptions), high scores reflect increasing levels of functional impairment. Specifically, elevations on the Paranoia and Schizophrenia clinical scales are associated with extreme cognitive impairment and thought disorder. High elevations on the Psychasthenia clinical scale or the Obsessiveness content scale suggest extreme preoccupation with disordered thinking, such as pathological rumination and obsessive–compulsive behavior.

2. *Mood and affect.* A patient's symptomatic behavior and mood are reflected in the MMPI-2 clinical and content scales. The mood scales indicate both the level and type of specific emotional states and are particularly relevant to the STS dimension of distress. Distress level is salient to later treatment planning, as described in the STS system. The interpretation of MMPI-2 scales should identify both the levels of specific moods and affects and the overall level of emotional distress and intensity.

Examination of the correlates for high scores on the Depression clinical scale (see Table 6.2) suggests that the high-scoring individual is likely to be depressed, unhappy, and dysphoric at the present time. These individuals show personality characteristics such as a pessimistic attitude about life, a self-deprecating self-concept, tendencies toward feeling guilty, and concern over failure on the job. In addition, they are usually introverted, shy, and timid, and tend to avoid interpersonal involvement. Substantial information on the empirical correlates of the MMPI-2 clinical scales has accumulated over the past 60 years (see Butcher, Rouse, & Perry, 2000; Gilberstadt & Duker, 1965; Graham, Ben-Porath, & McNulty, 2000; Lewandowski & Graham, 1972; Marks, Seeman, & Haller, 1974).

3. *Specific conflict areas.* The intensity of interpersonal conflicts are inversely correlated with the STS dimension social support level and are frequently indicative of high levels of resistance to external influence. Individuals with high levels of social conflict do not tend to generate social support, and they often resist assistance and help from others. These impairments around interpersonal relationships and the resulting social difficulties, moreover, are frequently transferred to the clinician who is providing treatment, especially if the patient's conflicts lead to resistance—that is, efforts to avoid being influenced by authorities or to complying with these authoritative demands.

In addition to the extensive information available on the symptomatic status of individuals from the MMPI-2 clinical scales, several of the supplemental scales provide information about specific problems (see Table 6.2). For example, several scales address possible problems with alcohol or drug abuse; one scale, the Marital Distress scale, focuses upon marital problems; and the Post-Traumatic Stress Disorder scales address symptomatic behavior related to this disorder. The TRT, a scale that is specifically designed to reflect level of treatment resistance, indicates when interpersonal resistance to authorities may interfere with treatment progress.

4. *Intra- and interpersonal coping styles.* The MMPI-2 provides several types of information related to interpersonal–intrapersonal functioning. Central to these descriptions is information on external and internal coping styles, as presented in the STS system. First, many of the MMPI-2 clinical scales have established empirical correlates that reflect the manner in which the individual deals with others. For example, the Psychopathic Deviate scale on the MMPI-2 is associated with interpersonal difficulty, aggressiveness, and the tendency to manipulate others for the subject's own gain (externalization). In addition, there are several specific indicators that address social deficits and internalizing defenses—for example, the Social Introversion (SI) and Psychasthenia (Pt) scales. High scores on the SI scale are characteristic of introverted, reclusive persons who have great difficulty in interpersonal contexts, whereas high scorers on the Pt scale indicate a worrisome and overcontrolled individual. Finally, interpersonal problem scales, such as the Family Problems content scale, can provide information as to specific interpersonal difficulties the individual may be encountering.

Dominant and enduring interpersonal patterns can be accurately classified by assessing the relative levels of externalizing and internalizing indices, as described in the STS system (Beutler, Clarkin, & Bongar, 2000). Coping styles, from this STS perspective, are identified by the presence of general personality dimensions, rather than indices of reactions that are only manifest during times of stress. Thus, "internalizing" tendencies include a propensity toward self-reflection as well as the more extreme patterns of self-criticism and self-punishment. This dimension also includes disruptions to emotional flexibility, as reflected in obsessive behaviors that constrain and overcontrol emotional responses, and the constriction of emotional expression. Finally, the internalizing dimension includes social patterns of withdrawal, constraint, and introversion. Thus, internalization is indexed by elevations on such scales as Hs (Hypochondriasis), D (Depression), Pt (Psychasthenia), and Si (Social Introversion) (see Beutler & Clarkin, 1990; Beutler et al., 2000; Gaw & Beutler, 1995).

In contrast to internalizing behaviors, "externalization" reflects a propensity to impulsivity, a relative absence of thought and planning, a tendency to feel controlled by circumstances rather than by self, and the denial of self-responsibility. This pattern is indexed on the MMPI-2 by elevations on such scales as Hy (Hysteria), Pd (Psychopathic Deviate), Pa (Paranoia), and Ma (Hypomania). The weight of these latter scales, relative to the internalizing scales, can provide a general index of the balance between, and salience of, internalization and externalization (Beutler et al., 2000; Fisher, Beutler, & Williams, 1999b; Gaw & Beutler, 1995).

5. *Diagnostic considerations.* Information is also available on the relationship between diagnostic classification and MMPI-2 scores. Diagnosis is an indirect indicator of level of the STS dimensions of functional impairment and chronicity/complexity. Although it is usually not a good practice to attempt to use MMPI-2 scores to signify a particular DSM code, some MMPI-2 profile types have been found to correspond fairly well with some DSM patterns (for examples, see Manos, 1985; Savasir & Erol, 1990). The value of the MMPI-2 in the diagnostic process is to provide likely behavioral correlates and symptom patterns for particular profile types.

Beyond simple diagnosis, however, it is important to determine the levels of dysfunction and chronicity attendant on patient problems. These factors bear heavily on predicting how quickly and how much change will occur. Chronic and severe problems resolve slowly and are subject to relapse. Thus indices such as the number of scales within the clinical range, the relative elevation of scales that suggest the presence of long-term problems (e.g., Sc, Ma, Si) relative to those that suggest the presence of acute distress (e.g., D, Pt, F) can serve to indicate the presence of complex and difficult problems that can be expected to impede the patient's prognosis. Social Introversion (Si) is a particularly valuable scale for indicating the level of social support available to the patient. Low levels of support are particularly strong impediments to achieving good posttreatment adjustments and allaying relapse.

Treatment Planning. The second task to be accomplished in the course of assessing patient behavior includes the determination of probable treatment response and the assignment of a specific treatment. The MMPI and MMPI-2 have been extensively used in treatment planning, and a substantial base of information is available on the use of the scales in predicting response to treatment. Numerous studies detailing the utility of the MMPI and MMPI-2 in treatment planning have been published (e.g., Apostal, 1971; Aronoff & Evans, 1982; Barron, 1953; Brandwin & Kewman, 1982; Butcher, 1990; Distler, May, & Tuma, 1964; Elliott, Anderson, & Adams, 1987; Haase & Ivey, 1970; Hollon & Mandell, 1979; Kuperman, Golden, & Blume, 1979; Moore, Armentraut, Parker, & Kivlahan, 1986; Pustell, 1958; Raab, Rickels, & Moore, 1964; Reich, Steward, Tupin, & Rosenblatt, 1985; Schofield, 1950, 1953; Shealy, Lowe, & Ritzier, 1980). In planning treatment that utilizes MMPI-2 results, the following types of information can provide a client with an important perspective on his or her problems:

1. The MMPI-2 scores provide objective, "outside" information that the therapist can employ in treatment sessions to bring into focus particular problems or personality characteristics relevant to the therapy.
2. The scale scores provide important problem summaries. When MMPI-2 content scales are used, the summaries are considered to provide "highly relevant" content themes that can be used to highlight the patient's problems and concerns (Butcher, Graham, Williams, et al., 1990).
3. The validity scales provide an appraisal of possible treatment resistance and other negative factors that could influence on the treatment process.
4. The validity and clinical scales provide an appraisal of the individual's motivation for treatment.
5. The clinical, content, and supplemental scales provide information about the client's need for therapy.
6. The MMPI-2 variables serve as an excellent mechanism for providing test feedback to clients in therapy—an important process that is described below (Finn & Martin, 1997).

Within the STS system, the MMPI-2 has been especially successful in identifying patient coping style and resistance levels. Although also useful for assessing levels of functional impairment and distress (e.g., Beutler, Kim, Davison, Karno, & Fisher, 1996), the results are less impressive and consistent.

Treatment plans that adapt intervents that are compatible with patient coping style and resistance levels have consistently resulted in more effective and enduring results (Beutler et al., 2000). Patients with externalizing defenses do best with treatments that focus on symptom change, whereas those with internalizing defenses do better with insight-oriented and aware-ness-based treatments. Likewise, patients with high levels of resistance tend to respond best to nondirective interventions, whereas those with low levels of resistance do well in therapist-controlled treatments (e.g., Beutler et al., 2000; Beutler, Engle, et al., 1991; Beutler, Mohr, Grawe, Engle, & Mac-Donald, 1991).

Content-Based Hypotheses

The third level of MMPI-2 interpretation involves an inspection of the content scales. These scales, which reflect similar themes based on manifest content, generally provide an overview of the areas that are identified by the patient as problematic.

Patients assessed in a mental health setting usually expect the mental health professional to pay careful attention to the content of their communications about their symptoms. With respect to the MMPI-2, in which patients are asked to share personal information about their symptoms and adjustment, clients expect that the information they share will be incorporated in their evaluation. The content of test-item responses can be viewed as direct communications between the patient and the clinician, at least when a person being assessed is motivated to participate in the evaluation. Patients, of course, will not be able to provide information they do not have; however, they are able to provide such information about themselves as whether they feel sad at times, whether they have been in trouble with the law, or whether they enjoy going to parties.

If clients are motivated to share personal information and have access to the information being requested, they are usually excellent testifiers to the presence or absence of their own mental health problems. In fact, patients generally hold the key to understanding their problems and, under appropriate conditions, can provide accurate, useful information about themselves. As described earlier, the MMPI-2 content scales provide a means of summarizing an individual's problems and attitudes in terms of important themes. The content scales provide an objective framework for appraising the major content dimensions represented in the MMPI-2 (see Table 6.3 for a discussion of the MMPI-2 content themes).

FEEDBACK CONSIDERATIONS

It is important for the psychologist to conduct a test feedback session with the client before therapy begins or as an integral part of the therapy. Elsewhere, Butcher (1990) has suggested guidelines for providing MMPI-2 feedback to therapy patients. Most practitioners who share MMPI-2 feedback with their patients early in the therapy are often very pleasantly surprised over the beneficial therapeutic impact such information can have on clients' progress in therapy.

What effect does test feedback have on the patient's behavior and adjustment? Finn and Tonsager (1992) showed that the test feedback process itself can be a powerful clinical intervention. They conducted a clinical study in which one group of patients from a therapy waiting list (n = 32) received MMPI-2 test feedback, according to a model developed by Finn (1990). The second group of patients (n = 29) from the waiting list was administered the MMPI-2 but not given test feedback. The results of the study were very informative: The authors found that individuals who were provided feedback on their MMPI-2 results showed a significant decline in reported symptoms and an increase in measured self-esteem, compared with the control group. Finn and Tonsager reported:

> This study provides support for the therapeutic impact of sharing MMPI-2 test results verbally with college age clients. Clients who completed an MMPI-2 and later heard their MMPI-2 test results reported a significant increase in their self-esteem immediately following the feedback session, an increase that continued to grow over the 2-week follow-up period. In addition, after hearing their MMPI-2 test results, clients showed a significant decrease in their symptomatic distress, and distress continued to decline during the subsequent 2-week period. Last, compared with clients receiving attention only from the examiner, clients who completed the MMPI-2 and received a feedback session showed more hopefulness about their problems immediately following the feedback session, and this persisted at the final follow-up. (p. 284)

The results of this study suggest that psychological test results can be effectively used more directly as a therapeutic intervention (Butcher, 1990; Finn & Martin, 1997; Finn & Tonsager, 1992)

CASE EXAMPLE

Let us now turn to an examination of how the information available in the MMPI-2 can be searched and organized within the STS dimensions, to bear on a particular case, using R.W. as our example, who was introduced in Chapter 3. We will not reiterate the description of R.W. here since it can be found in Appendix A, if the reader needs to review the particulars of this case.

R.W. was administered the MMPI-2 as part of the effort to respond to the consultation request for assistance with diagnosis and treatment planning. Because of elevations on the F scale (> 100), a question was raised about the validity of the profile. The MMPI-2 was readimistered a few weeks later, after discussing the profile with the patient. The two profiles were virtually identical. Thus the first profile was used for analysis; it is shown in Figures 6.1, 6.2, and 6.3. The computer-generated narrative summary from the Minnesota Report (Butcher, 1993) is given in Table 6.4.

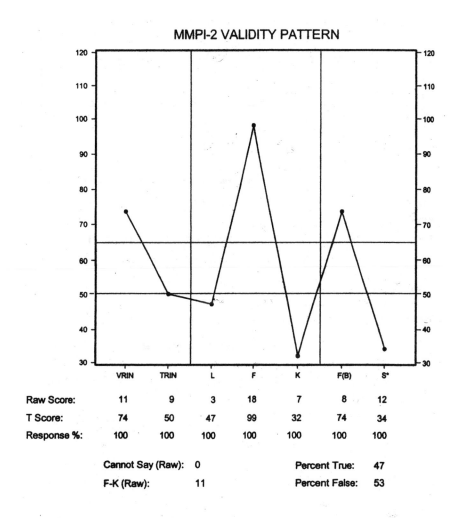

	VRIN	TRIN	L	F	K	F(B)	S*
Raw Score:	11	9	3	18	7	8	12
T Score:	74	50	47	99	32	74	34
Response %:	100	100	100	100	100	100	100

Cannot Say (Raw):	0		Percent True:	47
F-K (Raw):	11		Percent False:	53

*Experimental

FIGURE 6.1. MMPI-2 validity pattern for R.W.

MMPI-2 BASIC AND SUPPLEMENTARY SCALES PROFILE

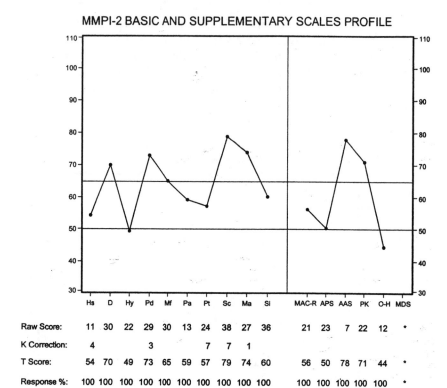

	Hs	D	Hy	Pd	Mf	Pa	Pt	Sc	Ma	Si		MAC-R	APS	AAS	PK	O-H	MDS
Raw Score:	11	30	22	29	30	13	24	38	27	36		21	23	7	22	12	*
K Correction:	4			3			7	7	1								
T Score:	54	70	49	73	65	59	57	79	74	60		56	50	78	71	44	*
Response %:	100	100	100	100	100	100	100	100	100	100		100	100	100	100	100	*

Welsh Code (new):	8942'5+0-671/3: F*"+-/L:K#
Welsh Code (old):	84"92'607-531/ F"-/L?K:
Profile Elevation:	64.40

*MDS scores are reported only for clients who indicate that they are married or separated.

FIGURE 6.2. MMPI-2 basic and supplementary scales profile for R.W.

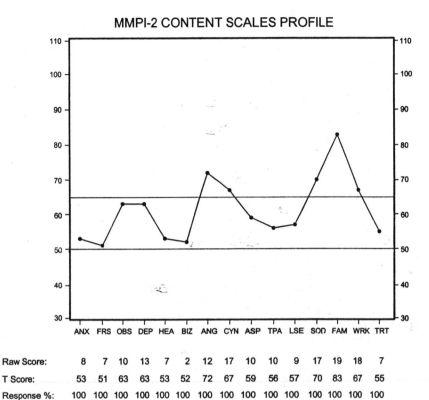

MMPI-2 CONTENT SCALES PROFILE

	ANX	FRS	OBS	DEP	HEA	BIZ	ANG	CYN	ASP	TPA	LSE	SOD	FAM	WRK	TRT
Raw Score:	8	7	10	13	7	2	12	17	10	10	9	17	19	18	7
T Score:	53	51	63	63	53	52	72	67	59	56	57	70	83	67	55
Response %:	100	100	100	100	100	100	100	100	100	100	100	100	100	100	100

FIGURE 6.3. MMPI-2 content scales profile for R.W.

TABLE 6.4. Minnesota Report for R.W.

Profile Validity

Her extremely elevated F score and low VRIN scale score suggest that her endorsement of extreme items is a result of careful item responding rather than an inconsistent response pattern. She apparently understood the item content and considers the symptoms descriptive of her current functioning.

Her self-description as extremely disturbed requires further consideration because she has claimed many more psychological symptoms than most patients do. Two likely possibilities require further evaluation. It is possible that she is exaggerating her symptoms in order to gain attention or services. Sometimes an individual involved in litigation will produce this exaggerated clinical scale profile in order to win his or her case. If an exaggerated response set can be ruled out, based on life circumstances, it may be that her extreme responding resulted from unusually severe psychological problems.

Symptomatic Patterns

This report was developed using the Sc and Ma scales as the prototype. The client's profile reflects a longstanding psychological adjustment problem. She appears to be somewhat impulsive, emotionally labile, and agitated. Sometimes excitable and hostile, she tends to be grandiose and boastful and may show poor judgment. Individuals with this profile may appear to be confused and disorganized, and they often experience stress from vocational or family problems. They may exhibit some evidence of a thinking disturbance and have problems with reality contact, including a tendency to withdraw into fantasy and to manifest paranoid behavior. The possibility of delusions and hallucinations should be evaluated. The client also may report symptoms of depression, tension, and anxiety. Her MMPI-2 clinical profile suggests a potential for excitable and unpredictable behavior. Personality and symptomatic features are likely to remain relatively constant.

In addition, the following description is suggested by the content of the client's item responses. She has endorsed a number of items suggesting that she is experiencing low morale and a depressed mood. She reports a preoccupation with feeling guilty and unworthy. She feels that she deserves to be punished for wrongs she has committed. She feels regretful and unhappy about life, and she seems plagued by anxiety and worry about the future. She feels hopeless at times, as if she were a condemned person.

According to her response content, there is a strong possibility that she has seriously contemplated suicide. The client's recent thinking is likely to be characterized by obsessiveness and indecision. She has endorsed a number of items reflecting a high degree of anger. She appears to have a high potential for explosive behavior at times. The client is alienated, feeling that she is getting a raw deal from life and that others do not understand her or are trying to do her harm. She seems quite hyperactive, impulsive, and excitable. She is easily bored and seeks stimulation to "stir up excitement." She endorses statements that indicate she has some inability to control her anger. She may physically or verbally attack others when she is angry.

Profile Frequency

Profile interpretation can be greatly facilitated by examining the relative frequency of clinical scale patterns in various settings. The client's high-point clinical

(continued)

TABLE 6.4. *(continued)*

---

scale score (Sc) is the least frequent MMPI-2 peak score in the MMPI-2 normative sample of women, occurring in only 4.4% of the cases. Only 2.2% of the women had Sc as the peak score at or above a *T*-score of 65, and less than 1% had well-defined Sc spikes. This elevated MMPI-2 profile configuration (8-9/9-8) is very rare, occurring in less than 1% of the MMPI-2 normative sample of women.

This profile also is relatively infrequent in various samples of outpatient women. In the NCS outpatient sample, 5.1% of the females had this high-point clinical scale score (Sc). Moreover, 4.4% of the women in the outpatient sample had the Sc scale spike at or above a *T*-score of 65, but only 1.7% had well-defined peak scores on Sc. Her elevated MMPI-2 profile configuration (8-9/9-8) occurs in 0.7% of the women in the NCS outpatient sample.

Profile Stability

The relative scale elevation of her highest clinical scale scores suggests some lack of clarity in profile definition. Although her most elevated clinical scales are likely to be present in her profile pattern if she is retested at a later date, there could be some shifting of the most prominent scale elevations in the profile code. The difference between the profile type used to develop the present report and the next highest scale in the profile code was 3 points. So, for example, if the client is tested at a later date, her profile might involve more behavioral elements related to elevations on D. If so, then on retesting, pronounced complaints of depressed mood and low morale might be more prominent.

Interpersonal Relations

She appears to be self-centered and immature, placing unrealistic demands on others and sometimes becoming hostile when these demands are not met. She does not relate well to others, fears emotional involvement, and avoids close interpersonal contact. Many individuals with this profile are so self-absorbed and unskilled in sex-role behavior that they never develop rewarding intimate relationships. Some never marry.

She is somewhat shy, with some social concerns and inhibitions. She is somewhat hypersensitive about what others think of her and is occasionally concerned about her relationships with others. She appears to be somewhat inhibited in personal relationships and social situations, and she may have some difficulty expressing her feelings toward others.

The content of this client's MMPI-2 responses suggests the following additional information concerning her interpersonal relations. She appears to be an individual who has cynical views about life. Any efforts to initiate new behaviors may be colored by her negativism. She may view relationships with others as threatening and harmful. She views her home situation as unpleasant and lacking in love and understanding. She feels like leaving home to escape a quarrelsome, critical situation and to be free of family domination. She feels intensely angry, hostile, and resentful of others, and she would like to get back at them. She is competitive, uncooperative, and tends to be very critical of others. Her social relationships are likely to be viewed by others as problematic. She may be visibly uneasy around others, sit alone in group situations, and dislike engaging in group activities.

(continued)

TABLE 6.4. *(continued)*

Diagnostic Considerations

Individuals with this profile are usually viewed as disturbed. They may receive a diagnosis that reflects a psychotic process, such as schizophrenic disorder or a major affective disorder. They may also be viewed as having borderline personality disorder. The alcohol or drug problems she has acknowledged in her responses should be taken into consideration in any diagnostic evaluation.

Treatment Considerations

Psychotropic medications are usually the primary form of treatment for individuals with this profile. The client is probably not very open to individual insight-oriented psychotherapy at this time, due to relationship problems and suspicious ideation. She is also likely to have difficulty concentrating and focusing on relevant issues in an interview.

The item content she endorsed indicates attitudes and feelings that suggest a low capacity for change. Her potentially high resistance to change might need to be discussed with her early in treatment in order to promote a more treatment-expectant attitude.

Examination of item content reveals a considerable number of problems with her home life. She feels extremely unhappy and alienated from her family. She reports that her home life is unpleasant and that she does not expect it to improve. Any psychological intervention will need to focus on her negative family feelings if progress is to be made.

In any intervention or psychological evaluation program involving occupational adjustment, her negative work attitudes could become an important problem to overcome. She has a number of attitudes and feelings that could interfere with work adjustment.

Her acknowledged problems with alcohol or drug use should be addressed in therapy.

Recommendations Based on the MMPI-2 Results

In this section, we review the characteristics of R.W. that relate to treatment planning through the lens of the six STS dimensions (Beutler et al., 2000). To reiterate, these dimensions include functional impairment, social support level, problem complexity/chronicity, coping style, resistance traits, and distress level.

Functional Impairment/Severity

Level of impairment is indexed on the MMPI-2 by the average elevation of scores as well as by the specific elevations of scores indicating more serious and chronic types of psychopathology (e.g., Sc, Ma, and various content scales). The MMPI-2 report observes that R.W. appears to be self-centered and immature, placing unrealistic demands on others and sometimes becoming hostile when these demands are not met. She does not relate well to others, fears emotional involvement, and avoids close interpersonal contact. Many individuals with this profile are so self-absorbed and unskilled in sex-role behavior that they never develop rewarding intimate relationships. Her poor level of functioning suggests that long-term treatment is likely to be needed, with the use of medication, in order to help her deal with the psychological problems she is experiencing. Her low self-esteem may lead her to make irresponsible social decisions.

Social Support Level

Level of social support is directly indicated on the MMPI-2 by elevations on the Si (Social Introversion) scale that indexes the degree of social contact, and less directly by scales such as Pd (Psychopathic Deviate) and Pa (Paranoia) that suggest the degree to which there are disruptions in the patient's ability to get close to or trust other people.

In this case, R.W. appears to be somewhat alienated from other people. Her MMPI-2 pattern suggests that she is likely to act out in impulsive ways that may add to her feelings of estrangement. An examination of her MMPI-2 item content reveals a considerable number of problems with her home life. She feels extremely unhappy and alienated from her family. She reports that her home life is unpleasant and that she does not expect it to improve. Any psychological intervention will need to focus on her negative family feelings if progress is to be made.

Problem Complexity/Chronicity

Chronicity is indexed on the MMPI-2 by, for one, the overall elevation of clinical scales. The F scale also indicates chronicity, as does the relative elevations of the Pt and Sc scales. Sc is a strong indicator of chronicity, whereas Pt and D are often affected by acute stress. Note that R.W.'s profiles are characterized by indicators of long-term psychological problems. She shows a high degree of immaturity, an impulsive lifestyle, and poor judgment in interpersonal relationships. She shows many features of severe personality problems, including possibly borderline personality features. She reports having problems with substance abuse.

Coping Style

Before drawing on the various individual scales comprising the general coping styles of internalization and externalization, the examiner should consider the general level of elevation in the profile. The overall elevation of the scales is within the clinical range and suggests that she is having trouble coping with her current situation. The high elevation of the F scale is particularly noteworthy and suggests that she is unconventional and inconsistent in her problem-solving efforts. She has difficulty separating realistic and unrealistic aspects of situations in which she finds herself. Interestingly, the elevation of her clinical scales vary and are not universally high. Analysis of scales that indicate externalizing and internalizing behaviors suggest a good deal of similarity in mean elevations, indicating a degree of instability in how she copes with problems and behaves interpersonally. The presence of both types of scales within the clinical range is ordinarily associated with a pattern of overcontrol, followed by acting out, then overcontrol. Thus, when problems arise, she may initially respond with internalizing tendencies (Hs, D, Pt, Si), becoming depressed, withdrawn, self-critical, and anxious. As she becomes overwhelmed with these feelings, she may erupt under pressure, displaying more impulsivity, anger, and resentment. Under the press of these externalizing tendencies (Hy, Pd, Pa, Ma), she may blame others for her problems, avoid taking responsibility for her acts, and resist authoritative control. Overall, she is likely to be emotionally labile and agitated. She tends to be grandiose and boastful and may show poor judgment.

Collectively, individuals with this profile may appear to be confused and disorganized (high F), and they often experience stress from vocational or family problems (D, Pd). They may exhibit some evidence of a thinking disturbance and have problems with reality contact, including a tendency to withdraw into fantasy and to manifest paranoid behavior. They may also report symptoms of depression, tension, and anxiety. R.W.'s MMPI-2 clinical profile suggests a potential for excitable and unpredictable behavior, again reinforcing the general view of an unstable, externalizing pattern. Personality and symptomatic features are likely to be difficult to treat and remain relatively intractable to treatment.

Resistance Traits

Resistance traits are generally indicated on the MMPI-2 by reference to such scales as Pd (Psychopathic Deviate), Pa (Paranoia), and TRT, the content scale that indicates readiness for treatment. Specific content scales that indicate problems with accepting authority (CYN) and hostility (ANG) are also important to interpret.

The general level of interpersonal conflict presented by this patient is reflected in specific scales, such as Pd and Pa, both of which suggest the level of noncompliance and resistance to authority to be expected in treatment. Both of these scales are in the clinically significant range for R.W., indicating her general resistance to treatment, suspiciousness of authorities, and difficulty establishing close relationships with others. These factors are likely to impair relationship with the clinician who provides treatment and, overall, indicate a considerable amount of interpersonal conflict around issues of authority and control.

Based on this patient's profiles and the accompanying report further, it can be assumed that she is likely to respond in the therapeutic relationship in a manner that is similar to her typical means of interacting in other relationships—that is, with resistance to therapist demands and implied control. On the MMPI-2 she acknowledged a resistance to suggestions from others and a tendency to place unrealistic demands on others. The item content she endorsed indicates attitudes and feelings that suggest a low capacity for change. Her potentially high resistance to change might need to be discussed with her early in treatment to promote a more treatment-expectant attitude. The therapist needs to be aware that she may become hostile when her demands are not met. She does not relate well to others, fears emotional involvement, and avoids close interpersonal contact. These long-term personality characteristics are likely to impact her treatment relationship and might result in treatment termination if therapy becomes "demanding" of her.

Distress Level

Personal distress levels are indicated on the MMPI and MMPI-2 by such clinical scales as D (Depression) and Pt (Psychasthenia), as well as by content scales indicating subjective anxiety and distress (e.g., ANX). In this case, the client shows clear personality and symptomatic features that are likely to remain relatively constant. She is likely to feel somewhat sluggish, for she has many somatic complaints, feels weak and tired much of the time, and reports having low energy. In addition to these symptoms of depressed mood, R.W. is likely to be prone to worry and to lack self-confidence.

Her reports of depression, tension, and anxiety must be considered in view of a clinical profile that suggests a potential for excitable and unpredictable behavior. At present, she shows a great deal of social and personality disorganization. She is presenting her problems in an extreme manner, indicating some effort on her part to obtain attention for her problems.

LIMITATIONS OF THE MMPI-2

The MMPI-2 can be used in a wide range of clinical situations for assessing clients. There are, however, some limitations or restrictions that should be considered in its use with clients. In some respects, the major strengths of the MMPI-2 can also be seen as possible limiting considerations.

The MMPI-2 is an empirically based instrument developed in a "blindly empirical" fashion, without regard to any theoretical orientation or guiding viewpoint. It provides observations that are not bound to any particular theoretical perspective. Some authorities have considered the lack of an underlying theory to be a major drawback of the MMPI. In the past, the MMPI has been criticized by therapy theorists from divergent camps—for example, behaviorists, psychoanalysts, humanistic psychologists, and nondirective theorists. Psychologists who follow a strict therapeutic discipline or school may find that the patient information provided by the MMPI-2 cannot be readily integrated into their particular doctrine.

The MMPI-2 is a verbal instrument and requires certain reading and comprehension skills to complete. Individuals with a very low reading level or severe intellectual impairment may not be able to complete an MMPI-2. Similarly, since the MMPI-2 items usually require some motor responding, such as marking an answer sheet or punching a computer keyboard, some accommodation may be necessary if an individual is unable to engage in such responding. For example, in the case of blind or deaf clients, it may be necessary to use special forms for item presentation and response recording.

As noted at several points in this chapter, the quality of the information presented through the MMPI-2 items is limited by the motivation of the client. If a client is motivated to provide a distorted picture on the test, he or she can readily do so. The answer to the question "Can the MMPI-2 be faked?" is "Yes!" If individuals want to appear psychologically disturbed, they can certainly endorse the items in an extreme manner to present many symptoms. If they do not wish to cooperate with the evaluation, they may simply deny any and all symptoms. There are certainly times and situations when the only information gained through an MMPI-2 is that the respondent has faked the test. We do not then know much about the person, except that he or she was uncooperative. In some situations, such as a forensic case, this may be important (though limited) information.

Although some patients and therapists alike may consider the MMPI-2 to be too long for a particular use, the opposite argument (that it does not contain enough range) can be made as well. The 567 items on the inventory address a broad range of problems and symptoms; however, there are areas in contemporary clinical practice that are not addressed. For example, the inventory is problem-oriented and does not contain many items that assess resources or strengths. Thus the MMPI-2 does not provide much information with respect to this important aspect of personality functioning.

The question as to how much of the information needed by clinicians for assessment is provided by the MMPI-2 must also be addressed. Can the MMPI-2 be used as the only instrument in the assessment, or should the inventory always be employed as part of a more extensive battery of tests? Answers to this question obviously differ. Some clinicians, for some applications, use only the MMPI-2 in their clinical work because of its objectivity, validity, and easy-to-use format; others employ the MMPI-2 as part of a test battery. Practitioners who employ a number of tests in their assessment study then need to integrate the results from differing tests into a integrated report. Practitioners interested in the issues of integrating psychological test results are referred to Butcher (1999), Tallent (1993), and Weiner (1993).

SUMMARY

The MMPI, originally developed by Hathaway and McKinley to aid in diagnostic screening, soon became the most widely used personality instrument in psychological assessment. Moreover, the MMPI has been adapted in numerous other countries, indicating strong generalization of validity across cultural settings. Though enormously successful, the MMPI's use became problematic as time went by and as the applications expanded beyond the original purpose of the instrument. In 1982 the test's publisher, the University of Minnesota Press, initiated a program of revision that resulted in the publication of two separate but overlapping and parallel forms of the MMPI, the MMPI-2 for adults and the MMPI-A for adolescents.

The MMPI-2 is a revised version of the original instrument, in which the clinical and validity scales have been kept relatively intact. In addition, a number of new scales for expanded clinical applications were developed. New norms, based on a large, representative sample of normal subjects, provide a more relevant comparison sample for today's test uses. A number of validity studies has documented the MMPI-2's effectiveness as a replacement for the original MMPI in the assessment of adults.

In interpreting the MMPI-2 in clinical practice, three major strategies are usually involved. First, careful consideration of the validity scale pattern is important, in order to ensure appropriate motivation for, and cooperation with, the assessment. If the test is considered valid and interpretable, the empirically derived behavioral correlates are surveyed. Finally, the MMPI-2 content scales are employed as direct communications between the patient and the clinician. Computer-generated clinical interpretation has been illustrated with a case, and personality description and treatment recommendations have been provided.

7

The Millon Clinical Multiaxial Inventory–III

Paul D. Retzlaff and Thomas Dunn

This chapter introduces the Millon Clinical Multiaxial Inventory (MCMI-III) (Millon, 1997). First, the MCMI-III's strengths and weaknesses are covered from a psychometric perspective, including the organization and content of the scales and a discussion of the reliability and validity of the test. Next, approaches to the interpretation and planning of treatment are introduced. Finally, an understanding of the use of the MCMI-III within the STS framework is provided through an application of the test and model to the case example.

DEVELOPMENT OF THE MCMIs

The various versions of the MCMI have integrated all three of the traditional approaches to test construction: clinical content, statistical homogeneity, and empirical validation. This sequential, multimethod integration is referred to as a domain construction approach (Nunnally, 1978; Suen, 1990). Clinical theory, understanding, and need determine what scales are developed. Items are developed and retained within scales based on their homogeneity and high reliability. Finally, validity analyses are conducted to demonstrate that the test will cross-validate and generalize.

MCMI-I Development

All MCMI revisions have been rooted in the original MCMI-I (Millon, 1977), and all have used approximately the same combination of test construction techniques. Content techniques were used for the development of an initial, large, item pool with face validity. Judges created items that they viewed as essential to the theoretical domains of each scale. Next, the initial item pool was reduced by clinician sorting. Naive clinicians were asked to sort each item into its appropriate domain(s). If an item was, "I like robbing 7-11s," and five out of the total eight clinicians put it into the antisocial domain, then it stayed. They also had a chance to put it in other domains, keyed either true or false. Because clinicians were used to sort the items, the items enjoy a broad base of consensual support (Gibertini & Retzlaff, 1988; Retzlaff & Gibertini, 1987).

Considerations of the internal statistical structure constituted the next phase. After patient groups endorsed these items, those items with the highest total correlations were retained. An "item total correlation" is the correlation of the endorsement of each item (zero for false, one for true) with the total score of the 40 or 50 initial items in that domain. Those items most central to that domain were retained, producing the attribute of *homogeneity* (i.e., internal consistency), which was operationalized by the Cronbach Alpha reliability statistic.

Next the empirical approach was utilized. Here 167 clinicians gave the test to, and completed diagnostic rating forms on, actual patients. The final MCMI-I included 175 items that were keyed 733 times.

MCMI-II Development

With the publication of the DSM-III–R, it was deemed appropriate to revise the MCMI. A provisional MCMI-II (Millon, 1987) of 368 items was developed, which included the development of two new scales: Sadistic and Self-defeating. All of the construction steps used for the MCMI-I were repeated for these two scales. Furthermore, other scales were strengthened by the addition and deletion of items.

At this time, a multipoint keying system was added, wherein an item was given a weight of 1, 2, or 3 points based on how the developers of the test judged it in relation to the various criteria-related hurdles. If an item was sorted well, had a very high item total correlation, and had a high validity correlation, it was given 3 points. Lesser quality items received 1 or 2 points. This multipoint scoring system has come under attack as unnecessary (Retzlaff, Sheehan, & Lorr, 1990).

After most of the development process had been completed, Desirability (exaggeration of positive qualities) and Debasement (exaggeration of negative qualities) scales were empirically derived. A number of graduate students were asked to go through the 175 items and endorse those they viewed as being either socially desirable or debasing. If the majority of these graduate students agreed on an item, it was added to that scale. These scales are not as strong as they could be, because of this construction method. They would be better scales if the composite items had been generated in an initial item pool and then subjected to the rigorous steps undergone by the rest of the scales.

MCMI-III Development

With the publication of the DSM-IV in 1994 (American Psychiatric Association), the MCMI was again revised. Sufficient items were added to develop a Depressive personality disorder scale and a PTSD scale. Ninety of the 175 MCMI-II items were changed. The item weighting procedure was reduced from a possible 3 points to 2 points. Finally, the number of items per scale was cut dramatically. Instead of having 35 to 45 items per scale, as on the Millon-II, there are only 16 or 17 items per scale in the MCMI-III (Millon, 1994, 1997). This pruning has resulted in far more specific scales.

DESCRIPTION OF THE MCMI-III SCALES

The MCMI-III is comprised of 175 items that are scored on 28 scales. The first four scales assess validity and response style. The first scale, labeled Validity, primarily assesses whether or not a patient read the items. The second scale, Disclosure, assesses the tendency to overreport or underreport psychopathology. The third validity scale, Desirability, is similar to social desirability scales commonly found in other psychological tests. The final validity scale, Debasement, assesses self-perception primarily in terms of self-esteem.

Scale Organization

Millon (1997) divides personality disorders into two types: Basic and Severe (see Table 7.1). Basic personality disorders include schizoid, avoidant, depressive, dependent, histrionic, narcissistic, antisocial, sadistic, compulsive, negativistic, and self-defeating. Individuals with basic personality disorders may experience mild-to-moderate levels of impairment in their ability to function socially or occupationally, but they may be able to maintain an intimate relationship and continue to work. In contrast, the three severe personality disorders—schizotypal, borderline, and paranoid—are usually considerably disabling. As a result, it is difficult for patients scoring high on these scales to function effectively in social, occupational, or academic areas.

TABLE 7.1. MCMI-III Scales

Validity Scales	Severe Personality Disorders
Validity	Schizotypal
Disclosure	Borderline
Desirability	Paranoid
Debasement	
	Basic Clinical Syndromes
Basic Personality Disorders	Anxiety
Schizoid	Somatoform
Avoidant	Bipolar
Depressive	Dysthymia
Dependent	
Histrionic	Alcohol Dependence
Narcissistic	Drug Dependence
Antisocial	PTSD
Sadistic	
Compulsive	Severe Clinical Syndromes
Negativistic	Thought Disorder
Self-defeating	Major Depression
	Delusional Disorder

The first 11 scales of the MCMI-III evaluate Millon's Basic Personality Disorders. These scales are a superset of the DSM-IV (American Psychiatric Association, 1994) personality disorders. The DSM-IV dropped the sadistic and self-defeating disorder diagnoses found in the DSM-III–R (American Psychiatric Association, 1987), while adding a depressive personality disorder diagnosis in the appendix. Although the MCMI-I and MCMI-II adhered to the prior editions of the DSM (American Psychiatric Association, 1980, 1987), the MCMI-III has retained all 11 of the personality disorders rather than stay in lockstep with the DSM-IV, which lists nine personality disorders. The MCMI-III, therefore, includes the Sadistic and Self-defeating personality disorders from the appendix of DSM-III–R as well as the new depressive personality disorder found in the DSM-IV. Finally, negativistic personality disorder, as it has been termed from the very first MCMI, continues as such in the MCMI-III. The DSM-IV has added the negativistic label to the passive-aggressive diagnosis.

The MCMI-III Severe Personality Disorders scales contains assessment questions related to the three personality disorders, schizotypal, borderline, and paranoid, that are severely impairing. This division of personality disorders into two categories reflects the hierarchical structure of the MCMI-III; these scales are viewed as largely superseding the Basic Personality Disorder scales and form their own block from an interpretation perspective.

As it does with the personality disorders, the MCMI-III breaks clinical syndromes into two categories: Basic and Severe. Basic Clinical Syndromes scales include anxiety, somatoform, bipolar, dysthymia, alcohol dependence, drug dependence, and posttraumatic stress disorder (PTSD). Again, individuals with elevations on the Basic Clinical Syndrome scales can probably function with only mild to moderate impairment.

The Severe Clinical Syndromes scales include thought disorder, major depression, and delusional disorder. These three scales are designed to reveal more severely debilitating and more complex clinical syndromes; the scales subsume elements of the Basic Clinical Syndrome scales. Distinguishing these three Severe Clinical Syndromes from the others aids interpretation. Within the clinical scales, the mild to severely impairing differentiation is less clear than within the personality disorder scales, as evidenced by the placement of bipolar and PTSD among the Basic Clinical Syndromes.

ADVANTAGES AND LIMITATIONS

Advantages

DSM Mapping

The MCMI-III does the best job of all major, commercially available psychological tests of mapping the diagnoses found in the DSM-IV, particularly the personality disorder diagnoses. Although many will complain that the MCMI-III does not do a perfect job of operationalizing the DSM-IV, it does a fairly good job, especially given the "moving target" quality of the DSM series. Comparing the changes made from DSM-III–R to DSM-IV, it becomes apparent that the DSM criteria are not "fixed in stone." The document is a working, organic model that does—and should—change, as more is learned about psychopathology. It would be wrong, however, to use this movement in criteria as a complaint about the MCMI-III. Conversely, "keeping pace" with the DSM does mean frequent revisions of the MCMI, which makes it more difficult to evaluate the psychometrics of the newest version.

The reason that concordance between the DSM and MCMI-III is important is that a clinician is able to conceptualize a case without having to switch back and forth between theories. The diagnoses and criteria of DSM are a fact of clinical and insurance life. As such, a test that works in the same vein allows the clinician to move easily from testing to diagnostics to treatment planning.

Integration

The MCMI-III offers an exceptional opportunity to integrate assessment with treatment. For the personality disorders, the test offers treatment approaches consistent with the majority of the philosophical schools within clinical psychology. As such, it is a rare assessment instrument. Practitioners are afforded an opportunity to integrate most aspects of clinical practice while retaining the flexibility to choose the type of therapy most suited to both patient and therapist.

Personality Disorders

In my opinion, the MCMI-III is simply the best way to assess the personality disorders (Choca & Van Denburg, 1997; Retzlaff, 1995). The personality disorders are diagnosed in highly varied ways across clinical practice. Some clinicians never diagnose a personality disorder, whereas others may diagnose most patients with one or more. Perhaps a more appropriate view of the personality disorders is that (1) they deserve more attention than is given in training and the DSMs, and (2) they are probably distributed clinically in logical patterns. The personality disorders deserve more clinical attention because they are often the true chief complaint. In my opinion, there is a clinical bias to establish an Axis I diagnosis. When wondering what is wrong with a patient, clinicians first go to the Axis I disorders. Is this a psychosis? Is this a depression? Is this an anxiety disorder? Again, in my opinion, patients additionally bias us toward Axis I disorders in the presentation of their symptoms; patients never come in and complain of a lifelong characterological problem. They come in and complain of depression, anxiety, marital problems, or occupational dysfunction. However, the true nature of many chief complaints is a personality disorder not an Axis I disorder. Indeed, many personality disorders are misdiagnosed as Axis I disorders. A patient will come in and complain of cycling mood, one minute happy, the next sad, the next angry. Too many of these patients are misdiagnosed as bipolar. Rapidly shifting moods is more likely a negativistic personality disorder or a borderline personality disorder. Other common errors include the affective chief complaints of borderline personality disorders. The patient reports dysphoria, difficulty concentrating, and suicidal ideation. This, depending upon the history, is just as likely a borderline personality disorder as a major depression. We, however, make the major depression diagnosis, refer for medication, and engage in lengthy and unrewarding psychotherapy. Proper diagnoses must be made to properly treat patients.

The second reason the personality disorders deserve more attention is that they often make the treatment of true Axis I disorders very difficult. Not all people with paranoid schizophrenia are the same, obviously, and the differences are often due to the comorbid personality disorders. A person with paranoid schizophrenia who is also schizoid and dependent behaves very differently from a patient who is sadistic and negativistic. The first will appear, at least, to be a model patient and cause little concern for inpatient staff. That patient will be compliant with medications and generally a successful treatment outcome. The sadistic and negativistic patient with paranoid schizophrenia, however, will be a source of untold difficulty for the treatment team and nursing staff. The patient's unpleasant behavior may even escalate to a level that is dangerous for staff and other patients. Medication regimes will not be followed and the patient will overutilize in-patient treatment. In short, the personality disorders will often impact treatment far more than the Axis I focus of treatment.

In addition to developing DSM-IV diagnoses, the MCMI-III is also useful in identifying important patient characteristics central to treatment planning. For example, the severity of a patient's difficulty would be indicated by high elevations as well as the presence of elevations on the severe personality disorder and severe clinical syndrome scales. A high level of resistance is indicated by elevations on the Negativistic, Paranoid, Sadistic, Antisocial, or Narcissistic scales. Thus clinicians can plan treatment based on formal diagnosis, client characteristics, or a combination of the two.

Limitations

Few Items, Many Scales

From a psychometric perspective, perhaps the greatest limitation of the MCMI-III is the number of scales scored from the number of items. Since the first version of the test, there have been 175 items. However, across the development process, the number of scales has grown to the current 28. There are only so many scales one can score from a certain number of items before the scales begin to lack specificity. The MCMI-III is close to that point. The scales would probably perform better if there were either 225 items or five fewer scales. This option, of course, presents a conflict. The 175 items are tolerated well by patients and quickly accomplished. It is therefore difficult to argue for more items. It is equally difficult to pick five scales to eliminate. The personality disorder scales are the strength of the test, so it is hard to argue for any eliminations there. Conversely, there are relatively few clinical scales, given the number of Axis I disorders.

Overdiagnosing and Overpathologizing

One of the most common complaints about the test is that it identifies too many pathologies through too many elevated scales. It is suggested that the test should only have a single high scale for any particular patient and that this scale should always be the correct diagnosis. This outcome would be very possible in a perfect psychometric world. Only two options in this situation are viable. First, the test could provide too *few* high scales, which would result in the clinician not being made aware of a possible problem and undoubtedly missing it. Second, the test could do as it does—provide three to five elevations for a particular patient—and allow the clinician to use additional techniques, such as interview, to confirm which elevations are correct. This second option is by far the better for the typical clinician.

Whereas researchers might strive for focal perfection, the typical clinician is looking for hypotheses to test.

PSYCHOMETRIC PROPERTIES

Reliability

Table 7.2 presents the number of items per MCMI-III scale and the reliability coefficient. The personality disorders scales include 15–24 items. From a traditional psychometric viewpoint (Nunnally, 1978), this should be a sufficient number of items to create psychometrically sound scales. The Clinical Syndrome Scales have generally fewer items: 12–17. Potential problem scales are those with the smallest number of items, especially Somatoform, with 12, and Bipolar and Delusional, with 13 each. Scales with fewer than 16 or so items often suffer from poor reliability, limited domain saturation, and coarse resolution.

Scales should have Cronbach alpha internal consistency reliabilities of .70 or greater (Nunnally, 1978). The Basic Personality Disorder scales generally have alphas in the .80s, which are excellent. The Narcissistic scale is low, with a .67, and the Compulsive scale is 1 point lower. The severe personality disorder scales are sound, with alphas in the mid-.80s.

The Basic Clinical Syndrome scales are also all in the .80s, with the exception of Bipolar, at .71, which could be related to its low number of items (13). Finally, the Severe Clinical Syndrome scales have excellent coefficients, ranging from .79 to .90.

In summary, the reliability coefficients of the MCMI-III scales, with the exception of perhaps one or two scales, are among the highest in the industry.

Base Rate Scores and Score Interpretation

One of the most confusing aspects of the MCMI tests is their base rate scores. Base rate scores utilize criterion, rather than normative, referencing. Norm referencing is utilized in most psychological tests (Retzlaff, 1992). In normative-based tests, scores reflect an individual's relative position within the normal population. For example, with intelligence tests, an IQ score of 100 reflects a performance at the population mean or the 50th percentile level. In contrast, when using criterion referencing, it is not important how far the patient scores from the mean of the normal population. Instead the patient's position in relation to a criterion is important. Criterion referencing attempts to model the prevalence of a disorder, syndrome, or diagnosis. If 10% of the population has major depression, is your patient part of that 10%?

Base rates reference the test scores to these diagnostic criteria rather than to the norm or the mean. Specifically on the MCMI, base rate scores of 85 (or greater) indicate the strongest possibility that the respondent has

TABLE 7.2. MCMI-III Numbers of Items
per Scale and Scale Reliabilities

Scale	No. of items	Alpha
Validity Scales		
Validity	3	na
Disclosure	na	na
Desirability	21	.85
Debasement	33	.95
Basic Personality Disorders		
Schizoid	16	.81
Avoidant	16	.89
Depressive	15	.89
Dependent	16	.85
Histrionic	17	.81
Narcissistic	24	.67
Antisocial	17	.77
Sadistic	20	.79
Compulsive	17	.66
Negativistic	16	.83
Self-defeating	15	.87
Severe Personality Disorders		
Schizotypal	16	.85
Borderline	16	.85
Paranoid	17	.84
Basic Clinical Syndromes		
Anxiety	14	.86
Somatoform	12	.86
Bipolar	13	.71
Dysthymia	14	.88
Alcohol Dependence	15	.82
Drug Dependence	14	.83
PTSD	16	.89
Severe Clinical Syndromes		
Thought Disorder	17	.87
Major Depression	17	.90
Delusional Disorder	13	.79

that disorder. A 75 base rate score, or greater, means that the patient (at least) has features or symptoms of that disorder. These two-cut scores were developed by comparing clinician ratings against the MCMI-III scores. Criterion referencing does not force distributions to a normal curve, and it does not require acceptance of constructs and domains as being normally distributed.

Figure 7.1 exemplifies this difference between normative and criterion referencing. In the top distribution (they are drawn as normal distributions to simplify comparisons between the two) is dependent personality disorder, with a prevalence of 17%. This designation means that in the construction phase of the MCMI-III, 17% of the patients had dependent personality disorder (an Axis II disorder), and it was their primary disorder. However, 38% of the sample had at least some dependent traits or features. In other words, there are two base rates: The first base rate is 17% and indicative of the primary pathology; the second base rate is 38% and indicative of at least some part of the symptom picture.

Base rate scores arbitrarily go from 0 to 115. The distribution of raw scores on the Dependent scale is from 0 to 24 (16 items with either a 1 or 2 weight). These raw scores are counted down from the high end of the normative distribution until 17% of the subjects have been identified. For male norms, anyone having a raw score of 15 or greater is part of that 17%. Continuing on down the distribution to the 38% point gives us a raw score

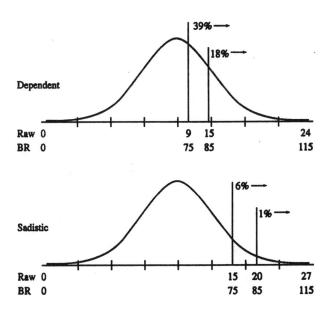

FIGURE 7.1. Base rate score assignment for Dependent and Sadistic scales.

of 9. The 85 base rate score is set (nonlinearly) at a raw score of 15, and the 75 base rate is set at a raw score of 9. The base rate scores thereby allow an optimized modeling of the diagnoses.

Compare the first distribution in Figure 7.1 with the second distribution. Sadistic personality disorder is found far less often. Indeed, the prevalence of having that disorder as a primary diagnosis is only 1%; having it as a primary *or* secondary diagnosis is only 6%. The base rates, again, vary between 0 and 115; the raw scores vary between 0 and 27. Now a raw score of 20 identifies the 1% of the subjects with a sadistic personality disorder. The 85 base rate score is mapped to that 20 raw score. Going down an additional 5% is a raw score of 15. The 75 base rate score is placed at that raw score of 15. Although Dependent and Sadistic scales have the same base rate cutoff scores of 85 and 75, representing a diagnosis and trait, respectively, these base rate scores lie at different points on the frequency distribution for the population. Thus, the base rate scores allow us to know whether or not a patient has a disorder without having to be aware of the specific prevalence or base rate of that disorder.

A brief comment on scores below 75 is warranted. Whereas in most scoring techniques, we look at the very high and very low scores, this approach is inappropriate with the MCMI-III. There is no interpretive difference between a base rate score of 0 and a base rate score of 60; they are both below the cutoff of 75 and, as such, should be viewed as differentially uninterpretable. In the pushing and pulling of the base rate scores, so that they map up with the raw scores, the base rate scores lose their ratio measurement characteristics.

In summary, the first salient interpretation is whether or not a patient scores between 75 and 84, which leads to an interpretation of the patient having that psychopathology at a trait or feature level. The second major interpretation is that a patient with a score of 85 or greater has scored at a disorder level and is probably impaired. The final interpretation is that a score of 74 or less imply that the patient does not have the pathology.

The response bias scales are scored somewhat differently and therefore interpreted differently. The validity scale does not have base rates scores; its raw-score range is 0–3. A raw score of 1 or more should be viewed as potentially invalidating the test. An example item is: "I have not seen a car in the last 10 years."

The Disclosure scale is the only scale where both ends of the base rate distribution should be interpreted. The Disclosure scores range from 0 to 100. If there is a score of 85 or more on the Disclosure scale, it should be seen as an overreport of symptoms. If there is a score of 35 or less on this scale, it should be viewed as an underreport of psychopathology.

Both the Desirability and Debasement scales range from 0 to 100. Theoretically, a score of 85 or more on either scale results in high levels of that particular construct.

Validity

Operating Characteristics

As stated earlier, the MCMI-III is not a traditionally norm-referenced test. Traditionally, newly constructed tests and scales are validated either by correlating them with an external scale of similar content or by comparing two or more groups. In criterion-referenced tests, it is far more important to identify the criterion hit rates; the term *operating characteristics* is used for these hit rates (Gibertini, Brandenburg, & Retzlaff, 1986; Retzlaff & Gibertini, 1994). Table 7.3 shows the five operating characteristics: prevalence, sensitivity, specificity, positive predictive power, and negative predictive power.

The first operating characteristic, *prevalence*, answers the question, "What is the percentage of patients in the group who has the disorder?" This characteristic is also the probability that an individual patient has a disorder prior to any knowledge of the case or clinical examination.

Sensitivity addresses the question, "Can this test identify a pathology when it is present?" An example from the MCMI-III would be "Of all the subjects in this group who have antisocial personality disorder, how many have scores above 85?" This is a classic statistic that we might use in research to determine how "good" a test is. Unfortunately, this characteristic requires us to know who is in the experimental and control groups, and it requires us to know, a priori, who is antisocial—because if we do not know who is antisocial, then we do not know how many people with antisocial personality disorder scored above 85.

TABLE 7.3. Operating Characteristics

Prevalence. The proportion or percentage of patients in the group who has the disorder.

Sensitivity. The proportion or percentage of patients known to have a disorder, who are identified by the test as having it (e.g., Of all the antisocials in this group, how many have scores above 85?).

Specificity. The proportion or percentage of patients known to not have a disorder, who are identified by the test as not having it (e.g., Of all the patients who are not antisocial, how many have scores below 85?).

Positive predictive power. The proportion or percentage of patients within a sample who are identified by a test as having a disorder, who actually have the disorder (e.g., Of all my patients who have a score above 85 on the Antisocial scale, how many actually are antisocial? What is the chance that the patient in front of me, with a 90 on the Antisocial scale, is actually antisocial?).

Negative predictive power. The proportion or percentage of patients within a sample who are identified by a test as not having a disorder, who actually do not have it (e.g., What is the probability that this patient in front of me, with a 40 on the Antisocial scale, is actually not antisocial?).

Specificity is the flip side of sensitivity. It asks: "How specific is this test to a single disorder in relation to the other disorders?" For the MCMI-III, it asks the question, "Of all the patients who are not antisocial, how many have a score below 85 on the Antisocial scale?" In most research paradigms the question would be: "Knowing my control group is non-antisocial college freshmen, how many scored below 85 on my test of anti-social personality disorder?" Here we obviously want the majority of the control group to have low scores. Again, however, we must know the com-position of the control group before the testing is conducted.

The last two operating characteristics are of far more importance in clinical assessment. *Positive predictive power* asks: "Only knowing that this person has a high score on the Antisocial scale, what are the chances that he or she is really antisocial?" This question comes closer to the condi-tions we typically encounter in clinical practice. We have no a priori knowl-edge of whether the person is in the antisocial group or the normal popula-tion group. Positive predictive power also can be viewed as answering the question, "How confident are we in this diagnosis?" Positive predictive power is very rarely used in psychological testing. Most psychological tests provide validity statistics with, for example, correlations of .37 or *T*-tests with *P* values of .001. Knowing a *T*-test had a probability of .001 tells us little about the probability of an individual patient in our office having a particular diagnosis. Positive predictive power, in contrast, indicates the probability that a patient with a base rate score of 85 or greater is antiso-cial. This probability is calculated by dividing the number of patients in the normative study who had a score above 85 and were diagnosed by the cli-nicians as having the disorder, by the number of patients who simply had a score above 85, regardless of actual diagnosis.

Negative predictive power answers the question: "Knowing that my patient had a score of less than 85, what are the chances that he or she re-ally does not have this disorder?" If the patient has a score of 40 on the An-tisocial scale, what is the chance that he or she is really not antisocial? Sur-prisingly, these statistics are usually quite high, in the 90% range, because negative predictive power capitalizes on the large prevalence of patients, in general, not being antisocial.

Positive Predictive Powers

Table 7.4 provides the positive predictive powers (validities) of the MCMI-III scales. By way of example, if a patient scores at 85 or above on the Schizoid scale, that patient has a .67 probability of actually having a schiz-oid personality disorder. A score of 85 or higher on Anxiety suggests a .75 probability of a diagnosis of an anxiety disorder. A score of 85 or higher on Drug Dependence results in an astounding .93 probability. Although some of the positive predictive powers are more modest, such as the .39 for the

TABLE 7.4. MCMI-III Validities

Scale	Positive predictive power
Validity Scales	
Validity	na
Disclosure	na
Desirability	na
Debasement	na
Basic Personality Disorders	
Schizoid	.67
Avoidant	.73
Depressive	.49
Dependent	.81
Histrionic	.63
Narcissistic	.72
Antisocial	.50
Sadistic	.71
Compulsive	.79
Negativistic	.39
Self-defeating	.30
Severe Personality Disorders	
Schizotypal	.60
Borderline	.71
Paranoid	.79
Basic Clinical Syndromes	
Anxiety	.75
Somatoform	.39
Bipolar	.58
Dysthymia	.81
Alcohol Dependence	.88
Drug Dependence	.93
PTSD	.67
Severe Clinical Syndromes	
Thought Disorder	.52
Major Depression	.66
Delusional Disorder	.33

Negativistic scale and .30 for the Self-defeating scale, the important point to remember is that these numbers are always above the chance base rate levels. The Dependent scale shows a positive predictive power of .81, which is much higher than the 18% prevalence rate (see Figure 7.1). Indeed, the administration of the test has resulted in a 4.5% increase over chance. Oddly, the .71 positive predictive power for the Sadistic scale provides even more incremental validity; with a 1% prevalence rate, this .71 rating represents a 71% increase over chance.

These types of validity statistics are rarely used and generally not well understood. There has also been debate in the literature over the appropriate magnitudes and methods (Retzlaff, 1999; Rogers, Salekin, & Sewell, 1999). When reviewing these data in the manual, consult the second edition from 1997; the study included in the first edition was flawed (Retzlaff, 1996).

Traditional Validities

The MCMI-III also has demonstrated validity in more traditional terms. The manual provides correlations between all of the MCMI-III scales and a number of other tests. These correlations are generally high and of a magnitude typically viewed as indicating scale validity. For example, the Beck Depression Inventory correlates with the Dysthymia scale at .71 and the Major Depression scale at .74. The Michigan Alcoholism Screening Test correlates with the Alcohol Dependence scale at .67. The State–Trait Anxiety Inventory correlates with the Anxiety scale in the .50's. Correlations are also high with the MMPI-2, indicating generally accepted levels of validity. The MMPI-2's 2 scale (Depression) correlates with Dysthymia at .68 and Major Depression at .71. Scale 7 (Psychasthenia) correlates with the MCMI-III Anxiety scale at .61, and scale 8 (Schizophrenia) correlates with the Thought Disorder scale at .61.

Although statistics comparing the MCMI-III scores to diagnoses and other tests are of interest, it is more important that a test actually predict something. We (Retzlaff, Stoner, & Kleinsasser, 2002) administered the MCMI-III to 10,000 inmates of the Colorado Department of Corrections and followed them for 2 to 3 years. Relative risk ratios against outcomes were very high against a number of variables. For example, inmates scoring 75 or higher on the Major Depression scale were 850% as likely as those scoring lower to be diagnosed with an Axis I disorder within 2 years of testing. Those scoring high on Borderline were 340% as likely as those scoring low to end up on a psychotropic medication within 3 years of testing. Finally, those scoring high on Thought Disorder were 410% as likely as those scoring low to require relatively high amounts of monthly therapy time. This study is an example of the types of work that are needed; real-life predictions of important outcomes.

ADMINISTRATION AND SCORING

Hand Scoring

It is possible to hand score the MCMI-III; there are, however, many reasons not to do so. First, although hand-scoring templates and forms are available from the test company, the materials are very expensive. Second, there are many overlay templates with the item weight for each item. Then the raw scores are converted to base rate scores through a series of transformation tables. After this, the formulae for the Disclosure scale and several correction algorithms (see below) must be followed. Finally, about half an hour later, the profile sheet is drawn. Of course, at this point, most of us have no confidence in our counting, math, transformations, or base rate scores. Hand scoring is discouraged by the author, test company, and anyone who has ever attempted it.

Internal Corrections

In order to better optimize the hit rates of the test, a number of internal corrections are necessary. In many ways, these corrections are similar to the use of the K correction on the MMPI, where a certain proportion of K is added to different scales to compensate for defensive reporting. In addition to a couple of minor algorithms and variations, the two major corrections in the MCMI-III are the correction for the Disclosure scale and one for the possibility of depression with anxiety.

A high Disclosure scale score results in all scales of the MCMI-III being reduced to some degree. Conversely, very low scores on the Disclosure scale result in additional base rate points for all scales on the MCMI-III. The logic here is that someone who overreports psychopathology will generally have artificially inflated scale scores across the entire test, which should be corrected. Similarly, profiles reflecting underreporting need to be corrected upward.

The high depression and anxiety correction algorithm is driven by high scores on Depression or Anxiety scale, coupled with a recent admission to a psychiatric hospital, and leads to a downward adjustment in base rate scores on the Avoidant, Self-defeating, and Borderline scales. This manipulation attempts to correct for situationally high affectively oriented personality disorder scale scores.

Computer Scoring

The test is best scored by computer. The test company will do the scoring by mail-in or phone-in method, but the easiest course of action is for clinicians to use their own computers. The software is part of the National Computer System's platform, which scores all of their tests, including the

MMPI-2. The software can be loaded on any number of computers; a small device (a "dongle") must be placed between the computer and printer. The dongle keeps track of how many administrations you have purchased. Carrying the dongle from one practice site to another allows for mobility of testing resources.

The computer scoring can include only the scores and profile sheet or, for an additional cost, a multiple-page interpretive output that offers a very interesting "consultation" on the case. Many find this enhancement a great help in the conceptualization of the diagnostics and treatment. Others prefer to "hand-craft" their interpretations. An important point to note, however, is that the computer scoring and interpretations tend to reject very few protocols as "invalid." The recommendations here are more conservative and result in a rejection of 10–15% of the protocols. In my opinion, just because the output identifies a specific diagnosis does not mean it is accurate. Always examine the raw scores before drawing clinical conclusions.

INTERPRETATION

Scale Interpretation

The content of the scales of the MCMI-III is an admixture of Millon's (1969, 1981, 1986a, 1986b, 1990) theory and DSM-IV criteria, honed during the construction of the test. A general interpretation of each scale is offered below, drawing from the test construction, the authors' clinical experience with the test, and Choca and Van Denburg's (1997) chapter on interpretation. Interpretations also can be expanded by referring to the descriptions of the specific domains (see section on "Domain-Specific Psychotherapy" and Table 7.6). We present a sample item from each scale to orient the reader to the scales of the MCMI-III.

Response Bias Scales

The response bias or style scales point to possible test-taking response problems (Retzlaff, Sheehan, & Fiel, 1991).

Validity. The first scale, Validity, is composed of only three items, each of which has extremely unusual content. An example is: "I was on the front cover of several magazines last year." Neither this item nor the other two should be endorsed by anyone in a clinical population. If patients answer true to any of these three items, it either implies that they could not, or did not, read it correctly or that they did not respond to the items appropriately. The scale, therefore, flags profiles where patients have either a reading or gross motivational problem.

Disclosure. The Disclosure scale is based upon a formula that is a function of the personality disorder scale scores. The assumption is that patients who present clinically should fall within a particular window of personality disturbance. If they report too much personality disturbance, such that they obtain elevated scores on seven or eight personality disorder scales, they are probably overreporting their psychopathology. Conversely, if they report no problematic personality traits, they are probably underreporting their psychopathology. This is a relatively unique approach to the assessment of response bias and works very well in clinical practice.

Desirability. The Desirability scale includes items such as, "I think I am a very sociable and outgoing person." This item captures more of a histrionic than a desirability theme. It seems, therefore, to lack face validity. We place little stock in this scale, given its development and content.

Debasement. The Debasement scale suffers from similar content validity problems. Here the item "People make fun of me behind my back, talking about the way I act and look" seems to tap more avoidant or schizotypal characteristics than it does debasement. As with the Desirability scale, we recommend against rigid interpretation or use of this scale.

Basic Personality Disorders

Schizoid. High scorers on the Schizoid scale are classic introverts with little affect. They are aloof and nonsocial by nature and are not concerned with their lack of social interaction. They are complacent and impassive. A prototypical item from the Schizoid scale is "I've always had less interest in sex than most people do." The lack of social connectedness and affect results in very difficult psychotherapy (see additional descriptors on the first row of Table 7.6; e.g., impassive, disengaged, impoverished cognitive style, etc.).

Avoidant. The Avoidant scale reflects social sensitivity and fear. These patients appear to be pathologically "shy." They have the social isolation features seen in the person with schizoid tendencies, but these individuals are upset about it, resulting in an affective anxiety component. This fragile anguish only makes social interaction more aversive for them as well as those with whom they interact. An example of an Avoidant personality disorder scale item is: "In social groups, I am almost always very self-conscious and tense" (see Table 7.6 for additional descriptors).

Depressive. The characterlogical nature of the Depressive scale differentiates it from the Dysthymia scale and the Major Depression scale. It encompasses the "dejection, gloominess, cheerlessness, joylessness, and unhappiness" (p. 732) of the DSM-IV criteria. This dysphoric affect is "part of them," melancholic in nature, and not viewed as ego-dystonic. Cognitions and social interactions include pessimism, worthlessness, and a depleted quality. A Depressive personality disorder scale item is: "I have been down-hearted and sad much of my life since I was quite young" (see Table 7.6 for additional descriptors).

Dependent. The Dependent personality scale includes items that reflect interpersonal submissiveness and feelings of incompetence. Those high on this scale appear incompetent and naive, seek others to care for them, and have low self-confidence in their own abilities. These attributes often lead to dysfunctional relationships with someone apparently much stronger. The representative Dependent personality disorder item is: "I am a very agreeable and submissive person" (see Table 7.6 for additional descriptors).

Histrionic. The Histrionic scale is often elevated in tests by "normal" people who are simply very sociable; it is the most commonly elevated scale for psychologists who take the test themselves. The high score is often a sign of ego strength and social ability and, as such, something of a marker for relatively good clinical outcomes. High scores should only be viewed as pathological if the clinical history indicates dramatic but shallow attention-seeking behaviors and a flighty, shallow affective quality. These patients are often flirtatious and "chatty." As such, the clinician must guard against extratherapeutic tracks. The Histrionic personality scale's first prototypical item is: "I think I am a very sociable and outgoing person" (see Table 7.6 for additional descriptors).

Narcissistic. In the Narcissistic personality disorder scale, we see the "grandiose sense of self-importance" (p. 661) suggested in DSM-IV. These individuals lack empathy and do not care what other people think or feel. They themselves feel special and superior. As with the Histrionic scale, however, a high Narcissistic scale is commonly found in high functioning "normal" people. For example, it is the most commonly found high score among Air Force pilots. At times, this confidence is adaptive. At other times and in other situations, an exploitive coping style with rationalized interpretations is apparent. Therapy is difficult, given these patients' confidence in themselves and their egocentric worldview. A representative item from the Narcissism scale is: "I know I'm a superior person, so I don't care what other people think" (see Table 7.6 for additional descriptors).

Antisocial. Acting out is obviously part of the Antisocial scale, as is impulsivity. Many see the scale as reflecting perhaps more competitive than criminal traits (Choca & Van Denburg, 1997). Here again, many non-patients have some elevation on this scale, and those elevations are best interpreted as adaptively reflecting assertiveness. Very high scores are indicative of an irresponsible unruliness. Indeed, in a sample of about 10,000 prison inmates in Colorado, more subjects scored above the 75 cut-score (29%) on this scale than on any other personality disorder scale (Retzlaff, Stoner, & Kleinsasser, 2002). The Antisocial personality disorder scale includes the item "As a teenager, I got into lots of trouble because of bad school behavior" (see Table 7.6 for additional descriptors).

Sadistic. DSM-IV has dropped sadistic personality disorder and, as such, there is less convergence on the meaning of the disorder and scale. The MCMI-III scale probably shares some of the "cruel, demeaning, and aggressive behavior" construct of the DSM-III–R appendix criteria (p. 371). Sadists have abrasive interpersonal interactions, enjoy cruelty, and are eruptive. These traits, in addition to dogmatism and combativeness, make psychotherapy extremely difficult. The Sadistic scale includes the item "I often criticize people strongly if they annoy me" (see Table 7.6 for additional descriptors).

Compulsive. People with compulsive personality disorder tend to lack a capacity for enjoyment and affective expression. As a result, they often have social difficulty, such as with spouses. A constricted affective and behavioral approach to life makes them difficult people with whom to relate. On the plus side, they are disciplined, respectful, and conscientious. The Compulsive personality disorder scale includes the item "I keep very close track of my money, so I am prepared if a need comes up" (see Table 7.6 for additional descriptors).

Negativistic. There is a pervasive angry quality to people who score high on the Negativistic personality scale. These patients tend to rely on others but simultaneously feel that others are untrustworthy. This internal bind leads not only to the anger but also to highly changeable behavior. Displacement is their defense mechanism of choice, and they displace their discontent on anyone in their environment. They are unhappy, irritable, and, as such, irritating. The Negativistic personality disorder scale includes the item, "If my family puts pressure on me, I'm likely to feel angry and resist what they want" (see Table 7.6 for additional descriptors).

Self-Defeating. As with the Sadistic scale, the Self-defeating scale was dropped for the DSM-IV; as such, there is a lack of concordance in professional opinion about its validity. An undeserving self-image, central to Millon's theory of this disorder, is manifested behaviorally by self-sabotage. The scale seems to capture the criteria included in the initial "options" draft of the DSM-IV (American Psychiatric Association, 1991): "perceives himself or herself as undeserving of being treated well" (p. R-19). Highly affective individuals may present with both anxious and dysphoric qualities, and clinicians will attempt to improve the affect, only to discover the underlying sabotage of progress. A Self-defeating personality disorder item is: "I often think that I don't deserve the good things that happen to me" (see Table 7.6 for additional descriptors).

Severe Personality Disorders

Schizotypal. Patients who score high on the Schizotypal personality scale are usually very dysfunctional and may appear schizophrenic. Indeed, this scale captures much of the schizophrenia symptoms and, at times, does a better job of identifying people with schizophrenia than does the Thought Disorder scale. As in DSM-IV, the scale attempts to reveal the "odd, eccentric, or peculiar" aspects of the behavior, and also has elements of the excessive social anxiety that the schizotypal individual may display. A Schizotypal personality disorder item is: "People make fun of me behind my back, talking about the way I act and look" (see Table 7.6 for additional descriptors).

Borderline. The Borderline personality disorder scale taps the anger, instability, and drama of the individual with borderline characteristics. High scorers experience instability of identity, cognition, affect, and behavior. They are seriously dysfunctional and are very difficult patients to treat. The clinician will often conceptualize such a patient as having a simple major depression, only to discover the manipulation, self-destructiveness, and paradoxical intentions later in therapy. A Borderline personality disorder scale item is: "Lately, I have begun to feel like smashing things" (see Table 7.6 for additional descriptors).

Paranoid. The Paranoid personality scale should not be interpreted as a "delusional disorder" scale. These patients are untrusting, suspicious, resistant, and secretive, but they are not delusional. This scale primarily taps Millon's cognitive suspiciousness element. They are often people with a decompensated narcissism, with similar control issues. Therapy is extremely difficult and is usually court-ordered, as these patients rarely see the need to change. The Paranoid personality disorder scale includes the item "People have never given me enough recognition for the things I've done" (see Table 7.6 for additional descriptors).

Basic Clinical Syndromes

Anxiety. The Anxiety scale does a very good job of discerning the autonomic aspects of an anxiety disorder. High scorers are classically anxious across physiology, affect, cognition, and behavior. The scale is often moderately high not only because it is a highly prevalent disorder, but also because relatively few item endorsements quickly elevate the scale. Very high scores are usually indicative of generalized anxiety disorder. An Anxiety scale item is: "Lately, I've been sweating a great deal and feel very tense."

Somatoform. The Somatoform scale is a weak scale and difficult to interpret. The sample Somatoform item, "I have a hard time keeping my balance when walking," is probably a poor item choice. Patients in nursing homes or on orthopedic units or even those with a simple inner ear infection will affirm this item as true without having somatoform features. Here the problem is that some domains and some constructs within psychology simply do not lend themselves to the development of items and the construction of scales. In essence, a somatoform disorder is an unconscious process driven by defense mechanisms and the morphological organization of the psyche. Yet it is the conscious mind of the patient that is asked to endorse these items. An item would have to be something like, "When I'm upset with my spouse, I tend to get headaches driven by unconscious needs for secondary gain." Patients are not likely to endorse such an item. The MCMI-III has done as good a job as is possible to construct this scale, but the unconscious origins of this disorder do not lend themselves to objective testing. We do not recommend the use of this scale at face value. The scale (too) broadly taps physiological symptoms indicative of (too) many disorders. *Do not base medical or medicolegal recommendations on this scale.*

Bipolar. The Bipolar scale tends to tap energy levels, in general. Hence the scale is best viewed as an energy scale, much as scale 9 of the MMPI-II is interpreted. Many "normal" individuals score high on this scale, simply because they are very energetic and involved in activities. Very rarely does this scale predict serious pathology. Very low scores, however, bode poorly for therapy. High scores indicate a need to harness and focus the patient's energy toward the desired therapeutic outcome. A Bipolar item is: "I enjoy doing so many different things that I can't make up my mind what to do first."

Dysthymia. The Dysthmia scale covers the affective sadness and behavioral elements of depression. The Dysthymia scale of the MCMI-III is an excellent scale of depression, in general. At low levels, it should be viewed as reflecting a situational dysphoria; at moderate levels, it is probably indicating a dysthymic condition; and at high levels, it is probably pointing to a major depression. Depressed patients do a very poor job of differentiating their depression across several scales and constructs on psychological tests. They do, though, do a good job of quantifying their depression. An example of a Dysthymia item is: "I began to feel like a failure some years ago."

Alcohol Dependence. Most of the Alcohol Dependence scale items are explicit behavioral statements. If patients want to deny that they are drinking, they can do so on interview by simply saying "No, I don't drink." They can also do so on a test such as the MCMI-III by answering "True" to the statement "I don't drink." Alcohol and drug dependence are so behavioral in nature that patients, if they want to lie to you, certainly can. This is a good scale, not for identifying whether or not someone is an alcoholic, but for quantifying the severity of whatever alcohol dependence they are willing to admit. Relatively low elevations are probably indicative of the need for brief, educational-based treatment. Moderate elevations suggest a possible need for group therapy. High elevations point to the need for inpatient treatment. One Alcohol abuse item is: "I have a drinking problem that I have tried unsuccessfully to end."

Drug Dependence. The same quantification approach goes for the Drug Dependence scale. The sample item, "My drug habits have often gotten me into a good deal of trouble in the past" is quite obvious. If someone wants to deny this, they can on an interview or on the MCMI-III. Again though, while the scale should not be used for identification, it can be used for quantification of the severity of the drug dependence assuming the person is open in disclosing their difficulties. Similarly, the level of the scale indicates the type of treatment indicated.

Posttraumatic Stress. A representative PTSD scale item, "The memory of a very upsetting experience in my past keeps coming back to haunt my thoughts," illustrates how this scale not only encompasses combat types of traumas but other physical and sexual types of traumas in a patient's past. Here again, though, is the double-edged sword of face validity. Patients who want to "prove" that they have PTSD, perhaps for financial gain, are probably going to be able to spot these items and endorse them as true. Hence an endorsement on this scale should be viewed only as a soft hypothesis until more objective additional data can be collected.

Severe Clinical Syndromes

Thought Disorder. The Thought Disorder scale has a more modest validity than many of the MCMI-III scales. Strong interpretations should not be made on its basis. The scale reflects disturbed thinking and behavior. The symptoms include atypical cognitions (especially rumination), severe dysfunction, and derealization. A sample item is: "Ideas keep turning over and over in my head, and they won't go away."

Major Depression. The Major Depression scale reveals the fatigue elements and perhaps some of the terminal insomnia components of the major depression symptoms. The scale tends to map the more vegetative elements of depression. When patients score high on the scale, they usually are severely depressed. Many with major depression, however, will not be identified by this scale but by the Dysthymia scale. A typical item is: "Lately, my strength seems to be draining out of me, even in the morning."

Delusional Disorder. The Delusional Disorder scale maps true delusional ideation of a paranoic nature. Patients with high scores believe others are "out to get" them, plotting against them, and attempting to control them. The scale is often high for people who have paranoid schizophrenia, and its items tap the paranoid delusions of this disorder. The Delusional Disorder scale's first item is: "Many people have been spying into my private life for years."

Interpretation Approach

There are a number of ways to interpret psychological tests. Usually, the fewer the scales on the test, the easier the interpretation. Unfortunately, with 28 scales on the MCMI-III, a more complex approach to interpretation is required. The interpretation of the Millon test uses blocks of scales, as described below, and is viewed as hierarchical, with the severe disorder scales dictating the interpretation of the basic disorder scales.

Validity Scales

The first block of scales to consider are the validity scales. It is important to examine these response bias scales before examining the content scales. The most fundamental of these is the Validity scale. If the patient endorsed even one of the three extremely unlikely items as true, the test should be viewed as uninterpretable. Next, the patient's profile should be analyzed for disclosure. Is the patient, in general, underreporting or overreporting psychopathology? If the Disclosure scale is below 35 or above 85, the profile is, in most clinical settings, technically invalid. Finally, examine the Desirability and Debasement scales for general style.

Personality Disorder Scales

At this point, look at the Severe Personality Disorder Scales. A high scale in this category should serve as an anchor for the rest of the personality disorder scales. A high score on a Severe Personality Disorder scale is usually accompanied by high scores on a number of the Basic Personality Disorder scales. If patients have schizotypal personality disorder, it is highly likely that they will have high scores on Schizoid and Avoidant scales and perhaps one or two other basic personality scales. The primary personality interpretation should focus on the severe personality scale, and that interpretation should be "fleshed out" with information from the Basic Personality Disorder scales.

If there is not a high severe personality scale, then the high 1- or 2-point code from the basic personality scale should be interpreted. Indeed,

Choca and Van Denburg's (1997) and Craig's (1993a, 1993b) books do a good job of providing common high-point code interpretations (Retzlaff, Ofman, Hyer, & Matheson, 1994).

Clinical Syndrome Scales

As when interpreting the personality scales, the first step in formulating results from the clinical syndrome scales is to examine the category of Severe Clinical Syndrome scales. A high scale score there indicates the anchor or pivot point of the clinical syndrome scales interpretation. If there is a high scale score within this block, there are probably elevated basic clinical syndrome scales as well. If a patient is high on Major Depression, he or she is probably high on Anxiety and Dysthymia. This deduction makes clinical sense and is consistent with the construction of the MCMI-III. Elevated scales are not contradictory but complementary. If there is no high Severe Clinical Syndrome scale, then the highest one or two Basic Clinical Syndrome scales should be interpreted.

Finally, it is common for profiles with elevated clinical syndrome scales to have elevated complementary clinical syndrome scales as well as some high personality disorder scales. For instance, if PTSD is high, one might expect Avoidant and Dysthymia to be high as well as possibly Alcohol Dependence. This interpretive process also involves considering what personality constellation comprises PTSD (e.g., Hyer & Associates, 1994). This personality constellation might include Schizoid, Avoidant, Antisocial, Sadistic, or Negativistic, as well as Borderline, in severe cases. Again, multiple high-point scales are not necessarily contradictory but hierarchical and complementary.

The final step in the interpretative process is to integrate what is learned from the MCMI-III with the patient and clinic history. What is the patient's chief complaint? What is his or her age, sex, and particular psychopathology history? Clinical interpretation also needs to consider the clinical setting in which the testing is conducted. What type of patient does the clinic normally attract? What are the diagnostic biases within your particular clinic? The MCMI-III and testing in general is strongest when suggesting a pathology that is particularly common in your clinic. Higher prevalences lead to higher positive predictive powers.

TREATMENT PLANNING

Domains of the Personality Disorders

Millon (1990, 1994) has hypothesized the existence of eight domains of personality that are relevant to the personality disorder: Expressive Acts, Interpersonal Conduct, Cognitive Style, Object Representations, Self-

Image, Regulatory Mechanisms, Morphologic Organization, and Mood–Temperament. Millon primarily created these descriptors to use in the factorial delineation of the personality disorders diagnostics. The desire was to go beyond the DSM criteria by encompassing a broader range of clinical phenomena that would facilitate better understanding of the personality disorders.

The domains are defined (Millon, 1994) in Table 7.5. *Expressive Acts* are seen as the overt behaviors of the patient and include physical actions as well as verbalizations (obvious and accessible). *Interpersonal Conduct* refers to the patients' interactions with others and includes the style of interactions, content of the interactions, as well as the outcomes of the interactions (including others' impressions).

Internal phenomena include *Cognitive Style*, which involves the perceptions, interpretations, and conclusions made by patients about their world. Of interest is both the manner in which these occur as well as the content of the cognitions. *Object Representations*, another internal phenomenon, have distinct processes and contents in people with personality disorders (generally, the memories and experiences of significant others) that form an internal structure. The *Self-Image* refers patients' sense of self: "Who" they are is comprised of attributes that may or may not be realistic.

Intrapsychic dimensions include the *Regulatory Mechanisms*, the classic defense mechanisms whose function is the amelioration of anxiety and conflict. Each personality disorder manifests a primary defense mechanism. The structure of these intrapsychic processes is the *Morphologic Organization*. This organization may be strong or weak, flexible or rigid, and consistent or inconsistent. It is the psychic "house" and its construction.

The sole biological dimension delineated by Millon is the *Mood–Temperament* domain. Here specific affects are associated with particular personality disorders. Although a lack of affect has been attributed to the personality disorders since the DSM-II (American Psychiatric Association, 1968), here a full emotional contingent is seen as part and parcel of all the personality disorders.

Domain-Specific Psychotherapy

Retzlaff (1995) provides a school-of-thought approach to the personality disorders and the MCMI-III. The eight domains above are presented by various authors with an eye to using the MCMI-III as a treatment targeting system. Table 7.6 (Millon, 1994) crosses the 14 personality disorders with the eight domains. The resulting cells indicate the symptom for each personality disorder by school of thought. For example, the antisocial person is seen as impulsive from an expressive acts/behavioral perspective. The dependent person is defenseless interpersonally. From a cognitive perspective the histrionic person is flighty. These traits may be useful "tags" when for-

TABLE 7.5. Clinical Definitions of the Domains

Expressive Acts. The observable aspects of physical and verbal behavior can be identified readily by clinicians. Through inference, these data enable us to deduce (1) what patients unknowingly reveal about themselves, or (2) what they wish us to think or to know about them. The criteria for this clinical attribute consists of both of these presented behavioral variants.

Interpersonal Conduct. Patients' style of relating to others may be captured in a number of ways, such as (1) the manner in which their actions impact on others, intended or otherwise; (2) the attitudes that underlie, prompt, and give shape to these actions; (3) the methods by which they engage others to meet their needs, or their way of coping with interpersonal tensions and conflicts.

Cognitive Styles. This domain includes some of the most useful indices for identifying patients' distinctive ways of functioning. Here it is learned how patients perceive events, focus their attention, process information, organize their thoughts, and communicate their reactions and ideas to others. The criteria for this clinical attribute represent some of the more notable styles in this functional realm.

Object Representations. Significant experiences from the past leave an inner imprint, a structural residue composed of memories, attitudes, and affects that continue to serve as a substrate of dispositions for perceiving and reacting to life's ongoing events. Both the character and content of these internalized representations of the past are evaluated.

Self-Image. Each person builds a perception of self as an identifiable being, an "I" or "me." Most people have a consistent sense of "who they are" but do differ in the clarity of their introspections into self and/or in their ability to articulate the attributes comprising this image. Clinical ratings, therefore, are likely to be somewhat speculative.

Regulatory Mechanisms. This clinical attribute represents internal and often unconscious processes that are difficult to discern and evaluate. Nevertheless, they are important in that they show how patients deny or distort painful feelings or incompatible thoughts, often setting into motion a sequence of events that intensify the very problems they may have sought to circumvent.

Morphologic Organization. The overall configuration of elements comprising the mind's interior world may display (1) weakness in organizational cohesion, (2) deficient balance and coordination, or rigidities or pressures. It is the structural strength, interior congruity, and functional efficacy of this intrapsychic system to which this clinical attribute pertains.

Mood–Temperament. The "meaning" of extreme affective states are easy to decode. Not so with persistent moods and subtle feelings that insidiously continue to color a wide range of patients' relationships and experiences. No matter how clear the criteria for this clinical attribute may be, the database for their deduction may call for more information than may be available observationally, especially during acute emotional periods.

TABLE 7.6. Symptoms of Personality Disorder by Domains

Disorder	Expressive Acts	Interpersonal Conduct	Cognitive Style	Regulatory Mechanisms	Self-Image	Object Representations	Morphologic Organization	Mood–Temperament
Schizoid	Impassive	Disengaged	Impoverished	Intellectualization	Complacent	Meager	Undifferentiated	Apathetic
Avoidant	Fretful	Aversive	Distracted	Fantasy	Alienated	Vexatious	Fragile	Anguished
Depressive	Disconsolate	Defenseless	Pessimistic	Asceticism	Worthless	Forsaken	Depleted	Melancholic
Dependent	Incompetent	Submissive	Naive	Introjection	Inept	Immature	Inchoate	Pacific
Histrionic	Dramatic	Attention seeking	Flighty	Dissociation	Gregarious	Shallow	Disjointed	Fickle
Narcissistic	Haughty	Exploitive	Expansive	Rationalization	Admirable	Contrived	Spurious	Insouciant
Antisocial	Impulsive	Irresponsible	Deviant	Acting out	Autonomous	Debased	Unruly	Callous
Sadistic	Precipitate	Abrasive	Dogmatic	Isolation	Combative	Pernicious	Eruptive	Hostile
Compulsive	Disciplined	Respectful	Constricted	Reaction formation	Conscientious	Concealed	Compartmentalized	Solemn
Negativistic	Resentful	Contrary	Skeptical	Displacement	Discontented	Vacillating	Divergent	Irritable
Self-defeating	Abstinent	Deferential	Diffident	Exaggeration	Undeserving	Discredited	Inverted	Dysphoric
Schizotypal	Eccentric	Secretive	Autistic	Undoing	Estranged	Chaotic	Fragmented	Distraught or insentient
Borderline	Spasmodic	Paradoxical	Capricious	Regression	Uncertain	Incompatible	Split	Labile
Paranoid	Defensive	Provocative	Suspicious	Projection	Inviolable	Unalterable	Inelastic	Irascible

mulating an interpretation of the personality disorder scales. For example, the entire row of descriptors to the right of Histrionic includes the following interpretive adjectives: dramatic, attention seeking, flighty, dissociation, gregarious, shallow, disjointed, and fickle.

These adjectives serve as useful descriptors of the disorders as well as targets of treatment. As such, the behaviorist would want to reinforce less impulsive behavior in the antisocial person; the group therapist would want to help the dependent person construct healthy defenses; the cognitive therapist would focus on the flighty thought processes of the histrionic patient.

This symptom-to-treatment planning matrix illustrates the integrative quality of the MCMI-III and how this test is suitable for use by all therapists, regardless of theoretical orientation.

An STS/MCMI-III Model

A valid MCMI-III profile can be integrated into the STS therapy approach. A number of the MCMI-III scales provide valuable data regarding the six STS dimensions. As Table 7.7 indicates, some of the scales provide a dichotomous high–low scoring in some of the dimensions, whereas others provide specific qualitative information regarding other dimensions. These adjectives are borrowed from the domain theory of symptoms and treatment targets of the MCMI-III (Retzlaff, 1995).

STS Dimension and MCMI-III Scales

Most of the MCMI-III scales can be used to assess the STS dimensions. Functional impairment is likely if any of the three severe personality disorder scales are elevated, as these three disorders tend to result in the most social and occupational dysfunction. It is hard to be married to or supervised by a person with a schizotypal, borderline, or paranoid personality disorder. Although these hypotheses of functional impairment are probably accurate within the STS framework, it is likely and common that the other personality disorders on a case-by-case basis will have functional impairment problems especially if scores are high and/or there is the presence of Axis I-related difficulties.

Low scores on the Schizoid and Avoidant scales are theoretically indicative of low levels of social support and general interaction, whereas elevated Dependent and Histrionic scores tend to suggest high levels of social support. These high levels may not be all that functional and positive, but at least they are involved, and that involvement can be used toward therapeutic ends.

A comorbid Axis I disorder is usually required for a case to be seen as highly complex. However, high scores on any of the three severe personality disorder scales (Schizotypal, Borderline, Paranoid) tend to indicate a

TABLE 7.7. An STS—MCMI-III Model

Disorder	Functional impair-ment	Social support	Complexity	Coping style	Resistance	Distress
Schizoid		Low	Moderate	Disengaged—internal	Passivity—low	Low
Avoidant		Low	Moderate	Fantasy—internal	Fretful—low	High
Depressive			Moderate	Pessimistic—internal	Pessimistic—low	High
Dependent		High	Moderate	Submissive—internal	Incompetent—low	
Histrionic		High	Moderate	Attention-seeking—external	Dramatic—high	
Narcissistic			Moderate	Exploitive—external	Rationalization—high	Low
Antisocial			Moderate	Deviant—external	Irresponsible—high	Low
Sadistic			Moderate	Dogmatic—external	Abrasive—very high	Low
Compulsive			Moderate	Disciplined—internal	Constricted—low	Low
Negativistic			Moderate	Displacement—external	Contrary—high	High
Self-defeating			Moderate	Deferential—internal	Underserving—high	High
Schizotypal	High	Low	High	Eccentric—internal	Secretive—high	
Borderline	High		High	Labile—external	Regression—very high	
Paranoid	High	Low	High	Suspicious—external	Defensive—very high	Very high

221

high degree of problem complexity. Moderate-to-high complexity also can be indicated by high scores on any of the personality disorder scales, especially with a comorbid Axis I disorder. This approach is logical and straightforward, given the structure of Millon's personality disorder theory and the organization of the test. However, the three severe personality disorder scales reflect the most impairment and complexity.

The STS coping element is more qualitative. High scores on any of the scales can provide the clinician with information about how patients cope. For example, a high score on the Antisocial scale would suggest that the patient may externalize his or her difficulties through, perhaps, criminality or drug use. This patient would be likely to respond to stress and anxiety by acting out or blaming others. A person with compulsive tendencies is typically rigid and disciplined, and these attributes intensify when the person is under stress. This person will use more internal means of coping by developing lists, rules, and rituals that are rigidly followed.

Similarly, elevated scales also can suggest how and to what degree a patient may resist treatment. Someone with a high score on the Sadistic scale, for example, may present with an abrasive interpersonal style, making it very difficult for the clinician to work with him or her. Conversely, a dependent person is more likely to overrespond to and internalize suggestions made by the therapist.

With regard to the STS distress dimension, it is probably best to include the clinical syndrome scales in this interpretation. The Anxiety scale, particularly, is a good indicator of distress. The personality disorder scales, however, might add to the interpretation. Specifically, low scores on the Schizoid, Narcissistic, Antisocial, and Compulsive scales would probably indicate that the patient feels low levels of personal distress about his or her situation. This low level of response bodes poorly for therapy, as there is little felt need to change. Conversely, higher levels of distress would be generally be associated with higher scores on the Avoidant, Depressive, Negativistic, and Self-defeating scales. Very high levels of distress are likely in a patient whose score on the Borderline scale is elevated. Indeed, in this case, the distress often overwhelms any therapeutic attempts to explore the causes of the distress.

CASE EXAMPLE

The case used throughout this book as an example is detailed in Chapter 3. In brief, the 22-year-old female presents with a chief complaint of panic attacks and social phobias. More disturbing history includes physical and sexual abuse early in life, "emotional changeability," "doing well, messing up, and then feeling depressed," self-destructive behavior such as promiscuity and drug use, identity confusion with "different people within her," and a relationship with a much older, married man.

MCMI-III

The MCMI-III base rate scores for the case example (R.W.) can be found in Table 7.8 (and also Appendix A). For ease of interpretation, we have highlighted scores from 75 through 84([a]), those from 85 to 94([b]), and those above 94([c]). Following the outline for the interpretation of an MCMI-III protocol above, we first consider the Validity scales. None of the three items of unusual content was endorsed; therefore, it is assumed that the patient could and did read the items. The Disclosure score is at 54, right in the middle of the valid range. This score indicates that the patient neither under- nor overreported her symptoms. The profile is seen as a fairly accurate reflection of her current functioning.

Examining the personality disorder scales first and specifically, the severe personality disorder scales, the 84 on the Borderline scale is of concern. Here we reality test the MCMI-III hypotheses against the case history and find many elements of the presentation that would suggest a borderline personality disorder. As such, we accept that as the possible working diagnosis. People with borderline personality disorder come in many forms, and the basic personality disorder scales allow for a coloring of this particular case. There is usually a high Negativistic scale score associated with a high Borderline scale score, and that correspondence is evident here and consistent with the anger and social difficulties described in the case presentation. What is atypical in this protocol is the very high Narcissistic scale. At this level, the clinician would have to wonder which scale, the Borderline or the Narcissistic, should take precedence. Narcissism is an interesting explanation for the reported social sensitivity the patient experiences when there is discord with her lover. This complaint could initially be seen as an avoidant type of process, but there is also an egocentrism to it. The Schizoid high point may reflect situational reactivity or be part of a narcissistic aloofness. Finally, the high Self-defeating score is consistent with many of this patient's behaviors, such as the "doing well, messing up, and then feeling depressed" cycle and repeatedly choosing less-than-appropriate men with whom to become involved.

None of the three severe Clinical syndromes is high. Indeed, even within the basic clinical syndrome block, only Anxiety is high and that is at a relatively low 75. A relatively low Anxiety score is atypical of most borderline protocols. Usually Anxiety and Dysthymia are quite high and secondary to the borderline personality disorder. An explanation may be found in the atypical narcissistic elevation in the personality section. People with narcissistic personality disorder rarely report much affect on an MCMI-III. It is likely that the narcissistic features are insulating this patient from much of the usual "felt" affective disturbance. This lack of affect, however, appears to contradict all the anxiety and dysphoria reported in the history by this patient. This discrepancy could indicate that the reported disturbance is something of a behavioral manipulation.

TABLE 7.8. MCMI-III Base Rate
Scores for R.W.

Scale	PPP
Validity Scales	
Validity	0
Disclosure	54
Desirability	35
Debasement	56
Basic Personality Disorders	
Schizoid	78[a]
Avoidant	72
Depressive	68
Dependent	60
Histrionic	60
Narcissistic	98[c]
Antisocial	68
Sadistic	64
Compulsive	20
Negativistic	79[a]
Self-defeating	86[b]
Severe Personality Disorders	
Schizotypal	63
Borderline	84[a]
Paranoid	73
Basic Clinical Syndromes	
Anxiety	75[a]
Somatoform	26
Bipolar	72
Dysthymia	47
Alcohol Dependence	63
Drug Dependence	64
PTSD	60
Severe Clinical Syndromes	
Thought Disorder	43
Major Depression	38
Delusional Disorder	65

In sum, this patient appears to have a somewhat atypical narcissistic–borderline clinical profile. Obviously, she would be a difficult patient to manage and treat.

MCMI-III Treatment Planning

The domain-oriented psychotherapy recommendations explained above and summarized in Table 7.6 require a specific therapeutic style as a starting point. If the patient were seen as having a borderline condition with narcissistic features, a behaviorist would want to treat the erratic aspects of the behavior. However, any endogenous behavioral regulation would require behavioral contracting to control. The difficulty with this tack would be evident not only in the patient's borderline qualities but also in the haughty behavior driven by the narcissism.

Moving to the interpersonal conduct realm, should this patient be placed in group therapy, the borderline and narcissistic qualities would be manifested by paradoxical and exploitive behavior that would be a highly disruptive scenario for a quiet hour of group work. Such paradoxical and exploitative interpersonal behavior should be addressed by the therapist and group in an attempt to minimize it.

Table 7.6 provides the guidelines for cognitive, psychoanalytic, and other therapeutic orientations. Again, the descriptors are both interpretive/descriptive as well as indicative of directions for appropriate theory-specific treatment goals.

STS Interpretation of the Case

From an STS perspective, the case is a complex one, given the multiple symptoms and longstanding characterlogical issues in the history. This complexity is confirmed by the MCMI-III with the Borderline personality disorder high-point score in the Severe Personality Disorder section. The social support element is mixed. Although the case history makes much of older partners and a pathological need for support, the patient obviously has a mixed pattern of relationships. There is the sense that her need for social support is more out of a borderline fear of abandonment than a true, positive social interaction quality. The STS functional impairment theme is obvious in her history of not finishing high school, not having a job, and not having a more functional social/love life. The coping style is impaired by the labile affective complaints and the overreliance on inappropriate males in her life. The resistance traits are multiple, also consistent with a borderline hypothesis. Using our matrix, traits of regression are apparent and the need for parent-like lovers. The rationalization of the narcissist is also seen with the odd-sounding fear of social disapproval over choice of lovers. She reports more concern over others' estimation of her life than her own estimation. Finally, the STS distress dimension is obviously very high, again consistent with a borderline personality diagnosis. The affect is pan and poly and appears to be the chief complaint. However, this is an example of how the Axis I chief complaint is often actually reflecting an underlying personality disorder.

STS Treatment Planning

Following Gaw and Beutler's (1995) suggestions for integrating the STS model into treatment planning, we have found that this client's problem has been identified as both complex and severe enough so that it is functionally impairing. When attempting to tackle her complex problems, therapy will likely be most beneficial if it works toward setting outcome goals related to thematic changes. For example, focusing on obtaining employment as a goal would increase functioning while giving the patient a certain degree of independence from older men. To reach this goal, treatment planning for her would likely require a combination of methods, including psychosocial and environmental interventions. Since she becomes affectively labile when attempting to cope with her difficulties, a behavioral or skill-building focus to improve her ability to cope would be warranted. As mentioned above, this client will likely display a significant amount of resistance in therapy. This resistance will most likely take the form of regression driven by the borderline elements, and rationalization driven by the narcissistic traits. Therefore, self-directed, nondirective, and paradoxical interventions may be of value. Finally, theoretically and by chief complaint, her level of distress is high, which would normally indicate the need for arousal reduction procedures. However, the lack of objective evidence on testing of anxiety or dysphoria as well as the high narcissistic traits suggest that this element of the STS model will probably prove to be less fruitful.

SUMMARY

In this chapter, we have shown that the MCMI-III is a well-built modern test of broad-based psychopathology. The test is consistent with DSM-IV as well as diverse theoretical philosophies. The emphasis on personality disorders is useful for both diagnosticians and therapists. We have presented treatment planning from both the MCMI-III perspective and the STS perspective. The MCMI-III is a robust assessment device and allows these diverse perspectives.

8

The California
Psychological Inventory

David A. C. Donnay and Timothy R. Elliott

The intellectual roots of clinical assessment lay in a tradition of psychometric theory and its application in measurement; however, an array of practice and training opportunities in psychiatric settings during the mid-20th century eventually turned the *focus* of assessment to the detection and description of psychopathology (Maddux, 2002). In reaction to this well-entrenched enterprise, the positive psychology movement has decried the limitations of the "disease" model of human behavior, and has advocated for a renewed interest and emphasis on the positive aspects of human behavior and development (Seligman & Csikszentmihalyi, 2000). Unfortunately, psychologists seem to have considerable difficulty recognizing the personal assets, resources, and potentials in clientele (Sheldon & King, 2001; Vaillant, 2000; Wright & Fletcher, 1982). The reliance upon a psychopathological model has restricted the professional nomenclature to the extent that positive attributes, such as *affiliation, humor,* and *altruism,* are construed as "defense mechanisms" in the leading diagnostic manual (Maddux, 2002, p. 15).

Instruments that have a strong heritage in psychometric theory and that are unencumbered by a psychopathological bias will prove essential in the positive psychology movement. The California Psychological Inventory (CPI) has held this unique distinction for decades, and its use is as relevant today as when it was first introduced. Counseling psychologists—who have long extolled a focus on human assets and potential development (Gelso & Fretz, 1992)—have often used the CPI for research and applied purposes. The CPI is structured much like the MMPI (Hathaway & McKinley, 1943a), but it was developed primarily for use with non-pathological populations, and it yields scores on positive attributes of personality that are much more congruent with the themes of positive psychology.

The stated goal of the CPI is to assess individuals by means of variables and concepts that ordinary people use in their daily lives to understand, classify, and predict their own behavior and that of others. The primary purpose is to color a true-to-life and useful picture of the person taking the inventory. The CPI was first published commercially in 1957 (Gough, 1957) and published in its third edition in 1996. The current edition of the CPI (Gough & Bradley, 1996) contains 434 items in total, 158 of which also appear on the Minnesota Multiphasic Personality Inventory–2 (MMPI-2; Butcher, Dahlstrom, Graham, Tellegen, & Kaemmer, 1989).

The advent of the CPI came out of Harrison Gough's determination to develop personality measures using healthy adult personality constructs. He began with developing nonclinical measures, such as Social Status, Prejudice, Dominance, and Responsibility, from the MMPI item pool. Because of the clinical nature of the MMPI items, Gough eventually expanded his work, using his own pool of items designed for nonclinical populations. The first published edition of the inventory contained 18 scales measuring familiar concepts such as socialization, responsibility, and dominance. Prior to publication, an early research version of the CPI was available in 1951 and contained 548 items measuring 15 scales. The current 434-item edition of the inventory includes 20 folk scales, 3 structural scales, and a number of special scales and additional indicators (see Table 8.1).

BACKGROUND

Development of the CPI closely followed the logic of five guiding principles. Gough has espoused these principles as critical to appreciating the CPI's goal of understanding, classifying, and predicting peoples' behavior. The first two principles communicate the intended aims of the CPI. The remaining three principles outline criteria inappropriate for the CPI: namely, a theoretical definition of the structure of personality, orthogonal measurement of personality, and the assessment of personality traits.

The first principle dictates that the concepts measured on the CPI should be familiar to most everyone, everywhere. The idea is that such "folk concepts" represent everyday understandings about personality that all people, everywhere, use in observing and making sense of human behavior. In other words, it was decided, early on, that the concepts measured on the CPI should be ones spoken about by ordinary people trying to under-

TABLE 8.1. List of Scales on the CPI

CPI scale	Scale description (measure of)
Folk Scales	
Dominance (Do)	Prosocial interpersonal power and influence
Capacity for Status (Cs)	Ambition for challenge and social status
Sociability (Sy)	Social participation
Social Presence (Sp)	Poise and comfort with attention and recognition
Self-acceptance (Sa)	Sense of personal worth and self-confidence
Independence (In)	Self-sufficiency and self-directedness
Empathy (Em)	Capacity to understand and respond to others' needs
Responsibility (Re)	Conscientiousness and follow-through
Socialization (So)	Conformance with social norms and customs
Self-control (Sc)	Cautiousness and self-regulation
Good Impression (Gi)	Tact and positive self-presentation
Communality (Cm)	Conventionality of behavior and attitudes
Well-being (Wb)	Overall sense of health and optimism
Tolerance (To)	Open mindedness and respect for others
Achievement via Conformance (Ac)	Motivation within organized settings
Achievement via Independence (Ai)	Motivation within unstructured settings
Intellectual Efficiency (Ie)	Comfort with intellectual and conceptual matters
Psychological Mindedness (Py)	Analytical insight into the motivations of others
Flexibility (Fx)	Adaptability and comfort with change
Femininity/Masculinity (F/M)	Personal and interpersonal sensitivity
Vector Scales	
Externality–Internality (v. 1)	Extroversion versus introversion
Norm doubting–Norm favoring (v. 2)	Rule-following versus rule-questioning
Ego integration (v. 3)	Fulfillment of personal potential
Special Purpose Scales	
Managerial Potential (Mp)	Inclination for supervisory responsibilities
Work Orientation (Wo)	Sense of dedication to work
Creative Temperament (CT)	Individualization and capacity for innovativeness
Leadership (Lp)	Initiative and effectiveness in leading others
Amicability (Ami)	Cooperation and friendliness
Law Enforcement Orientation (Leo)	Conventional and practical values
Tough-mindedness (Tm)	Objective and rational decision making
Anxiety (Anx)	Nervousness and negative affectivity
Narcissism (Nar)	Grandiosity and feelings of entitlement

stand themselves and their interactions with others. This first principle also implies a degree of cultural universality. Consistent with this principle, the CPI has been translated and researched in nearly three dozen languages.

The second guiding principle states that the inventory is to remain an "open system." This principle means that scales may be added, or dropped, from the inventory, as deemed appropriate. A decision to add or drop a scale is based strictly on the ability of an individual scale or some combination of scales to predict important nontest criteria. The open system thereby allows for new scales to be added to the inventory if an important real-world behavior is not adequately predicted from the current scales or combinations of scales. Likewise, a scale may be dropped if it is found, over time, that it does not add substantially to the prediction of such criteria. At present, Gough (1996) contends that the 20 folk scales on the current CPI represent a sufficient number of constructs to predict "any consequential, recurring form of interpersonal behavior" (p. 2).

The third guiding principle concerns the instrumental approach of the CPI. According to this approach, each scale on the inventory must accurately predict what people will say and do in a given situation. In addition, each scale also must be able to identify how an individual would be described by an objective other who knows him or her well. By these two criteria, the "instrumental approach" sets the intention of the CPI as an inventory primarily concerned with the pragmatic goals of predicting the behavior of an individual and how he or she is seen by others. This intention is in contrast to what Gough (1996) calls the "definitional approach" to scale construction that tends to be more focused on academic constructs and blind adherence to psychometric criteria, such as internal consistency and orthogonality.

The fourth guiding principle addresses how the scales on the CPI relate to one another. According to this principle, the topography of the inventory should resemble how individuals use these concepts in the everyday language of describing people and their behaviors. The scales on the inventory, therefore, should relate to one another in a pattern that approximates, as a map would, the use of the folk concepts by ordinary people. Specifically, the intercorrelations of scales on the CPI should reflect the correlations between these same concepts in the natural world. Because of this topographical principle, the scales on the CPI are not psychometrically independent but rather naturally interrelated.

The fifth guiding principle deals with the intensification of measurement. In relation to the CPI, this principle means that classes or groups of scales represent higher-order structures for interpretation and that the individual folk scales reflect more nuanced measurement. Pushing this concept further, the fifth principle emphasizes that the individual scales of the CPI measure complex concepts (rather than unidimensional traits) to predict what people will say and do in specific contexts and how they will be perceived by others. The interpreter of the CPI is encouraged to attend to whole sections on the profile or to meaningful clusters of scales across the inventory for broader manifestations, and to the individual but multifaceted scales for important subtleties.

ADVANTAGES AND LIMITATIONS

This brief introduction to the CPI underscores some of its major advantages. The test is designed for normal populations, assesses important aspects of interpersonal relationships, can be used to evaluate an individual's strengths, and uses everyday folk concepts. As a result, the domains it measures are of interest to a wide range of individuals. Since the scales measure folk concepts, it also enables practitioners to provide feedback easily to participants. In contrast, assessments like the MMPI-2 require much more effort to translate scale score results into meaningful language. A further feature is that the CPI does an excellent job of measuring an individual's strengths. This arena may include such variables as the participant's degree of empathy, tolerance, or the extent to which he or she feels a sense of community with others. Thus, providing feedback is not only easy due to the use of folk concepts, but is also facilitated by the fact that discussing client strengths is more likely to increase rapport and acceptance than discussing the client's problem areas.

One of the main assets of the CPI is that it has been used extensively and, as a result, is extremely familiar in the field. A sample review of the literature reveals nearly 1,000 published studies of the CPI referenced in PsychINFO. Recent studies have addressed topics such as those listed in Table 8.2. Gough (2002) has collected nearly 2,000 published and unpublished studies of the CPI. The reader is also encouraged to see Groth-Marnat (in press-a) for a more in-depth review of studies related to educational, vocational, and clinical assessment.

A further asset of the CPI is that research efforts have paid close attention to making relevant real-life predictions. These predictions include such diverse areas as how effectively the person will function as a manager, how well he or she will perform in training programs (medical school, police training), likelihood of criminal recidivism, or simply the likelihood that others will describe him or her in a certain manner. Many of these predictions can be assisted with the use of regression equations or prediction indices from the existing literature.

One of the most frequent criticisms of the CPI is that there is extensive item overlap among the many scales, meaning that the scales measure somewhat similar constructs. A psychometric "purist" might argue that the scales should have been developed to measure constructs that were more clearly differentiated. The primary rebuttal to this criticism is that the

TABLE 8.2. Recent Research on the CPI

Research focus	Researchers
Academic achievement	Gough & Lanning (1986)
Job performance	Day & Bedeian (1991); Dyer (1987); Gough, Bradley, & McDonald (1991); Sarchione, Cuttler, Muchinsky, & Nelson-Gray (1998)
College student adjustment	Konson, Steurwald, Newman, & Widom (1994); Schroer & Dorn (1986)
Career assessment	Gough (1995a); Murray (1980)
Personality development	Helson & Roberts (1994); Helson, Stewart, & Ostrove (1995); Helson & Wink (1992); Loehlin (1997)
Social and political attitudes	Agronick & Duncan (1998)
Personnel selection	Hargrave & Hiatt (1989); Hough (1988)
Creativity	Helson & Pals (2000); Helson, Roberts, & Agronick (1995)
Depression	Holliman & Montross (1984)
Therapeutic responsiveness	Friesen & Andrews (1982)
Social intelligence	Sipps, Berry, & Lynch (1987; Sternberg, Wagner, Williams, & Horvath (1995)
Leadership	Gough (1990)
Marital and family relationships	Hooley & Hiller (2000); Wink & Helson (1993)
Cross-cultural personality assessment	Davis, Hoffman, & Nelson (1990); Yang et al. (1999)
Gender socialization	Helson & Picano (1990)
Employee retention	Haddad (1990)
Military success	Blake, Potter, & Slimak (1993); Campbell (1995)
Moral development	Gibson (1990)
Managerial potential	Gough (1984); Rawls & Rawls (1986)
Substance abuse	Alterman et al. (1998); Kadden, Litt, Donovan, & Conney (1996)
Stress management	Adams (1994)
Criminality	Collins & Schmidt (1993); Gough & Bradley (1992)
Personality disorder	Standage (1990); Standage, Smith, & Norman (1988)

scales reflect folk concepts, and the reality of these folk concepts is that, in real life, the concepts *do* overlap. For example, a person who is dominant is also likely to have a high capacity for status. This correspondence increases the likelihood of item overlap between scales seeking to measure these constructs. However, it is the subtle nuances between the scales that refine scale meanings. Importantly, these nuances in meanings accurately reflect real-life descriptions.

The second rebuttal to the criticism is that research on the CPI has been less concerned with scale refinements than whether or not the scales (and patterns of scales) can usefully predict real-life behaviors (e.g., success in graduate school; the likelihood of early resignation from a job). Thus the CPI should be judged on its instrumental characteristics—in other words, by the utilitarian criteria of how well it predicts what people say and do and what others will say about them. Critics have often failed to recognize this important differentiation, tending to compare the CPI against definitional criteria that better fit tests such as the Sixteen Personality Factor Questionnaire (16PF; Cattell, Eber, Tatsouka, 1970). The 16PF represents a definitional test, given its factorial construction, and as such displays slightly higher internal reliability and greater orthogonality. However, the CPI was never intended to meet these criteria. Rather, the CPI is intended to serve as a practical and useful measure of personality. The CPI does not define the traits or structures of personality, but it does include the necessary and sufficient concepts to provide an accurate and useful personological study of the individual.

A further criticism of the CPI is that insufficient research has been conducted on various patterns of scales. Often interpretation is based on a rational understanding of scale patterns rather than empirically derived knowledge. For example, it can be assumed that an individual who has a high score on the Dominance scale but a low score on the Empathy scale will have a leadership style that is highly task- (rather than person-) oriented and may be somewhat abrasive (especially if there is additional support from other rationally considered scales). In contrast to the CPI, the MMPI-2 has undergone extensive research on scale patterns (see code types, Butcher & Williams, 2000) that facilitate profile interpretation. The best source on CPI configurations to date is McAllister's *Practical Guide to CPI Interpretation* (1996).

PSYCHOMETRIC PROPERTIES

Reliability

Since the scales have been developed to approximate folk understandings of personality, they naturally have a multifaceted quality that might potentially result in lower internal consistency reliabilities. Nevertheless, the alpha coefficients of reliability are consistent with those usually found for self-report personality inventories. The alpha coefficients from the normative sample of 6,000 men and women range from .62 for Psychological Mindedness to .84 for Well-being, with an average of .75 for the 20 folk scales. The alpha coefficients for the three vector scales are .82, .77, and .88 for vectors 1, 2 and 3, respectively. The alpha coefficients for the nine most commonly used special purpose scales range from .49 for Anxiety to .88 for Leadership, with an average of .72. The intercorrelations from the normative sample of 6,000 show a preponderance of nonzero positive correlations, as would be expected. For example, the correlation coefficient of .75 between Dominance and Self-acceptance reflects the natural confluence of increasing ability to exert authority with increasing confidence in self-judgments.

The test–retest reliabilities suggest a reasonable degree of stability over time. For women over a 1-year period, the average correlation coefficient is .56 for the folk scales, .68 for the vector scales, and .58 for the special purpose scales. For men over a 5-year period, the average correlation coefficient is .60 for the folk scales, .68 for the vector scales, and .60 for the special purpose scales.

Validity

As noted, the CPI has been used extensively to make predictions of relevant behavior. The research has thus focused extensively on evaluating predictive validity. For example, law enforcement officers who exhibited dysfunctional behaviors scored relatively low on the CPI scales of Responsibility, Conscientiousness, and Self Control (Sarchione et al., 1998). In addition, CPI regression equations, based on patterns of scale scores, have been used to predict such variables as college grades (Gough, 1964; Gough & Lanning, 1996) and parole success (Gough, Wenk, & Rozynko, 1965; see Gough, 2000, and Groth-Marnat, in press-a, for more extensive reviews).

Even though the CPI was not designed using factor analysis, studies have supported a two-, four-, and five-factor solution. For example, Megargee (1972) found that a two-factor structure comprised of interpersonal effectiveness and internal control accounted for most of the variance. In contrast, Gough and Bradley (1996) found a five-factor solution (outlined in the Interpretation section; see level 3, "interpret scale groupings") consisting of ascendance, dependability, conventionality, originality, and masculinity–femininity. The factors of ascendance and conventionality correspond to the first two CPI vectors (Externality/Internality and Norm-doubting/Norm-focusing, respectively). Finally, various patterns of CPI scales correspond with the five-factor model of personality (neuroticism, extroversion, openness to experience, agreeableness, and conscientiousness; Johnson, 2000; McCrae, Costa, & Piedmont, 1993).

Openness to experience, for example, correlated with Flexibility (.42) and Independence (.41), Capacity for Status (.38), and Social Presence (.42; McCrae et al., 1993). The one exception: Agreeableness was only minimally represented. Overall, however, this research supports the CPI's validity as an instrument of relevant real-life predictions as well as a measure of core aspects of personality.

ADMINISTRATION AND SCORING

The CPI can be administered in one of the following three ways: (1) as a paper-and-pencil instrument for scanning or mail-in scoring, (2) as a computer-administered instrument on a local system, or (3) via the Internet. No hand-scoring templates are available for the latest edition of the CPI. Irrespective of the method used for administration, the same 434 items are used to generate one of three reports. The reports include the *CPI Profile Report* (Gough, 1995c), *CPI Narrative Report* (Gough, 1995b), and the *CPI Configural Analysis Report* (Gough & McAllister, 1995). The *CPI Profile Report* is an organized snapshot of the individual's CPI type, level, folk scale, and special purpose scale results. The *CPI Profile Report* provides standardized (i.e., mean = 50, standard deviation = 10) *T*-score results using both gender-specific and gender-neutral (combined) norms. The *CPI Narrative Report* provides written interpretation of each of the type, level, and scale results on the inventory. The report includes the graphic profiles from the *CPI Profile Report* and interprets and elaborates on that information in a readable, comprehensive format. The *CPI Narrative Report* also includes a listing of all 100 California Q-sort statements, ranked from the most to the least descriptive, which help to describe the individual in a knowledgeable, objective manner. The *CPI Configural Analysis Report* provides an even more complete interpretation that considers the separate CPI scales in combination. This report includes all of the information from the *CPI Profile Report* and *CPI Narrative Report* and builds on that information by providing interpretations based on combinations of two or more scales.

Studies of reliability and validity in numerous conditions, ranging from formal to informal testing sessions or even take-home or mail-survey administrations, have consistently shown similar, satisfactory results. When administering the test to persons who have severe mobility impairments, arrangements can be made for them to read the item quietly and respond to a technician with the item number and the response. Evidence indicates that this nonstandardized application with persons who have severe physical disabilities (e.g., persons with spinal cord injuries; Kemp & Vash, 1971) can result in profiles that are valid and meaningful. Nevertheless, standard supervised testing conditions are recommended, particularly when the results will be used for evaluative rather than developmental or research purposes.

The inventory is appropriate for most individuals above 13–14 years of age or with a reading level at or above seventh grade. For younger individuals, some of the 434 items may be somewhat difficult to understand or may be irrelevant to their life experiences. Questions concerning the simple meaning of a word or phrase should be explained; however, questions concerning interpretation of an item should be handled by encouraging the individual to use his or her own best judgment. The protocol may be scored if some items are left blank, but caution should be used if more than 30 of the items are left unanswered.

The inventory consists of 434 true–false items. The amount of time typically required to complete the inventory is approximately 45–60 minutes. Computer and Internet administration has actually proven to slightly shorten the duration of the testing sessions. The individual should be directed to read the instructions on the inventory, or the instructions may be read aloud to him or her. The instructions direct the respondent to consider each statement carefully and respond by indicating that the statement is either true or not true about him or her. In addition, better results are usually obtained when the individual is provided with a preface addressing the purpose of the testing and how the results will be used.

INTERPRETATION

The established method for interpretation of the CPI is a five-step process that moves from the overall clinical picture to the specific details of the measured scales and their interactions. Note that the remainder of this chapter, including our case study of R.W., follows this pathway from the general to the specific. The following is a listing of the five steps:

1. *Determine profile validity.* The interpretive process should begin with an assessment of the validity of the profile. A general impression of validity can be discerned from a perusal of the Good Impression, Communality, and Well-being scales. A more actuarial approach is also described in this chapter and is available to those using the computer- or Internet-scored versions of the instrument.

2. *Interpret vector scales.* The second step is to classify the profile based on the three vector scales into one of four types or general lifestyles, and by the level of realization of this type.

3. *Examine scale groupings.* The third step is to examine the overall profile and consider the different groupings of scales. Profiles with scores generally at or above 50 typically suggest positive functioning, whereas lower overall elevations indicate the possibility of some problems in adjust-

ment. Comparing the average elevations of the different groupings or classes of scales adds further accuracy to this type of impressionistic reading of the profile.

4. *Examine each of the individual scales, special purpose scales, and predictive indices.* The fourth step in interpreting the CPI is to examine each of the individual scales. Scores above or below 50 can be interpreted as relatively higher or lower levels of the particular attribute, respectively. In general, attention should be directed first to scores near 60 and above and to scores of approximately 40 or below. These score ranges, one standard deviation above or below the mean, can be interpreted with a fairly high level of confidence. However, a person's occupational, educational, and personal background should be taken into account when considering whether or not a score is high or low. For example, an attorney with "average" scores ($T = 50$) on Intellectual Efficiency may rate quite low when compared with others within his or her profession. Special purpose scales and predictive indices also can be used to refine the meanings of the 20 folk scales as well as provide additional information.

5. *Interpret interactions of the individual scales (configural interpretation).* The final step is to conduct a configural analysis of the profile by looking at the interactions of the individual scales. This concluding step encourages the interpreter to elaborate or adjust the meaning of a specific finding based on how the other scales moderate it. McAllister's guide (1996; *A Practical Guide to CPI Interpretation*) can be an extremely useful source to assist the examiner in interpreting the interactions between two or more scales. This step also might involve calculating and interpreting known actuarial equations used for making specific predictions related to areas such as achievement, college attendance, job performance, leadership, and parole success (see Groth-Marnat, in press-a).

Determine Profile Validity

A decision about whether or not a profile is sufficiently valid to make a reasoned interpretation is a matter of professional judgment. Ideally, such a judgment should be made in the context of knowledge of (1) the testing circumstances, (2) the individual's motivation for taking the test, (3) observational data, and (4) the larger configuration of the profile. Interpreting whether or not a profile is valid involves considering the overall larger context of the assessment in addition to examining the scores per se. The CPI has a number of features that attempt to help the user control for the validity of responses and resulting profiles. The origination of much of this work is found in the MMPI, with which the CPI shares many items.

In 1954, the author of the CPI identified 74 items on the MMPI that could be used to detect dissimulation or faking (Gough, 1954). For the CPI, Gough used 31 of these dissimulation items to score the CPI Well-being scale. The dissimulation items from the MMPI that were not included in the Well-being scale were those that indicate more extreme psychopathology. The Well-being scale is also scored in the reverse direction from the Dissimulation scale on the MMPI, in correspondence with the CPI's emphasis on positive psychological functioning and human strengths. Low scores at or below 30 on the Well-being scale may suggest that the individual is exaggerating personal distress or providing a fake–bad profile.

The Good Impression scale consists of 40 items that show significant differences when a respondent is attempting to be judged as admirable and praiseworthy (Gough, 1952). High scores at or above 70 on Good Impression suggest extremely positive response characteristics consistent with a fake–good profile. This profile generally occurs when the respondent is trying to make a positive impression on the test, such as in a job application or other such evaluative setting. Low scores at or below 30 suggest a more negative response bias and the possibility of a fake–bad profile.

The Communality scale is very similar to the F scale on the MMPI. The Communality scale contains 38 items that respondents almost always identify in a given direction. In other words, the scale is made up of a subset of items to which a very high percentage of respondents answers true, and another subset of items to which a very high percentage of respondents answers false. The Communality scale measures the extent to which an individual has answered the CPI in a typical or modal fashion. High scores at or above 50 on this scale suggest a standard approach to the inventory; low scores at or below 30 indicate the possibility of random responding, inability to read, errors in marking, or a fake–bad profile.

For more precise classification of fake–good, fake–bad, and random profiles, three equations have been developed (Lanning, 1989) and are available to the interpreter. The three equations improve classification by combining the three validity indicators already discussed plus the addition of other scales from the CPI profile. The following three linear equations use raw scale scores:

$$\text{Fake good} = 41.225 + .273\text{Do} + 198\text{Em} + .538\text{Gi} - .255\text{Wb} - .168\text{Fx}$$

$$\text{Fake bad} = 86.613 - 1.000\text{Cm} - .191\text{Wb} + .203\text{Ac} - .110\text{Fx}$$

$$\text{Random} = 34.096 = .279\text{Gi} + .201\text{Wb} + .225\text{Py} + .157\text{Fx}$$

The results of the three equations are applied in a decision-tree format. If the fake–good score is equal to or greater than 60.60, the profile is considered fake–good. If the score on fake–bad is equal to or greater than 59.50, and if the score on random is less than 48.01, the profile is considered fake–bad. Lastly, if the score on fake–bad is equal to or greater than 59.50, and the score on random is equal to or greater than 48.01, the profile is considered random. All other profiles are considered normal.

Interpret Vector Scores

Considerable efforts were taken to identify orthogonal dimensions within the inventory that might provide a parsimonious model for interpretation. Through a series of factor and spatial analyses of the folk scales, Gough (1987) identified three primary themes or dimensions. The three themes concern orientation toward people, orientation toward societal values and rules, and orientation toward self. Gough (1987, 2000; Gough & Bradley, 1996) has frequently compared the three themes within the CPI to the work of Philip Vernon. Vernon (1953) surveyed the personality literature and identified two primary dimensions arising out of the factor analytic studies done by that time. The two dimensions Vernon pinpointed were dependability–undependability and extroversion–introversion. These dimensions are indeed very similar to the CPI's themes toward societal values and rules and orientation toward people.

In constructing a parsimonious model for interpreting the CPI, Gough (1987) conducted a tedious review of item-correlation matrices, with various experimental markers ultimately revealing pools of items to represent the three themes. The items were chosen for each dimension based on contribution to the content of an individual theme and minimal correlation with items representing the other two themes. The resulting three-vector model has come to consist of three vector scales. The three scales are externality–internality (v. 1), norm-favoring versus norm-doubting (v. 2), and ego integration (v. 3) (see Figure 8.1).

In using the three-vector model for interpretation of the CPI, the three scales, v. 1, v. 2, and v. 3, are best considered in concert. Considered together, the v. 1 and v. 2 scales define four types or lifestyles unique to the CPI: The four lifestyles are termed Alpha, Beta, Gamma, and Delta. The third scale, v. 3, is a measure of self-realization within each lifestyle, indicating the degree to which the person has maximized the potentiality of his or her own style. Results on v. 3 range from malfunctioning and risks for psychopathology to psychological competence and potential for superior ego integration. Seven levels exist within v. 3; level 1 represents *poor* realization; level 2 represents *distinctly below-average* realization; level 3 represents *below-average* realization; level 4 represents *average* realization; level 5 represents *above-average* realization; level 6 represents *distinctly above-average* realization; and level 7 represents *superior* realization of style.

Description of the four lifestyles varies depending on the level to which the style has been realized by the individual (see Table 8.3). At higher levels of realization, Alpha styles are exhibited by socially oriented and ambitious individuals who tend to meet external expectations and readily accept responsibility for themselves and others. They can be charismatic and productive leaders. "Alphas" may also be referred to as implementers. Alphas who have not realized their potential are likely to be described as authori-

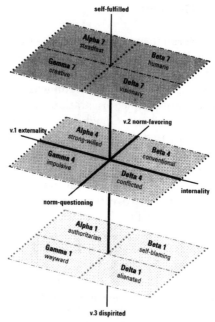

Figure 2.3 Schematic Representation of the Three-Vector or
Cuboid Model of Personality Structure Showing
Cross-Sections at Levels 1, 4, and 7 of Ego Integration

FIGURE 8.1. Schematic representation of the three-vector model of personality, with cross-sections at levels 1, 4, and 7 of functioning. Modified and reproduced with special permission of the Publisher, Consulting Psychologists Press, Inc., Palo Alto, CA 94303 from the CPI Manual, Third Edition, by Harrison Gough, PhD. Copyright 1996 by CPP, Inc. All rights reserved. Further reproduction is prohibited without the Publisher's written consent.

TABLE 8.3. Adjectival Descriptors for Each Lifestyle at Lower and Higher Levels of Functioning

Lifestyle	Lower functioning	Higher functioning
Alpha (implementer)	Self-centered, manipulative	Interpersonally oriented, productive, task-focused, ambitious, accepts responsibility for leading others
Beta (supporter)	Overly conforming, rigid, unresponsive	Well-controlled, dependable, comfortable in the role of follower
Gamma (innovator)	Rebellious, selfish, skeptical, disruptive	Individualistic, engaged, innovative
Delta (visualizer)	Self-defeating, withdrawn, vulnerable, prone to decompensation, detached	Private, reflective, imaginative, creative

tarian, self-centered individuals who tend to criticize others and manipulate situations for their own advantage.

At higher levels of realization, Beta styles are exhibited by internally focused, dependable individuals who adhere to, and protect, social norms and values. "Betas" can be strong models of virtue, are often inclined to support the needs of others. Betas may be referred to as supporters. Betas who are not well realized may be seen as inhibited, rigid individuals who are unresponsive to their environment.

Higher-level Gamma styles are exhibited by engaged, creative individuals who tend to question traditional norms and values. "Gammas" can be innovative, cutting-edge leaders. Gammas may be referred to as innovators. Gammas who have not realized the potential of their style are frequently described as self-centered and disruptive individuals who tend to rebel in impulsive, nonproductive ways.

Delta styles at higher levels are exhibited by reserved, reflective individuals who tend to think and act privately on their own terms. "Deltas" can be imaginative, artistic contributors, even visionary leaders. Deltas may also be referred to as visualizers. Deltas who are not well realized are likely to be seen by others as withdrawn and self-defeating individuals who live primarily in their own private world of thoughts and fantasies.

Examine Scale Groupings

The 20 CPI folk scales are typically organized around the classes described in this section. Factor analysis of the scales has provided an alternate arrangement, which will also be discussed. The organization of the scales into the following classes or factors provides a conceptual framework that assists with interpretation of the instrument:

Scale Classes

The 20 folk scales on the CPI are usually presented as four separate groups or classes of scales. The four classes of scales are organized according to conceptual or rational decisions about the folk use of the scales and not according to any statistical measure of similarity.

Class I scales measure interpersonal aspects of the self, such as self-confidence, poise, ascendancy, and social effectiveness. The seven scales in this first class are Dominance, Capacity for Status, Sociability, Social Presence, Self-acceptance, Independence, and Empathy. Scores consistently above 50 on these scales suggest outgoing, socially competent persons. Lower scores are indicative of a more socially reticent, nonassertive style.

Class II scales assess internal values and normative expectations such as personal values, self-control, maturity, and sense of responsibility. The seven scales in this class are Responsibility, Socialization, Self-control,

Good Impression, Communality, Well-being, and Tolerance. Taken together, elevations on all or most of these scales suggest a cautious, controlled type of person. In contrast, lower scores suggest a more carefree, action-oriented person who may also have problems with controlling his or her impulses.

Class III scales measure achievement needs and cognitive tendencies, including motivation, persistence, and organization. The three scales included in this class are Achievement via Conformance, Achievement via Independence, and Intellectual Efficiency. Consistently high scores, above 50, on these three scales suggest a driven person with superior ability to access his or her intellectual resources under a variety of environmental circumstances. Lower scores suggest a reluctant individual with less ability to draw on his or her own resources, except in the most concrete and tangible of matters.

Class IV scales assess stylistic preferences for attributes such as insightfulness, adaptability, and sensitivity. The three scales in this grouping are Psychological Mindedness, Flexibility, and Femininity–Masculinity. High scores (above 50) on these three scales are indicative of someone who could be described as perceptive, open-minded, and attuned to his or her surroundings. Scores below 50 on these scales suggest someone with a more closed stance who functions best in a stable, predictable environment.

Scale Factors

Factor analysis has provided an alternative approach to the class groupings. The intercorrelational matrix of the 20 folk scales has been examined on several occasions (see discussion in Gough & Bradley, 1996), typically yielding a five-factor solution (e.g., Burger, Pickett, & Goldman, 1977).

Ascendance, the first factor, is represented by the same seven scales as found in class I scales: Dominance, Capacity for Status, Sociability, Social Presence, Self-Acceptance, Independence, and Empathy. Not surprisingly, this factor appears to measure assertiveness, poise, self-assurance, initiative, and interpersonal effectiveness. Consistently high scores, above 50 on the scales of this factor suggest a confident, outgoing, charismatic, and ascendant person. Lower scores here are suggestive of individuals who are more withdrawn and prefer to maintain a low profile.

Dependability, the second factor, appears to measure overall personal adjustment and sense of well-being and is represented by as many as seven scales. The scales making the largest contribution to this factor are Self-control and Good Impression, but Responsibility, Socialization, Well-being, Tolerance, and Achievement via Conformance also lend meaning to this factor. Consistently high scores, above 50, on the scales of this factor suggest a person who could be described as stable, well-socialized, and reasonable. Lower scores are indicative of those who are more influenced by their emotions and may occasionally be seen as erratic or impulsive in their behaviors.

Originality, the third factor, is represented by five scales: Achievement via Independence, Flexibility, Tolerance, Intellectual Efficiency, and Psychological Mindedness. This factor appears to measure degree of independent thought and action. Consistently high scores (above 50) on these scales suggest a person described as autonomous, open-minded, and creative. Lower scores are indicative of more conventional thought and action.

Conventionality, the fourth factor, is most centrally represented by Communality, but Responsibility, Socialization, and Well-being contribute. Together, the four scales of this factor measure the degree of adherence to social norms. Higher scores (consistently above 50) on these scales suggest a person who could be described as conforming and socially responsible. Lower scores are indicative of a more unconventional individual, with a tendency to act with less regard for social expectations or rules.

Sensitivity, the fifth factor, is defined primarily by the Femininity–Masculinity scale. This remaining factor measures general sensitivity, aesthetic interests, and tender- versus tough-mindedness. Consistently high scores of above 50 on this scale are indicative of individuals described as sensitive to others' emotions, interested in artistic expressions, and generally tender-minded. Lower scores suggest action-oriented individuals who could be described as pragmatic and tough-minded.

Examine Each of the Folk Scales, Special Purpose Scales, and Predictive Indices

Below are descriptions of each of the 20 folk scales. It should be noted that they are also organized according to the four different classes described above. Tables summarizing the scale descriptors are included and similarly organized around the classes. For example, Table 8.4 summarizes the descriptors for each of the seven scales comprising the first class; Tables 8.5–8.7 summarize the descriptors for classes II–IV.

Class I Scales

Dominance (Do). The 36-item Dominance scale was empirically constructed with the purpose of assessing attributes related to prosocial interpersonal dominance. The scale has been shown to consist of the following four factors: leadership, self-mastery, authority, and obligation. The Dominance scale is a useful measure of leadership ability, assertiveness, verbal fluency, persuasiveness, and social poise. It can be used to assess the extent to which a person is likely to take charge and persist to achieve a social good.

TABLE 8.4. Adjectival Descriptors for Low/High Scores for Each of the Class I Scales

Class I scale	Low scores	High scores
Dominance (Do)	Unassuming, reticent, mild, submissive	Confident, assertive, persuasive, task-centered
Capacity for Status (Cs)	Unsure of self, dislikes direction, noncompetitive, pessimistic, silent	Ambitious, wants to be a success, likes the good life, outgoing
Sociability (Sy)	Shy, feels uneasy in social situations, prefers to stay in the background, worries about making decisions	Sociable, active, optimistic, socially competent
Social Presence (Sp)	Cautious, hesitant about stating own views, reserved, inhibited	Self-assured, spontaneous, not easily embarrassed, witty
Self-acceptance (Sa)	Self-doubting, readily assumes blame when things go wrong, often thinks others are better, withdrawn	Has good opinion of self, self-confident, views self as talented, outspoken
Independence (In)	Lacks self-confidence, seeks support from others, defers to others, often nervous	Self-sufficient, resourceful, detached, strong-willed
Empathy (Em)	Uneasy in social situations, unempathic, defensive, not good at judging other people	Likeable, feels comfortable about self, understands the feelings of others

Capacity for Status (Cs). The 28-item Capacity for Status scale was empirically derived with the purpose of measuring personal qualities that are associated with, and that lead to, high social status. The scale is comprised of items that largely adhere to the following four factors: poise/self-assurance, aesthetic/cultural interests, optimism, and recognizing the advantage of status and success. The Capacity for Status scale is useful in assessing people who view themselves as having high status and who are self-assured. It is not a measure of people who have high status from an objective standpoint, but rather reflects an absence of anxiety and a high degree of social confidence.

Sociability (Sy). The 32-item Sociability scale was empirically constructed to measure degree of social interaction. The following four factors comprise the scale: comfort/self-assurance, enjoyment of social functions, self-confidence, and enjoying attention. The purpose of the Sociability scale is to identify people who are outgoing, socially affiliative, and who enjoy social participation. The scale was originally developed to predict the extent to which people participate in social activities. It has since been generalized and found to differentiate usefully between outgoing and shy people.

Social Presence (Sp). The 38-item Social Presence scale was developed using rational scale construction with the purpose of measuring social poise and charisma. The items hold together well within the following three-factor model: self-confidence/self-assurance, self-assertion/liking attention, pleasure seeking/zest for new experiences. The Social Presence scale is useful for identifying people characterized by feelings of self-assurance, confidence in dealing with others, and versatility. It measures poise, feelings of personal worth, confidence, sense of accomplishment, and spontaneity in social situations.

Self-acceptance (Sa). The 28-item Self-acceptance scale was constructed using a rational approach to scale construction with the purpose of measuring feelings of personal worth and accomplishment. The following three factors represent the variance of this scale: comfortable/confident in dealing with others, willingness to admit self-serving/self-centered behavior, and positive self-evaluation. The Self-acceptance scale can be used to identify persons with high self-regard and a strong sense of personal esteem.

Independence (In). The 38-item Independence scale was empirically constructed as a measure of the extent to which people strive for vocational and interpersonal autonomy. The following three factors are important to this measure: resoluteness/perseverance/feeling competent, self-confident/assured under scrutiny, and self-sufficient/willingness to follow own judgment despite disagreement from others. The purpose of this scale is to assess the twin elements of psychological strength and interpersonal detachment.

Empathy (Em). The 38-item Empathy scale was empirically constructed to measure the ability to perceive and feel the experiences of others. The scale has the following four primary factors: personal flexibility, accommodating to others' feelings, social interest/leadership skills, and interests in intellectual activities. The purpose of this scale is to identify persons with affective insight (i.e., a talent for understanding how others feel or think). It is also a useful measure of related social skills such as confidence, leadership, social awareness, and extroversion.

Class II Scales

Responsibility (Re). The 36-item Responsibility scale was empirically derived in order to measure the acceptance of social rules. Responsibility, as measured by this scale, contains the following four factors: feelings of re-

TABLE 8.5. Adjective Descriptors for Low/High Scores for Each of the Class II Scales

Class II scale	Low scores	High scores
Responsibility (Re)	Unconcerned about duties and responsibilities, tends to be careless and lazy, immature, rebellious	Responsible, circumspect, takes duties seriously, dependable
Socialization (So)	Resists rules and regulations, finds it hard to conform, unconventional, tends to blame others for problems	Conservative, sincere, comfortably accepts ordinary rules and regulations, finds it easy to conform
Self-control (Sc)	Impulsive, willing to take risks, has strong feelings and emotions and makes little attempt to hide them, speaks out when angry or annoyed	Avoids risks, peaceable, tries to control emotions and temper, takes pride in being self-disciplined
Good Impression (Gi)	Skeptical, frank, individualistic, insists on being him- or herself even if this causes friction or problems	Tactful, compliant, wants to make a good impression, tries to please others
Communality (Cm)	Moody, sees self as different from others, preferences and ideas often differ from others, has given unusual answers to many items on the test, moody	Stable, practical, fits in easily, sees self as an average person
Well-being (Wb)	Complaining, anxious, concerned about health and personal problems, worried about the future	Optimistic, cheerful, feels in good physical and emotional health, copes well with pressures and demands
Tolerance (To)	Distrustful, self-centered, resentful, not tolerant of others' beliefs and behaviors	Fair-minded, reasonable, clear thinking, tolerant of others' beliefs even when different from own

sponsibility, dependability, civic responsibilities for others, and positive attitudes toward education and self-improvement. The Responsibility scale is useful in identifying persons who are aware of societal rules and who can and do comply with them, when appropriate. In fact, the scale appears to tap into the type of person that has a true understanding of the need and purpose for such rules. It assesses social responsibility, conscientiousness, and dependability.

Socialization (So). The 46-item Socialization scale was empirically constructed primarily to assess the degree to which societal norms have been internalized and become autonomously operational within the individual. Four factors comprise the Socialization scale: self-discipline and rule-observing behavior; optimism, self-confidence, and positive emotionality; good upbringing and favorable family memories; and interpersonal awareness and reflective temperament. The Socialization scale is a useful measure of adherence to social norms, maturity, integrity, delinquency, and antisocial behavior.

Self-control (Sc). The 38-item Self-control scale was rationally constructed as a measure of the degree to which an individual can self-direct his or her own behavior. The following four factors comprise this scale: self-control, modesty, denying of rule-breaking tendencies, and suppression of hedonistic and aggressive feelings. The purpose of the Self-control scale is to identify persons with strong, effective, mechanisms of ego control and societal constraint. The scale is a useful assessment of internalized social norms, social values, and of the ability to self-regulate and maintain freedom from impulsive behavior.

Good Impression (Gi). The 40-item Good Impression scale was developed using a combination of empirical and rational scale construction methods. The scale measures the degree to which an individual is prone toward trying to make a good impression. The scale has at least four factors, including denying self-serving or egotistic motives, claiming equanimity and absence of moodiness or irritability, willingness to accept supervision and work under strict rules, and expressing faith in ethics and goodwill. The primary purpose of the Good Impression scale is to identify CPI protocols too strongly characterized by social desirability and thereby detect invalid or dissimulated profiles. The scale is interpretable, however, as a measure of a more generalized self-presentation style that emphasizes ingratiation and compliance.

Communality (Cm). The 38-item Communality scale was developed using a combination of empirical and rational scale construction methods. The scale is essentially a measure of random responding. However, four interpretable factors have been identified: disagreeing with negative views of human nature, optimism about self and society, recognizing benefits that accrue from life experiences, and admitting to ordinary emotionality and affect. The primary purpose of the Communality scale is to identify protocols with too many deviant or unusual responses to permit ordinary interpretation of the instrument for that individual. Interpretation of this scale also allows for assessment of good socialization, conformity, optimism, denial of neurotic characteristics, and conventionality of behavior and attitudes.

Well-being (Wb). The 38-item Well-being scale was developed using a combination of empirical and rational scale construction methods. The scale is primarily a measure of a person's adjustment. The scale is comprised of the following four factors: feelings of wholeness and ability to withstand stress, trust in others and feelings that life is fair, good relations with others and absence of extreme irritation, and happiness and good morale. The purpose of the Well-being scale is to assess feelings of physical and psychological well-being. Extremely low scores also suggest that individuals are feigning emotional disturbances or faking bad responses.

Tolerance (To). The 32-item Tolerance scale was developed empirically as a measure of nonjudgmental social beliefs (high scores) and intolerant attitudes (low scores). The four factors of this scale are integrity and goodwill, feelings of being treated fairly, concern for others, and belief in the ideas of fairness and equity. The Tolerance scale was constructed to assess attitudes of tolerance, patience, and respect for others. It is a measure of the degree to which persons are socially intolerant versus the extent to which they are accepting, permissive, and nonjudgmental in their social beliefs and attitudes.

Class III Scales

Achievement via Conformance (Ac). The 38-item Achievement via Conformity scale was empirically constructed to measure positive orientation toward achievement in clearly structured situations. The following four factors are important in understanding this scale: ability to concentrate and think in order to persevere, acceptance of rules and conformity, expression of liking for school, and planfulness and orientation toward the future. The purpose of the Achievement via Conformity scale is to assess achievement potential within well-defined academic and vocational environments. It is a useful measure of need for structure and organization as a means for harnessing achievement motivations.

Achievement via Independence (Ai). The 36-item Achievement via Independence scale was empirically constructed as a measure of achievement based on attributes of autonomy and independence. The scale has four important factors: independent beliefs, confidence in self and in the future, breadth of interests, and denying common fears. The purpose of the Achievement via Independence scale is to assess achievement potential in open, minimally defined situations. It is predictive of superior performance in settings requiring independent planning and effort.

Intellectual Efficiency (Ie). The 42-item Intellectual Efficiency scale was empirically derived to measure intellectual resources and endurance. The scale has the following four interpretable factors: good morale and confidence about the future, denial of common fears and worries, partici-

TABLE 8.6. Adjectival Descriptors for Low/High Scores for Each
of the Class III Scales

Class III scale	Low scores	High scores
Achievement via Conformance (Ac)	Easily distracted, an underachiever, has difficulty doing best work in settings with strict rules and regulations, does not like to conform	Industrious, efficient, has strong drive to do well in school and elsewhere, likes to have goals clearly defined
Achievement via Independence (Ai)	Apathetic, lacks initiative, has difficulty doing best work in situations that are vague and lacking in clear-cut goals, wants others to specify objectives and methods	Insightful, versatile, has strong drive to do well in any situation, likes work that requires initiative and independent thinking
Intellectual Efficiency (Ie)	Lacks confidence, has limited interests, easily discouraged, prefers dealing with tangible matters rather than concepts or abstractions	Verbally fluent, foresighted, makes good use of intellectual abilities, thinks easily about abstract ideas

pation in intellectual activity, and enjoyment of science. The purpose of the
Intellectual Efficiency scale is to assess the degree to which intellectual resources are efficiently utilized over time. It is a useful measure of personality factors related to degree of conceptual ability, efficient use of cognitive
ability, and good sense in general living.

Class IV Scales

Psychological Mindedness (Py). The 28-item Psychological Mindedness scale was empirically constructed to measure interest in psychological
phenomena. The scale includes these four factors: ability to direct and
maintain intellectual functions, indifference to minor conventions and personal neatness, liking for intellectual endeavors, and ability to maintain
nonjudgmental stance until all facts are known. The purpose of the Psychological Mindedness scale is to identify people who think psychologically
and have a knack for figuring out how people think and feel by attuning to
their needs, motives, and experiences. It is an assessment of an analytic, rational, conceptualizing approach to understanding people.

Flexibility (Fx). The 28-item Flexibility scale was developed using rational scale construction methods to measure adaptability and comfort
with change. The four factors of the scale are tolerance for ambiguity,
noncompulsiveness, admitting bias and prejudgment, and absence of severe

TABLE 8.7. Adjective Descriptors for Low/High Scores for Each
of the Class IV Scales

Class IV scale	Low scores	High scores
Psychological Mindedness (Py)	Feels misunderstood by others, tends to complain, poor at predicting how others will feel and react, looks more at what people do than at what they think	Understands people's feelings, forms impressions quickly, good at detecting flaws and self-deceptions of others, avoids close relationships
Flexibility (Fx)	Careful and deliberate in new situations, well-organized, uncomfortable with ambiguity, programmatic and planful	Changeable, imaginative, likes change and variety, easily bored by routine and everyday experience
Femininity/ Masculinity (F/M)	Aggressive, tough-minded, action-oriented, somewhat insensitive to others' feelings	Sensitive to criticism, tends to interpret events from a personal perspective, tries not to hurt others' feelings, often feels vulnerable

or punitive constraint. The purpose of the Flexibility scale is to assess a continuum from resistance to change and from novelty to fluidity. It is a useful measure of abilities related to flexible and adaptable thinking, behavior, and temperament.

Femininity/Masculinity (F/M). The 32-item Femininity/Masculinity scale was empirically constructed to measure the continuum from femininity to masculinity. The scale consists mainly of the following four factors: preference for traditional masculine occupations, feelings of vulnerability, preference for traditional female occupations, and dislike of horseplay and practical jokes. The purpose of the Femininity/Masculinity scale is to assess a continuum from individualistic to sensitive, nurturant beliefs and values.

Special Purpose Scales

Over the years, and in keeping with the test's open system, a number of scales has been developed from the CPI item pool for use in specific applications. The following is a brief review of the most frequently used of these scales.

Managerial Potential (Mp). The 34-item Managerial Potential scale was empirically constructed to measure behavioral effectiveness, self-confidence, cognitive clarity, and goal orientation. The primary purpose of this scale is to identify individuals with an interest in supervisory or managerial positions. The scale has been shown to be a useful predictor of good performance in management (Gough, 1984; Jacobs, 1992).

Work Orientation (Wo). The 40-item Work Orientation scale was developed empirically to measure degree of dedication to work and the likelihood of performing well, even in the most routine or unheralded positions. Its primary purpose is to identify individuals with a disciplined will to work versus those lacking a strong work ethic.

Creative Temperament (CT). The 42-item Creative Temperament scale was empirically constructed as a measure of creativity in a broad sense and includes such themes as individualized and nonconventional values, enjoyment of the unpredictable and improbable, and progressive social attitudes. The Creative Temperament scale is useful in identifying individuals with the potential to generate original and inventive ideas. Scores are generally found to correlate with observers' ratings of creativity.

Leadership (Lp). The 70-item Leadership scale was empirically developed to identify individuals whom others view as having the characteristics and requisite skills of a leader. The Leadership scale is a useful measure of the extent to which an individual is able to gain the admiration and cooperation of others. It also appears to tap into related attributes of leadership, such as confidence, resilience, resourcefulness, and initiative.

Amicability (Ami). The 36-item Amicability scale was empirically constructed as a measure of the degree to which an individual can be described as cooperative and friendly. The purpose of the scale is to identify individuals who are socially responsive and considerate in their dealings with others.

Law Enforcement Orientation (Leo). The 42-item Law Enforcement Orientation scale was developed empirically to measure characteristics such as organization and conscientiousness that are strongly related to success in the world of work generally and to positive outcomes in law enforcement work specifically. The intended purpose of this scale is to identify individuals with an orientation toward law enforcement and with a likelihood of success in such work.

Tough-Mindedness (Tm). Based on works by William James (1907) and Eysenck (1944), the 36-item Tough-mindedness scale was rationally constructed as a measure of the extent to which an individual is tough-minded versus tender-minded in his or her thinking. The purpose of the scale is to identify persons who are independent and objective thinkers.

Anxiety (Anx). The 22-item Anxiety scale was developed (Leventhal, 1966) to parallel the Anxiety scale on the MMPI. The scale measures an individual's degree of nervousness or tension. The purpose of the scale is to identify anxious, pessimistic individuals.

Narcissism (Nar). The 49-item Narcissism scale was rationally developed in order to measure exaggerated self-esteem and narcissism, including the additional themes of devaluation of others, feelings of entitlement, and dissatisfaction with present level of status. The purpose of the Narcissism scale is to identify individuals with a tendency toward self-centeredness and egotism.

Predictive Indices

In addition to the special purpose scales (e.g., Managerial Potential, Creative Temperament), clinical use and ongoing research have contributed special indices for predicting important nontest behaviors. The Leadership Potential Index, Social Maturity Index, and Creative Potential Index are examples of these types of indices available within the extensive CPI literature.

Leadership Potential Index (Lpi). The Leadership Potential Index was derived to identify potential leadership, foresight, and decisiveness. The index has been used a number of times in the literature, including its introduction in 1969 (Gough) and in a study of personological dynamics of leadership in 1978 (Hogan).

Social Maturity Index (Smi). The Social Maturity Index was developed (Gough, 1966) to assess self-discipline, good judgment, and sensitivity to moral and ethical issues.

Creative Potential Index (Cpi). The Creative Potential Index was derived (Weiss, 1981) through a multigroup analysis of the personality patterns involved in creative processes. It is useful in identifying persons motivated to work innovatively, create new ideas and products, and deviate from customary practices.

Interpret Interactions of the Individual Scales (Configural Interpretation)

It is critical to the purpose of the CPI—that is, "to furnish information to the interpreter from which a veridical (true-to-life) and useful picture may be drawn of the person taking the test" (Gough & Bradley, 1996, p. 1)—that the interactions among the scales on the profile be considered. However, the meaning of pairs or combinations of scales on the CPI is not as well researched as MMPI code types. Future research on the meaning of specific pairs or combinations of CPI scales is probably central to a greater use of this tool. McAllister (1996) outlined 152 different configural combinations of CPI scales with varying levels of empirical, clinical, and rational bases. Specific scale combinations are noted below with respect to the STS model.

SYSTEMATIC TREATMENT SELECTION

The CPI was designed primarily for use with nonpatient populations such as individuals in vocational settings. However, a number of inferences can be made in accordance with the STS model, and this information might be relevant to the treatment of patients entering psychotherapy.

Degree of Functional Impairment

The domain of *functional impairment* in the STS system refers to the degree to which clients can function in an adaptive manner. The CPI makes this type of assessment from a strengths perspective. A number of CPI scales indicate the degree to which respondents are able to draw on their intrapersonal and interpersonal capacities. At the same time, the CPI is not a diagnostic test and therefore does not diagnose specific symptoms or clusters of symptoms (disorders).

The v. 3 scale is the most obvious indicator of functioning on the CPI; this scale provides data on how well individuals use their psychological capacities and realize their potentialities. The continuum of functioning, from full ego integration to psychological incompetence, is also assessed. The v. 3 scale should be interpreted as a general assessment of functioning that taps into overall attributes of psychological and physical well-being, interpersonal maturity, and cognitive capacity.

In addition to the v. 3 scale, the overall level of the CPI profile is indicative of maladjustment versus healthy functioning. A profile with scores consistently above 50 suggests positive adjustment. A profile with scores consistently below 50 suggests the likelihood of poorer functioning. Three specific scales also should be consulted for a more delineated understanding of the individual's level of ego strength. (1) The Self-acceptance scale taps into sense of personal worth. Higher scores are generally related to a greater degree of fulfillment and optimism, whereas lower scores are related to a lack of self-confidence. Persons with lower scores on this scale are less likely to persevere in the face of difficulties and are more likely to withdraw. (2) The Communality scale was developed as a way of identifying invalid protocols marked by randomness, carelessness, or misinterpretation. The scale also can be used to clarify the degree of ego integration in an individual with lower scores; poor morale, self-doubt, feelings of alienation, and general instability may be differentiated with this scale. (3) The Well-being scale measures sense of physical and psychological well-being. Higher scores suggest positive functioning and a tendency to minimize complaints or problems. Lower scores suggest feelings of victimization, worry, and a tendency to emphasize or even exaggerate complaints and problems.

Level of Social Support

In general, high scores on class I and II scales indicate individuals who are interested in interacting with people and can do so in a socialized, well-controlled, and responsible manner. As a result, they would be more likely to have a good network of *social support*. However, elevations within these classes are particularly important to note. Individuals with high scores on the class I scales of Sociability and Empathy are likely to have extensive social support, since they are outgoing and understand the feelings and concerns of others. In contrast, low scores on Sociability and Empathy, combined with elevations on Dominance, Capacity for status, and Social Presence, indicate that even though the individual is interested in others, this interest will be more likely to be concerned with control issues than with fostering closeness. As a result, this person's social support may not be particularly high. The class II scales that are most likely to indicate high social support are: Good Impression, Communality, and Tolerance. High scores on Responsibility, Socialization, and Self-control may *not* necessarily indicate that the person has high social support, since these scales measure internal control rather than an ability to connect with others in a meaningful manner. Still, significantly low scores on these three scales are likely to indicate chaotic or even violent relationships whereas high scores indicate dependability.

Degree of Problem Complexity/Chronicity

The domain of *problem complexity/chronicity* refers to the presentation of thematic versus symptomatic problems. A few specific folk-scale configurations on the CPI profile can be helpful in making this discernment. The Socialization scale is a measure of adherence to social norms. As such, it measures a continuum from social maturity, integrity, and rectitude to delinquency, criminality, and aggressiveness. Low scores on the Socialization scale can be very indicative of complex problems. Lower standing on the Socialization scale generally means that the individual likely experienced a chaotic and unhappy family life and may suffer from dysphoric mood and pessimism. Very low scores on the Socialization scale are associated with personality disorders, especially borderline and antisocial personality disorders. Scores on the other class II scales affect interpretation of low scores on the Socialization. For instance, elevated scores on Responsibility, Self-control, and Communality, along with a low score on Socialization, suggest a high level of conflict between the individual's inner desires and outward expressions. Such a pattern is predictive of a very guarded and defensive personality that may be prone to explosiveness under stress. Furthermore, the configurations of the Self-acceptance and Well-being scales are critical to understanding the complexity of the presentation. CPI profiles on which both Self-acceptance and Well-being are low suggest current feelings of distress coupled with longstanding feelings of incompetence. Low scores on Self-acceptance in the absence of lowered Well-being point to a more thematic pattern in which the individual is generally insecure about his or her own worth but may or may not be particularly troubled at the present time. Low scores on Well-being in the absence of lowered Self-acceptance may suggest more transient problems that have not compromised the individual's self-esteem or personal optimism.

Coping Style

Coping style refers to a continuum of coping patterns ranging from internalizing to externalizing. The three vector scales of the CPI potentially provide a wealth of information about coping style. More specifically, the v. 1 scale is a measure of internalizing versus externalizing tendencies, and the v. 2 scale is a measure of norm-following versus norm-doubting tendencies. Alpha types are externalizing and norm-following; they cope through active, socially sanctioned means but may come across as opportunistic, manipulative, or hostile toward others. Beta types are internalizing and norm-following; they cope privately and tend to blame themselves for any misfortune. Gamma types are externalizing and norm-questioning; they cope outwardly in a unique, rebellious, or potentially disruptive fashion. Delta types are internalizing and norm-questioning; they are likely to keep to themselves and tend to be reflective, detached, or alienated.

Resistance Potential

Resistance potential refers to the likelihood of reactance or opposition to therapeutic intervention. A number of scales on the CPI is likely to be useful in predicting how open an individual will be to intervention. For instance, higher scores on the Independence scale are indicative of a more self-sufficient and detached style that does not easily accept external influences. Seeking support from others about how to do things is much more characteristic of individuals with lower scores on the Independence scale. Low scores on the Tolerance scale suggest that the individual will likely present as cynical, defensive, distrustful, and closed-minded. In contrast, high scores on the Tolerance scale suggest a more cooperative and reasonable stance. High scores on the Flexibility scale are also suggestive of receptiveness to change, whereas low scores on it suggest rigid, overcontrolled behavior. The Good Impression scale can suggest difficulties at both the low and high end. Low scores on the Good Impression scale suggest resistance to the expectations of others and a tendency to be skeptical and aggressively indifferent to what others think or feel. On the other hand, individuals with very high scores on the Good Impression scale have such a pervasive need to make a good impression that they may minimize their negative traits and deny their problems.

Combinations of folk scales are also important in considering an individual's reactance potential to treatment. High scores on the Responsibility and Self-control scales accompanied by low scores on Socialization are indicative of individuals who may be very guarded and defensive and prone to explode violently. Individuals with high Self-acceptance scores and low Well-being scores are likely to rely on their own judgments and distrust the advice of others. A high score on Dominance with a low score on Good Impression suggests argumentativeness. High scores on Self-control and Good Impression along with low scores on Socialization and Self-acceptance are indicative of a repressive, overcontrolled manner. Overall, consistently low scores across both class II and class III scales are suggestive of a more resistant, uncooperative orientation.

Distress Level

The domain of *distress level* refers to the degree of subjective distress experienced by the individual. The Self-acceptance, Communality, and Well-being scales can help the clinician assess level of distress and the degree of psychological capacity. Low scores on Self-acceptance generally mean that the individual has less time, energy, or positive affect for ego-enhancing activities. Low scores on Communality indicate poor morale and a sense of isolation. Low scores on Well-being generally mean that an individual is excessively aware of his or her personal problems, does not know what to do about them, and experiences a perceived lack of support. Very low scores on Well-being indicate an extreme level of distress or perhaps a tendency to feign physical or psychological illness.

In addition to these three scales, scores on the class III scales of Achievement via Conformance, Achievement via Independence, and Intellectual Efficiency can also be helpful in determining the degree to which individuals are able to draw on their own resources and improve their condition. Consistently low scores across the class III scales suggest feelings of dejection, incapacity, and a lack of resourcefulness.

CASE EXAMPLE

Interpretation of the CPI should be done in the context of the individual and his or her presentation. In this case, R.W. has presented a complex picture marked by mood and thought disturbances, anxiousness, and impaired interpersonal functioning (see Figure 8.2).

As discussed, the established method for interpreting the CPI involves a five-step sequence that begins with an assessment of the validity of the profile. Clinical assessment of validity should take into account the individual's approach to the test and his or her resulting scores on the Good Impression, Communality, and Well-being scales. Duration of the testing session and the number of omitted or corrected items on the answer sheet may provide meaningful information about the individual's capacities or degree of conscientiousness. Scores on the Good Impression scale carry much import regarding how the profile should be interpreted. Scores above 70 on Good Impression are generally indicative of a fake–good profile; scores below 35 suggest a fake–bad profile.

Scores below 30 on either the Communality or Well-being scale are also critical to the validity of the profile. Low scores on Communality suggest random responding, extreme distintegration, or the possibility of faking bad. Scores below 30 on Well-being also suggest the possibility of a fake–bad profile but may be indicative of significant feelings of dysphoria. For more precise measurement of fake–good, fake–bad, and random profiles, the series of equations described previously (and included in the computer-generated reports provided by the test publisher) can be used.

The profile for R.W. (see Appendix A for actual scores) appears valid, but her marginal scores (below 40) on Good Impression and Well-being indicate worry, poor morale, feelings of dysphoria, and a negative self-concept. Although not faking bad, R.W. appears to be dispirited and may be crying out for help. Her level of distress appears to be high. Given the symptom presentation and cultural background of R.W., her score on Communality is important; furthermore, it suggests that she was indeed able to comprehend and respond in a typical manner to the items on the CPI.

The second step in interpreting the CPI is to consider the three-vector model of personality structure. R.W. scored on the introverted and internalizing side of the v. 1 scale, and on the norm-questioning side of the v. 2 scale. In combination, this scoring on v. 1 and v. 2 means that R.W. is best characterized by a Delta lifestyle on the CPI. As a Delta, R.W. will tend use a coping style best described as internally focused and detached from oth-

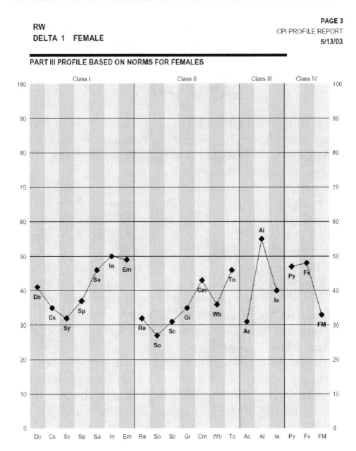

FIGURE 8.2. CPI profile for case example: R.W. Modified and reproduced by special permission of the Publisher, CPP, Inc., Palo Alto, CA 94303 from the CPI Manual, Third Edition, by Harrison Gough, PhD. Copyright 1996 by CPP, Inc. All rights reserved. Further reproduction is prohibited without the Publisher's written consent.

ers. She is likely not capitalizing fully on the strengths of her Delta lifestyle, as indicated by her low score on the v. 3 scale. This result suggests that she may be self-defeating, withdrawn, vulnerable, and prone to decompensation. The low score on the v. 3 scale highlights her relatively high level of functional impairment. R.W.'s difficulty in controlling her frustration and anger is also predicted by her Delta lifestyle on the CPI. Unless R.W. can learn to better tap into the intellectual and creative potentialities of her lifestyle, she will continue to be at risk for disturbances in ego functioning and for lashing out at self, others, and the community.

The third step in interpreting the CPI is to examine the overall profile and consider the different groupings of scales. The overall level of R.W.'s CPI profile is largely below 50. The relatively low level of her profile is consistent with the adjustment difficulties with which she presented. In fact, 12 of the 20 folk scales fall at, or below, 40. Among the class I scales, Dominance, Capacity for Status, Sociability, and Social Presence are at, or below, 40. These scores further confirm R.W.'s tendency to shy away from social interaction. The more moderate scores on the two class I scales of Independence and Empathy suggest some potential for resourcefulness and some understanding of the thoughts and feelings of others, despite the overall implication of her class I scores that she is detached and prefers to "go it" alone.

The class II scales are all below 50, suggesting an opportunistic, carefree approach to making decisions and judgments. R.W. is likely to take risks, to see things very differently from other people, and to feel alienated from others and the culture, in general. The combined low elevations on the class I and class II scales pinpoint a perceived lack of social support and a deficit of meaningful connections with others. The class III scale scores range from 31 to 51. The 20-point difference between her Achievement via Conformance and Achievement via Independence scores (with Achievement via Independence more elevated) is important to note; this pattern suggests creativity and an inclination to act in unconventional ways. Furthermore, R.W. is likely to dislike or even resist structure, and her score of 39 on Intellectual Efficiency suggests that she is insecure about her intellectual ability and may deal poorly with stress and trauma. Each of the three class IV scales are below 50, indicating a tendency to accept things at face value, resist change, and remain emotionally independent.

An alternative synthesis of the test's findings is to focus on CPI factors. In R.W.'s case it is helpful to consider the factor II scales as a grouping. All 7 of the scales on factor II are below 50. In fact, 6 of the 7 are below 40. These low scores on factor II suggest impulsivity, a poor mental outlook, and a tendency for R.W. to be influenced by her emotions in decision making.

The fourth step in interpreting the CPI is to examine each of the individual scales. At this point, the general dynamics of R.W.'s personality have been well illuminated. However, it may be helpful to emphasize the strengths or weaknesses of her personality profile. Of greatest concern is the particularly low score on Socialization. Her score of 28 suggests the possibility of a personality disorder and a high degree of problem complexity/chronicity. R.W. is the product of a chaotic and unhappy family life. Scores below 30 on Socialization are expected among those who experienced conflict at home, underachieved at school, and who were sexually precocious and disruptive among their peers. Of greatest hope are R.W.'s more moderate scores (between 40 and 51) on Self-acceptance, Independence, Empathy, Achievement via Independence, Communality, Tolerance, Psychological Mindedness, and Flexibility. These scores suggest that, with encouragement, she may be able to gain insight into her feelings and those of others. R.W.'s detachment and distrust suggest a strong potential for resistance, which will make it difficult to work with her. However, her level of independence is not so high as to preclude a willingness to tolerate, and be influenced by, others.

The fifth and final step in interpreting the CPI for R.W. is to conduct a configural analysis of the profile by looking at the interactions of the individual scales. Given the number of scales and the acceptable practice of interpreting both high and low scores on the CPI, configural interpretation of the profile is a complicated process. A thorough configural analysis would begin with Dominance and move systematically through each of the scales on the instrument, considering the configural meaning when (1) the target scale and one or more other scales are high, (2) the target scale is high and one other scale is low, (3) the target scale is high and two or more other scales are low, (4) the target scale and one or more others scales are high and one or more other scales are low, and (5) the target scale and one or more other scales are low. To simplify this process, the interpreter may choose to focus the configural analysis on a few scales that appear to have particular import to the profile or clinical situation. A configural interpretation reference chart is available (McAllister, 1996) to provide assistance in identifying particular CPI scale configurations.

In the case of R.W., the majority of important configural interpretations focus on combinations of low scores. Her relatively low scores on Dominance and Good Impression suggest that she may be seen by others as moody and touchy. The further combination of low Dominance and low Intellectual Efficiency means that R.W. is probably not a self-starter and may need prodding if positive changes are going to happen in her life. The combination of low scores on Capacity for Status, Self-control, and Well-being pinpoint the fact that R.W. may be feeling overwhelmed and will likely evidence further errors in judgment without intervention.

A very telling configuration for R.W. is her moderate score on Self-acceptance combined with a low score on Well-being. This configuration suggests that her tendency toward self-reliance is likely to be more from a sense of alienation from others than any great degree of self-confidence. Low scores on Responsibility, Socialization, and Self-control indicate that R.W. can be excitable and aggressive. Her low impulse control is confirmed by this pattern on the CPI and greatly complicates her clinical picture. R.W.'s low score on Femininity/Masculinity further confirms an action orientation. Low scores on Responsibility, Achievement via Conformance, and Intellectual Efficiency suggest immaturity and lack of discipline, as well as a lack of commitment to anyone other than herself. The key in working with R.W. will be to engage her in the process and draw out her own potential for creativity and action.

SUMMARY

The CPI provides a true-to-life and useful picture of the person completing the inventory. It is unique in its distinction as a well-established assessment of human assets that is congruent with the themes of positive psychology. The CPI is appreciated by a wide range of users for its ability to understand, classify, and predict peoples' behavior within the broadly defined normal range of human activity.

The CPI was designed primarily for use with nonpatient populations. However, an extensive amount of insight regarding the STS model can be gained from interpretation of its contents. The established method for interpretation of the CPI is a five-step process that moves from the overall clinical picture to the specific details of the scales and their interactions. The five-step process includes determination of profile validity, interpretation of the three-vector model, examination of the scale groupings, examination of each of the individual folk scales, special purpose scales, and predictive indices, and lastly, configural analysis of the interactions among the individual scales. Clinical interpretation emphasizes both the strengths and developmental needs of the individual; as a result, the CPI is often relevant to the treatment of patients entering psychotherapy.

9

The Rorschach

Radhika Krishnamurthy and Robert P. Archer

The Rorschach inkblot test was originally conceived as a test of perception, but it is typically classified as a projective technique to distinguish it from personality measures that utilize more direct or self-report forms of assessment. The test was developed by Hermann Rorschach, a Swiss psychiatrist, and published in 1921. The use of inkblots and other ambiguous visual forms for evaluating psychological processes had existed prior to Rorschach's work, dating to the latter part of the 19th century. These stimuli had been applied toward measuring various cognitive–intellectual processes, including imagination and creativity. Hermann Rorschach's unique contribution consisted of systematically employing a series of standardized inkblots to (1) investigate perceptual processes, (2) develop an empirically derived system for scoring the responses of normal and psychiatric patients to the inkblots, and (3) adopt a norm-based method for interpreting these responses.

Rorschach developed his inkblot test for the practical purpose of rendering psychiatric evaluation more reliable and objective than was possible through clinical observations. The test was based on the assumption that there was a meaningful association between an individual's perception and his or her underlying personality. Rorschach initially used 40 inkblots in a comparative investigation of nonpatients' and schizophrenic patients' responses in order to classify prominent response characteristics. His studies led him to conclude that the inkblot method permitted assessment of personality styles as well as diagnosis of psychopathology. Prior to his untimely death at age 37, Hermann Rorschach succeeded in printing a series of 10 inkblots as the Form Interpretation Test and published a monograph, *Psychodiagnostik*, describing his method (see Rorschach, 1921). His technique was perpetuated by three of his colleagues—Emil Oberholzer, Walter Morganthaler, and Georgi Roemer—who elaborated on his scoring procedures, but it received limited attention in Europe for several years.

Rorschach's test began to gain some interest and attention in the psychological community in the 1930s subsequent to its introduction in the United States. Specifically, it began to gain recognition through the works of Samuel J. Beck, Marguerite Hertz, and Bruno Klopfer, who each developed a system of scoring the test. A historic rivalry developed between Beck, who developed an empirical–normative approach that emphasized structural aspects of personality, and Klopfer, who evolved a content-based qualitative approach to interpretation. Additional Rorschach systems were developed by Zygmunt Piotrowski and David Rapaport, such that five different and overlapping Rorschach systems were in existence by the mid-1950s.

The history of the Rorschach test has been marked by various shifts in emphases, ranging from its description as a test of perception to a projective technique, which have been the source of considerable controversy and criticism. Moreover, there was substantial confusion over the appropriate method of scoring and interpreting the test during the first five decades of its use. Each of the different Rorschach systems recommended different test-administration procedures, employed different codes for scoring the responses, and produced different interpretive yields. The identification of the test as a projective method fueled additional skepticism during the era when Behaviorism dominated the field of psychology and unconscious processes were considered suspect and/or irrelevant to the study of human behavior. To date, disagreements about the definition of the Rorschach test continue, and the test continues to be variously described as a personality test, a semistructured interview, and a technique or method rather than a test (Exner, 1997).

In 1969, John Exner presented a comparative analysis of the five Rorschach systems that was undertaken to identify their relative standing in terms of empirical robustness and clinical utility. Exner's investigation served as the foundation for the development of the Rorschach Comprehensive System (CS). Exner found that each system had its merits as well as flaws, and he undertook an integration of the more defensible features of each system to create a unified approach to Rorschach assessment. The CS was published by Exner in 1974 and originally contained 69 variables. The system included an adult normative data set as well as a separate set of norms for children ages 5 through 16 years. In recent years, the CS has undergone expansion and refinement with the development of new variables and constellations, and minor modifications in administration procedures and validity criteria have also been instituted. The CS is currently the most widely accepted standard of Rorschach assessment, although alternative content–interpretation approaches also are available and can serve as useful supplements to the structurally based methodology of the CS.

Within the parameters of the CS, the Rorschach is described as a problem-solving task in which the subject's basic requirement is to misidentify the blots as something other than inkblots. This "forced misidentification" activates a number of decision-making and response-delivery processes. Moreover, the task is conceptualized as one in which projection *may* occur, particularly when movement is perceived and reported. However, projection is neither crucial nor inevitable in the perceptual–cognitive process of the Rorschach respondent (Exner, 1993). Exner (1997) adds that the test provides "a source from which many personality features can be evaluated . . . by the study of clusters of scores and the enhancement of objective findings with careful thematic analysis" (p. 41).

Despite its controversial history, the Rorschach has enjoyed a noteworthy level of popularity among clinicians, reflected in survey findings that report the frequency of its usage. For example, earlier surveys (e.g., Lubin, Larsen, & Matarazzo, 1984; Lubin, Wallis, & Paine, 1971; Sundberg, 1961) consistently reported that the Rorschach was used in more than 80% of surveyed clinical settings. More recent surveys (e.g., Archer & Newsom, 2000; Camara, Nathan, & Puente, 2000; Piotrowski & Keller, 1989; Watkins, Campbell, Nieberding, & Hallmark, 1995) have indicated that the Rorschach ranks steadily among the top 10 assessment instruments used across settings and age groups. Furthermore, recent surveys of training programs have indicated that 85% of APA-approved graduate programs teach competence in the Rorschach (Piotrowski & Zalewski, 1993), and the test ranks among the top three assessment instruments regarded by internship training directors as essential for current and future practicing psychologists (Piotrowski & Belter, 1999). Butcher and Rouse (1996) reported that the Rorschach was the second most frequently researched personality test during a 20-year period from 1974 to 1994, and recent reports indicate that there are more than 200 published books and between 8,000 and 9,000 published articles on the Rorschach (Exner, 1997). In all respects, then, the Rorschach is a widely used personality assessment measure. Indications point to the conclusion that the test will continue to hold an important position as a clinical assessment tool, and that the Comprehensive System will continue to evolve to address current and future assessment needs.

ADVANTAGES AND LIMITATIONS

The standardization of Rorschach assessment practice engendered by the development of the CS represents a major asset of the test. Specifically, the confusion related to the use of multiple Rorschach systems of assessment, and the associated arbitrary differences among clinicians in administering, coding, and interpreting the Rorschach, have been largely eliminated. The integrative and empirical approach used in CS development achieved substantial standardization of test administration, coding, and interpretation. Psychometric investigations of the reliability and validity of Rorschach variables and research-based efforts to revise and refine test variables have provided additional scientific credibility to the test. The current usefulness of the Rorschach, however, can be attributed largely to the vast research findings and descriptive literature that provide the foundation for the test.

The Rorschach has some unique advantages related to its relatively unstructured, performance-based methodology. The ambiguity of the task, coupled with the minimal directions provided to the respondent, gives him or her an extensive response range that permits considerable self-revelation. Moreover, because the information is acquired indirectly, through a transformation of the verbal responses into coded data, it is not dependent on conscious awareness or necessarily directed by the individual's self-conceptions, and may even bypass conscious control. Consequently, the Rorschach can be effective for assessing underlying personality characteristics, tendencies, and schemas, assuming that there is a reasonable level of task engagement (Meyer, 1997).

This advantage of the Rorschach methodology has been extended to claims that the test is not susceptible to malingering or denial of disturbance. Exner (1991) provided a detailed discussion of findings concerning attempts to malinger schizophrenia and depression. He cautioned that the results of the current body of research are not conclusive, and suggested that some characteristics of distress are potentially fakable. On the other hand, he reported that the simulation of positive adjustment is more difficult to achieve on the Rorschach, and that significant problems in personality and adjustment are likely to be revealed despite efforts by the respondent to conceal them. Some recent empirical investigations have lent support to the conclusion that although exaggeration of psychopathology on the Rorschach can occur, it can often be detected and discriminated from honest responding. For example, Frueh and Kinder (1994) evaluated the ability of coached malingerers to fake combat-related posttraumatic stress disorder (PTSD) symptoms, using comparisons with honest protocols obtained from undergraduate students and Vietnam veterans with actual PTSD. They found that individuals who were instructed to malinger PTSD on the Rorschach were able to alter their test records in a direction consistent with the records of patients with PTSD. However, malingerers were distinguished by their higher frequency of highly dramatic, less complicated, and emotionally unconstrained responses, and they scored in a more pathological direction on reality-testing indices than did the patients with PTSD.

A central advantage of the Rorschach test is the depth and breadth of information generated from this method of assessment. The test provides information concerning personality structure (i.e., enduring traits, situational states, and customary styles of reacting) as well as dynamic processes (e.g., underlying needs and conflicts that are relevant to diagnostic and treatment decisions). These issues are clearly articulated by Weiner (1997), who states that "the Rorschach is a multifaceted method of generating structural, thematic, and behavioral data that can be applied in both quantitative and qualitative terms and can be interpreted from many different theoretical perspectives" (p. 6), and by Exner (1997), who comments that "[the Rorschach] permits the study of personality from both nomothetic and idiographic perspectives" (p. 40). Clinicians using the Rorschach recognize that it yields an extensive array of information concerning a person's thought processes and problem-solving operations, emotional states, psychological stressors and disturbances, coping ability, self-image, and interpersonal capacities. Thus an enormous amount of clinically relevant data can be obtained in a relatively short time period and used for diagnostic, descriptive, and treatment-planning purposes.

The clinical use of the Rorschach for treatment planning and evaluation constitutes the largest area of its application. Weiner (1997) notes that test variables aid in (1) identifying primary targets of psychological intervention, (2) discerning potential barriers to treatment progress, (3) selecting suitable treatment modalities, (4) monitoring treatment progress, and (5) evaluating posttreatment gains. Rorschach studies of treatment-related change (e.g., Exner & Andronikof-Sanglade, 1992; Weiner & Exner, 1991) have provided evidence of the utility of the test in measuring treatment progress among outpatients receiving brief, short-term, and long-term psychotherapy. Exner (1995) presented preliminary data from an ongoing investigation using Rorschach data to track features of patients who were undergoing one of five modes of outpatient psychotherapy and who had terminated treatment within 8 weeks (*n* = 73) or demonstrated very favorable progress during a 4-month treatment duration (*n* = 123). These findings suggest a direction for using Rorschach data in treatment-planning decisions, particularly in regard to selecting methods of interventions suited to patients' personality characteristics and detecting potential dropouts.

Rorschach data may be usefully integrated with results of other personality and psychological tests to produce a comprehensive assessment of an individual. Combining Rorschach data with findings from self-report personality inventories such as the Minnesota Multiphasic Personality Inventory (MMPI) potentially offers a more detailed and nuanced depiction of an individual's functioning than may be obtained from a single instrument. Archer and Krishnamurthy's (1993a, 1993b) reviews of MMPI and Rorschach interrelationships in adolescent and adult samples indicated that conceptually similar indices across the two tests bear little-to-no relationship with each other. These findings are interpreted by several Rorschach researchers as reflecting the unique contributions of each test in personality description. As articulated by Weiner (1993), for example, apparent discrepancies between MMPI and Rorschach results can be generative, because each instrument measures different levels of conscious awareness, and these differences also can serve to mitigate the effects of false negative findings. Meyer (1997) suggested that a comprehensive personality assessment should include the use of both instruments because neither method can consistently represent the full range of a personality construct. Finn (1996a) discussed four scenarios involving combinations of high and low disturbance patterns across the MMPI-2 and Rorschach. He proposed that attention to these test-result patterns may provide incremental therapeutic utility, particularly in the course of providing test feedback to clients. In recent years, there has been increasing recognition of the potential utility of the Rorschach test as part of neuropsychological assessment, and findings concerning the Rorschach results of closed head-injury patients (e.g., Exner, Colligan, Boll, Stischer, & Hillman, 1996) and patients with Alzheimer's dementia (e.g., Perry, Potterat, Auslander, Kaplan, & Jeste, 1996) have offered promising directions for the integration of Rorschach and neuropsychological tests in clinical assessments.

The clinical application of the Rorschach has also been usefully extended to forensic contexts. In this regard, some authors have reported that the Rorschach is generally well received in the courtroom and meets legal, scientific, and professional standards for admissibility as part of expert testimony. For example, Weiner, Exner, and Sciara (1996) surveyed 93 clinicians who had testified in a total of 7,934 federal and state court cases across the country. They found that the credibility of the Rorschach was challenged in only .08% of the cases, and Rorschach testimony was deemed inadmissible in only .01% of the cases. McCann (1998) observed that the Rorschach meets current criteria of admissibility: It is a published test with extensive peer-reviewed research support, has a standardized methodology and norms, demonstrates evidence of psychometric adequacy, has established error rates, and achieves general acceptance in the field. Additionally, the relevance, helpfulness, and falsifiability of the Rorschach were deemed acceptable when inferences are appropriately drawn by the expert witness and when the testimony is based on empirically established indexes from the CS.

The Rorschach method, with its ambiguous stimulus and minimal directions, has the added advantage over more direct forms of personality assessment of cross-cultural and multicultural applicability, although local norms are required for accurate interpretation. The Rorschach is used extensively in several European and Asian countries, many of which have national Rorschach associations and offer comprehensive training programs. Norming projects and cross-cultural validation studies have been undertaken in several countries and have demonstrated important similarities and differences in comparison to the U.S. normative expectations (Meyer,

2001; Weiner, 1997). Among minority groups within the United States, marked similarities between African American and Caucasian American subgroups of the normative sample have been found for most Rorschach variables, providing some support for the clinical use of the Rorschach with African American clients (Presley, Smith, Hilsenroth, & Exner, 2001).

Despite its substantial assets, the Rorschach method is not without its liabilities and limitations. One of the prime difficulties associated with the Rorschach is that it is a complex and difficult method to learn and use effectively. The test user must effectively apply a large number of codes, which are then transformed into ratios and derivations and interpreted in the context of normative data. The initial step of coding the data requires considerable accuracy, and it is not uncommon to find important discrepancies between the codes obtained from different raters. Rorschach interpretation is a complicated undertaking that requires (1) systematic progression through a series of clusters comprised of a multitude of variables, and (2) substantial conceptual sophistication to arrive at accurate findings. Learning to administer, code, and interpret Rorschach data requires extensive graduate-level academic and practical training, and a single graduate course is typically insufficient for learning the method effectively. Hilsenroth and Handler's (1995) survey of 156 psychology graduate students revealed that although 53% of the respondents rated a graduate course as excellent for learning Rorschach administration, only 31% found it adequate for learning test interpretation. Moreover, approximately one-fourth of a smaller sample of 77 students who had completed a second, advanced course reported their training as inadequate for using the Rorschach in report writing.

Another significant limitation of the Rorschach comes from research findings indicating that Rorschach variables are not uniformly reliable and valid. Test–retest stability, interrater reliability, external validity, and incremental validity of many CS variables have all been questioned in recent critiques (e.g., Wood, Nezworski, & Stejskal, 1996). Several of these criticisms are discussed further in the following section. These criticisms have led some contemporary researchers to question the utility of the test, whereas other researchers have been motivated to revise and improve test variables. Overall, recent publications have provoked a reexamination of the view extended by Rorschach proponents that the CS rests on a firm empirical foundation.

Research studies have also revealed limited evidence of validity on several test indices. For example, the Depression Index (*DEPI*), which was developed in 1986 to facilitate diagnostic determination of depression and revised in 1990 to improve its sensitivity to depressive conditions, was originally reported to be useful in distinguishing depressed from non-depressed psychiatric patients. Whereas some research studies reported promising results for this index for diagnostic and descriptive purposes (see Exner, 1993, for a description), others have reported insufficient discriminative power in adult samples (e.g., Meyer, 1993; Viglione, Brager, & Haller, 1988) and particularly weak discriminative power in child and adolescent samples (e.g., Archer & Gordon, 1988; Archer & Krishnamurthy, 1997; Ball, Archer, Gordon, & French, 1991; Krishnamurthy & Archer, 2001). The utility of the *DEPI* in evaluating child/adolescent depression, and probably adult forms of depression, is therefore not supported currently. Other indices, particularly newer ones such as the Obsessive Style Index (*OBS*), Hypervigilance Index (*HVI*), and the recently released Perceptual–Thinking Index (*PTI*), have been subjected to minimal independent investigation of their effectiveness and should consequently be used with substantial caution in clinical and forensic settings.

PSYCHOMETRIC PROPERTIES

Norms

The original set of norms for the CS was based on the coded responses of a national sample of 600 nonpatient adults collected from the Northeast, South, Midwest, Southwest, and West. This sample was stratified by geographic distribution and also partially stratified based on socioeconomic levels. In addition to this norm set, data from comparison samples of 320 inpatients with schizophrenia, 210 inpatients with depression, and 200 adults with character disorders were provided as diagnostic comparison groups to facilitate interpretation. A separate set of child and adolescent norms was developed based on a national sample of 1,580 nonpatients, ages 5 through 16 years, to permit the use of the test with younger age groups. In 1990, the adult normative data was updated by increasing the sample size to 700 nonpatient adults, and descriptive statistics were provided for an increased set of 111 Rorschach variables. Descriptive statistics were also provided separately for adults with introversive, extratensive, and ambitent characteristics based on partitioning the adult sample in terms of participants' Erlebnistypus (problem-solving) style. A concurrent revision in the child and adolescent normative sample involved a reduction of the norm sample size to 1,390 nonpatients, with the elimination of records containing fewer than 14 responses.

Exner's norms for the CS have been in use for several years and, until recently, provoked little discussion about their representativeness. However, Rorschach research with adult nonpatients, conducted by Shaffer, Erdberg, and Haroian (1999), has yielded reference data that differ substantially from the CS normative data. These researchers provided descriptive statistics for a sample of 123 nonpatient volunteers from central California. Their sample was reasonably matched to 1996 census data, had a mean age of 36.75 years, and an average educational level of 14.03 years.

Among the important discrepancies observed, their sample produced higher values for *Lambda*, Distorted Form (*X–%*), and the Weighted Sum of 6 Special Scores (*WSum6*) variables. Thus the Shaffer and colleagues sample could be viewed as more guarded and exhibiting greater disturbances in thinking than Exner's sample, but it appeared to be similar to contemporary nonpatient samples employed in other research studies.

Further fueling the controversy concerning the accuracy of the original CS norms, Wood, Nezworski, Garb, and Lilienfeld (2001) undertook an evaluation of 14 CS variables investigated in 32 Rorschach studies involving nonpatient adults, and found that the aggregated means for all 14 variables differed significantly from CS norms. They concluded that the CS norms for these variables are not representative of contemporary American nonpatient adults and were inaccurate from the inception. Exner (2001a) suggested that some of the obtained differences (e.g., in *X–%*) may be attributed to revisions in Form Quality coding guidelines over the last two decades and argued that these differences would not produce a mismeasurement of psychopathology. Meyer (2001) added the observation that expected normative shifts may have occurred over time, which would heighten the differences between the original CS normative samples and current nonpatient samples.

The adequacy of the original adult norms is also currently under question by Rorschach critics, because Exner (2000a) recently reported discovering more than 100 duplicated records in the original normative data set. The current (5th) edition of the CS workbook provides norms based on a reduced data set of 600 adult nonpatient records, subsequent to the elimination of the duplicated records. While the debate over the norms continues, a renorming project directed by Exner is currently in progress and should eventually address the continuing questions about the adequacy of the CS norms (Exner, 2002).

Reliability and Validity

The psychometric adequacy of a psychological test is evaluated in terms of the two central concepts of reliability and validity. As noted in an earlier chapter, *reliability* refers to the consistency of test scores as revealed by evidence of temporal stability, internal consistency, interrater agreement, and/or equivalence of alternate forms of the test. Among these four basic types of reliability, issues of temporal stability and interrater reliability are pertinent to the Rorschach. *Validity* is generally defined as the totality of empirical evidence concerning the extent to which a test is useful in assessing the traits or characteristics that it purports to assess. Validity is reflected in the accumulated body of validity-related research on the psychological assessment instrument, including how adequately the test samples a domain of interest (content validity), how test scores relate to scores from other measures of similar constructs (concurrent validity), and how scores predict future performance on a criterion of interest (predictive validity). Validity is also affected by the reliability characteristics of a measure. For example, a Rorschach variable that cannot be coded with adequate levels of reliability cannot demonstrate high levels of validity.

The initial selection of variables for the CS was based on the criterion that retained measures demonstrate a minimum .85 level of interscorer reliability (Exner, 1986). Moreover, the development of the CS was accompanied by reports of the reliability and validity of CS variables (Exner, 1974, 1986, 1993, 2002). For example, Exner (1993) reported that greater than 30 temporal consistency studies were completed in the first decade of the CS's development. In adult nonpatient samples, long-term retest coefficients ranged from .26 to .86 for single variables over a 1-year retest interval, and from .64 to .91 for ratio and percentage data. Over a 3-year retest interval, the coefficients ranged from .23 to .87 for single variables and from .72 to .90 for ratios and percentages. The lower stability coefficients were obtained typically for variables measuring state characteristics that were expected to change as a function of time (Exner, 1993). Stability indices for child samples are also reported to be high when the retest interval does not exceed 1 month. However, Exner and Weiner (1995) caution that changes in scores on Rorschach variables, paralleling developmental changes, should be expected among younger clients even over short time periods, because many Rorschach variables do not produce stable values until adolescence.

The adequacy of Rorschach interrater reliability has received renewed attention in recent years. For example, Wood and colleagues (1996) argued that percentage of agreement, which had been used as the index of interrater reliability in Rorschach research, was an inadequate and misleading measure. They noted that inflated agreement rates tended to be produced for variables coded with low frequency. Furthermore, they observed that evidence of interrater reliability had not been provided for several Rorschach variables, such as constellations and content scores.

A recent study by Acklin, McDowell, Verschell, and Chan (2000) addressed some of these concerns by furnishing evidence of interrater reliability using improved statistical indices. Acklin and colleagues' investigation was based on a sample of 20 nonpatient protocols and 20 clinical protocols. Reliability of coding was assessed using the intraclass correlation coefficient (ICC) for protocol-level data consisting of structural summary variables, ratios, percentages, and derivations; the kappa coefficient was used to evaluate response-level reliability. They found that 41% of the variables in the nonpatient sample and 47% of the variables in the clinical sample demonstrated excellent reliability, reflected in kappa values ≥ .81. Furthermore, substantial reliability (kappa .61–.80) was found for 36% and 44% of the nonpatient and clinical sample codes, respectively. At the protocol level, excellent ICC values (≥ .81) were found for 55% and 62% of the variables evaluated for the nonpatient and clinical samples, respectively, and substantial (.61–.80) reliability was found for 29% and 28% of the variables, respectively. Acklin and colleagues concluded that the majority of CS codes, coding decisions, and summary scores yielded acceptable and, in many instances, excellent levels of reliability. They felt that their findings provided strong evidence for the reliability of CS data, but they acknowledged that a subset of CS variables demonstrated less than acceptable (kappa or ICC < .61) levels of interrater reliability. We identify some of these latter variables in our cautionary statements in a following section of this chapter.

A considerable amount of controversy and debate continues to surround the reliability of the Rorschach coding system. Advocates of the Rorschach generally maintain that adequate levels of reliability have been clearly demonstrated for trait characteristics of individuals in adult populations. In contrast, critics of the Rorschach method continue to point out that Rorschach reliability studies have typically addressed few of the comprehensive array of variables used in test interpretation. This debate will undoubtedly continue until more data is collected on the issue. It is also useful to note that the interrater reliability established in carefully controlled research studies using well-trained coders may be substantially different from the coding accuracy demonstrated by clinicians in their use of the Rorschach in applied settings. Therefore, an important source of data, largely absent to date, should be based on field studies of coding accuracy as demonstrated by "typical" clinicians in their everyday clinical practice with this instrument.

Given the controversy surrounding the reliability of the Rorschach, it is not surprising that a broad range of opinions also exists concerning the validity and utility of the Rorschach method. Hunsley and Bailey (1999) observed:

> The Rorschach has the dubious distinction of being, simultaneously, the most cherished and the most reviled of all psychological assessment tools. . . . The Rorschach is held in great esteem by many psychologists for its ability to access intrapsychic material, whereas others point to the Rorschach as a prime example of unscientific psychological assessment. (p. 266)

Illustrating this controversy, *Psychological Assessment*, the *Journal of Personality Assessment*, *Assessment*, and the *Journal of Clinical Psychology* have all published special sections within the last few years devoted to exchanges on the utility of the Rorschach. A review of this literature underscores a striking diversity of opinion. Hunsley and Bailey (1999), for example, concluded that there was no scientific evidence to justify the clinical use of the Rorschach in psychological assessment, and Garb (1999) concurred with this viewpoint and called for a moratorium on the use of the Rorschach in clinical and forensic settings "until we have determined which Rorschach scores are valid and which ones are invalid" (p. 313). In contrast, Viglione (1999) concluded that the evidence clearly warranted the use of the Rorschach in clinical and forensic practice, and Weiner (1999, 2001) felt there was compelling evidence of the usefulness of the Rorschach method, including pervasive evidence of incremental validity.

Early validity studies provided support for the clinical use of CS variables through empirical demonstrations of the capacity of CS variables to discriminate between nonclinical and various types of clinical samples. The current research base for the CS includes several independent studies that have examined the psychometric adequacy of the CS and have produced mixed findings. The most widely cited evidence for the reliability and validity of the Rorschach comes from a meta-analytic study by Parker, Hanson, and Hunsley (1988). These researchers examined reliability and validity findings for three of the most widely used psychological tests: the Rorschach, the MMPI, and Wechsler Adult Intelligence Test (WAIS). Parker and his colleagues reviewed published data on these tests for a 12-year period and concluded that the instruments were essentially equivalent in terms of overall evidence of reliability and validity. Garb, Florio, and Grove (1998) subsequently reanalyzed the Parker and colleagues' Rorschach and MMPI data, performing several new analyses, and observed that the weighted mean effect sizes for the MMPI were substantially higher than those obtained for the Rorschach.

Most recently, Meyer and Archer (2001) undertook a detailed reexamination of the Parker and colleagues data set and also provided a summary of four other meta-analyses in this area, concluding that, overall, the reliability and validity data support the use of each of these popular tests, and that each test may produce relatively higher validity results for specific purposes, as reflected in particular predictor–criterion relationships. For example, the MMPI may produce higher validity coefficients when distinguishing psychiatric patients from control groups; IQ tests may be better at differentiating patients with dementia from control groups; and the Rorschach may produce higher validity estimates when utilized to detect psychiatric patients with psychotic diagnoses. Viewed from this perspective, sweeping conclusions concerning the overall validity of a particular measure, independent of the particular assessment tasks or criterion, may be of very limited usefulness. Although Meyer and Archer did not concur that a moratorium should be imposed on the clinical use of the Rorschach, they did propose that it be used selectively, based on the nature of assessment questions, and that certain applications of the Rorschach (e.g., use of the *DEPI* to diagnose depressive disorders in either adolescents or adults) were clearly not supported by the empirical literature.

A specific issue in the debate over the validity of the Rorschach involves questions about the incremental validity of the test. As noted by

Weiner (2001), *incremental validity* refers to the extent to which the inclusion of scores from a particular instrument is likely to increase the accuracy of predictions derived from other sources of information, including scores on other test instruments. Hunsley and Bailey (1999) concluded that the Rorschach has demonstrated little evidence of incremental validity. They based their conclusions on Garb's (1984) findings that the Rorschach did not add to the accuracy of personality assessment beyond information gathered from demographic or self-report sources; and on findings by Archer and Gordon (1988) and Archer and Krishnamurthy (1997), who reported that the Rorschach added little to the diagnostic accuracy obtainable through the use of MMPI results. Garb (1999) also recently concluded that results from the limited research on the incremental validity of the Rorschach offered little support for the view that the addition of Rorschach to other types of data leads to an increase in descriptive or predictive accuracy.

In contrast, Weiner (2001) has argued that most clinicians who use the Rorschach and MMPI conjointly are familiar with numerous cases in which the Rorschach has added important and unique information to the clinical assessment task. Meyer and Archer (2001) acknowledged that incremental validity is an important standard to apply in evaluating psychological assessment instruments, but they questioned whether a demonstration of incremental validity was necessarily a requirement in determining the overall utility of the test. Further, they observed that if incremental validity was considered a crucial standard in determining a test's usefulness, it should be applied to *all* test instruments and assessment procedures. Thus the MMPI-2 would be required to show incremental validity over other forms of objective personality assessment. Meyer and Archer also noted that incremental validity, like the broader construct of validity, is a criterion-specific issue. Since psychological tests are useful for multiple purposes, it is difficult to ascertain the incremental validity of a test in general and much more useful to discuss the incremental validity of an assessment instrument in terms of a specific purpose or criterion.

In summary, Archer (1999) has advocated for a balanced and comprehensive perspective on the Rorschach debate. Problems in reliability and validity are certainly manifested by the Rorschach but are in no way unique to this assessment instrument. Although other assessment instruments have been subjected to substantial criticisms concerning the various aspects of reliability and validity, these criticisms have typically stopped short of questioning the overall utility of the instrument or its appropriateness for general clinical use. It is certainly important to hold the Rorschach accountable to the traditional measures of reliability and validity published for all instruments, but it is also important to remember that all psychological assessment techniques have inherent flaws, limitations, and areas of needed improvement.

Cautionary Concerns

In the interpretation, treatment planning, and clinical case description sections that follow, standard interpretive statements are provided for CS variables and indices. Rather than qualifying many of these statements with cautions regarding the limited or contradictory nature of the research foundation for some of these variables and indices, the reader is generally reminded that substantial caution is applicable to the interpretation of many CS variables. Although much research has already been conducted on the Rorschach, more research is needed to fully validate the usefulness of clinical inferences based on Rorschach findings.

More specific cautions are appropriate for a number of CS variables that have demonstrated substantive problems either in reliability or validity, to enable the prudent interpreter to exercise particular caution in drawing inferences from these variables. As discussed in the previous section, the Depression Index or *DEPI* has been the subject of substantial debate and has generally failed to show a consistent and meaningful relationship to the diagnosis of depression in either adolescent or adult populations. The Schizophrenia Index (*SCZI*) also has shown a relatively mixed pattern of relationship to schizophrenic diagnoses, including a high rate of false positive classifications, and has recently been replaced by the Perceptual–Thinking Index (*PTI*) in the current edition of the CS. The *S-CON* or Suicide Constellation also appears suspect because of the problems in reliability for nonpatient samples noted by Acklin and his colleagues (2000), and because the *S-CON* deals with prediction to a very low baserate behavior (a psychometric task usually doomed to failure) and may consequently be of little practical value to most clinicians. The *S-CON* also may be subject to dangerous misinterpretations when inappropriately used to rule out the potential for suicidal behavior.

Additionally, a number of relatively new CS variables or indices clearly require further empirical study before they can be considered reliable contributors to the interpretive process. These variables involve the *PTI*, Coping Deficit Index (*CDI*), Hypervigilance Index (*HVI*), Obsessive Style Index (*OBS*), the Good Human Representation (*GHR*) and Poor Human Representation (*PHR*) variables, and the Form Appropriate–Extended (*XA%*) and Form Appropriate–Common Areas (*WDA%*) indices.

Acklin and colleagues (2000) identified a number of variables as producing interrater reliability results that are below acceptable limits. These variables involve several Special Scores, including Deviant Verbalizations (*DV*), Deviant Response (*DR*), Fabulized Combination (*FABCOM*), Incongruous Combination (*INCOM*), and Inappropriate Logic (*ALOG*)—all of which displayed significant reliability problems in nonpatient samples, clinical samples, or both populations. The Difference (*D*) and Adjusted Difference (*Adjusted D*) scores also exhibited significant reliability limitations in clinical and nonpatient samples, respectively, and Texture (*FT, TF, T*) and Vista (*FV, VF, V*) responses displayed substantive reliability problems in nonpatient samples. Additionally, the Unusual Form (*Xu%*) variable appeared to be unreliable in both patient and nonpatient samples, and the Form–Color Ratio Index (*FC:CF+C*) displayed similar reliability problems in both populations. Since variables that cannot be coded reliably cannot be useful in terms of providing meaningful inferences about extra-test correlates, these latter variables also should be viewed with particular caution.

At the present time, we have attempted to illustrate the use of the Rorschach CS by utilizing the full set of Structural Summary variables. A promising direction for the future of the CS would involve excluding variables that are demonstrated across multiple studies to be unreliable or have questionable validity. This method, a discussion of which is beyond the scope of this chapter, would result in a reduced set of relatively strong variables furnishing increased confidence in the interpretive findings.

ALTERNATIVE INSTRUMENTS

There are many other tests and methods that share the Rorschach's "projective" approach to personality assessment. Some of these methods use inkblot stimuli similar to the Rorschach; others rely on pictorial stimuli, sentence-completion methodologies, and drawing techniques. Among inkblot techniques, the most recognized alternative to the Rorschach is the Holtzman Inkblot Technique (HIT; Holtzman, Thorpe, Swartz, & Herron, 1961). This technique contains two parallel forms, each consisting of a series of 45 inkblots in addition to two practice blots. The HIT measures characteristics such as ego boundaries, anxiety, hostility, and various aspects of perception and thinking aimed at identifying psychopathological conditions. The test has standardization data and norms as well as a collection of research studies that offers support for the use of the test. One psychometric advantage of the HIT over the Rorschach is that it involves obtaining only one response per inkblot. This standardization of response frequency eliminates the complicating influence of response rate that is seen with the Rorschach.

The most popular alternative to the Rorschach, however, is the Thematic Apperception Test (TAT; Morgan & Murray, 1935). The TAT has a long history of use as a projective measure of personality dynamics and is typically ranked among the most widely used instruments in surveys of test usage. The TAT consists of a series of 31 cards, including 30 pictorial cards and one blank card. It utilizes a storytelling methodology, requiring the examinee to construct a story that describes the observed scenes, addresses the thoughts and feelings of the figures in the pictures, and proposes an outcome. The basic assumption is that personal apperceptions are revealed in the course of the narrative, which impart important information concerning personality features, including possible fears, anxieties, insecurities, interpersonal needs, conflicts, and defenses. Several scoring systems have been developed for the TAT over the course of its history, including Bellak's (1947) scoring system, which is the most widely used system for scoring and interpreting the test. More recently, Cramer (1991) has developed a system of scoring defense mechanisms, and Westen (1991) has developed a system for evaluating interpersonal object relations, which offer promising applications of the test for clinical assessment. The TAT also has a substantive research literature that includes clinical diagnostic studies. Moreover, the development of alternative versions of the test for children (Children's Apperception Test [CAT]; Bellak & Bellak, 1949) and older adults (Senior Apperception Technique [SAT]; Bellak & Bellak, 1973) has extended its use to broader age groups. Despite these developments, the TAT continues to lack a unified method of scoring and interpretation and is best considered a supplement to, rather than a substitute for, the Rorschach.

ADMINISTRATION

The Rorschach Comprehensive System requires the examiner to follow standardized procedures and instructions in its administration. Substantial variation from these administration procedures precludes the use of the test norms for interpretation, which renders the test of little value for deriving reliable conclusions. Rorschach administration generally takes approximately an hour to an hour and a half, but test administration time would vary depending on the number of responses produced by the examinee and the examiner's speed of recording the responses. The test administrator should anticipate that a lengthy protocol, resulting from the production of an abundant number (≥ 30) of responses and/or highly elaborated articulations of responses, would require a longer testing session. Conversely, an insufficient response production (fewer than 14 responses) requires test readministration (and, consequently, additional time).

Rorschach administration is divided into two primary phases: response and inquiry. Similar to all other psychological testing, Rorschach test administration begins with establishing rapport and explaining the purposes of testing. This rapport and clarity are particularly important in Rorschach testing because the ambiguity of the test is frequently anxiety provoking and may have an inhibitory effect on clients who are uncertain or uninformed about the intent of the testing.

Setting Up the Testing Session

The test administration is preceded by an interview that has multiple purposes. First, the interview is designed to obtain relevant background information that provides a context for meaningful interpretation of test findings. The pretesting discussion should also be directed toward setting the client at ease and enlisting his or her active participation in the testing process. Furthermore, it provides an opportunity to inform the client of the reason(s) for the testing, provide an overview of what the testing session entails, and discuss the eventual applications of the test results for treatment planning and goal-setting purposes. The examiner is advised to take as much time as needed to address any misconceptions held by the examinee about the test and to establish a collaborative relationship around the testing experience.

The CS workbook (Exner, 2001b) recommends introducing the test by stating, "One of the tests we will be doing is the inkblot test, the Rorschach. Have you ever heard of it, or have you ever taken it?" (p. 3). A client who reports knowing little about the test would be informed, "It's just a series of inkblots that I'll show you and I want you to tell me what they look like to you" (p. 3). The examiner should avoid discussion of the nature of the task or the characteristics measured beyond indicating that the test provides useful information about personality and psychological functioning.

Test Materials

The basic stimulus materials consist of the series of 10 cards that are administered in chronological order. The examiner should also have two or more location sheets at hand to record the response locations during the inquiry phase of testing. Finally, the examiner requires several sheets of paper or a legal pad to record the verbalized responses. These sheets should be sectioned into two main columns—"Response" and "Inquiry"—with additional columns or designated spaces, as needed, to record the card number, response number, and rotation of the card (upright, inverted, or side rotations) for each response.

Test Administration Procedure

Before administration begins, the examiner stacks the cards facedown, with Card I on top of the stack. The stacked cards are arranged in the correct order and in a position so that they are in an upright position when handed to the examinee. The examiner also arranges the location sheets facedown on the table, and has the recording sheets and pens or pencils on hand.

A crucial consideration in Rorschach administration concerns the seating arrangement, which consists of side-by-side seating in contrast to the traditional face-to-face seating position used for most tests. This former position prevents the examiner from providing nonverbal cues, while enabling him or her to view the card (including its position and any aspects of the blot to which the examinee points) as it is held by the examinee.

The response collection phase of the test administration involves handing each card, in sequence, to the examinee and asking, "What might this be?" The examiner provides minimal direction during the testing, permitting the response process to unfold without undue influence. However, the examiner can offer brief answers to commonly asked questions, such as whether the cards can be turned and whether the entire blot needs to be used ("It's up to you"). The client's responses are recorded verbatim, preferably with few responses recorded on a page to prevent overcrowding. The workbook for the Comprehensive System (Exner, 2001b) provides a list of standard abbreviations that can be used by the examiner to expedite the process of recording responses.

Since Rorschach administration requires a minimum of 14 responses to the 10 blots in order to be deemed interpretable, Exner (2001b) has recently recommended a procedure for ensuring that a sufficient number of responses is obtained. Specifically, the examiner prompts for additional responses if only one response is given to Card I. If the client continues to deliver only one response each to Cards II, III, and IV, and if the examiner is convinced that an insufficient record will result, the client is prompted once again to take more time after the response to Card IV is offered. If a Rorschach record of fewer than 14 responses is obtained despite these interventions, the inquiry phase of testing is revoked. Instead, the response collection phase is repeated with the instruction to give more responses, with the provision that previously delivered responses could be given again in the readministration. However, card rejections are not accepted at any point during the testing session. If a rejection occurs at the early stages of testing, efforts to establish greater rapport are indicated; if a rejection occurs at a later point, encouragement to persist in producing a response is recommended.

Conversely, an excessively lengthy response record is unnecessarily time consuming and has been found to provide no incremental interpretive value (Exner, 2001b). In fact, an unusually long record interferes with effective utilization of normative data for interpretation, because the values obtained in the client's record for several variables are likely to be skewed. Exner (2001b) recommends intervening after five responses are delivered to Card I, and more appear to be forthcoming, to interrupt the client's responding to Card I. The examiner would then proceed to Card II. This procedure is repeated on Card II, and each subsequent card, if the same level of response productivity continues. The intervention is discontinued when fewer than five responses are given to a card, after which it is not reinstated, even if the earlier set reappears (i.e., the subject resumes producing more than five responses to one or more cards).

After all responses to the 10 cards have been recorded, the inquiry phase begins with the verbatim delivery of a standard explanation (**boldface** added for emphasis):

Now we are going to go back through the cards again. It won't take very long. I want to see the things that you said you saw and make sure that I see them like you do. We'll do them one at a time. I'll read what you said and then I want you to show me **where** it is in the blot and then tell me **what** there is there that makes it look like that to you, so that I can see it too, just like you did. Is that clear?" (Exner, 2001b, p. 15)

The inquiry is the most crucial phase of test administration and serves as the foundation for accurate coding and interpretation of the responses. During this phase, the examiner again presents the cards to the client in chronological sequence. Each response is read to the client in verbatim form, and the client is given the opportunity to elaborate on the response in order to permit accurate coding by identifying the location, determinants, and contents of the response. The examiner records the responses verbatim and also uses the location sheet(s) to mark the location of each response. When the location is unclear, the client can be asked to run his or her finger around the part of the blot used for the response. Inquiry questions should be nondirective, and a standard set of neutral queries/statements (e.g., "What makes it look like a _____?" or "I'm not sure I see it as you do") can be employed by the examiner to elicit clarification. It is crucial to avoid leading questions (e.g., "Is it the shading that makes it look like that?"), which can affect the spontaneous verbalizations of the examinee and potentially alter or bias the test findings. The examiner should antici-pate that the inquiry phase may become frustrating for some clients, who may become defensive or resistant when their elaboration appears to be in-sufficient. These negative reactions are often reduced when a skillful in-quiry is undertaken to achieve the necessary clarification without excessive and unnecessary questioning, but the examiner may also need to reassure and calm clients who feel particularly perturbed or threatened.

SCORING

From a technical standpoint, Rorschach responses are "coded" rather than scored. Specifically, all response segments are first converted into a series of codes based on categories of information that are deemed meaningful. These codes are subsequently transformed into ratios and percentages that compose the Structural Summary of the Rorschach Comprehensive System and are interpreted with reference to normative values for each test vari-able. Table 9.1 presents a summary of the basic coding categories that con-stitute the sequence of scores for the Comprehensive System's Structural Summary, and the specific codes that can be derived within each category. Variables in this table that displayed less than acceptable levels of interrater reliability in the research by Acklin and colleagues (2000) are delineated by the use of footnotes.

TABLE 9.1. Summary of Rorschach Comprehensive System Codes

Coding category	Description	Codes
Location	Whole	W
	Common Detail	D
	Unusual Detail	Dd
	Space	S
Developmental Quality	Synthesized	+
	Ordinary	o
	Synthesized–Vague	$v/+^c$
	Vague	v
Determinants	Form	F
	Movement	
	Human	M
	Animal	FM
	Inanimate	m
	Chromatic Color	
	Pure Color	C
	Color–Form	CF^a
	Form–Color	FC
	Color Naming	Cn
	Achromatic Color	
	Pure Achr. Color	C'
	Achr. Color–Form	$C'F$
	Form–Achr. Color	FC'
	Shading–Texture	
	Pure Texture	T^a
	Texture–Form	TF^a
	Form–Texture	FT^a
	Shading–Dimension	
	Pure Vista	V^a
	Vista–Form	VF^a
	Form–Vista	FV^a
	Shading–Diffuse	
	Pure Shading	Y^a
	Shading Form	YF^a
	Form–Shading	$FY^{a,b}$
	Form Dimension	FD
	Pairs	(2)
	Reflections	
	Reflection–Form	rF
	Form–Reflection	Fr

(continued)

TABLE 9.1. *(continued)*

Coding category	Description	Codes
Form Quality	Ordinary–Elaborated	$+^a$
	Ordinary	o
	Unusual	$u^{a,b}$
	Minus	$-$
Contents	Human	
	Whole	H
	Whole, Fictional or Mythological	(H)
	Detail	Hd
	Detail, Fictional or Mythological	(Hd)
	Human Experience	Hx
	Animal	
	Whole	A
	Whole, Fictional or Mythological	(A)
	Detail	Ad
	Detail, Fictional or Mythological	(Ad)
	Anatomy	An
	Art	Art
	Anthropology	Ay^a
	Blood	Bl
	Botany	Bt
	Clothing	Cg
	Clouds	Cl
	Explosion	Ex
	Fire	Fi
	Food	Fd
	Geography	Ge
	Household	Hh^b
	Landscape	Ls
	Nature	Na^a
	Science	Sc
	Sex	Sx
	X-ray	Xy
Populars		P
Organizational Activity (Z-score)	Whole (ZW)	
	Adjacent Detail (ZA)	
	Distant Detail (ZD)	
	White Space Integration (ZS)	

(continued)

TABLE 9.1. *(continued)*

Coding category	Description	Codes
Special Scores	Deviant Verbalizations	
	Deviant Verbalization	$DV^{a, b, c, d}$
	Deviant Response	$DR^{a, b, d}$
	Inappropriate Combinations	
	Incongruous Combinations	$INCOM^a$
	Fabulized Combinations	$FABCOM^{a,c}$
	Contamination	$CONTAM$
	Inappropriate Logic	$ALOG^b$
	Perseveration	PSV^a
	Special Contents	
	Abstract Content	AB
	Aggressive Movement	AG
	Cooperative Movement	COP
	Morbid Content	MOR
	Human Representational Responses	
	Good Human Representation	GHR
	Poor Human Representation	PHR
	Personalized Answers	PER
	Special Color Phenomena	
	Color Projection	CP

Note. From Exner (2001b). Copyright 2001 by the author. Adapted by permission.
[a] = kappa < .61 for nonpatient sample in Acklin et al. (2000); [b] = kappa < .61 for clinical sample in Acklin et al. (2000); [c] = ICC < .61 for nonpatient sample in Acklin et al. (2000); [d] = ICC < .61 for clinical sample in Acklin et al. (2000).

Location and Developmental Quality

One of the basic aspects of Rorschach coding is determining *where* the perceived object is seen in the blot. Identifying the response locations results in four coding possibilities. First, the percept may be based on the entire blot, as is commonly found when clients perceive a bat or butterfly on Cards I and V, resulting in the Whole Response (W) code. The coding of nonwhole location areas is facilitated in the CS by numerical designations of Common Detail, Unusual Detail, and White Space areas. A Common Detail (D) response code is used when the response is located in one of the 82 areas designated in the Comprehensive System as a common detail area. The designation of a portion of a blot as a common detail area is based on the criterion that at least 5% of the subjects in two large psychiatric and nonpsychiatric samples gave at least one response to the D area (Exner, 1993, 2001b). Locations used with a frequency of less than 5% by these subjects define Unusual Detail (Dd) areas; any response that is not coded W or D receives a Dd code by default. The White Space (S) code is used when a white space area is integrated with other blot areas (e.g., the *DdS30* areas on Card I reported as eyes of an animal when the entire blot represents the animal face), or when it alone constitutes the perceived object (e.g., spaceship in the *DS5* area of Card II). The *S* code does not stand alone in either scenario, but would be coded as either *WS*, *DS*, or *DdS*.

The Developmental Quality (DQ) of the response refers to the qualitative and integrative sophistication of the response. Essentially, the articulated response can range from a simple, concrete, or unorganized level to a high level of specificity and complexity. The four DQ codes of the CS are as follows:

Synthesized (+) response, involving two or more separate objects with specific form features that are described as related

Ordinary (*o*) response, where single objects with specific form demand are described

Synthesized–Vague (*v/+*) response, in which the separate and related objects lack specific form demand

Vague (*v*) response, in which objects without specific form demand are described in a diffuse manner.

The DQ symbol is affixed to the Location symbol to render the determination of response location complete.

Determinants and Form Quality

Identifying and coding the determinants of the response, which involve clarifying *what* made the perceived object look like it did to the client, is one of the most crucial and complex aspects of Rorschach CS coding. At the most basic level, the response may be based on form features that are articulated in terms of the shape, size, or contours of the object. In addition, human, animal, and inanimate objects may be perceived in movement, resulting in codes of *M*, *FM*, and *m*, respectively. All three types of movement are further designated as active or passive. Activities such as talking, looking, and sitting are considered passive movement, whereas fighting, running, and exploding reflect active movement. Rorschach responses also may involve the use of color. Use of the Chromatic Color symbols—*C*, *CF*, and *FC*—reflects the extent to which (1) color use is the sole determinant of the response (e.g., "It looks like blood because it is red") or (2) is considered along with form features. The Color Naming (*Cn*) code is given in the relatively rare circumstance when colors are simply named (e.g., *red*, *green*) as opposed to being used to delineate or describe a specific object. Similar in concept to the Chromatic Color codes, Achromatic Color codes are used when the response is based on the black, white, or gray features of the inkblots either exclusively *(C')*, *or in combination with form features to a greater or lesser extent (FC' vs. C'F).*

Shading determinants in the CS are coded when the light and dark shading components of the blot are utilized in forming the percept. Diffuse shading (*Y*, *YF*, and *FY* codes) is identified when these shading components are reported, for example, in forming impressions of clouds, smoke, or fog. Shading also can be used to imply tactile characteristics such as hard, rough, or furry, resulting in a Texture (*T*, *TF*, or *FT*) code. Alternatively, the light and dark features can be used to create impressions of objects perceived as having depth or dimensionality, such as a tunnel or cavern, which is coded as Vista (*V*, *VF*, or *FV*). Shading determinants are distinct from Achromatic Color determinants and warrant careful attention by the coder to differentiate perceptions of black, white, and gray colors from light and dark shading features. Moreover, an important distinction is made between the Vista determinant and the Form Dimension (*FD*) determinant, the latter involving perceptions of depth or dimensionality based on form features such as size, shape, and position and which do not involve the use of shading.

Another important set of determinants in the CS involves perceptions of identical objects derived from the symmetrical features of the blot. One type, referred to as Pairs (*2*), is coded when equivalent images are reported as two identical objects, such as two human figures in the *D9* areas of Card III. The other type, known as Reflections (*rF* or *Fr*), is coded when the symmetrical objects are reported as mirror images or reflections of a single object.

The coding system for the CS also recognizes that multiple determinants may be involved in a single percept, which is denoted as a Blend. In these instances, each relevant determinant is recorded for the response and is separated by a period. For example, the response to Card II, "two dogs attacking each other; the red puddle below their legs is blood from their wounds" would have the determinant code of $FM^a.CF$.

The coding of Form Quality (FQ) accompanies the determinant code for each response. Form quality refers to the "goodness of fit" between the perceived object and the blot area in which it is seen, and has been a component of Rorschach scoring since the inception of the method (Exner, 1993). At the most basic level, form quality was differentiated into "good" and "poor" form in all the major Rorschach systems, with as many as six separate codes assigned in some earlier systems. In the CS, four FQ codes are assigned: "+" when there are detailed and precise articulations of form features that produce qualitative enrichment of the verbal production without compromising perceptual accuracy; "*o*" when relatively obvious form features are described without overelaboration; "*u*" when uncommon responses are given that can be seen fairly easily and do not violate basic form contours; and "−" when form use is distorted, arbitrary, and inappropriate for the blot area used. Form Quality coding is done by cross-referencing the perceived object against the detailed listing of responses by card and location area provided in the CS workbook.

Contents and Populars

Rorschach responses also are coded for the contents represented in the response, which commonly include whole- or part-animal (*A, [A], Ad, [Ad]*) and human (*H, [H], Hd, [Hd]*) figures perceived as actual or fictionalized objects. In a recent revision of the CS (Exner, 1993), the Human Experience (*Hx*) code was added to depict attributions of human emotions such as sadness or fear, and sensory experiences such as sounds and feelings, to the object perceived in the blot. A variety of other commonly reported contents also are categorized, as seen in Table 9.1, including anatomical features, art and anthropological contents, features from the natural environment such as clouds, fire, botany, nature, and landscapes, and objects of clothing, science, and household items. The Sex (*Sx*) content code is also a relatively recent addition to the CS, developed to reflect perceptions of sexual organs and activities. Contents that do not easily fit the 26 content categories are coded as Idiographic (*Id*) contents. Rorschach content is also differentiated into primary and secondary contents when multiple contents are involved in a response, although this differentiation is not maintained in the interpretive process.

The CS continues the tradition of the previous Rorschach scoring systems of coding Popular (*P*) responses, which consist of 13 percepts across the 10 inkblots that are frequently reported in various psychiatric and nonpsychiatric samples. "Populars" are fairly straightforward to code: Only responses that *exactly* fit the criterion image qualify for the code of *P*.

Organizational Activity

In contrast to the previously described codes, the coding of Organizational Activity in the CS involves assigning a numerical code, known as a *Z* score, for each response that involves perceptual organization. The individual *Z* scores have interpretive significance only after they are subsequently tallied and transformed into Structural Summary indices. Responses that involve form may receive a *Z* score under one of four conditions: (1) ZW if it is a Whole response with an acceptable Developmental Quality code (excluding vague responses); (2) ZA if it involves two or more separate objects perceived in Adjacent Detail areas that are described in a meaningful relationship; (3) ZD if it involves two or more separate objects in Distant Detail areas that are described in a meaningful relationship; and (4) ZS if White Space is actively integrated into other blot areas in forming the response. The CS workbook provides a table of *Z*-score values for each of the four types of organizational activity by card, which is used in assigning the appropriate *Z* score. When more than one *Z* score is applicable (e.g., when both Whole and White Space Integration criteria are met), the higher *Z*-score value is assigned to the response.

Special Scores

The last coding category in the CS concerns the Special Scores that are used to record a variety of important response characteristics. Some of the codes in this category identify problematic perceptual–cognitive processes, whereas others denote phenomena that are likely to involve projection. Special Scores, like the Determinants, are among the most challenging codes to derive and require careful attention to the client's verbalizations. Even experienced coders may have difficulty reliably assigning Special Scores.

The first set of Special Scores, called Unusual Verbalizations, encompasses Deviant Verbalizations, Inappropriate Combinations, and Inappropriate Logic, all of which are marked by dysfunctional cognitive processes ranging from milder forms of cognitive slippage to more serious levels of cognitive disarray. Deviant Verbalizations are further differentiated into two codes: (1) Deviant Verbalization (*DV*), resulting from use of neologisms or redundant words, and (2) Deviant Response (*DR*), involving departures from the task by use of inappropriate or irrelevant phrases or by engaging in circumstantial verbalization. Inappropriate Combinations are divided into three types: (1) Incongruous Combinations (*INCOM*), which are coded when blot images are condensed into a single object (e.g., a man with four eyes); (2) Fabulized Combinations (*FABCOM*), involving an inconceivable relationship between two objects (e.g., "two tigers playing basketball") or dubious transparencies (e.g., "a man eating and you can see his food being processed in his stomach"); and (3) Contamination (*CONTAM*), involving serious reality distortions by means of fusing images into a single response (e.g., "the head of a pig-owl"). *DV*, *DR*, *INCOM*, and *FABCOM* codes are additionally differentiated into Levels 1 and 2, reflecting milder and more serious levels of cognitive disruption, respectively, denoted by a numerical suffix of "1" or "2." The Inappropriate Logic (*ALOG*) Special Score is coded when strained reasoning, reflecting a concrete and poorly developed form of thinking, is used to account for a response (e.g., "It must be an angry butterfly because it is red").

Perseverations (*PSV*) represent another set of Special Scores that reflect cognitive rigidity and/or extreme levels of psychological preoccupation that prevent shifts in cognitive set. *PSV*s are divided into three types: (1) within-card perseveration, in which the same coding is produced for consecutive responses; (2) content perseveration, in which a perceived object is identified as the same object seen previously in another response or another card; and (3) mechanical perseveration, found in severely neurologically impaired individuals who tend to report the same object repetitively and in a mechanistic manner.

The CS permits coding of four types of Special Content characteristics. The Abstract Content (*AB*) code is assigned when a description of formless human sensory or emotional experiences comprises the sole response content (e.g., "It looks like depression"), or when a symbolic representation (e.g., "It is a white flag representing peace") is articulated in the response. The Aggressive Movement (*AG*) code is provided for human, animal, or inanimate movement responses involving aggressive actions in progress, such as fighting, hunting, or glaring. The Cooperative Movement (*COP*) Special Score is provided for movement responses involving explicitly positive or cooperative actions between two or more objects. Finally, the Morbid Content (*MOR*) code is given for responses involving either dead, destroyed, and damaged objects or attributions of dysphoric features to perceived objects.

The latest revision of the CS (Exner, 2001b) has incorporated a new set of variables known as Human Representational (HR) responses, developed to measure the capacity for effective interpersonal functioning. HR responses are differentiated into good (*GHR*) and poor (*PHR*) responses that are coded by using a sequence of progressive steps described in the CS workbook. All responses containing human content coding, human movement determinants, and *COP* or *AG* Special Scores receive either a *GHR* or *PHR* Special Score. Two additional types of Special Scores are coded to register the presence of defensive operations. The Personalized Answers (*PER*) code is given when the respondent invokes personal knowledge or experience (e.g., "I have one like it at home") to justify the response and avert any further questioning. The Color Projection (*CP*) code is assigned when chromatic color is described on achromatic blots.

It should be noted that multiple Special Scores may be applicable to a given Rorschach response. For example, a response may meet criteria for *FABCOM*, *PER*, and *GHR* codes, or for other Special Scores that are independent of each other. However, for a smaller set of six interrelated Critical Special Scores, caution should be exerted during coding decisions to avoid duplication. For example, a response that meets criteria for both a *DV* and *DR* code will only receive the *DR* code, and a response that meets criterion for a *CONTAM* code should not receive *DV*, *DR*, *INCOM*, *FABCOM*, or *ALOG* Special Scores, even when the latter codes appear applicable.

Structural Summary

When Rorschach coding is completed, the coded data are used to develop the Structural Summary. The coded responses are listed in the Sequence of Scores page of the Structural Summary booklet and are used to obtain the frequency data presented in the upper section of the Structural Summary page. Specifically, the upper section contains tallies of each type of Location, Developmental Quality, and Form Quality code, as well as a listing of Blends, Single Determinants, Contents, and Special Scores. The Location section includes three types of Organizational Quality entries: (1) the Z frequency *(Zf)*, which is a tally of the total number of Z-score occurrences in the record; (2) the *ZSum*, which is a numerical sum of the weighted *Z* scores in the record; and (3) the estimated weighted Z-Sum (*Zest*), which is obtained from a table of estimated *Z* scores for each value of *Zf*, presented in the CS workbook. In the Special Score section, Level 1 and Level 2 Special Scores are recorded separately, adjacent to their respective weights. The Raw Sum6 value is the total number of cognitive Special Scores obtained in the record, and the Weighted Sum6 value is computed as the sum of the six Special Scores multiplied by their respective weights. Finally, the upper section of the Structural Summary page contains space to record the Approach Summary, or the sequence of location choices used for each card.

The lower section of the Structural Summary page contains the ratios, percentages, and derived scores that collectively form the nucleus of interpretation. This section is subdivided into several sections: Core, Affect, Ideation, Mediation, Processing, Interpersonal, and Self-Perception. The Core section contains the frequency entries of *R* (total number of responses) and total numbers of the determinants *FM, m, SumC'*, ΣυμT, Συμς, and *SumY*, inclusive of the occurrence of these determinants in Blends. It also contains the following nine ratios and derivations:

1. Lambda (*L*) is computed as number of Pure *F* determinants divided by *R–F*.
2. Erlebnistypus (*EB*) is presented as a ratio of Sum *M* determinants to the Weighted Sum Color (*WSumC*). In determining the *WSumC*, progressively higher weights are assigned to *FC, CF*, and *C* determinants, respectively.
3. Experience Actual (*EA*) is the sum of *M* and *WSumC*.
4. EB Pervasive (*EBPer*) is calculated only when *EA* is 4 or greater, *L* is less than 1, and the two sides of the *EB* differ substantially. This latter difference must be at least 2 points when *EA* is in the 4–10 range and at least 2.5 points when *EA* is greater than 10 points.
5. Experience Base (*eb*) is the ratio of *FM+m* to *SumC''* + *SumT* + *SumY* + *SumV*.
6. Experienced Stimulation (*es*) is the sum of the two sides of the *eb*.
7. Difference score (*D Score*) is computed in a two-step process whereby the difference between the *EA* and *es* score is first obtained and a conversion table is used to derive the corresponding *D Score* value.
8. Adjusted *es* (*Adj es*) involves a recalculation of the *es* subsequent to eliminating all *m* and *Y* values in excess of 1 each.
9. Adjusted Difference Score (*AdjD*) is obtained by a two-step process of subtracting the *Adj es* from the *EA* value and using the *D Score* conversion table to find the corresponding *D Score* value.

The Affect cluster of the Structural Summary includes tallies of the number of *Pure C, S*, and *CP* responses in the record. It also contains (1) the Form–Color Ratio of $FC:CF+C$, (2) the Constriction Ratio of $SumC'$: $WSumC$, (3) the Affective Ratio (Afr) computed as the number of responses to Cards 8, 9, and 10 divided by the number of responses to the first seven cards, and (4) the Complexity Ratio of $Blends:R$.

The Ideation section of the Structural Summary contains frequency data for the variables of MOR, $RawSum6$ and $WSum6$, $Level\ 2$ Special Scores, $M-$ responses, and formless M ($Mnone$) responses. Additionally, it contains two ratios: the ratio of all movement responses (M, FM, and m) that are active versus passive ($a{:}p$), and the ratio of active to passive Human Movement responses ($Ma{:}Mp$). It also includes the Intellectualization Index that is computed as $2AB+Art+Ay$.

The Mediation section contains frequency scores for the number of Popular (P) responses and the number of Space responses with a minus Form Quality ($S-$). It also includes five additional indices:

1. Form Appropriate Extended ($XA\%$): This variable has been introduced in the latest edition of the CS and is calculated as the sum of responses with FQ codes of +, o, or u, divided by R.
2. Form Appropriate–Common Areas ($WDA\%$): This is also a new variable, calculated as the sum of $W+D$ responses that have an FQ coding of +, o, or u, divided by the sum of $W+D$.
3. Distorted Form ($X-\%$) is calculated as the sum of minus FQ responses in the entire record ($FQx-$), divided by R.
4. Conventional Form ($X+\%$) is calculated as the sum of FQx + and o, divided by R.
5. Unusual Form ($Xu\%$) is obtained by dividing the sum of $FQxu$ by R.

The Processing cluster of the Structural Summary contains frequency tallies of Zf, PSV, $DQ+$, and DQv. It also includes three indices known as the (1) Economy Index and represented by the ratio of $W{:}D{:}Dd$, (2) Aspirational Ratio of $W{:}M$, and (3) the Processing Efficiency (Zd) Index, obtained by subtracting the $Zest$ from the $ZSum$ value with notation of the appropriate sign.

The Interpersonal section contains a total of 10 entries. Six of these, consisting of COP, AG, $Food$, $SumT$, $Pure\ H$, and PER are frequency data transferred from the upper section of the Structural Summary. Additionally, a Human Content total is tallied to reflect the $H+(H)+Hd+(Hd)$ frequencies. Two ratio scores—$GHR{:}PHR$ and $a{:}p$—are also provided in this section, and the Isolation Index ($Isolate/R$) is computed from content scores using the formula $Bt+2Cl+Ge+Ls+2Na/R$. The Self-Perception variables of the Structural Summary include frequency data concerning Reflections ($Fr+rF$), $SumV$, FD, $An+Xy$, and MOR. This section also contains the Egocentricity Index ($3r+[2]/R$), calculated as the total number of Reflections multiplied by 3, plus the total number of Pairs, divided by R.

The final set of entries on the Structural Summary involves data concerning six special indices: Perceptual–Thinking Index (*PTI*), Depression Index (*DEPI*), Coping Deficit Index (*CDI*), Suicide Potential Index (*S-CON*), Hypervigilance Index (*HVI*), and Obsessive Style Index (*OBS*). These indices are computed after all other computations are completed because they utilize the numerical values recorded in the lower section of the Structural Summary. Obtaining the values for the indices also requires the use of a Constellations Worksheet, which presents a series of empirically derived criteria for each index. A numerical score reflecting the number of criteria met for each index is obtained for the *PTI, DEPI, S-CON,* and *CDI,* whereas the *HVI* and *OBS* are evaluated in terms of a Yes/No threshold criterion. It should be noted that the cutoff values for two criteria on the *DEPI* and one criterion on the *PTI* are not applicable to younger clients (ages 16 or 13, depending on the criterion), and these latter two indices require the use of an alternative, age-adjusted table of values.

INTERPRETATION

Rorschach interpretation is best undertaken in the CS as a multistep process that uses nomothetic and idiographic aspects of the test record to yield a conceptual understanding of personality structure and processes. Procedurally, the interpretive process for the CS begins at the level of the Structural Summary and consists of a complex, configural analysis that furnishes the highest level of confidence in test findings. The interpretation proceeds to the level of the Sequence of Scores where patterns and sets can be identified, and ends in an analysis of the actual verbal responses. The verbalizations constitute the level at which projection and idiographic reactions can be identified, but they also represent the level where inferences are more speculative and warrant use of cautious conservatism.

Structural Summary Interpretation

A Rorschach record is deemed interpretable when a minimum of 14 responses is obtained across the 10 stimulus blots. However, the average number of responses for nonpatients is 22.32 (*SD* = 4.40), and records with substantially fewer responses may be relatively lacking in detail, consequently limiting the scope of interpretation.

Interpreting the Rorschach Structural Summaries of adults requires use of the nonpatient adults norms that are provided in the CS workbook. Specifically, the test interpreter consults the table of descriptive statistics for the mean and standard deviation values for each variable, and evaluates the degree to which the values in the client's record deviate from normative expectations. The median and modal values also should be considered, as many Rorschach variables are not normally distributed. To improve the accuracy of interpretations, the test interpreter could additionally examine the normative data tables for Introversives, Extratensives, and Ambitents, utilizing the table that is appropriate, based on the client's *EB* style. This procedure is useful because the normative values for some Rorschach variables are quite different across these groups. For example, although the mean *EA* value for nonpatient adults is 8.66 (*SD* = 2.38), the mean value is somewhat higher for Introversives (mean = 9.61, *SD* = 2.17) and Extratensives (mean = 9.04, *SD* = 1.82) and lower for Ambitents (mean = 7.64, *SD* = 2.53). Moreover, as expected, Extratensives tend to obtain markedly higher values than Introversives on color variables and substantially lower values on the *M* variable. Unlike these two groups, the mean *D score* value for Ambitents tends to be a negative value. These data suggest that exclusive reliance on the general nonpatient sample norms may produce over- or underinterpretation for selected variables in some cases. In general, Exner (2000b) cautions against the concrete use of normative data and/or overemphasis on deviation findings, suggesting instead that a series of hypothesis be developed and evaluated by progressively cross-checking normative reference points for multiple variables and modifying findings. A final step in the normative evaluation could include examining the descriptive statistics provided separately for outpatients, inpatients with depression, and inpatients with schizophrenia, for relevant comparisons based on the client's diagnostic/treatment setting status.

The Structural Summary contains a series of eight interpretative clusters relating to Capacity for Control and Stress Tolerance, Situational Stress, Affect, Information Processing, Cognitive Mediation, Ideation, Self Perception, and Interpersonal Perception. Each cluster contains a number of variables that illuminates different facets of the psychological domain represented by that cluster. Exner (1991, 2000b) has formulated a systematic approach to Rorschach interpretation involving the use of empirically determined key variables to organize the sequence in which the eight clusters are addressed. Each key variable has a cutting score defining the values needed to clarify that variable as positive. For example, a criterion score of greater than 3 points on the Perceptual–Thinking Index indicates that it is a positive variable in the client's Rorschach record. The search routine to be employed in this instance begins with the Information Processing cluster, followed by Mediation, Ideation, Capacity for Control, Affect, Self Perception, and Interpersonal Perception, respectively. Additionally, the Situational Stress cluster is reviewed when there are positive findings in this domain.

The search methodology is based on the recognition that each Rorschach record is unique in terms of the personality characteristics that are important for the individual client, and it permits appropriate emphasis on the salient aspects of his or her test record. A list of 12 key variables is provided in the *Primer* (Exner, 2000b); if none of the key variables is positive, an alternative list of tertiary variables may be used to determine the interpretive sequence. Regardless of the search sequence employed, all of the seven major clusters of the Structural Summary are interpreted. Exner has further facilitated the interpretive routine by identifying a series of steps to be followed for within-cluster interpretation of variables, which ensures an exhaustive examination of pertinent variables. The end point in a structural approach to interpretation involves integrating the findings to yield a comprehensive description of the individual.

Capacity for Control and Stress Tolerance

This cluster contains the *D score* and *Adj D score* that reflect the balance between the stressors experienced by the individual and his or her use of psychological resources to manage those stressors. Specifically, the *D score* reflects the current control capacity of the individual, whereas the *Adj D score* reflects the individual's longer-term coping and control abilities when the effects of acute stressors are eliminated. *D/Adj D* scores of 0, which are the modal values for these variables among the CS's nonpatient normative sample, indicate adequate control capacities. Negative values for these variables indicate a vulnerability to loss of control and the potential for becoming disorganized and overwhelmed by stress. Positive values generally suggest superior coping capacity. In clients undergoing psychological services, however, positive scores may indicate that states of stress are chronic and ego-syntonic. A positive (≥ 4) *CDI*, reflecting social ineptness and an unrewarding or chaotic interpersonal history, suggests vulnerability to coping difficulty regardless of the values of *D* and *Adj D*, but the former variable has received relatively little empirical evaluation at present.

Other variables to be considered in the Controls and Stress Tolerance cluster include (1) the *EA*, which serves as an index of the internal psychological resources available for coping and control functions, and (2) the *EB*, which represents the characteristic problem-solving style of the individual. The *EB* is an important, well-researched, and stable variable relevant to several clusters of the Structural Summary. *EB* values are categorized into three styles: Introversive, Extratensive, and Ambient. Introversives tend to "think through" problems by relying on internal judgments. In contrast, Extratensives utilize a trial-and-error approach that depends on feedback received from their actions. Both styles are reasonably comparable in their effectiveness, particularly when they are flexibly employed. The Ambient style, however, is considered a liability because it reflects the absence of a reliable and consistent approach to problem solving.

The Controls and Stress Tolerance cluster also requires an examination of the value of *Lambda*. An elevated *L* score indicates use of a minimizing and simplifying strategy that renders the coping world more manageable, whereas a low L score suggests a tendency to be drawn into complexities and nuances of experiences, which may complicate coping tasks when vulnerabilities are present in other aspects of personality. Finally, the Suicide Constellation (S-CON) may be examined for indications of risk factors. The 12 criteria of this index encompass indicators such as self-criticism, confused emotions, emotional reactivity, and unconventional thinking. Although an elevated S-CON score may serve to alert the clinician to make further inquiries about the client's potential for suicide, the index has been found to produce false-positive and false-negative problems in different populations. Low range S-CON values should not be used to rule out the possibility of suicide risk.

Situational Stress

The presence of situational stress is broadly identified on the Rorschach by the es and Adj es variables. The es variable is a composite of the two sides of the eb ratio, consisting of FM and m on the left side and C', T, V, and Y variables on the right side. FM and m represent cognitively based stressors stemming from unmet needs (FM) and situational stress that is experienced as worry, frustration, and disrupted thinking (m). C', T, V, and Y collectively represent emotionally based stressors when their frequencies exceed normative values. These latter stressors involve unnatural affective constraint (C'), interpersonal distancing or neediness (T), painful negative self-appraisal (V), and anxiety (Y). An examination of these specific variables reveals aspects of the nature of difficulties experienced by the individual.

The D and Adj D scores also have some bearing on situational stress assessment; the relative magnitude of experienced situational stress is likely to increase progressively with the degree to which the Adj D $score$ value exceeds the D $score$ value. Finally, the presence of blends with m and Y determinants and the occurrence of color-shading blends signal complicated and confused emotional experiences, respectively, that contribute to overall stress.

Affect

The recommended procedure for interpreting the Affect section on the Structural Summary involves examining the $DEPI$ and CDI constellations as a starting point for positive values of ≥ 5 and ≥ 4, respectively (Exner, 2000b). As mentioned earlier, however, the $DEPI$ has received equivocal research support, and few studies have been conducted on the CDI, warranting particular caution in interpreting these indices. The four central variables related to affect consist of the FC:$CF+C$ ratio, Pure C, Afr, and S. FC responses represent a greater level of affective control than CF or C responses. A higher FC than $CF+C$ value, which is expected for nonpatient adults, indicates that affective expressions are reasonably well regulated. However, excessively high *FC* values suggest emotional overcontrol, whereas high *CF+C* values, relative to *FC*, suggest poor affective modulation. Furthermore, the occurrence of any Pure *C* determinants reflects propensities toward unrestrained emotional displays.

These color-related determinants are best viewed in the context of the *Afr*, which measures the individual's degree of affective responsiveness or willingness to respond to affective material. For example, a Rorschach record containing a high *FC* value combined with a low *Afr* suggests that there is discomfort with emotions, dealt with by avoidance and overcontrol maneuvers. An excessive number of Space responses in a Rorschach record indicates levels of negativism and anger that are likely to have a disruptive influence on various aspects of a person's functioning.

In addition to these four variables, some variables previously examined in the Controls/Stress Tolerance and Situational Stress clusters, including *EB*, *L*, and right side *eb*, are relevant to the evaluation of affect and offer a new interpretive nuance in this context. For example, CS findings indicate that *EB* Introversives do not permit emotions to influence their decisions and tend to exert control over their emotional displays, whereas *EB* Extratensives utilize emotions to guide decisions and are prone to express emotions more freely. In contrast, emotions play an inconsistent role in the decisions and behaviors of *EB* Ambitents. Furthermore, high *L* individuals tend to avoid affect, whereas low *L* individuals may be excessively drawn into affective complexities. A higher value for the right side *eb*, compared to the left *eb*, points to the presence of emotional discomfort. Other affective variables in the Rorschach Structural Summary include Color-Shading blends indicative of confused emotional experiences and shading blends signaling painful emotions, neither of which has received sufficient research attention in CS studies.

Next we turn our attention to three clusters—Information Processing, Cognitive Mediation, and Ideation—that provide a comprehensive overview of the individual's perceptual and cognitive operations.

Information Processing

The individual's information-processing style is examined in the context of the *EB* and *L* styles that reveal, for example, a propensity to use trial-and-error methods (*EB* extratensive) or a preference for an economical and simplified approach to dealing with information (high *L*). The *OBS* and *HVI* variables, developed to measure preoccupations with details and hyperalertness, respectively, are also located in this cluster as contextual variables, but should be used minimally until further empirical support is available for these measures. Key information-processing variables include *Zf*, *W:D:Dd*, *W:M*, and *Zd*. Additional variables that offer some supportive information include *PSV* and DQ quality. *Zf* reflects the degree of effort put into information-processing activity, ranging from excessive to minimal attempts to absorb new information. The *W:D:Dd* ratio reflects the extent to which the processing method involves striving (*W*), economy (*D*), or an atypical focus on details (*Dd*). The *W:M* ratio has been considered an index of aspiration, reflecting the balance between achievement strivings (*W*) and the functional capacities of the individual (*M*). Deviations from norms in the *W* > *M* direction suggest that achievement goals exceed capacities and possibly lead to experiences of frustration, whereas the reverse direction reflects an orientation toward relatively low aspirations and underachievement. *Zd* is a measure of processing efficiency that can range from underincorporation (< –3.0) to overincorporation (> 3.0) of information. Exner (1991, 2000b) suggests that underincorporation of information, resulting from hasty and unsystematic methods of inspecting the environment, is apt to have an adverse impact on decision-making processes. Overincorporation is advantageous when thoroughness is necessary but may become a liability under conditions that require rapid and efficient information processing.

The *PSV* Special Score identifies the types of difficulties in shifting attention usually experienced by individuals with neurological impairments, but it is also found in cognitively unimpaired individuals who have inflexible perseverative styles. Finally, the *quality* of information processing is reflected in the DQ distribution, ranging from sophisticated (DQ+) to immature (DQv) levels.

Cognitive Mediation

The Cognitive Mediation section of the Structural Summary addresses the degree of reality orientation maintained in the process of translating information into coherent ideas. Important variables in this cluster include *P*, *X+%*, *X–%*, *Xu%*, and *S–* frequency. The two new variables of *XA%* and *WDA%* are also located in this cluster. *P* responses constitute the typical or acceptable responses to obvious blot features and reflect the ability to produce conventional responses. *P* values can range from excessive conventionality (high *P* frequency) to excessive individuality (low *P* frequency). *X+%* has a normative value of 0.77 (*SD* = 0.09) and is a robust variable with high temporal consistency that measures the degree of conventionality involved in interpreting information. It is counterbalanced by *X–%*, which signals distortions in thinking involving distortions of reality; and *Xu%*, which represents idiosyncratic thought processes. A low *X+%* indicates problems with reality testing when coupled with a high *X–%*, but it reflects a less critical departure from socially accepted forms of thinking when coupled with a high *Xu%*. *XA%* and *WDA%* also measure the intactness of reality testing; at present, they can be considered as less informative adjunctive data until shown to provide incremental interpretive yield. The S– frequency, however, offers unique interpretive information relating to perceptual inaccuracies associated with negativism or anger.

Ideation

The Ideation cluster reflects the central concepts formed by the individual, which serve as the basis for decisions and actions. EB and L continue to be of relevance in this regard, identifying if the individual is (1) prone to emphasize use of logic (EB Introversive) versus intuition (EB Extratensive) during decision making, (2) inconsistent in the development and application of conceptual thinking to problem solving (EB Ambitent), or (3) prone to avoid decision making (high L). Moreover, an elevated m frequency suggests that goal-directed thinking is likely to be disrupted by intrusive thoughts generated by stress. Significant variables in the Ideation cluster include $a{:}p$, $Ma{:}Mp$, the Intellectualization Index, $RawSum6$ and $WSum6$, M– and $Mnone$, and MOR. The HVI and OBS indices also may be examined in this section, though with caution, to determine if perfectionistic or distrusting cognitive sets are in operation, with the recognition that these variables require further validation.

The $a{:}p$ ratio provides data concerning the flexibility or rigidity of an individual's ideas and concepts. The more discrepant the values of the ratio, the more likely it is that the individual finds it difficult to modify existing attitudes and opinions. The $Ma{:}Mp$ ratio is interpretively significant only when Mp exceeds Ma, indicating a propensity to defensively replace reality with fantasy in highly stressful situations. The Intellectualization Index also identifies a defensive process, in this case involving maneuvers to neutralize or deny emotions by use of distorted concepts. The Sum6 variables identify the presence of cognitive malfunctioning that can range along a continuum of severity, depending on the specific types of Special Scores involved. For example:

DVs involve milder forms of cognitive slippage.
$INCOM$s reflect concrete thinking and problems in differentiation.
DRs reflect indecisiveness at Level 1 and dysregulated ideational impulses at Level 2.
$FABCOM$s indicate an irrational synthesis of ideas and flawed judgment.
$ALOG$s represent strained reasoning.
$CONTAM$s indicate the most disorganized and bizarre type of conceptual reasoning.

The $RawSum6$ value represents the frequency of any type of cognitive lapse, whereas the $WSum6$ reflects the severity of the ideational disruption.

The Human Movement (M) response provides another important set of data concerning the cognitive processes of reasoning and imagination. This variable has been widely researched in the various Rorschach systems and has been linked to intellect and abstract thinking. From a clinical perspective, poor M quality has been associated with psychological disturbance, confirming Hermann Rorschach's original view that the test identifies psychopathology. $M-$ responses signal peculiarities in ideation, and $Mnone$ responses suggest that thought processes are not adequately rooted in reality. The MOR score, which is also considered in the Self Perception cluster, suggests proneness to pessimistic forms of thinking.

Rorschach evaluation of perceptual and cognitive processes has typically also involved examination of the Schizophrenia Index ($SCZI$). The $SCZI$ was developed by Exner in 1984 to facilitate diagnostic assessment of thought disorder. However, clinical applications and empirical evaluations of the $SCZI$ revealed that it yielded high false-positive rates. The index also received criticism for its label because it appeared to measure broad forms of psychotic thought processes rather than the specific characteristics of schizophrenia. As noted, the $SCZI$ has been revised and relabeled the Perceptual–Thinking Index (PTI) in the current edition of the CS. PTI values are interpreted along a continuum of severity ranging from 1 to 5. Given the recency of its development, the PTI index requires research evaluation before it can be used accurately in clinical assessment.

Self Perception

The Self Perception cluster primarily involves a review of Reflections, the Egocentricity Index, FD and V, $An+Xy$, MOR, and the $H:(H)+Hd+(Hd)$ ratio. A high score on Reflections is associated with a heightened state of narcissism, manifested in an elevated sense of self-worth that requires constant validation from others and is sustained through the use of defensive mechanisms. An elevated Egocentricity Index, on the other hand, indicates an inordinate degree of self-involvement that may be related to high self-regard or, in the absence of reflections, indicates strong self-concern. A low Egocentricity Index is associated with deficits in self-esteem that may forebode depressive experiences.

FD and V responses both relate to introspective tendencies but are qualitatively different from each other. The presence of FD is generally favorable and reflects the ability to view oneself with perspective, whereas V is invariably associated with negative emotions arising from critical self-evaluations. $An+Xy$ is viewed as the body concern index that may also indicate a sense of physical and/or psychological vulnerability; however, it is not a robust CS variable. MOR responses are associated with negative self-attributions and pessimistic self-perceptions.

The Human content variables offer rather direct information about self-image. A higher value for *H* in relation to *(H)+Hd+(Hd)* suggests that the self-image is derived from life experiences as opposed to being subjectively construed or misconstrued. Other qualitative aspects of *H* and *M* responses may reveal important data concerning self-perceptions. In addition to these central variables, a perceived sense of vulnerability is implied by a positive *HVI*, and underlying insecurity may be hypothesized to exist in cases of a positive *OBS*.

Interpersonal Perception

The Interpersonal Perception section of the Structural Summary contains seven central variables for interpretation: *T*, Human contents, Pure *H*, *PER*, *COP*, *AG*, and the Isolation Index. The *T* determinant, originally investigated in pre-CS Rorschach systems, has been related to relational and affectional needs and dependencies. The modal value among nonpatient adults is 1, indicative of an appropriate degree of openness to relating to others. Higher values of *T* are associated with strong needs for closeness, possibly arising from experiences of loneliness or acute emotional loss, and include manifestations of dependency. In contrast, the absence of *T* suggests interpersonal caution, guardedness, and distancing.

Human content scores serve as a means of gauging interest in people, with Pure *H*—in comparison to *(H)* or *(Hd)* scores—serving as a measure of whether these interests are grounded in reality. The *PER* Special Score reflects tendencies to justify one's self-concept in interpersonal interactions; these individuals are likely to alienate others by their defensive and argumentative expressions and may have difficulty sustaining meaningful relationships. *COP*, reflecting positive views or expectations of relationships, and *AG*, reflecting hostile attitudes or impulses, are best interpreted jointly in terms of whether a largely positive or largely negative view is held of relationships. High *COP*/low *AG* individuals are viewed as gregarious and amicable, whereas low *COP*/high *AG* individuals are believed to be forceful and contentious in their interactions with others. The Isolation Index identifies the degree of social interaction or isolation, indirectly revealing the extent of social support available to the individual.

In addition to these variables, the *CDI*, *HVI*, *a:p* ratio, *Fd* content, and *GHR:PHR* offer ancillary data concerning interpersonal functioning. Exner (2000b) reports that a positive *CDI* is suggestive of social immaturity and interpersonal ineptness, and is associated with histories of unsatisfying relationships. A positive *HVI* is found to be associated with interpersonal suspiciousness, guardedness, and distancing. The *a:p* ratio is notable when $p > a$, indicating passivity in relationships, and the *Fd* content is associated with dependency needs. The new variables of *GHR* and *PHR* were developed to measure effectiveness of interpersonal functioning, with the normative data indicating that nonpatients produce a *GHR* value that is approximately three times the value of *PHR*. These variables appear promising but require further empirical study before they are assigned interpretive significance.

Interpreting the Sequence of Scores

An analysis of the Sequence of Scores includes attending to the quality of the first and last responses (i.e., the "sign in" and "sign out") in the record to evaluate the person's reaction to task initiation and conclusion. For example, the examiner might note a response process that began conservatively and progressed to displays of deteriorated thought processes, or a pattern in which the early responses evoked processes of defensiveness or oppositionality, revealed by *PER* and *S* codes. Examination of the Approach Summary may reveal the presence of a consistent method of perception (e.g., uniformly progressing from Whole to Detail locations of each blot) or, conversely, an apparently random approach lacking a coherent strategy.

Analysis of Verbalizations

At the final level of interpretation, an Analysis of Verbalizations includes evaluating the qualitative features of the responses, including embellishments and comments that fall outside codable categories. For example, responses may contain histrionic overtones (e.g., "Wow, these bright colors are pretty!" or "That one looks like an outpouring of unending love"), or a self-denouncing quality (e.g., "I guess I'm crazy for seeing such strange things" or "I'm not good at this kind of test") that may not be adequately represented in the Structural Summary indices concerning affect and self-perception. Moreover, responses that receive a Special Score may vary widely along a descriptive continuum (e.g., "a bleeding finger" and "a pet rabbit that has been disemboweled" are both coded *MOR*), indicative of problems at different levels of clinical significance. Noting these characteristics of the verbalizations provides important supplementary data that may support, qualify, or extend the interpretation derived from the structural variables and indices.

An Alternative Organization for Interpretation: Use of the Systematic Treatment Selection Model

A beneficial approach to Rorschach interpretation involves use of the Systematic Treatment Selection (STS) model to organize Rorschach data into meaningful themes that are relevant to treatment considerations. As discussed in Chapter 3 (see also Beutler, Clarkin, & Bongar, 2000; Beutler &

Harwood, 1995), use of this model involves organizing the test data to evaluate an important set of client characteristics, labeled predisposing variables, that have been empirically related to treatment outcome. These variables include (1) problem-relevant factors such as major symptoms, problem severity, and problem complexity; (2) personality traits and state characteristics manifested in level of distress, coping style, self-esteem, interpersonal reactivity, and amenability to change; and (3) environmental variables of stress and social support that interact with client variables and may produce impairments in functioning or serve to foster functional adaptation. Rorschach variables can be arranged into six clusters to address the six components outlined in the STS model: functional impairment (severity), social support level, complexity/chronicity, coping style, resistance traits, and distress level. These categories are discussed further in the following section to illustrate their use for treatment planning.

Functional impairment is predominantly assessed by constellations developed to serve as markers of significant cognitive (*PTI, OBS*), emotional (*DEPI, S-CON*), and interpersonal (*CDI, HVI*) dysfunction. Although these indices require further empirical support and should not be used to derive specific diagnoses, they may be used as a starting point for further investigation of impaired functioning. A negative *D* and/or *Adj D score* suggests the likelihood of loss of control and disorganized functioning, and the Rorschach interpreter would examine the Affect, Cognitive, and Interpersonal clusters to determine the area(s) of greatest impairment.

A number of Structural Summary variables permit inference concerning the individual's access to *social support*. The *CDI* may be considered in this regard, because the likelihood of an unsuccessful interpersonal history is associated with a positive *CDI* and implies that adequate social support has been inconsistently available. Indices of interpersonal distancing and isolation, including the absence of *T*, an elevated Isolation Index, and a low *H* frequency, suggest that the individual is not oriented toward seeking supportive connections with others. This finding is strengthened when the frequency of *COP* is low, suggesting that relationships are not typically viewed as positive or rewarding. Social support is also likely to be inadequate for individuals who have elevated *PER, Fr+rF,* or *AG* scores, because their interpersonal behaviors are likely to estrange them from others.

Identifying the *chronicity* of problems is facilitated by comparing the *D* and *Adj D* scores in the Rorschach Structural Summary. A negative value for the *Adj D score* implies that problems are chronic and likely to be recurrent, whereas a negative *D score* with an *Adj D score* of 0 or higher suggests that acute situational stressors are the primary source of difficulty. Conversely, a positive *Adj D score* in a client presenting for treatment suggests that the individual may have become accustomed to a state of stress overload, and further investigation to validate this hypothesis would be indicated. Additionally, a significant *CDI* suggests that there are longstanding interpersonal difficulties that are likely to produce recurring problems in adjustment. *Problem complexity* is suggested by an elevated number of blends in the protocol, particularly blends containing a variety of shading elements and color-shading combinations. The presence of an *EB* Ambient style further suggests that the individual is likely to have repetitive experiences of coping difficulty.

The predominant indicator of *coping style*, or characteristic patterns of problem solving and decision making, is the *EB* variable. As discussed earlier, Introversive and Extratensive styles are distinctly different in terms of the approach to problem solving. Introversives are more likely to use an internalizing coping style, whereas as Extratensives depend more on externalizing strategies. Both styles may be effective when problem severity and functioning impairment are low, and when psychological resources (*EA*) are adequately accessible for coping functions. However, the presence of an Ambient style indicates the absence of a reliable mode of problem solving and increases the potential for problems in adjustment. A high *L* style indicates a characteristic mode of defensive constriction that is most likely to impair thought processes. Other defensive approaches to coping are suggested by an elevated Intellectualization Index, high *PER*, and a low *Afr*.

Several of the variables discussed previously also may be used to identify client characteristics that serve to rebuff treatment interventions and resist change (*resistance*). For example, the presence of Reflection responses, in conjunction with a high Egocentricity Index, suggests that the individual is strongly invested in maintaining an inflated self-image and may resist treatment attempts that encourage revising the self-view or promoting greater consideration of others' needs. The presence of *V* responses indicate self-critical, ruminative tendencies that present barriers to examination of personal strengths; the individual may be particularly resistant to positive self-examination when the Rorschach record also contains several *MOR*s. A client with a high *L* style of functioning and a underincorporative *Zd* mode is not easily amenable to examining facets of experience that are typically overlooked. Moreover, elevated Intellectualization Index scores and other forms of defensive maneuvers to avoid negative affect impede the development of insight. Resistance to treatment intervention also may be found for a client with a *T*-less Rorschach record, resulting from a failure to develop a trusting relationship with the therapist.

The presence of *distress*, which may serve as a motivator for treatment-related change, is identified by *es* and further differentiated by the examination of the *C'*, *V*, *T*, and *Y* variables that evaluate different facets of emotional distress, including discomfort, anxiety, guilt, and loneliness. As discussed earlier, negative and confused emotions are detected by the presence of Shading and Color-Shading blends. The *FM* and *m* variables also aid in identifying stress experienced as disrupted concentration and a sense of struggle.

TREATMENT PLANNING

A predominant application of Rorschach assessment is to assist in the development of an appropriate treatment plan. Ideally, the assessment should be tailored to address specific questions about a particular client, including issues concerning the client's current level of functional impairment and distress, factors contributing to his or her maladaptation, psychiatric diagnosis, prognosis for treatment-related improvement, and selection of appropriate type(s) of treatment. Integrating Rorschach assessment with the STS model is a useful method of focusing the assessment process, rendering Rorschach findings meaningful, and systematically employing the test findings to construct effective treatment plans.

Presenting problems can be categorized as either acute or chronic in nature. When Rorschach data reveal the presence of acute or situational problems involving symptom formation, as suggested by a negative D score, elevated es, and corresponding elevations in m or Y variables, the treatment plan should be oriented toward providing symptomatic relief. In this context, the therapist may be able to utilize a short-term framework that promotes restoration of normal functioning. Supportive treatment approaches and/or relatively straightforward behavioral techniques in the course of outpatient psychotherapy are likely to be useful in this scenario.

The presence of chronic and recurrent problems, identified by a negative $Adj\ D$ score and/or a positive CDI, warrants consideration of long-term treatment involving interventions that promote broader changes in personality and functioning. The specific nature of the problem and its level of complexity further help to focus the treatment plan. For example, clients with elevated CDI scores require a treatment plan that would effectively address interpersonal conflicts and struggles, whereas clients with elevated m and Y variables require a central focus on internal processes of anxiety, worry, and helplessness. Complex reactions to problems, suggested by a high frequency of blends, warrant efforts to simplify psychological experiences by, for example, cognitive techniques of labeling and categorizing. In general, identifying problem chronicity and complexity with the Rorschach aids determination of the proposed type, intensity, and length of treatment.

The lack of social support has been associated with longer treatment duration and reduced durability of therapeutic benefits (see Chapter 3 and Beutler et al., 2000; Groth-Marnat, 1999b). Rorschach indicators of low social support offer guidelines concerning specific types of interventions to be incorporated into the treatment plan. For example, clients producing no T, a low frequency of COP, or a high HVI value are prone to interpersonal cautiousness, possibly due to experiences of being "burned" in previous relationships, and are likely to have few relational sources of support. As a result, they may have considerable difficulty developing a therapeutic alliance. These clients often require substantial time and effort in the early phases of treatment to facilitate their development of trust in the therapist and in the treatment process. They may also require repeated assurances and demonstrations of therapist reliability and support before they can engage meaningfully in the treatment process.

Such clients would benefit from an individual psychotherapy format, and the development of a trusting relationship should be regarded as a long-term goal in their treatment plans. They may eventually be transitioned into family therapy or group therapy formats that would enable them to receive broader forms of social support and be gradually encouraged to cultivate supportive relationships within their living environment. Indeed, a positive *HVI* is a contraindication for group psychotherapy and also signals that therapist expectations regarding the client's engagement in treatment should be informed by an appreciation of the client's sense of vulnerability. Group psychotherapy would also be a poor fit for clients with elevated *PER*, *AG*, *Fr+rF*, and Egocentricity Index scores, because these individuals are prone to provoke others into rejecting them or withdrawing support. These clients may benefit from social skills training, offered within an individual therapy modality, in the earlier stages of a long-term treatment. In contrast, when the Interpersonal cluster of the Rorschach Structural Summary is predominantly marked by a low *H* frequency and an elevated Isolation Index, the use of group therapy may be beneficial in helping the client to establish connections with people and thereby reduce his or her social isolation.

Evidence of marked functional impairment on the Rorschach protocol provides important guidelines for treatment planning. For example, indications of severe cognitive impairment in the Mediation and Ideation clusters, including low *X+%*, high *X–%*, high *RawSum6* and *WSum6* scores, *M–*, and high *PTI* scores, suggest that treatment approaches that rely on complex insight-oriented methods would be unproductive. Rather, a concrete, reality-testing approach should be maintained, and the treatment plan may need to incorporate adjunctive pharmacological interventions. The combined use of psychological and pharmacological treatments is also indicated for clients with severe affective disturbance (positive *S-Con*, *DEPI*, and *CDI*, high *C'*, *V*, *m*, *Y*, Shading blends, and Color-Shading blends) and functional disorganization (significantly negative *D* score). In these circumstances, hospitalization and monitoring of suicide risk are also important treatment considerations.

A Rorschach record with a low Egocentricity Index, high *MOR*, and high *V*, indicating markedly low self-esteem, also warrants ongoing examination of self-destructive potential and use of ego-supportive measures to foster a more favorable self-image. As discussed by Beutler and colleagues (2000), high levels of problem severity generally suggest the need for more restrictive forms of treatment of longer durations and a higher frequency of treatment sessions. Often the treatment will emphasize initial treatment goals of symptom reduction and stabilization and involve the use of psychiatric medications to facilitate this stabilization. In contrast, lower levels of problem severity often can be treated successfully through psychosocial interventions provided in an outpatient setting.

Rorschach indicators of coping and problem-solving style, principally involving the *EB* variable, provide useful guidance in selecting appropriate treatment interventions. In general, Introversives are likely to benefit from cognitive and analytic treatment approaches, whereas Extratensives benefit from behavioral approaches that involve hands-on tasks. Exner (1996) reported that Introversives are generally rated more favorably by therapists using psychodynamic and cognitive treatment models, and Extratensives tend to be rated more favorably by therapists using short-term directive treatment models. The *EB* style also may help identify other qualitative aspects of therapy response and guide therapist expectations. For example, Exner (1995) noted that in conditions of elevated distress, Extratensives are more likely than Introversives to internalize pain and exhibit emotional confusion. Distraught Introversives, however, are less prone to self-degradation than distraught Extratensives, despite showing higher levels of self-focus. For Ambitents, a central treatment priority should be the acquisition of a dependable and consistent coping style.

One important consideration for all *EB* styles concerns whether the client has sufficient psychological resources (i.e., *EA*) to facilitate coping, or whether these resources would need to be developed in the course of treatment. Coping styles also may be conceptualized as falling on a continuum ranging from externalizing to internalizing modes (see Chapter 3). A Rorschach record characterized by a low *Afr*, high *FC*, high Isolation Index, high Intellectualization Index, and high *C' and V* scores shows evidence of internalizing tendencies. On the other hand, an externalizing mode is suggested by elevated scores on *PER*, *AG*, *HVI*, *S*, and the Egocentricity Index. Internalizers benefit from methods that emphasize insight and self-awareness, whereas techniques of anger management, assertiveness training, social skills training, and contingency management are likely to be useful for externalizers (see Chapter 3 and Beutler et al., 2000; Groth-Marnat, 1999b). The Rorschach record also can identify whether the coping methods are defensive in nature, as suggested by a high *L*, Intellectualization Index, and *PER*; these indicators would aid formulation of treatment goals for learning and applying positive coping methods.

The development of an effective treatment plan frequently rests on obtaining an understanding of the client's potential responsiveness to various treatment interventions. Clients differ in their motivation for change, and many clients present with characteristics of resistance and avoidance that may sabotage the treatment process. Resistance to change may be inferred when clients' Rorschach data reveal anger and oppositionality (high S), strong self-involvement and corresponding disregard for others' opinions and reactions (high Egocentricity Index coupled with Reflections), or entrenched patterns of thinking and behavior (high L, high OBS, high HVI, disparate $a:p$ ratio). When there is a high level of egocentric self-focus, the client's self-image is likely not easily amenable to change. The use of confrontational techniques is likely to be unsuccessful with these clients; a nondirective treatment approach that emphasizes the attainment of personal benefit, including acceptance from others, is more likely to be productive.

When defensive and rigidly maintained patterns of intellectualization, avoidance, or hypervigilance are evident, these maneuvers should be tackled gradually, and such clients may need to learn relaxation and other anxiety-reduction techniques before they can release their grip on these defenses. Some treatment-resistant clients also may benefit from paradoxical interventions that are not likely to be experienced as ego-threatening. The treatment plan for clients with ruminative and self-critical tendencies (i.e., high V or MOR) may include use of thought-stopping and cognitive restructuring techniques. Dependent or needy clients (e.g., with high T, FM, and Fd) and highly distressed or overwhelmed individuals (i.e., with negative D $score$, high es) are more inclined to follow therapist directions and comply with treatment-related tasks. These clients are likely to benefit from structured, therapist-led activities ranging from behavioral contracting and therapeutic assignments to the provision of interpretation and advice.

A final important consideration in treatment planning concerns the level of distress experienced by clients when they present for treatment. Moderate levels of distress frequently provide crucial motivation for change, but excessive distress tends to have a disruptive or immobilizing influence. Long-term trait-like variables such as C' produce a sustained or chronic level of emotional distress that requires long-term treatment. State-anxiety variables, such as m and Y, are more amenable to change in a shorter duration. The presence of V, reflecting painful self-reviews that are not conducive to positive change, is considered an unfavorable sign for all clients and would require a treatment plan involving extensive supportive therapy. In summary, Rorschach assessment enables identification of the type and level of emotional distress, which are important issues to be considered during treatment planning.

Exner (1995) reported the results of preliminary analyses concerning the Rorschach features of patients who responded favorably to dynamic, cognitive, behavioral, short-term, and brief psychotherapies. He found, for example, that Introversives responded well to dynamic and cognitive therapies, and Extratensives showed progress in short-term and brief-therapy formats. Progress was observed for most forms of therapies when the patients' Rorschachs contained a higher right side eb (Sum Shading) than left side eb ($FM+m$), suggesting that experiences of emotional distress serve as a motivational force for change regardless of the type of treatment approach used. Similarly, a D $score$ < 0 with an Adj D ≥ 0 was related to progress for all but behavioral and brief therapies. A T > 1 score was associated with progress in dynamic, short-term, and brief therapies, suggesting that interpersonal neediness facilitates treatment progress in interpersonally centered therapies.

As might be expected, progress in cognitive therapy was achieved for patients with $RawSum6$ < 4 and M > 3, indicating that clear thinking and reasoning capacities are necessary and beneficial when using this therapy approach. Interestingly, S > 2 was associated with progress in short-term and brief therapies, suggesting that the level of autonomy associated with a moderately high S score is well-suited to these approaches. Exner also found that $Fr+rF$ > 0 and Egocentricity Index > .32 was associated with premature termination from dynamic, short-term, and cognitive therapies, as was a T = 0 score, suggesting that narcissistic self-focus and interpersonal distancing interfere with effective treatment participation. Further studies are needed to establish empirical relationships between Rorschach variables and treatment approaches, but these findings provide encouragement that the Rorschach can be usefully applied to develop effective treatment plans.

FEEDBACK CONSIDERATIONS

Conducting a Rorschach assessment for treatment planning is most effective when it is undertaken collaboratively with the client and when test feedback is provided in a manner that, in itself, constitutes a therapeutic intervention (see Chapter 12). When clients are fully involved in the testing process and have input into the uses of test findings, they are more likely to be active participants in their assessment and treatment. Additionally, clients are likely to experience symptom reduction, improved self-esteem, reduced feelings of isolation, greater hope and self-understanding, and higher motivation for treatment when they receive test feedback (Finn & Butcher, 1991). It appears that the experience of receiving test feedback is very meaningful to clients and reduces their anxiety, even when the feedback deals with negative aspects of their functioning (Finn, 1996b).

The Rorschach yields an extensive array of information that must be skillfully integrated, organized, and condensed to render it comprehensible for the client receiving the feedback. Finn (1996b) has proposed in his feedback model that this goal may be partly accomplished by developing a limited set of questions, *with the client*, to be addressed by the testing. For example, the Rorschach could be used to answer the question, "Why do I feel so overwhelmed in my day-to-day life?" A response to this issue could be based on data from the Controls and Stress Tolerance cluster, describing the imbalance between the individual's experienced stressors and his or her coping capacities, the nature and intensity of felt stressors, and/or the limited access to coping resources. Another appropriate question for Rorschach testing might be, "Why am I unable to stay in a relationship?" This issue could be addressed by using data from the Interpersonal cluster, Self Perception cluster, and Constellations to examine if the client is distrustful of others, is excessively needy, or shows other maladaptive behaviors, such as anger and self-centeredness, that disrupt relationships. Rorschach findings also can identify client strengths that may otherwise be unknown to them, such as indicating the presence of a well-developed problem-solving style, availability of psychological coping resources, effective information-processing methods, and balanced affective reactions. Test findings of client resources set a positive direction for using the client's personal assets toward developing psychotherapy goals and gauging treatment progress.

Effective test feedback should contain a limited set of core points to be discussed systematically with the client. Excessive detail should be avoided, as most individuals can meaningfully assimilate only a moderate amount of information in a single session. Examiners also should avoid the use of technical terms or psychological jargon in their communications. If a concept is not phrased in a language readily understandable by the client, it will be of little value as feedback. Beginning the feedback with positive aspects of the client's personality and functioning would likely reduce his or her apprehension about what was revealed in the testing. Lower levels of apprehensiveness, in turn, often enable the client to attend fully to the feedback and participate in a discussion about it. The central aspects of the feedback could be organized in the order indicated by the search strategy used for test interpretation. For example, when the interpretation strategy involves starting with the Self Perception cluster and proceeding to the Interpersonal, Controls, Ideation, Information Processing, Cognitive Mediation, and Affect clusters, respectively, based on a positive *MOR* variable, the prefeedback questions could be arranged to give precedence to questions related to self-concept. The feedback session should be interactive, as noted, with the clinician offering opportunities for the client to comment on each point made and to offer supporting or refuting examples.

A unique advantage associated with Rorschach testing is that the client's actual verbalizations can be used to personalize and heighten the test feedback. As discussed by Finn (1996a), the Rorschach provides a metaphorical language for the feedback communication. For example, a client who reports seeing a "black cloud, dense and weighted, ready to produce a downpour" on Card IV, and whose Rorschach indicates negative and painful affect, considerable affective constraint, and tenuous controls over affective expressions, may be told something like the following:

> "Your emotions are a source of much pain and confusion for you. You seem to be holding a lot of troubled feelings within, perhaps because you are used to doing so and haven't found good ways of releasing or expressing these emotions. These feelings are like a *black cloud* hovering over you that keeps you in a state of uneasiness. One thing that happens when feelings are held back for long periods of time is that they suddenly break through in unexpected ways, producing a *downpour* of feelings that may feel overwhelming."

During the segment of the test interpretation involving analysis of the verbalizations, the examiner should note key words or phrases to be used in this manner in the feedback session, particularly noting phrases that seem to contain projected material.

A prime consideration in providing Rorschach feedback is to link the feedback to treatment goals and plans. For example, when the test findings indicate ineffectual coping patterns, the clinician providing the feedback would discuss, with the client, the important treatment goal of developing an effective coping style, and suggest some methods that could be used to achieve this goal. When social support is found to be deficient, the client could be told that developing supportive relationships would be a focal issue in individual therapy, or that a group therapy format is recommended based on this finding. In summary, Rorschach feedback should be provided in a manner that promotes a dialogue between the examiner and the client, dispels the client's doubts and fears, engenders a sense of hope and direction, and facilitates a smooth transition to the work of psychotherapy.

CASE EXAMPLE

R.W.'s background and presenting concerns, discussed previously in this text, provide an important context for interpreting her Rorschach. Specific points to note include her symptomatic presentation of panic attacks, social anxiety, and depression. Her interpersonal history is characterized by experiences of physical and sexual abuse, feelings of maternal abandonment, perceptions of disapproval and rejection from others, and current reliance on her boyfriend as her sole social support. Her reports of "internal voices" and "three different people within [her]" are also noteworthy. Behaviorally, her history is marked by alternating patterns of social isolation and acting out, the latter expressed through episodes of sexual acting out and substance abuse.

This Rorschach protocol is deemed valid and interpretable because R.W. produced 18 responses (note that R.W.'s complete Rorschach responses and summary of coded responses are included in Appendix A). Her L score of .80 is also within acceptable limits, reflecting adequate responsiveness to the stimulus blots. The absence of S responses to the first blot suggests the absence of a negative or oppositional set at the onset of the Rorschach administration. Together with the presence of multiple determinants and special scores, these findings indicate that she was actively engaged by the Rorschach task. A review of key variables in this client's Structural Summary identifies her $PTI > 3$ score as the dominant variable, resulting in the following search strategy for examining the clusters: Ideation, Cognitive Mediation, Information Processing, Controls, Affect, Self Perception, and Interpersonal Perception. This sequence indicates that cognitive disruption and perceptual distortions represent the most critical aspect of her test profile.

R.W.'s Rorschach protocol shows evidence of severe impairment in thinking, marked by incoherent, illogical, and peculiar thoughts (*RawSum6*, *WSum6*, *M*–). Her ideas are poorly differentiated and frequently synthesized in a manner that is not reality-bound (*INCOM*, *FABCOM*). Specific examples of these processes are seen in the content of responses 14 (butterfly with cat whiskers), 15 (girls with monkey mouths), and 16 (whales with bird beaks and mouse tails) where various percepts are randomly combined, producing a confused report of unrealistic images. Moreover, an examination of the Sequence of Scores shows poor cognitive control at the onset of the task, revealed by a minus Form Quality and *INCOM2* Special Score on the first response. The progressive deterioration across her responses is indicated by an increased frequency of multiple Special Scores and numerous minus Form Quality scores. She does not "recover" effectively from these losses of cognitive control; in response to Card IX she produces a minus Form Quality, and a blend with unusual Form Quality follows for Card X. In addition to evidence of pervasive cognitive disturbance (Ideation cluster), R.W.'s thinking is likely to be particularly primitive and/or distorted in the interpersonal context (*M*– on Cards II and VII). She is prone to engaging in passive fantasy as a substitute for facing unpleasant realities (*Ma:Mp*), and this fantasy life may include magical thinking or even active delusions. Because of her stylistic tendency to rely on thinking to guide problem-solving and decision-making efforts (*EB* Introversive), her thought disturbance is very likely to impair her decisions significantly. The magnitude of her disorganized thinking, indicating serious psychopathology, will likely produce very poor and inconsistent judgments and significantly compromise her adaptation. From a diagnostic perspective, the presence of a psychotic disorder should be considered.

Further evidence of problems with reality testing is seen in the Mediation cluster, which shows that R.W. distorts reality to a significant degree ($X+\%$, $X-\%$ $WDA\%$, $XA\%$), despite her capacity to recognize more obvious or commonly perceived aspects of reality (P). She is prone to misperceive events, misinterpret people's actions, and form erroneous conclusions about her life experiences. These misconstructions occur despite considerable efforts to collect and organize information in complex ways (Zf and $W{:}M$ in the Processing cluster), the relatively sophisticated quality of her information-processing methods ($DQ+$ and DQv), and her tendency to try to respond to the entire stimulus (W responses shown in the Summary of Approach pattern). In light of her disrupted cognitive functioning, however, R.W.'s aspirations are unrealistically high. She is expending excessive time and energy in information-processing efforts that are ineffective and exceed her available resources ($W{:}M$).

The breadth of R.W.'s distortions and her basic confusion of reality with fantasy will likely produce chronic and wide-ranging adjustment difficulties in her life. Impaired reality testing of the magnitude seen in her Rorschach can be functionally disabling, and people with this degree of impairment are often unable to manage basic aspects of daily living, such as employment or child-care responsibilities, without assistance. Based on the data interpreted thus far, it is reasonable to conclude that R.W.'s difficulties are severe and are likely to produce considerable functional impairment.

R.W. has relatively limited coping resources available to her for contending with the psychological and practical demands of daily living (EA), and her affective resources seem to be especially impoverished ($WSumC$). However, her current psychological stressors are being held at a manageable level (es), and she is maintaining an apparently stable psychological balance by keeping disturbing thoughts and feelings out of her conscious awareness (D score, m, C', T, Y). She may give the appearance of being able to manage stressors and be relatively free from disabling levels of anxiety and tension (D score, $Adj\ D$ score). People with her Rorschach scores typically lead restricted lives that are limited to routine and nontaxing activities, and they stay within familiar environments and confine their interactions to familiar people. Within these carefully delineated conditions, they see little need to change and are unlikely voluntarily to seek psychological help. When stress levels rise to even average levels, however, their functioning becomes easily distressed and disorganized. In the context of her history and presenting problems, R.W.'s Controls/Stress Tolerance cluster scores suggest that she has established a degree of psychological equilibrium, possibly due to her 1 year of psychotherapy, but also due to defensive maneuvers that include affective and social restriction (Afr). Nonetheless, as discussed earlier, significant lapses in control are occurring that manifest primarily in the disorganization of her thought processes. In the affective domain, a salient Rorschach finding concerns the magnitude of her withdrawal from affectively toned situations, which borders on affective aversion and avoidance (*Afr*). This withdrawal is exemplified in her verbal response to Card IX, where she comments during the inquiry, "*You can't show feelings because someone could see . . . I don't feel emotions and don't feel that I should try to.*" Although there are no apparent indications of significant depression, she shows self-critical attitudes that are likely to generate emotional pain and serve as a precursor to depressive experiences (*V*).

Data from the Self Perception cluster indicate that R.W. displays an average degree of self-focus but is attentive to negative aspects of herself to a degree that reflects pessimistic thinking (*MOR*). She shows some introspective inclinations (*FD*) that are, however, slanted toward a critical self-evaluation and ruminations about her undesirable qualities (*V*) and are likely associated with poor self-regard and a sense of failure. Her self-concept is largely based on imagined or fantasized features that are not well integrated into a holistic image of self (*H: [H]+Hd+[Hd]*) and that likely result in an unclear and diffused identity. R.W.'s protocol also reveals unusual preoccupations with anatomical features and bodily functioning (*An+Xy*) that suggest a sense of fragility, embellished by verbal responses that imply feeling exposed (response 17: " . . . *you can see all his insides* . . . "). Additionally, she is preoccupied with sexual matters (*Sx*), and the content of her responses (e.g., "*a vagina that has blood coming out of it,*" "*dicks,*" "*he grabs the penis,*" "*connected at the butt*") suggest negative sexual imagery, sexual hostility, and masochism. Although interpretive inferences based on sexual content on the Rorschach should be carefully limited, the historical information concerning R.W.'s promiscuity and history of sexual abuse provides a reasonable context in which to understand these responses.

In the Interpersonal domain, R.W.'s protocol suggests a limited capacity for developing close attachments to other people (*T*, *COP*, Pure *H*). This finding may be related to her disrupted family history and reports of abandonment by her mother, abuse by her stepfather, and censure from others in her social environment. She does not appear to expect comfort or nurturance from others (*T*) and is generally uneasy when dealing with people. She has a reasonable amount of interest in people (Sum *H*) but does not have a realistic understanding of them (*H:[H]+Hd+[Hd]*). She is inclined to view others in distorted and somewhat dehumanized ways (e.g., percepts of android, wolf people, girls with monkey mouths). In particular, response 3 to Card II suggests a perception of men as difficult to see and understand ("*most of his face is covered with hair*") and as aggressive and taunting "wolves." Although interpersonal relationships may not be completely avoided, she is prone to detached and distant styles of relating within this domain (*T*). R.W. appears to view relationships as being more combative than cooperative (*AG* vs. *COP*), which likely contributes to her fear of social situations, and she seems to lack the requisite elements for developing healthy and mature relationships (*GHR:PHR*).

In summary, this Rorschach protocol reveals the presence of considerable psychopathology involving a seriously impaired capacity for coherent and reality-based thinking and tenuously held control and coping capacity. She displays affective constriction and avoidance, an inadequately developed and poorly organized self-concept, and extensive disturbances in interpersonal functioning marked by distorted views of people and self-protective detachment. From a diagnostic perspective, the possibility of a schizophreniform disorder or emerging schizophrenia is strongly suggested, although bipolar disorder should be ruled out in light of her report of emotional highs and lows, depressive episodes, and episodes of acting out. A secondary diagnosis of social phobia is also indicated by her history and test results. The prognosis for benefiting from psychotherapy is guarded. Positive features of R.W.'s personality and functioning, seen in her Rorschach protocol, include her capacity for control, her interest in people, her introspective disposition, and her extensive efforts to integrate and make sense of the information she encounters. The absence of prominent self-destructive features (*S-CON*) is also a favorable finding but should not be used to rule out possible suicidal actions in the present or future.

With reference to treatment planning, it should be recognized that R.W.'s symptoms and problems are severe and complex. These problems extend across multiple facets of functioning and include her reports of auditory hallucinations. Her history also indicates that her problems are chronic and recurrent, beginning during her teenage years and involving progressive deterioration in functioning by early adulthood. She has a notable lack of social support, having insulated herself from social contact, except for her dependence on her boyfriend. R.W.'s cognitively based problem-solving style is significantly compromised by her disordered thinking, and her current coping methods are fundamentally defensive in nature. The overall level of functional impairment is substantial.

These findings suggest a need for long-term psychological treatment involving ego-supportive and skill-development methods, combined with the probable use of antipsychotic medication. R.W.'s treatment plan should incorporate methods that furnish structure, support, and active assistance in dealing with existing symptoms and new problems that may arise. Treatment planning also should provide for the possible need for crisis intervention or brief inpatient services. It should be noted that R.W.'s Rorschach indicates a relatively low level of current distress that may provide insufficient motivation for treatment-related change. Furthermore, her affective constriction and interpersonal cautiousness suggest that treatment resistance is likely to take the form of withdrawal, and trust and openness within the therapy relationship will be slow to develop. These features underscore the importance of a consistent, predictable, and nurturing therapist–client relationship and give further support for the need for long-term individual psychotherapy.

SUMMARY

The Rorschach inkblot test, originally developed by Hermann Rorschach in 1921, has had a long and controversial history, with professional opinions ranging from strong espousal of its merits to vehement denouncement of its validity and utility as a measure of personality. It has, however, enjoyed the status of being the second most widely researched personality test, and has experienced new vitality with the development and ongoing improvement of Exner's Comprehensive System. The current (2001) norms for the test, based on refinement of the original CS adult normative data, provide a reference point for standardized interpretation of Rorschach protocols, and the development of new, contemporary norms is currently in progress.

Rorschach interpretation using the CS emphasizes the structure of personality and involves examination of a series of variable clusters related to capacity for control and stress tolerance, situational stress, affect, information processing, cognitive mediation, ideation, self perception, and interpersonal perception. The structural summary interpretation is augmented with an analysis of sequences of scores and content of the verbalizations. Rorschach structural data may be alternatively organized, using the STS model, to address issues of problem complexity and chronicity, access to social support, degree of functional impairment, coping style, resistance traits, and level of distress, in order to facilitate effective treatment planning. The latter method is demonstrated in this chapter with use of a case example.

10

Integrative Personality Assessment in Special Settings

Ronald A. Stolberg, Bruce Bongar, and Gary Groth-Marnat

As described in Chapter 1, psychological assessment addresses questions that pertain to six clinically relevant domains of behavior. Since the demands and responses to consultation vary from one type of setting to another, it is important to consider these questions within the context of the setting from which they arise. To answer referral questions, it is necessary to distinguish between normal or usual behavior and abnormal or pathological behavior. Conducting an evaluation into such matters is a difficult task under the best of circumstances, but for the professional asked to make these assessments in a variety of special settings, additional factors must be taken into account. The purpose of this chapter is to highlight some of the particular demands of forensic, psychiatric, general medical, vocational, psychological clinic, as well as a variety of other specific settings where personality assessment has become an integral part of an individual's treatment and future.

When a referral for personality assessment is received, the practitioner should immediately seek to clarify how the referral decision was reached, why the consultation is being sought, and what is expected to happen as a result of the findings. Often the referral is the result of a perceived discrepancy between the referred patient's behaviors, attitudes, or interpersonal interactions in some situation or environment and some more optimal level of functioning desired and defined by the referral source. The discrepancy may result from a conflict between one or more perspectives that conceptually define acceptable and unacceptable behavior (Knoff, 1986).

WORKING IN SPECIAL SETTINGS

Psychologists conducting personality assessment in any setting are repeatedly asked to exercise their professional judgment in response to the sometimes problematic behavior of their patients, and in the best interest of those patients. They accept the responsibility for delivering recommendations that will affect the lives of their patients as well as patients' families (Bennett, Bryant, VandenBos, & Greenwood, 1990).

In order to accomplish these tasks effectively, the practitioner must learn to listen, analyze, and speak with exceptional skill and sensitivity, and to do so in an environment that often is permeated with conflict, misunderstanding, and error. In that direction, Bennett and his colleagues (1990) proposed that psychologists must make decisions based on three distinct considerations:

1. The practitioner's primary humanitarian mission, which is to bring all of his or her training, skill, judgment, and commitment to the treatment of the patient.
2. The practitioner's personal ethics and the ethical principles for psychologists that he or she is obliged, by legal and professional codes, to maintain.
3. The practitioner's professional and legal liability for the nature and quality of care delivery, which represents the practitioner's point of exposure to civil lawsuits and to the requirements of laws regulating conduct as a licensed professional.

The relationship among these considerations for professional practice is complex, especially as the psychologist shifts roles from one setting to another. However, inseparable from all decisions must be the primary ethical principle guiding the conduct of the clinician: the practitioner's duty to the patient. The ethical commitment to duty and justice remains a guiding force even when the client is not the patient, as when the psychologist is an agent of the court or a consultant to an agency. Because roles differ, however, the balancing act among these principles frequently becomes very complex. The reality of practicing as a psychologist is that this balancing act is not always successful (Bennett et al., 1990). Inevitably, there will be times when a patient, a client-agency, or a patient's family is not satisfied with the results of an evaluation or of the ensuing recommendations. In such instances, prudent practitioners can be consoled by the knowledge that they acted within a prescribed set of guidelines, determined both by their codes of ethics and by established or accepted standards of good practice. Within the application of these guidelines, psychologists must endeavor to ensure reliable and valid applications of their assessment instruments, and to act in the best interests of the patient. This duty to the good of the patient is paramount even when the patient is not the psychologist's client and when this patient's good contrasts with the wishes of the client.

It is important to remember that each setting is governed by a particular set of procedures, expectations, laws, regulations, and acceptable practices, be it a hospital, a local, state, or federal facility, the criminal justice system, a school, a business, or any other facility wherein personality assessment is conducted. Thus it is essential that practitioners become familiar with the structure and procedures of the institutions that request their services so that they can provide efficient, effective service within these distinctive environments.

Forensic Assessment

Forensic psychology can generally be defined as addressing the interplay of law and psychology. This hybrid field covers a wide range of problems seen in both civil and criminal courts and involves such diverse topics as jury selection, evaluation of rehabilitation programs, evaluation of defendants to determine their competency to stand trial, making recommendations for or against the reunification of families and neglected or abused children, and so on (Blau, 1998; Maloney, 1985; Otto & Heilbrun, 2002). The role played by forensic psychologists in the definition, assessment, and reporting of forensic conditions is often ambiguous and controversial. Although the court ultimately determines whether a defendant is legally competent and responsible for his or her own behavior, the psychologist must provide the court with the information required for such a decision (Blau, 1998; Grisso, 2002; Woody, 1980). This information is drawn from the assessment process and relies on the validity of the assessment techniques selected and employed by the psychologist.

Expert Testimony

When psychologists and other mental health professionals are used as "expert witnesses," they conduct evaluations for use in civil and criminal legal proceedings (Blau, 1998; Heilbrun, 2001; Melton, Petrila, Poythress, & Slobogin, 1997). *Expert* witnesses differ from what are called *percipient* witnesses, who are assumed to have direct knowledge about the facts—

what happened, when, where, and so on. They are allowed to report these facts but cannot add their interpretations. Experts, in contrast, provide opinions and interpretations, based on certain assumptions about the "facts." Experts cannot testify directly to the facts of a case, but they can provide probable meanings in those matters that pertain to their field of expertise.

Experts may be called by either the defense or prosecution (in criminal cases) or by plaintiffs and defendants (in civil cases). Thus attorneys may "shop" for experts who will present the most favorable case. In some jurisdictions, however, experts may be appointed directly by the court (i.e., the judge) as "friends of the court," as a way of reducing the problems of multiple and contradictory expert witnesses. Experts may also be called to provide testimony in various kinds of cases. The following paragraphs review some of the peculiarities of these different demands.

Civil and Criminal Jurisdictions

Civil and criminal law pertain to different types of jurisdictions and sentences. Civil sentences typically involve distribution of money (e.g., personal injury or liability), responsibility (e.g., child custody), or property (e.g., divorce), whereas the outcomes of criminal proceedings involve *sentences* that impose fines, restriction of freedom (e.g., prison, probation, or parole), and even termination of life. Among the most common referrals for assessment in the forensic context are those designed to determine an individual's competence to stand trial, the harmfulness of various acts, and the assignment of criminal responsibility. In this context, "competence to stand trial" refers to the defendant's current ability to care for or control his- or herself, to understand legal proceedings, and to assist his or her lawyer in planning and conducting a defense. Questions of competence arise in both civil and criminal actions.

In the civil arena, expert testimony regarding competence may be involved in answering questions about "grave disability," child custody, personal injury litigation, and "dangerousness." Thus civil commitment to a mental hospital, the appointment of a caretaker to help manage an individual's resources (i.e., a fiduciary), apportionment of money based on the amount of psychic harm incurred by an act, and assignment of a parent or guardian to a dependent child or gravely disabled adult are all possible consequences of the psychologist's expert testimony.

In criminal matters, the major questions addressed revolve around determining the defendant's motive for a criminal act (e.g., self-defense), assigning criminal responsibility (also called *insanity*), and determining mitigating factors related to sentencing. These questions address the defendant's mental state prior to, or at the time of, the alleged offense (Borum &

Grisso, 1995), or even at the time of the trial or subsequent sentencing. In making these determinations, it is important to note that the standards of proof (i.e., the criteria by which guilt is judged) typically differ in criminal and civilian actions. In criminal court the standard required for conviction is generally the presence of evidence sufficient to judge guilt *beyond a reasonable doubt*. This means that, in a criminal court, a person cannot be convicted of a crime unless the judge or jury is convinced of the defendant's guilt with 95% certainty. This criteria requires that the decision, therefore, must be unanimously held among the jurors. If there is more uncertainty than this about the defendant's guilt, based on the evidence presented, no conviction can take place.

In many civil suits, such as personal injury claims, where the findings of the court determine liability and restitution, the standard by which guilt is judged is more lenient and is much easier to meet. In a civil suit, only a *preponderance of the evidence* (i.e., more than 50%) must point to the guilt of the accused. This standard requires that a judge or jury weigh the evidence presented by both disputing parties to see which side is more believable. In some courts, a third standard, that of "clear and convincing evidence," is required. This standard mandates that 67–75% of the evidence (depending on the laws of a particular jurisdiction) favors guilt. In both the cases (i.e., "a preponderance of the evidence" and "clear and convincing evidence") unanimous verdict is not always necessary. Sometimes a simple (or substantive) majority opinion among the jurors suffices.

In a related fashion, the "burden of proof" also varies among different jurisdictions. That is, the law of a jurisdiction defines which side of a dispute bears the responsibility for "proving" a point. If the evidence for and against guilt is found to be less than the standard of proof set by the jurisdiction, then the party that bears the burden of proof cannot win. Whereas in criminal action, the prosecution bears the burden of proving guilt (an accused person is guilty until proven innocent), in many criminal and civilian matters, particular judgments may shift to become the burden of the defense. For example, in some states and jurisdictions, the defendant who invokes a plea of "not guilty by reason of insanity" has the responsibility for presenting evidence that "proves" (by whatever standard is applied) that the accused is "insane." In other words, in this peculiar situation, the defendant must prove him- or herself innocent (not guilty by reason of insanity). In other jurisdictions, when such a plea is entered, it is the prosecution that carries the burden of offering proof that the accused is "sane." The variation in standards of proof and the assigned burden of proof, from court to court and state to state, requires practitioners to seek information about the specifics they will encounter before they enter the courtroom. Typically, the practitioner becomes familiar with the law by talking, at length, with the attorney whose side has requested his or her services as an expert.

Phases of the Legal Procedure

Psychologists may be asked to consult during jury selection and discovery processes as well as during evidentiary hearings. During the investigation or "discovery" phase of a court proceeding, psychologists might assist in determining the quality of a witness's testimony or the quality and accuracy of a practitioner's evaluation and treatment in previous testimony. An attorney might wish a psychologist to evaluate the extent to which a client has been injured (i.e., presence of posttraumatic stress disorder or extent of cognitive deficit following a head injury) or a client's competency to stand trial. A penal officer or judge might request a psychological evaluation to assist with sentencing or treatment planning. While in prison, a client might be assessed to determine his or her level of depression or need for special case management (i.e., danger to other inmates).

Each phase of the legal procedure may require attention to different questions and, correspondingly, may require adjustments in assessment and reporting procedures. For the needs of some phases of the proceedings, such as during jury selection, written reports are not usually used. Brief, verbal reports, heavy with conclusions, are required, whereas during discovery and evidentiary periods, one may gather extensive material and develop lengthy written opinions.

The audience to whom the psychologist addresses his or her opinions differs as a function of the phase of the legal procedure. During jury selection, the psychologist's audience is only the attorneys who are relying on psychological opinion to make decisions. During later phases, the psychologist's audience is the judge and jury, for whom extensive written reports are often necessary. These reports must be adjusted to the length and language of those who will be utilizing them in the legal process.

Standards of Practice

Expert witnesses base their opinions either on the knowledge of their field or on direct examination of other witnesses, the accused, or the plaintiff. Forensic evaluations to develop an opinion about an accused person, for example, are requested by attorneys and judges in both civil and criminal courts. However, there are few consensually accepted standards of practice that can guide the clinician in performing these assessments (see Borum & Grisso, 1995; Essig, Mittenberg, Peterson, Strauman, & Cooper, 2001; Melton et al., 1997). One of the most difficult problems facing clinicians who practice forensic psychology is that this work requires the combination of two complex and distinct types of professional activities. For instance, on one hand, clinicians must be knowledgeable about a complex and often contradictory set of laws that govern municipal, state, and federal court systems. Even within a given jurisdiction, complex legal codes may be interpreted differently (Heilbrun, 2001; Robbins, Waters, & Herbert, 1997). Indeed, it is almost impossible to find a specific definition of such things as "criminal responsibility" or "dangerousness" that would satisfy all the parties in a legal matter or that would translate across jurisdictions.

On the other hand, psychologists must be familiar with the strengths and shortcomings of a variety of psychological tests in relation to the specific requirements of the legal system—no easy task, given that there is considerable controversy in the field of forensic assessment regarding the appropriate manner and extent to which psychological tests should be used (Blau, 1998; Fowler & Matarazzo, 1988; Heilbrun, 2001; Ziskin, 1995). For example, Matarazzo (1990) has strongly supported the use of psychological assessment procedures and devices in the courtroom, whereas Ziskin (1995) has expressed doubts about whether any such instruments can be used validly in these settings (Borum & Grisso, 1995). Although many psychologists have identified the potential for misuse and abuse of psychological test data in forensic settings (Podboy & Kastl, 1993; Wakefield & Underwager, 1993), these controversies rage in the relative absence of empirical evidence on the subject (Heilbrun, 1992, 2001).

Numerous studies have examined patterns of test use in forensic settings. These include tests used for (1) general forensic evaluations (Holub, 1992), (2) assessment of child custody (Keilin & Bloom, 1986), (3) criminal evaluations (Lees-Haley, 1992; Rogers & Cavanaugh, 1983), (4) assessment of competence to stand trial (Borum & Grisso, 1995), and (5) forensic neuropsychology (Essig et al., 2001). The results of these surveys have established a baseline of use of specific assessment instruments across a number of settings and for a variety of uses. As described elsewhere in this chapter, a clinician using any instrument in a setting for which it was not normed, standardized, or intended, needs to examine existing literature and consult with colleagues to determine its usefulness. These studies provide valuable information about many of the most popular forensic instruments and their uses.

One important controversy involves the question of who should be considered an expert witness in matters of behavioral performance. Traditionally the courts have accepted physicians as expert witnesses in mental health matters, often without regard to whether or not they have had psychiatric training (Melton et al., 1997). Psychiatric social workers are often accepted in court as experts in juvenile and family matters, and marriage and family therapists are accepted for domestic disputes. So, just who is an expert? Historically, that question has been answered by examining educational credentials, particularly with respect to profession and specialty (Melton et al., 1997; Otto & Heilbrun, 2002). But does the possession of educational credentials qualify every psychologist to present his or her assessment data and findings as an expert witness? Currently, in most courts, yes. However, we would encourage clinicians from any discipline who testify as experts in court to examine not only their degree but their level of knowledge about the specific forensic matter to which they are testifying. Training as a mental health clinician, by itself, is insufficient to guarantee a specialized knowledge of forensic mental health (Melton et al., 1997; Otto & Heilbrun, 2002). Ideally, those clinicians who participate in forensic work would seek out consultation from other experts and obtain advanced training in various areas of forensic practice, earning certificates of completion and competence in these types of advanced work. They should also show evidence that they read appropriate journals in the field, and when possible, that they seek peer reviewed membership in associations promoting and protecting the science of their given specialty.

Important criteria to which clinicians must adhere when presenting psychological assessment material in legal settings are commonly known as the *Frye* and *Daubert* rules. Until 1993, the dominant method of evaluating the expertise of those who offer clinical testimony in federal court and many state courts was the *Frye* rule, named after the 1923 case *Frye v. The United States*. That decision held that scientific evidence must be sufficiently established to have gained general acceptance in the particular field to which it belongs (Melton et al., 1997; see also Otto & Heilbrun, 2002) in order to be admissible. That is, evidence was judged on the basis of its popularity or common acceptance among those within a given field. However, the *Frye* rule tended to exclude some reliable but new evidence and even some sciences whose members could not achieve a common perspective. Facts that were not yet widely accepted or known were not admissible. At the same time, the court accepted into evidence the validity of some unvalidated and even harmful practices simply because these practices were popular or common. Obviously problems arose from this definition. In 1993 the U.S. Supreme Court ruled, in *Daubert v. Merrell Dow Pharmaceuticals*, that expert opinions must be based on an inference or assertion derived by the scientific method and whether the reasoning or methodology underlying the testimony is scientifically valid and whether that reasoning or methodology can properly be applied to the facts at issue (Melton et al., 1997).

In their writings the justices offered criteria to use in forming such opinions, including the "testability" of the theoretical basis for the opinion and the error rate associated with the methods used. The justices statement is that the focus must be solely on the principles and methodology, not on the conclusions that they generate (Melton et al., 1997). When presenting assessment evidence and conclusions in court, the clinician's duty is to be able, when asked, to inform the court about the methodology, error rate, and scientific conclusions as garnered from the evidence. Thus the *Daubert* ruling meant that scientific evidence and methods replaced clinical opinions or informed hunches as the basis for determining the value of expert testimony. This criterion places added responsibility on clinicians who testify in court to select instruments whose validity is already accepted or easily defended from a scientific perspective. However, it is important to remember that not every state has accepted or applies the *Frye* and *Daubert* rules in the same way; some jurisdictions have developed their own ways of defining what and how scientific evidence is admissible. Psychologists must be careful to learn the rules that are practiced within the state or jurisdiction in which they testify.

In the face of the *Frye* and *Daubert* rules for the introduction of psychological assessment data, there has been a movement toward developing specialized forensic assessment instruments (Heilbrun, 2001). Many of these, however, have questionable psychometric properties. Among the interview schedules, surveys, and tests, the examiner will find instruments that pertain to specific legal issues. Topics include competence to waive *Miranda*; competence to stand trial; legal insanity; child custody/parental fitness; guardianship/conservatorship; and competence for medical treatment decision making. (See Table 10.1 for a list of popular assessment instruments by specialty.) These tests seek to address narrow and specific questions with reliable face valid questions and answers. Clinicians conducting forensic assessments will likely need to become familiar with new instruments as they become available.

Correctional Settings

There are now well over one million people incarcerated in state and federal prisons in the United States. Although a slew of new prisons have been built and expanded, overcrowding has become such a problem that some offenders are released before their sentences are complete, simply to make room for new offenders (Megargee, 1995).

Toward resolving this problem, personality assessment can provide an important tool for addressing the overcrowding. The National Advisory Commission on Criminal Justice Standards and Goals (NACJSAG) stated that "a good classification system . . . enables a correctional agency to utilize its limited manpower to maximize its impact on offenders . . . through a grouping process based on needs and problems . . . administrators [can] . . . make more efficient use of limited resources and avoid providing resources for offenders who do not require them" (NACJSAG, 1973, p. 201). Although the NACJSAG states that classification should be based on the assessment of individual offenders' needs and problems, the present system still relies primarily on age and gender as primary classification and placement determinants (Megargee, 1995).

As is the case in all "special settings," personality assessment techniques used in correctional settings need to be evaluated for their reliability and validity within this highly specific population and context. The courts

TABLE 10.1. Popular Personality Assessment Instruments
by Setting and Purpose

Forensic/correctional instruments for malingering

Test of Memory Malingering (TOMM)
Structured Interview of Reported Symptoms (SIRS)
Validity Indicator Profile (VIP)
Minnesota Multiphasic Personality Inventory—2 (MMPI-2)

Forensic/correctional instruments for competency

Revised Competency Assessment Instrument (RCAI)
MacArthur Competency Assessment Tool—Criminal Adjudication (MCAC-CA)

Forensic/correctional instruments for risk assessment

Hare Psychopathy Checklist—Revised (PCL-R)
Violence Risk Appraisal Guide (VRAG)
Historical Clinical Risk (HCR-20)
MMPI-2 and the MMPI-2 Criminal Justice and Correctional Report

Hospital and health settings

MMPI-2 and the MMPI-A Alcohol and Drug Treatment Report
Millon Clinical Multiaxial Inventory–III (MCMI-III)
Millon Behavioral Health Inventory (MBHI)
Battery for Health Improvement–2 (BBI-2)
Substance Abuse Subtle Screening Inventory (SASSI-3)
State–Trait Anger Expression Inventory–2 (STAXI-2)

Career counseling

16 PF Fifth Edition
Campbell Interest and Skills Survey (CISS)
Career Thoughts Inventory (CTI)
Occupational Stress Inventory—Revised (OSI-R)
Vocational Preference Inventory (VPI)

place a high level of importance on assessment in correctional settings, as it relates to the management and treatment of offenders. Clements (1982) noted, "Inadequacies in the classification process have been major contributing factors to the finding of unconstitutional prison conditions" (p. 37).

Psychiatric Settings

Traditionally, psychiatric settings have been the major ones in which clinical psychologists function. In these settings, those professionals who request psychological consultation occupy two somewhat different roles. These roles include administrator and treatment manager. Each role embodies different issues and therefore requires different types of information in order to be effective. In their role as an administrator, referring professionals are mainly concerned with decisions related to case management. They may make decisions that address suicide potential, danger to others, determining the importance of inpatient treatment, judging the ability of the patient to function independently, selecting methods of therapy, or selecting the type of ward to which a patient should be admitted. Since these questions often relate to the safety of society or custody decisions regarding the patient, the administrator needs to consider a number of legal ramifications. Ultimately, the administrator will be the primary person having responsibility for these decisions. Thus he or she will depend on information from a wide variety of sources to help make these decisions, of which the consulting psychologist will typically be an important one.

In contrast, a mental health practitioner who is administering medication or conducting psychotherapy with a patient will have a number of issues that are different from those of the administrator. Knowing a client's diagnosis and level of impairment might be particularly important for planning his or her medical treatment. At the same time, knowing patient personality characteristics as well as such particulars as the level of insight of which the patient is capable, the likelihood of acting out, and the level of expected resistance might be essential for selecting the format of, and managing, the psychotherapy relationship. This information can generate guidelines on the type of treatment that is likely to be most beneficial as well as provide a "road map" of the types of challenges that might occur during the course of therapy. Prognostic information might be especially relevant for the treating practitioner.

Two noteworthy areas of concern might be present in these roles. First, the nonpsychologist clinician may be functioning in both roles at once: as a ward administrator for patients and as their treating practitioner. One result of these multiple roles is that patients may come to feel that they cannot disclose information freely to the clinician for fear that the information might be "used against them" via administrative priorities (i.e., to extend their hospital stay longer than they wish) rather than treatment priorities. Thus the consultation for "assessment" might be most useful if it highlights this conflict and suggests ways in which such boundary issues might be handled.

A second potential concern arises when a patient is referred for assessment in the middle of therapy. This referral may be occasioned by the presence of difficulties in the therapeutic relationship, such as unrealistic expectations by the therapist, competition between treating practitioners, or anxiety in the psychiatrist about working with "this type" of client. In either of these two types of cases, merely identifying and elaborating on various personality features of the client will not be particularly useful. Instead, identifying and specifying the dynamics of these larger contextual and relational issues will be a more productive approach to the situation.

It is important for psychological consultants, in responding to all of these requests, to approach their task in a way that bridges different conceptual ways of understanding the patient. Psychiatrists and other medical practitioners are likely to take a much stronger biological position, with a resulting higher use of medication and other biologically based treatments (such as electroconvulsive therapy) than that preferred by nonmedical practitioners. Consulting psychologists, in contrast, are far more likely to focus on psychosocial aspects of the client than on biological ones. An important strategy in working with these conceptual differences between the referrant and the consultant is to understand the practical considerations that the referring psychiatrist might be facing, such as the level of danger and risk posed to self or others or the need to broaden the number of options available for making treatment decisions.

General Medical Settings

The various fields of medicine have become increasingly aware of the psychosocial components of illness (Pruit, Klapow, Epping-Jordan, & Dresselhaus, 1999). In some cases a physician who refers a patient to a psychologist might be interested in determining possible psychosocial complications of a clearly diagnosed medical condition. In other situations, a physician might refer a patient who presents with a confusing array of symptoms that are suspected to be solely or partially the result of psychosocial factors. These scenarios are consistent with the repeated finding that approximately two-thirds of patients who seek services in general medical settings are experiencing primarily psychosocial difficulties (Asaad, 2000; Katon & Walker, 1998; McLeod, Budd, & McClelland, 1997; Mostofsky & Barlow, 2000). Despite these statistics, psychosocial difficulties are typically not diagnosed accurately and, even if diagnosed, patients are often not referred for treatment to mental health professionals ("Introduction," 1999; Mostofsky & Barlow, 2000).

The roles played by psychologists in medical settings are varied and multiple. For example, a professional psychologist may be asked to serve as a consultant to one or more physicians in order to assist them in improving their sensitivity to psychiatric problems. This assistance might involve training the physician in interviewing techniques and the use of screening instruments or more in-depth formal assessment measures. Psychologists often can provide important perspectives on how to determine whether a patient has a true medical condition or a psychosocial problem that is being expressed through somatic features. There are many cases, for example, in which medical and psychological symptoms are intertwined. Patients with panic disorder, for example, typically present with dizziness, numbness, disorientation, and heart palpitations. These can, and typically are, confused with neurological or cardiac conditions. Another patient might be having seizures with no known organic basis. Personality assessment helps refine and clarify the cause and contributors to the patient's symptoms, thereby clarifying the actual diagnosis. The result can be the development of appropriate treatment plans for the patient, which in turn, result in an improved quality of life. Detecting, referring, and effectively treating such "somatizing" patients has been demonstrated to result in significant cost savings to the health care system (Chiles, Lambert, & Hatch, 1999; Cummings, 1999; Groth-Marnat & Edkins, 1996; Sobel, 2000).

Even patients with known medical conditions frequently need to be assessed to determine the presence of complicating psychosocial factors. For example, most chronic pain patients report significant levels of depression (Gatchel & Weisberg, 2000). Assessing the extent and nature of this depression can be crucial in treatment planning, since the depression and pain exacerbate one another. Relevant assessment might include a determination of (1) the severity or frequency of catastrophizing cognitions, (2) the level of emotional vulnerability, (3) the presence of positive emotions, (4) the degree to which the patient is invested in a purely physical explanation for his or her pain, and (5) the degree to which the patient may be receptive and responsive to psychosocial intervention.

There are multitudes of brief screening instruments appropriate for use in general medical contexts to deal with situations like those described (see Maruish, 2000). Frequently used measures are the General Health Questionnaire (Goldberg, 1972) Symptom Checklist-90-R (SCL-90-R; Derogatis, 1994), and the Beck Depression Inventory (Beck, Steer, & Brown, 1996). Physicians also may want to conduct structured interviews using an instrument such as the Primary Care Evaluation of Mental Disorders (Spitzer et al., 1994; PRIME-MD) that involves a brief series of questions (average 8.4 minutes), the answers to which enable the physician to make common DSM-IV diagnoses. Alternatively, a semistructured procedure, such as the Systematic Treatment Selection Clinician Rating Form described in Chapter 3 (STS-CRF; Fisher, Beutler, & Williams, 1999a), may be used. This instrument provides information on severity and impairment and identifies the patient's status in relation to the treatment planning dimensions described in Chapter 1.

Assessing various lifestyle factors in cardiovascular illness also might be important in designing a treatment plan. Such a plan might involve adherence to an exercise routine, dietary changes, smoking cessation, as well as modification of personality styles that might exacerbate the illness. A variety of instruments are available (Maruish, 2000), such as the Millon Behavioral Health Inventory (Bockian, Meagher, & Millon, 2000; Millon, Green, & Meagher, 1982) and the Sickness Impact Profile (Bergner, Bobbitt, Carter, & Gilson, 1981).

Bennett and colleagues (1990) suggest that psychologists working in hospital and other health settings routinely assess *themselves* for how well they adhere to the following suggestions:

- Understand the nature of the services provided by others on staff at all levels and understand how the services you provide support or impact others.
- When making oral or written reports that others will utilize, use terminology that those who are not mental health professionals can understand.
- Know the limits of your assessment instruments as they pertain to the specific population or individuals with whom you are working.
- Remember that hospital and other health settings depend on teamwork and the ability to intervene directly and immediately to resolve patients' problems.
- Periodically review the laws and regulations that govern ownership and access to client files and psychological reports. Once a psychological report is entered into the medical record, you have lost the ability to regulate who will have access to it.
- When possible, discuss the results and recommendations of a psychological evaluation directly with the patient. The results of the assessment are now part of a permanent record that often follows patients from facility to facility, and can be used to make critical decisions about their future.

The process of identifying the questions to be addressed, selecting the instruments to be used, evaluating the findings, and presenting the report varies from setting to setting. Psychologists working in these medical settings should become familiar with those who provide referrals and learn their biases and expectations about the nature of psychological consultation. This information will prove helpful in identifying and refining the questions being asked, the consequences to be expected from the assessment, and even selecting the particular instruments and procedures to be used. For example, it would not ordinarily be wise to select instruments about which the primary referrant has particular, negative biases. The instruments used and valued in different settings vary by reputation and the familiarity of the referring professionals.

Several lines of evidence demonstrate how personality assessment may be useful in a medical hospital. Using the MMPI-2, Cort, Kappagoda, and Greene (2001) were able to identify individuals likely to drop out of a cardiology rehabilitation program, which would place them in elevated risk for further, life-threatening heart disease. A model was developed from MMPI-2 scores to predict classification (compliers and noncompliers) with an overall accuracy of 93%. The researchers then applied their model to the next incoming treatment group and were able to replicate their findings with an overall accuracy of 90%, meaning that steps were taken to ensure that those patients with an elevated risk of noncompliance were given additional support to increase the effectiveness of the program for them. Cort and colleagues conclude that long-term management of patients with chronic coronary arteriosclerosis should be based upon a multidisciplinary approach to patient care that includes exercise training, dietary management and education, and psychological management. Compliance is a major problem in these complex programs because patients are required to make extreme lifestyle changes. It is not difficult to see that the appropriate use of personality assessment data can result in increased compliance and more discriminating use of resources in a variety of medical/health settings.

Neuropsychological assessment, also frequently used in general medical settings, is concerned with the evaluation of brain dysfunction, particularly with the development, standardization, and validation of techniques to assess behavioral manifestations of such dysfunction. Neuropsychological assessments employ batteries of tests to evaluate major areas of functioning, not only to provide information for a differential diagnosis but also to assess levels of impairment as part of planning a treatment and rehabilitation program for patients (see Groth-Marnat, 2000; Lezak, 1995). A typical neuropsychological assessment includes measures of memory/learning, attention/concentration, abstract reasoning, verbal abilities, visuospatial abilities, and the ability to plan, initiate, and monitor behavior (executive functions). Often personality functions are also essential to assess, since these can have important implications for the patient's overall functioning, ability to benefit from treatment, and predictions related to recovery.

Typical referral questions for neuropsychological evaluation include distinguishing between organic and psychological factors, describing the nature and extent of a known organic dysfunction, establishing the degree to which the patient can function independently, and designing an optimal treatment program. An example of a typical referral issue is differentiating between dementia of the Alzheimer's type, dementia due to a general medical condition, and dementia secondary to major depressive disorder. This differentiation requires an assessment of medical status, mental status, personality, social functioning, and the like. Another referral might be to determine the extent to which a patient has experienced impairment as the result of a motor vehicle accident. This information might then be used to design a treatment plan (i.e., psychotherapy to improve awareness of deficit, aids to compensate for memory problems) or, within a legal context, to determine the degree of compensation that might be awarded. As is the case with most specialties, we suggest that a clinician who wishes to practice in this arena should obtain advanced training, education, and supervised experience prior to practicing independently as a neuropsychologist. In fact, we suggest that interested parties obtain a certificate in neuropsychology, which is available at many universities and in the form of advanced continuing education.

The Vocational Setting

Clients are often self-referred or referred by a third party, such as an insurance company, to develop options and determine suitability for possible vocations. For example, clients who are self-referred due to dissatisfaction with their current job are seeking advice about the underlying causes of this dissatisfaction as well as knowledge about other types of work that might be more suitable to them. Often this type of assessment involves not only considering interests and abilities but also more subtle aspects of personality, such as the degree to which they feel comfortable in leadership positions. This level of comfort might relate more to the client's family of origin than the match between the person's abilities and the requirements of the job. Clients also might be referred for an evaluation to determine who would be the most appropriate candidate to take a position directing a company. This type of assessment would require establishing the degree of congruence between the person's managerial and coping style with the organization's culture and future direction. Yet another scenario might involve evaluation of a client with a psychiatric or neuropsychological disability to determine the type of work that might be suitable. A related but more global question would be whether or not the person can even return to part- or full-time employment.

Personality assessment is usually one of the core elements of a vocational assessment. For example, the client's level of extroversion and introversion must be matched with the social demands of the job. Whereas the social demands of the field of education or management require some degree of extroversion, the social support and demand for extroversion among computer programmers, novelists, or lab technicians is very low. A degree of introversion and introspection would benefit a person working in one of these professions. A person with a pragmatic orientation, who deals with the world in a concrete, direct manner, might do well as an engineer or plumber but may do less well as a philosopher or writer.

Additional functions that are crucial to evaluate in a vocational assessment include level of cognitive ability, level of achievement, nature of interests, preferred working environments, as well as typical styles of coping (Lowman, 1991; Lowman & Carson, 2000). The implications of the scores on tests of these variables can then be compared with the requirements of a job. This step requires the clinician to conduct a job analysis to determine the skills required for the job. Then the degree of match between client and potential jobs or careers can be determined. This information can then be given to the client, so that he or she can determine the aspects of the vocation that would be compatible versus those that might lead to dissatisfaction.

In order to perform effective vocational assessment and provide useful feedback to the referring professional, crucial knowledge external to the immediate assessment situation is needed. Psychologists must know what is required by various professions and jobs in terms of training (6-month training program, 4-year college degree), as well as being familiar with community resources to which a client can be referred. Sometimes schools and libraries have computer facilities that allow clients to gain additional information about jobs. Referring a client to talk with a person who is already working in a particular vocation can often be very helpful.

Finally, a market analysis is often helpful to determine the degree of demand for the types of jobs in which the client is interested. This type of analysis is particularly warranted during times of economic transitions, when some job markets are expanding and others are contracting. Effective vocational assessment requires not only the measurement of relevant variables but also working with the client to integrate the implications of this information for possible future directions (Lowman & Carson, 2000).

The Psychology Clinic

Often clinics are established in settings that are run primarily by psychologists. These clinics are common in training settings, private practice settings, and public service agencies. In such clinics, it is typically psychologists who make the administrative and treatment decisions. As a result, psychologists seek answers to questions that they themselves have posed. In contrast, in legal, medical, psychiatric, and vocational settings, psychologists serve as consultants to others who make the administrative and treatment decisions. As a result, in the psychological setting, psychologists need to be particularly aware of the possible legal and ethical implications that accompany the responsibility of making these decisions and assuming dual—and sometimes competitive—roles.

Most clients who seek services from psychological clinics are self-referred and in search of relief from emotional pain. Most of these clients do not require formal assessment beyond a semistructured interview or, if they do, it is usually in the form of brief, targeted assessment instruments to determine to which interventions they will be most likely to respond. These instruments also might be useful for monitoring and evaluating treatment (Maruish, 1999). If the clinician is confused by the client's array of symptoms, or if it is unclear why treatment is not progressing, then an in-depth assessment might be used. For example, patients with dissociative symptoms are often misdiagnosed because they typically report symptoms of depression or anxiety but not difficulties related to dissociation. Unless these symptoms are diagnosed in a more focused and in-depth evaluation and then addressed in treatment, the client typically does not progress. Other clients might have undiagnosed medical conditions and need to be referred for specialized and intensive evaluation and treatment. Still others might have extensive legal problems that need to be addressed through special procedures conducted by relevant specialists.

Other Settings

There are many examples of less researched settings where personality assessment has become commonplace. The important concept here is that psychologists need to obtain specialized training prior to practicing in any specialized setting. Practitioners are advised to determine (1) which personality assessment instruments have been used for the specific population being examined, and (2) to what extent each instrument's validity, reliability, and norms hold true. The American Psychological Association, in conjunction with several other groups, published a booklet entitled *Responsible Test Use: Case Studies for Assessing Human Behavior* (American Psychological Association, 1993). The booklet illustrates more than 75 cases from a wide variety of settings and perspectives, and can be used as a valuable resource.

For example, personality assessment is often used in the screening of entry-level law enforcement officers. In general, the goal of psychological screening is to identify candidates who are well adjusted and have good coping skills (Scogin, Schumacher, Gardner, & Chaplin, 1995). Beutler and his colleagues (Beutler, Storm, Kirkish, Scogin, & Gaines, 1985) found that in-service behaviors such as interpersonal ability, commendations, and suspensions could be predicted from scores on a test battery that included the MMPI. In the same direction, Scogin and his colleagues (1995) found that a personality evaluation that included, among other instruments, the MMPI-2 was able to identify potential officers who would evidence poorer job performance.

Another study examined 16 male commercial airline pilots who underwent independent psychological evaluations after the completion of a treatment regime for substance abuse. The pilots knew that the results of the assessments would be taken into account by their employers and the Federal Aviation Administration (Ganellen, (1994). As expected, the subjects responded in a defensive manner, as assessed by the MMPI validity scales. Yet, in spite of defensive test taking, the pilots were able to produce valid Rorschach protocols that suggested emotional distress, self-criticism, and difficulties with interpersonal relationships not found on the MMPI.

The military utilizes personality assessment in a variety of ways. For instance, Carbone and his colleagues (Carbone, Cigrang, Todd, & Fiedler, 1999) were able to use personality assessment data to predict, with close to 70% accuracy, which personnel referred for psychological evaluation would be able to return to basic military training and graduate. Bloom (1993) published a thorough review of practical approaches to using psychological assessment data to assess eligibility for security clearances, special access, and sensitive positions. The article addresses such topics as techniques, tests, and writing of the report. Santy and her colleagues (1993) propose and review an assessment battery in the evaluation of NASA astronaut candidates. They report that, until recently, there was no structured procedure for this process, which simply consisted of two separate interviews and recommendations. The procedure became known as a medical/ psychiatric "select-out" process; it determines the history and/or presence of a disqualifying mental disorder, based on NASA medical standards (Santy et al., 1993).

SPECIFIC TEST DIFFERENCES

Before selecting which tests or assessment instruments will be included in any evaluation, the examiner must first determine if he or she is competent to administer and/or interpret them. The American Psychological Association (APA) has developed guidelines to determine test-user qualifications. These guidelines refer to the combination of knowledge, skills, abilities, training, experience, and practice credentials that the APA has determined important for the responsible use of psychological tests (Turner, DeMers, Fox, & Reed, 2001). The APA's purpose in developing the guidelines is to inform all interested parties (clinicians, test users, and the public) about the qualifications that promote high professional standards in the use of psychological tests (Turner et al., 2001). An important component of the guidelines involves the selection of the best test or test version available for the specific questions being asked. Interested readers can consult the December 2001 *American Psychologist* (Vol. 56, No. 12) or contact the APA directly to obtain a copy of the guidelines (*www.apa.org*).

Conducting personality assessment in most settings often involves using the MMPI-2 and/or the Rorschach inkblot method. These two tests are examined in depth here, including a wide variety of applications and limitations of their use. As noted, Table 10.1 lists many of the most popular personality instruments by setting and use.

MMPI-2

According to Greene (2000), the setting in which the MMPI-2 is administered can have significant impact on whether the various scales are or are not elevated. The MMPI-2 is routinely used to screen police officers, firefighters, clergy, pilots, and many other groups for the presence of psychopathology. In these personnel screening situations, people generally understand that the presence of anything negative decreases the probability of their selection. Consequently, they minimize reporting symptoms of psychopathology and significantly lower the overall elevation of their MMPI-2 profiles (Greene, 2000).

The MMPI-2 is also used frequently in forensic evaluations in which there may be motivation to acknowledge (criminal cases where the individual pleads not guilty by reason of insanity) or not acknowledge (child custody evaluations; parole evaluations) psychopathology, which results in elevations or reductions on several key scales and the MMPI-2 profile in general. The results of differences in motivation are illustrated by comparing a sample of child custody litigants (Bathurst, Gottfried, & Gottfried, 1997) with a sample of personal injury plaintiffs (Lees-Haley, 1997). The results approach two standard deviations on some clinical scales (L, 1(Hs), 2(D), 3(Hy), 7(Pt), and 8(Sc)).

The MMPI-2 is also routinely used in medical and psychiatric settings. Patients in medical settings tend to elevate scales 1 (Hypocondriasis), 2 (Depression), and 3 (Hysteria). When the profiles of psychiatric patients (Caldwell, 2000) were compared to those of medical patients (Colligan & Offord, 1986), nearly 50% of the MMPI codetypes in the medical patients were contained within the combinations of scales 1, 2, and 3, whereas less than 25% of the codetypes in psychiatric patients were among these scales. Additionally, pain patients (Caldwell, 2000) showed mean T-scores on scales 1, 2, and 3 that were one standard deviation higher than the psychiatric patients. For a comparison of the effects of setting on the MMPI-2 in personnel screening, forensic settings (including child custody litigants, personal injury plaintiffs, and inmates) and medical/psychiatric settings, the interested reader is directed to Greene (2000, p. 494).

Finally, Greene (2000) suggests that clinicians would be well served to determine the mean profile for their specific setting as well as frequency of MMPI-2 codetypes. He adds that this information facilitates the interpretation of the MMPI-2 because the scales can be very sensitive to the effects of the setting in which the test is administered.

Rorschach

Exner (2002) cautions examiners to "exercise good judgement" in regards to when it is, and is not, appropriate to administer the Rorschach. He adds that when referrals are made, it is the lack of flexibility in decision making concerning the scheduling of an assessment that is often problematic. This lack of flexibility appears to be most common in inpatient psychiatric settings, where the need to formulate a diagnosis and subsequent treatment intervention requires that data be gathered shortly after admission. Although the idea is to begin treatment based on assessment results, there are instances in which the patients who are tested in actively psychotic or toxic states will produce results that, although reflecting their current state, are marked by considerable evidence of bizarreness and/or disorientation (Exner, 2002). Such results tend to be misleading; they present a more dismal picture of the basic personality than may have been the case if the testing were deferred until the subject had made some adjustments to the situation and the psychotic or toxic episode had subsided.

Clinicians in a hospital setting often encounter the lore that it is preferable to administer the tests before medication, especially when high-potency antipsychotics, are "in the wings." Exner (2002) indicates that the Rorschach data yield the clearest information when the subject is cooperative and coherent. He adds that pharmacological intervention will have relatively little impact on most Rorschach variables, and no significant impact on those variables associated with core features of the personality structure. Furthermore, it is suggested that those clinicians using the Rorschach in inpatient/medical settings make intelligent decisions about when the test should be administered and when an administration is best delayed in the interest of the patient and treatment planning.

Clinicians should be aware that there is some disagreement about the validity of using the Rorschach inkblot method with clinical and forensic patients. Garb and his colleagues (Garb, Wood, Grove, & Stejskal, 2001) have raised numerous questions about the methodology used to develop Exner's Comprehensive System. They point out that there are unanswered questions regarding control groups, criterion contamination, selective reporting, and alpha levels. As noted in a previous chapter, Garb (1999) even went as far as calling for a moratorium on the use of the Rorschach in clinical and forensic settings, until it is determined which of the Rorschach scores are valid. These researchers are currently a small minority, but they raise important issues about this, and any assessment instrument, especially in light of the *Frye* and *Daubert* rules (discussed earlier in this chapter). Although the call for a moratorium has for the most part gone unanswered, it has generated a healthy discussion among personality assessment researchers and will likely result in additional, sound, peer-reviewed research on the Rorschach and its scoring systems. The interested reader is directed to two recent "Special Sections" on this debate covered in depth in *Psychological Assessment* (Vol. 11, No. 3, and Vol. 13, No. 4).

Basic Referral Questions

In all settings, the process of personality assessment begins with the referral. An appropriate referral will include questions about a patient that need to be answered in order to maximize treatment planning for the individual. However, it is often the case that no specific question can be discerned from the referral source, or commonly the request may simply be one for "diagnostic clarification." When faced with ambiguous requests, the clinician must decide which instruments to use to maximize the yield of pertinent information. One sure strategy is to keep in mind six basic referral questions that a practitioner is likely to encounter: (1) diagnosis; (2) etiology; (3) prognosis; (4) differential treatment; (5) functional impairment; and (6) strengths and adaptive capacities. These basic referral questions are discussed in other chapters in this book and form the foundation of personality assessment.

CASE EXAMPLE

Systematic Treatment Selection (STS; Beutler, & Clarkin, 1990; Beutler, Clarkin, & Bongar, 2000) is a general model for identifying patient dimensions that may contribute to predictions of treatment outcome and treatment planning. The STS model proposes four levels of intervention: (1) patient predisposing qualities; (2) context of treatment; (3) therapist activity and relationship; and (4) match of levels 1 and 3.

In the first level of the STS model the practitioner is directed to examine, via the personality assessment results, the patient's problem (symptoms, intensity/severity, complexity/chronicity), the patient's personality (coping style, defenses, subjective distress, motivation for change) and the patient's environment (degree of functional impairment, level of social support, presence of strengths). It is in this first level that the setting-specific personality assessment plays a vital role in that the following levels are directly dependent on the findings and results of the assessment to this point. Questions about such matters as restrictiveness of care and intensity, mode, and format of treatment are directly influenced by the individual's particular combination of strengths and weaknesses. The therapist's role will be influenced directly by the individual's needs in the form of therapist–patient matching and personal fit. Lastly, the assessment information leads directly to an attempt to match or fit the intervention to each individual patient (Beutler et al., 2000).

Throughout this text authors examine the case of R.W., a hypothetical client but one with a very real need. R.W. was referred for evaluation in order to clarify the diagnosis and assist in treatment planning. Her history indicates that she has developed a fear of going out into public, has fainted, and sometimes experiences panic attacks. Furthermore, the client appears to experience emotional fluctuations, isolation, and some degree of thought confusion, and she has acted out sexually and engaged in substance abuse.

The assessment, report writing, and treatment considerations for R.W. can be found in Appendix A. What is of concern here is the various other settings in which care, evaluation, and/or treatment of R.W. may occur. For example, patients experiencing panic attacks sometimes end up in hospital emergency rooms with symptoms that appear to be extremely disturbing but which are generally treated effectively and quickly with medication. R.W. has a history of "acting out" with both drugs and alcohol and certainly could find herself involved with the police, if not careful. The corrections department would want to assess the degree and history of her substance use problem, screen for self-harm indicators, and refer her to an appropriate treatment setting (not to mention prescribing the consequences for any crime committed, such as driving under the influence of alcohol/illicit substances).

Clinicians may also find R.W. in a psychiatric hospital for symptoms ranging from depression to self-harm, or to rule out a psychotic disorder. While in the psychiatric hospital, R.W. may be given a full personality assessment in order to determine her correct diagnosis and begin her on a medication trial. Finally, it seems reasonable that R.W. may find herself in a substance treatment center. Here she would be assessed for history and severity of substance disorders, evaluated for eligibility in a support group or program, and educated about the physiological effects of substance use.

Finally, any clinician, in any setting, should quickly and competently evaluate clients such as R.W. for elevated risk of self-injury and suicidal thoughts, given that she presents with elevated risk criteria such as substance use, impulsive behavior, depression, possible thought disorder, and little social support.

SUMMARY

This chapter has addressed how personality assessments in special settings may differ from those conducted in traditional places such as an outpatient private practice. However, it is important to note that there are similarities as well. One of these is the principle that the patient be understood within his or her context. In this regard, good potential matches between patient predisposing qualities and treatment dimensions would be expected to include the following areas of fit: (1) level of functional impairment; (2) level of support, strengths, and assets; (3) complexity/chronicity of the problem; (4) patient coping style; (5) level of resistance; and (6) level of subjective distress and willingness to change (Beutler et al., 2000).

The purpose of this chapter is to describe various special settings in which clinicians are likely to be asked to conduct personality assessment. In providing this information, we do not intend to imply that these are the only settings or that the clinical methods and tests presented in this chapter are appropriate for answering all questions. The information presented is purposefully general so that it can be generalized to settings and situations not specifically addressed.

One of our important messages is that test data need to be evaluated not only against general norms but for setting-specific norms as well. For example, prison inmates and hospital patients are likely to endorse items on the tests indicative of paranoia, in that there really are people watching them, and anxiety, in that their situations are precarious for one reason or another. These test results need to be interpreted with an understanding of the context as well as the person. As illustrated throughout this text, it is useful for clinicians to develop and use a consistent framework and method for identifying and conceptually discriminating among various types of conflicts found in their various employment settings.

11

Integrative Personality Assessment with Older Adults and Ethnic Minority Clients

Forrest Scogin
and Martha R. Crowther

In the United States both older adults and people of racial and ethnic minorities are experiencing a remarkable rate of growth. By the year 2030, it is expected that older adults will comprise approximately 20% of the population (Cheeseman, 1996). The racial and ethnic minority population is exceeding the rate of growth of the white population. This is evident in the projected decrease in whites as a percentage of the population from 74% in 1995 to 72% in 2000, 64% in 2020, and 53% in 2050 (Cheeseman, 1996). In response to the changing demographic profile of the United States, it is important to establish the reliability, validity, and utility of various personality assessment instruments and techniques used with nonwhite and older populations. This chapter focuses on the use of such procedures to optimize benefits from psychosocial interventions via the Systematic Treatment Selection model.

KEY CONCEPTS

Arriving at workable definitions of the constructs *elderly* and *ethnic minority* is not a simple undertaking (Beutler, Brown, Crothers, Booker, & Seabrook, 1996). Consistent with most, we define older adults based on chronological age. Most use 60 or 65 years of age or greater to define the population of older adults. However, chronological age ignores biological, social, and psychological aspects of age and thus does not reflect the tremendous heterogeneity that exists in persons over 60 years of age.

It is important to keep in mind that at least two generations are included in the older adult cohort, with different experiences and historical perspectives: the young-old and the oldest-old (Berger, 1994). The phrase "oldest-old" refers to adults 85 years and over. The division between young-old and oldest-old has helped change the perception of older adults from that of a homogenous population to a heterogeneous population with varying social, health, and long-term care needs (Crowther & Zeiss, 2002). However, some researchers have voiced concern that the distinction may cause stereotyping of the oldest-old group (Binstock, 1992). This possibility raises an important consideration, given that chronological age is not the only factor that determines how persons adjust to aging. State of mind, health habits, and general social and psychological outlook on life also determine adjustment to aging.

The definition of age is further confounded with the often disparate concepts of "mental age," "social maturity," "chronological age," and "developmental age." Especially among the young and the mature, differences in responses to social systems, interventions, and stressors are less dependent on chronological age than upon the more nebulous concept of developmental or maturational level (Murphy & Longino, 1992). Nonetheless, of the demographic labels conventionally presented, age is the one that is imbued with the least controversy and, correspondingly, with the least conflict.

The nature of ethnicity/race and age/development distinctions can partially be reduced to a question of whether we are talking about a biological or a social construct. For example, the debates regarding racial differences, as typified by the work of Jensen (1980) and then Rushton (1995), are really debates about what is biological versus social—immutable versus changeable. Indeed, the debate is most heated when it comes down to whether the differences observed point to genetic superiority/inferiority of certain races (Helms, 1992; Yee, Fairchild, Weizmann, & Wyatt, 1993).

For whatever reason, it is clear that people representing different demographics are not treated evenly in the mental health system, partly because of the confusion between what is social and what is biological. Interestingly, this lack of evenness provokes a social outcry when ethnicity/race is the reason, but no such outcry is apparent when age is the factor. Differences noted in performance levels and patterns among different age groups are accepted as biologically based and, hence, beyond debate. Not so for other demographics about which there is disagreement. Such an imbalance in which demographics are tolerated as topics of debate discourages research in areas that are not politically correct.

Thus there is ample reason to question the validity of the assumption that demographic categories reflect identifiable, stable, and biological qualities of people. More specifically, consider the issue of race versus ethnicity. Those who use the term *race* tend to imply that the existence of a finite set of psychological qualities that is bound to genetics. However, literature does not support this assumption (Entwisle & Astone, 1994; Good, 1992; Yzaguirre & Perez, 1995; Zuckerman, 1990). Good (1992b) found that as much as a 46% disparity exists in the identification of race as a function of whether measurement derives from self-report or external raters. Self-reports are not stable and depend heavily on how many, and what kinds of, categories are made available to the respondent.

In 1950 a panel of experts declared the term *race* to be archaic and recommended that it be replaced with the term *ethnicity* (Yee, 1983). This group contended that the latter term was less emotionally laden and biased, was less subject to stereotypical views, and shifted the emphasis from physical characteristics to sociocultural influences and potentialities. Accordingly, *ethnicity* has been used by social scientists to reflect the psychological characteristics, attitudes, and cultural processes that are assumed to be characteristic of an individual's cultural identification. These aspects are expected to be more psychologically relevant, amenable to psychological measurement, and alterable than those associated with biological race.

The term *ethnic minority* is deceptive. It is easy to believe that people of ethnic minorities comprise a discrete number of groups that can be discussed in a clear and concise manner. According to the U.S. Census, Caucasian, African American, American Indian, and Asian and Pacific Islander are considered racial groups, whereas Hispanic is considered an ethnic group. For the purposes of clarity in this chapter, we use the term *racial and ethnic minority* to encompass African Americans, Hispanic Americans, Asian and Pacific Islander Americans, as well as American Indian and Alaska Natives. We also want to make note of the tremendous amount of diversity within each of these racial and ethnic groups. For example, there are over 30 Asian American/Pacific Islander ethnic groups that comprise the category *Asian American*.

Older adults and people of ethnic and racial minorities comprise two diverse special populations. They can differ in general status, acculturation level, language, religion/spiritual beliefs, cultural traditions, values, and gender roles. Given the diversity, mental health practitioners must understand the traits and qualities that exist within a particular culture and how those traits and qualities are manifested in an individual by examining the interaction between cultural, social, biological, environmental, and psychological factors.

GENERAL ASSESSMENT ISSUES

Use of the Mental Health System by Elders

Older adults and people of racial and ethnic minorities are among the groups that do not receive or seek the services that are available (at least, ostensibly). Until recently, outpatient mental health care services were underutilized by older adults, despite 1975 legislation mandating specialized services for older adults within community mental health centers. The majority of elders who receive mental health services are seen as inpatients during a hospitalization in a psychiatric hospital or a nursing home. Possible explanations for this underutilization include the idea that, within this cohort, there is a stigma attached to receiving mental health services, but this hypothesis has not been supported by research (e.g., Rokke & Scogin, 1995). Alternatively, mental health professionals have displayed a form of "professional ageism" dating back to Freud, who was pessimistic about the possibility of psychological change or the benefits of therapy in later life (Freud, 1905/1953). Finally, Medicare reimbursement for psychological services in the United States is very limited. The majority of the money spent goes toward psychopharmacology as opposed to psychotherapy.

However, usage patterns of psychological services by older adults are changing. Successive cohorts of older persons have higher levels of education and a greater acceptance of psychology. Rokke and Scogin (1995), for example, showed that older adults considered cognitive therapy to be more credible and acceptable than drug therapy for depression. Similar results have been reported by Landreville and colleagues (Landreville, Landry, Baillargeon, Guérette, & Matteau, 2001). Interestingly, many older adults are becoming receptive to mental health services—which suggests that the time is right for mental health practitioners to take an active role in reaching out to older adults to provide services.

Use of the Mental Health System by Minority Group Members

Evaluating the use of the mental health system by people of racial and ethnic minorities is a complex issue. Racial and ethnic minority group members enter into treatment at a lower rate than whites, and people from these groups are more likely to be hospitalized or to receive more restrictive and less individualized services than those typically afforded to majority participants (Rogler, Malgady, & Rodriguez, 1989; Sue, Fujino, Hu, Takeuchi, & Zane, 1991). Although these facts are typically interpreted as an indication that minority group members are differentially restricted from gaining access to the individualized and nonrestrictive services—that is, they receive a lower standard of care—the interpretation is seriously flawed by virtue of several contaminating variables that occur in naturalistic and epidemiological methods. For example, from clinical data it is clear that racial and ethnic minority group members generally, and Asian and Latino Americans specifically, enter treatment with higher levels of distress and disturbance than do whites (L. E. Beutler, personal communication, December 19, 2001). Additionally, racial and ethnic minority group members tend to seek treatment from different sources than majority group members. Specifically, (1) observed differences in access to care may reflect different rates of treatment seeking and differential availability of racial and ethnic minority providers; (2) differences in quality of care rendered to minority and majority individuals may reflect a tendency among minority members to avoid treatment until needs are very great and a different level and type of service is necessary than is true for less distressed/disturbed majority members; and (3) minorities may likely seek nontraditional sources of treatment, such as religious counseling.

SYSTEMATIC TREATMENT SELECTION DIMENSIONS: RELEVANCE TO OLDER ADULTS AND RACIAL AND ETHNIC MINORITY ADULTS

The Systematic Treatment Selection (STS) model (Beutler, Clarkin, & Bongar, 2000) provides a framework with which the impact of aging and racial and ethnic minority status can be evaluated in personality assessment. In the following section we discuss the components of the STS model and their relevance to these special populations. The case of R.W. (see Appendix A), a young Mexican American woman, is interwoven into our comments on ethnic and gender factors. However, the hypothetical age of this woman precludes her case from providing much assistance in illustrating the problems associated with aging. We note that although one of the four samples archived by Beutler and colleagues (2000) was comprised of older adults, few studies of STS constructs have specifically addressed issues of ethnicity. Most studies have included both men and women and a small number of nonwhite patients. To the degree that it can be determined by inspecting the results of disaggregating these samples, the STS dimensions appear to cut across age, sex, and ethnic boundaries. However, further research is needed to firmly establish the finding that paying attention to the STS components maximizes efficacy and effectiveness of treatment for older adults and people of racial and ethnic minorities.

Table 11.1 provides examples of instruments and methods that may be used to address the STS dimensions when working with older adults.

Functional Impairment

The functional impairment dimension of the STS model is a crucial focus when planning treatment for older adults. The major differences in working with older and younger clients tend to revolve around two areas: cognitive status and health issues (Gallagher-Thompson & Thompson, 1996; Scogin, 2000). Together, cognitive and health status largely determine functional impairment. Clients who present with age-related changes in cognitive functioning or mild-to-moderate indicators of dementia require interventions that are sensitive to their ability to process information. Likewise, knowledge of health conditions presented by older adults is central to understanding symptom presentation and prognosis (among other factors).

Assessment of functional status among older adults has a long tradition. Generally, this type of assessment includes appraisal of activities of daily living (commonly referred to as ADLs). ADLs are comprised of basic self-care activities such as bathing, feeding, and toileting. More complex tasks have been described as IADLs (instrumental activities of daily living) and include financial management, meal preparation, and transportation

TABLE 11.1. Instruments That Address the STS Dimensions Specific or Adaptable to Older Adults

Instrument	STS dimensions					
	Functional Impairment	Motivational Distress	Problem Complexity	Resistance	Coping Style	Social Support
GDS	×	×				
MMPI-2	×	×	×	×	×	
MMSE	×					
SCL-90-R/BSI	×	×	×			
SCID/SCID II	×		×			
ADL/IADL	×		×			
Duke Social Support Index/ REACH 26-Item Form						×
Clinical Indicators	×	×	×	×	×	×
Therapeutic Reactance Scale				×		

use. Assessment of ADL/IADLs is frequently a part of comprehensive evaluations of older adult clients. For these purposes, we have used the Physical Self Maintenance Scale and the IADL Scale (Lawton, 1988; Lawton & Brody, 1969). In composite, the scales consist of 25 items rated from 1 (not impaired) to 5 (severely impaired).

Assessment of cognitive functioning is also a routine aspect of a comprehensive evaluation of older adults. For brevity, an instrument such as the MMSE (Mini-Mental State Examination; Folstein, Folstein, & McHugh, 1975) is often used; this scale yields a total score that is relatively sensitive to overall cognitive impairment. (A score of 24 or higher is often selected as the marker for entry into psychotherapy clinical trials.)

Aggregated information on comorbid health status, functional abilities, and cognitive impairment can provide useful information on the STS dimension of functional impairment severity. Of course, mental disorders serve to exacerbate concurrent functional impairments, which is why older adults presenting for treatment are often experiencing excessive disability. Treatment of disorders such as depression can often reduce excessive disability.

Although assessment of functional impairment in older adults is based primarily on their physical and cognitive status, the assessment of functional impairment in people of ethnic minorities is based on knowledge of the individual's culture. Determining the degree to which an individual's style interferes with his or her functioning in a variety of settings is important. For example, the individual may be functioning well in his or her culture but having difficulty at work, which would suggest problems adjusting to mainstream society.

In the case of R.W., for example, having less than a high school education may reflect a low emphasis on education for Mexican American girls in a traditional culture. Likewise, many of her fears may be exaggerated by a culturally based reliance on external opinion and approval. However, most aspects of R.W.'s clinical presentation would represent an identifiable problem regardless of the culture in which she was raised. She presents with emotional instability, social anxiety, panic attacks, and troubled relationships. The panic attacks, disturbed intimate relationships, and fears cannot be attributed to cultural factors. It may be interesting to determine, however, if the "highs and lows" would be tolerated more easily within a close-knit Latino culture than in a Euro-American majority culture. In either culture, the symptoms presented by this woman's reduced mobility and avoidance are likely to be seen as indicating moderate impairment.

Many scales are available for measuring the cultural characteristics or levels of acculturation in people of racial and ethnic minorities. Among them are the Suinn–Lew Asian Self-Identity Acculturation Scale (SL-ASIA) developed for the assessment of acculturation of Asian Americans (Suinn, Rickard-Figueroa, Lew, & Virgil, 1987). The measure is a 21-item multiple-choice instrument modeled after the Acculturation Rating Scale for Mexican Americans (ARSMA; Cuellar, Arnold, & Maldonada, 1995; Cuellar, Harris, & Jasso, 1980). Scores on this latter scale, if they were available, may have helped us determine the degree to which cultural factors were exacerbating the patient's avoidance of disapproval and criticism.

As noted in Chapter 6, the MMPI is an objective measure that can be used to assess functional impairment in people of ethnic minorities. The MMPI has been used extensively with ethnic groups in the United States and was usefully applied in Chapter 6 to R.W. Several researchers have found that ethnic differences can occur at the item or profile level (Dana, 1993; Gray-Little, 1995). However, in clinical situations scale elevation and profile interpretation are the most common. The majority of the research examining ethnic differences using the MMPI has focused on African American–white comparisons. The MMPI has been criticized for its inability to differentiate severe pathology from moderate to normal reactions, as well as problems in distinguishing among clinical groups. Some have argued against its use with people of racial and ethnic minorities because of the lack of norms among minority groups or because of interpretive bias (e.g., Dana, 1993). It is important to note that criticisms of the original MMPI have not been empirically replicated with the MMPI-2 (Okazaki & Sue, 1995). Researchers also have noted the difficulty of renorming the MMPI in ethnic populations within the United States, given within-group heterogeneity and changing sociocultural contexts (Okazaki & Sue, 1995). Additionally, socioeconomic status is often a mediating factor in a person's cultural experience of his or her racial or ethnic minority status, such that established assessment measures may be more valid for those who have achieved middle-class status. Given the criticisms of the MMPI, we suggest that a multimethod approach be used for personality assessment: That is, the clinician should (1) administer the MMPI or other personality assessment instrument, (2) conduct an in-depth interview with the client, and (3) if possible, obtain secondary source information from other health professionals and/or family members of the client. The multimethod approach facilitates the gathering of extensive historical and background information on the client, which is important when placing the person (and his or her personality assessment responses) in the proper cultural or sociocultural context.

Level of Social Support

Social support has become an important construct in gerontological studies. Knowledge of an older client's positive and negative social variables can inform key intervention issues for older clients and their caregivers (Blieszner, 1995; Pearlin, Mullan, Semple, & Skaff, 1990). Thus inclusion of the social support dimension in the STS model is timely and of much relevance to work with older adults and their families. Not surprisingly, a number of assessment tools is available for evaluating the degree of social support available to elders. Given the multifaceted nature of social support, we have used an instrument developed by investigators involved in the National Institute on Aging's REACH (Resources for Enhancing Alzheimer's Caregiver Health) project. This 26-item form is a compilation of several instruments and measures social networks (family, friends, confidants), type of social support received and satisfaction with that support (emotional, tangible, informal), and negative interactions.

Not surprisingly, social support is also an important variable in the mental health of people from racial and ethnic minorities. The social support an individual receives from family, friends, and the community is an important component of the person's coping resources. For people of racial and ethnic minorities who are recent immigrants to the United States, these resources contribute to their ability to cope with the transition to a new culture. Often ethnic communities help these individuals make the transition to the new environment. In addition, the family system can promote resilience and the ability to cope with the pressures of racial and ethnic minority status in the United States.

In the case of R.W., for example, the absence of social support systems, other than the relationship with her "boyfriend," may induce considerable stress. The Latino cultures tend to emphasize family ties and to place strong emphasis on cultural attachments. R.W. has been deprived of these contacts and sources of support because of her unacceptable relationship. The disparity between cultural values and experience may exacerbate the effects of this low level of social support and probably makes the level of impairment more significant in her treatment. Certainly, a treatment that focused on enhancing support and reenfranchising R.W. within her family and cultural group would be helpful. This latter recommendation has received partial support from evidence that some people may be at greater or lesser risk as a result of the family-based definitions of their roles in society (Newman, 2001). Expectations and criticism of extended family members play an especially strong role in the sense of well-being among Latinos/Hispanics, African Americans, Asian American/Pacific Islanders, and American Indians (Boyd-Franklin, 1989; Sue & Sue, 1990). Persons who are not biologically related but are considered relatives, referred to in the literature as "fictive kin," are also considered a strong part of the social support system for many people of racial and ethnic minorities (Paniagua, 1994).

There are several good measures of social support used with racial and ethnic minority populations. We have used the Duke Social Support Index (DSSI; Hughes, Blazer, & Hybels, 1991), which measures instrumental and emotional support. We also have found that the scale captures the quality of the support being received as well as the number of persons in the support network. Based on her description, we would expect that this measure, had it been used with R.W., would confirm the low level of support she experiences, perhaps even elevated over that expected of a woman from the majority culture who had only one significant love relationship.

Problem Complexity/Chronicity

Pervasive and enduring issues characterize this domain. The factor of chronicity is often striking when working with older adults who, for example, report depression and anxiety disorders of 60 or more years in duration. In other respects, older clients are much like younger adult clients in patterns of complexity. We have found the Symptom Checklist–90–R (SCL-90-R)/Brief Symptom Inventory (BSI) to be a useful instrument for assessing problem complexity as well as other facets of the STS. The BSI has been used in a number of studies with elders and has norms for older adults as well as evidence of reliability and validity. Elevations across subscales, particularly those less overlapping, are an indication of problem complexity (Gaw & Beutler, 1995). Personality disorders also are an indication of both complexity and chronicity and are salient factors because of the known role they play in attenuating treatment efficacy in older adults (Zarit & Zarit, 1998). Interestingly, some personality disorders seem to be more prevalent among older psychotherapy patients. Dependent personality disorders and other Cluster C disorders tend to be seen more often (Kennedy, 2000). We suggest use of the Structured Clinical Interview for DSM—Personality Disorders (SCID-P; Spitzer, Williams, Gibbon, & First, 1990) as an efficient instrument to assess for the presence of personality disorders among older adults.

Evaluating the degree of problem complexity and severity in people of racial and ethnic minorities entails (among other factors) accurate communication and understanding between the clinician and client. The examiner needs to know how to interact with people from racial and ethnic minorities in a manner that conveys respect and creates a positive connection. The research that has examined mental health differences among ethnically diverse groups has found that race/ethnicity can play a large role in an individuals' conceptualization of their mental health and the manifestation of mental disorders (e.g., Shiang, Kjellander, Huang, & Bogumill, 1998). For example, schizophrenia is often diagnosed in African Americans. This diagnostic frequency could reflect misunderstanding and misinterpretation in the assessment of people whose cultural roots stem from an ethnic minority population. This cultural misunderstanding may be a factor in R.W.'s previous experience with the mental health field, wherein her presentation, which shows many signs of disturbances in cognition and judgment, may have been misinterpreted.

Minority clients (especially Asian Americans and Latinos) may present diffuse and vague physical/somatic symptoms as representations of unexpressed psychological conflicts and struggles. Psychological problems are not well tolerated in many minority cultures, so that members may find more support by focusing on and expressing their struggles as if they were physical and medical expressions of dysfunction. Such expressions may delay the verbal clarification and identification of more central problems of a social, interpersonal, and psychological nature. Thus the incorporation of specific cultural beliefs and behaviors into standard clinical assessment is suggested (Shiang et al., 1998) to differentiate between primarily medical and psychological problems. Such an assessment of R.W. may help prioritize the focus of treatment and help us determine if additional medical treatments are indicated. Identifying the degree to which cultural values and attitudes may prevent supportive contact with family and friends, thereby intensifying the patient's sense of loss and isolation, may also help us better estimate how impaired the patient is within a cultural norm. Once again, the results are likely to emphasize the importance of treatment that focuses on social support and facilitating social attachments.

For persons who immigrate to the United States, another assessment issue that arises in determining symptom severity is immigration history. Topics to be explored in this area include (1) what brought the individual (or his or her family) to the United States, (2) the length of time in this country, (3) the subsequent experience of cultural change, and (4) the current level of acculturation. For example, recent research has found that Mexican-born Mexican Americans had significantly lower prevalence rates across a wide range of disorders then U.S.-born Mexican Americans (Hansen, Pepitone-Arreola-Rockwell, & Greene, 2000).

Coping Style

The STS framework places coping style on a continuum from more internally to more externally oriented ways of coping. As suggested in the general literature on STS, the MMPI-2 can be used to evaluate status on this continuum (Gaw & Beutler, 1995; see Chapter 3). Scales indicating externalizing tendencies are Pd, Pa, and Ma, whereas D, Pt, Si suggest more internalizing tendencies. A number of clinical indicators may indicate a preference for internal or external methods of coping. For example, older adults who evidence introverted, withdrawn, and denying ways of coping may be better-suited for more insight-oriented treatments. Those who evidence more blaming, aggressive, and manipulative behavior may respond more readily to treatments emphasizing behavior and symptom change. Although it is true that most of the work examining the relation between the MMPI and STS variables has been done on the MMPI-1, several recent studies have used the MMPI-2 (Beutler et al., 2000; Beutler, Harwood, Alimohamed, & Malik, 2002; Karno, Beutler, & Harwood, in press).

Coping styles are often tied to cultural belief systems: The culture often dictates the manner in which individuals should respond to a given situation (Shiang et al., 1998). For example, does the situation call for an externalized coping style? The resources of the individual and his or her family/extended family, the resources available through the larger community, as well as the specific cultural group all contribute to the individual's ability to cope with adversity. It is likely that different coping styles characterize different cultural groups. Asian Americans may be more likely to use internalizing styles of coping, whereas Latinos and African Americans may be more inclined toward externalizing ones. Placing R.W.'s coping style within such a cultural framework would suggest that she may receive less support for some of her coping tendencies (e.g., withdrawal and isolation) than for others. These less-supported patterns may be indicative of higher levels of impairment than would be indicated by test scores alone. The need for intensive and continuing treatments would therefore be indicated.

Resistance

Resistance refers to the tendency to defend against control and intrusion from outside forces. This construct presents interesting issues when considered in relation to older adults. On the one hand, we (and others) have observed that many older adults are fiercely independent and prefer to take care of matters on their own. These individuals may never make their way to traditionally offered mental health services but, if they do, they may present with some resistance tendencies. Conversely, but often in concert, many older adults respond to mental health professionals with deferential tendencies. This deference seems to be related to generational developmental experiences, also known as cohort effects, that tended to elevate professionals to positions of great respect. A cautionary note: These are clearly generalizations, and individual cases will vary as greatly as they do with younger adult populations.

Some writers have discussed the possibility of older adults resisting treatment from providers much younger in age (Newton, Brauer, Gutmann, & Grunes, 1986; Newton & Lazarus, 1992). I (FS) have termed this the "Sonny boy" phenomenon, as in "Sonny boy, how would you know about that?" It is also possible that clinicians may induce resistance by responding to older clients in a somewhat paternalistic fashion. I (FS) can recall supervising a student therapist who, without any conscious awareness on her part, talked to her older client differently from her middle-aged client—more specifically, she verged toward "baby talk" with the older client.

Beutler, Moleiro, and Talebi (2002) reviewed the literature on the topic of resistance in psychotherapy and its assessment. Based on this review, the Therapeutic Reactance Scale (TRS) can be used as an instrument to assess this construct. This scale has been used reliably with older adults (Beutler et al., 2000). We also suggest attention to client behavior as a method of gathering important converging evidence. Beutler, Moleiro, and Talebi (2002) suggest that trait-like resistant behavior may be indicated by a history of difficulty in taking direction, tendencies toward stubbornness and obstructiveness, and difficulties in working cooperatively in groups. More state-like manifestations of resistance spawned by therapy may include anger or resentment expressed toward the therapy or therapist, low compliance with suggestions, or avoidance of difficult therapeutic issues.

Many people from racial and ethnic minorities have had negative interactions with social service agencies and view therapy as an extension of "the system." There is also a need to render mental health services for people from racial and ethnic minorities more culturally competent. For example, understanding the definitions of health and disease in a particular ethnic group would promote competence. In the case of R.W., it would be advantageous to learn how her family and "boyfriend" perceive the mental health system in order to know whether the intensive, continuing treatment that is indicated would be tolerated and supported.

It is noteworthy that the DSM-IV addresses many of these ethnic and cultural issues in establishing a diagnosis, including the role of culture in the expression and evaluation of symptoms and the impact of culture on the therapeutic relationship (American Psychiatric Association, 1994). It does not speak at length, however, about the relationship of these factors to treatment. In contrast, the TRS, drawn from the MMPI-2, is specifically developed to assess readiness for, and receptivity to, treatment. This instrument may work well with people from racial and ethnic minorities as well as older adults, indicating when they are ready to enter into a therapeutic relationship and to commit to a course of treatment.

Distress Level

Evaluation of distress level is important to the STS process because clients with low levels of distress may have little motivation for change, and those overly high levels may be unable to engage in therapeutic activities. We have mentioned the BSI and MMPI-2 as evaluative tools previously; these yield information on levels of distress, as described in previous discussions of this domain. Additionally, we recommend the Geriatric Depression Scale (GDS; Yesavage et al., 1983) as a useful instrument for measuring distress in older adults. The GDS comes in the original 30-item yes–no format, as well as briefer iterations, including a four-item short form. The GDS has evidenced good reliability and validity as a measure of depression and would probably show high association with summary scores such as the Global Severity Index of the BSI (see Scogin, Rohen, & Bailey, 2000 for a review of the GDS).

Assessing distress in people of racial and ethnic minorities is a multifaceted task. In discussing race, ethnicity, and psychopathology, Gray-Little

(1995) posits that when race and ethnic groups are thought of as distinct cultural groups, there is little reason to believe that particular levels of distress and psychopathology are inherent to the cultural features themselves. Thus there is no rationale for assuming that one group's culture causes psychopathology more than another, although cultural values and expectations may help shape the nature and course of the problems. However, when members of an ethnic group are differentiated from others in the same society and occupy a subordinate position, they are considered to be part of a minority group. To the extent that minority groups are thought of as having disadvantaged status in the social structure, individual members might be expected to have higher levels of distress. Thus culture and ethnicity are separated by the subjugation of a group, and this subjugation may lead to distress (Gray-Little, 1995; Shiang et al., 1998). This factor undoubtedly will complicate the treatment of R.W.: She is disenfranchised by virtue of her ethnic background, and she is all the more disenfranchised because she is isolated even within this group.

The assessment of acculturation level is also important to determine. The concept of acculturative stress (Berry & Annis, 1974) indicates that certain behaviors often occur during the process of acculturation, such as anxiety and depression, feelings of marginality and alienation, heightened psychosomatic symptom level, and identity confusion. A mental health practitioner must be aware of these possible cultural-related stress reactions as they may affect the clinical picture.

The clinical interview has been suggested as the appropriate place to determine the impact of ethnicity on level of distress (see Chapter 4). However, many argue that diagnosticians and clinicians are not familiar with manifestations of distress and coping in people from racial and ethnic minorities. The American Psychological Association has attempted to address this lacuna by providing guidelines that list the knowledge and skills needed to provide effective assessment and intervention to diverse populations (American Psychological Association, 1990).

Assessment of Additional Characteristics

A number of other topics have been identified as worthy of consideration in the assessment of older adults and people from racial and ethnic minorities. Two excellent sources that cover issues of older adults include Lichtenberg's (1999) *Handbook of Assessment in Clinical Gerontology* and Zarit and Zarit's (1998) *Mental Disorders in Older Adults: Fundamentals of Assessment and Treatment*. We have chosen to highlight two factors encountered in assessing some older adults: fatigue and cognitive impairment. Assessing the dimensions of the STS model with older clients will almost certainly occasion consideration of these issues. In regard to people from racial and ethnic minorities, we focus on three major components of assessment: ethnic identity, understanding the role of culture, and determining the appropriate methods to assess personality.

Fatigue in the Elderly

The variability in health status among older adults is considerable. For some robust elders, completing a comprehensive assessment of STS relevant dimensions, using separate instruments for each dimension, will present no real challenge. However, as physical frailty increases, so does the likelihood that fatigue will become an issue. In our work, we regularly plan for multiple sessions of assessment for frail elders. A comprehensive assessment of STS factors would probably entail two 1–1.5-hour assessment sessions. This estimate assumes the use of separate instruments for determining the status of each dimension. One alternative is to give the self-contained form of the STS, which requires no more than 40 minutes of patient or clinician time (see Chapter 3). Of course, in any of these cases, the clinician performing the assessment should closely monitor the person for signs of fatigue. Furthermore, efforts should be made to minimize unnecessary effort by the older respondent. Measures that offer simplified response formats, enlarged typeface, and brief versions are recommended.

Cognitive Impairments in the Elderly

Age-related changes in episodic and working memory are a fact of life (e.g., Salthouse, 1996). However, the degree of change experienced by older adults varies greatly. For those elders experiencing mild and moderate cognitive impairment, certain adaptations can facilitate the assessment process. As mentioned earlier, selecting instruments with simple response formats is recommended. Classic examples of this simplicity are the Geriatric Depression Scale (GDS; Sheikh & Yesavage, 1986) and the Beck Depression Inventory (BDI; Beck, Ward, Mendelson, Mock, & Erbaugh, 1961). The BDI uses a multiple-response format that can prove confusing for elders with age-related cognitive impairments. We have witnessed some older adults become locked in a repetitive loop of rereading the response options on the BDI, because they could not simultaneously read and recall. In contrast, the GDS uses a yes–no response format. Few older adults have difficulty in responding to yes–no or true–false formats. The major complaint we hear from older respondents regarding the GDS is that the response format is *too* limiting, as in "My answer is somewhere between yes and no—I can't say yes *or* no." For such persons, a more detailed measure such as the BDI may be best.

Another compensation we often use with older adults is oral presentation of material. This format is particularly helpful for respondents who have impairments in working memory, vision difficulties, and/or poor literacy. We offer respondents a copy of the instrument to follow along, if they wish, and we have a placard available with the possible responses (e.g., yes–no, true–false, Likert-type scale). This format requires skill on the part of the assessor. He or she must be able to pace the reading properly, create a comfortable atmosphere for ease in responding to troubling items, and be able to redirect loquacious responders. Oral presentation also requires less effort by the older respondent, thus producing fewer issues with fatigue.

Special Considerations with People of Ethnic Minorities

Several questions arise as our discussion considers the impact of ethnicity on personality assessment. What constitutes membership in an ethnic group? How do we address the relation between culture and racial and ethnic minority status in assessment? What types of personality assessment instruments and techniques yield the best information regarding personality assessment of people from racial and ethnic minorities?

Ethnic Identity. It is difficult to determine the impact of ethnicity on personality assessment, in part, because there is still debate in the literature over what constitutes ethnicity (Phinney, 1996). Currently, ethnicity is determined by self-identification. This means is problematic because persons from a particular ethnic group may differ in how fully they identify with their ethnic group. Several investigators have developed models of ethnic identity and instruments that accompany their theories. The models and scales were developed for either one ethnic group or were developed to apply across all ethnic minority groups. Some examples of ethnic identity theories that have accompanying scales are the following: White Racial Identity Development Theory (Helms, 1990), the White Racial Identity Scale (Helms & Carter, 1990), the Nigrescence Identity Model (Cross, 1978, 1991), and the Cross Racial Identity Scale (Vandiver, Cross, Worrell, & Fhagen-Smith, 2002). There is also the Minority Identity Development Model (Atkinson, Morten, & Sue, 1983), developed to apply across ethnic groups, and the Multigroup Ethnic Identity Measure (Phinney, 1992), developed to assess ethnic identity across all ethnic groups. Despite the increase in instruments that measures ethnic identification, there is debate regarding how well the existing scales achieve their objectives. Often the scales have not been fully developed or have not found widespread use in clinical practice. As a result, to date, there are no instruments that indicate whether ethnic identification is central to understanding personality in a given person.

Understanding the Role of Culture. Culture is another key concept in the personality assessment of older adults and people from racial and ethnic minorities. Everyone is raised within a culture. Thus culture influences each one of us by shaping how we see ourselves and others. Culture has been defined in a variety of ways; Betancourt and Lopez (1993) examined the study of culture in American psychology and found over 100 definitions of culture. We like Shiang and colleagues' (1998) definition of culture as "a shared belief system, a set of values, a common his/herstory, symbols, as well as preferred ways of behaving" (p. 184). Culture is passed to us through family and community. Multiple cultural layers, from of our immediate environment, which includes family, to the larger society in which we live, influence us. Personality assessment should emphasize the uniqueness of the individual and the diversity within racial and ethnic minority groups by its incorporation of different cultural views and values as well as sociocultural milieus (Okazaki & Sue, 1995).

Assessment Methods. As previously discussed, researchers are often displeased with the instruments available for assessing personality; however, there are few empirically derived alternatives. Personality assessment measures are developed to provide objective information about personality. There is an implicit assumption that personality instruments are designed to yield valid information regarding personality constructs across all racial and ethnic groups (Gray-Little, 1995). Dana (1993), in his discussion of multicultural assessment issues, divides assessment instruments into those representing emic and etic perspectives. An *emic* approach evaluates behaviors within a culture, using rules derived from that culture, whereas an *etic* approach applies a single, universal standard across groups. A criticism of the etic approach is that a "true" universal standard is not applied. In fact, instruments that use the etic approach were developed for use with middle-income Caucasians and subsequently applied to people from racial and ethnic minorities. Dana advocates for the use of more measures that use an emic approach. Unfortunately, the instruments Dana identifies are projective measures, such as picture–story techniques, inkblots, and drawings. These projective measures, rely on subjective interpretation and require extensive training; thus they are susceptible to the same biases as the etic measures. It is beyond the scope of this chapter to review all of these personality assessment measures. However, it is important to state that a particular test is not inherently culturally sensitive or biased. The skill of the assessor/interpreter and the use of the measure must be considered.

SUMMARY

In this chapter we have discussed how the Systematic Treatment Selection model can be used with special populations, in particular, older adults and people from ethnic and racial minorities. We suggest that researchers as well as practitioners need to be alert to defining the populations they serve in ways that are appropriate and respectful. To this end, we define key concepts such as age and ethnicity. We also highlight the diversity within and between both special populations. Additionally, we cover an important component of working with special populations: use of the mental health system. Older adults and people from racial and ethnic minorities are considered to use the mental health care system less often than others. The relation between utilization and access and is a complicated issue, however. There has been a stigma attached to using mental health services in both populations. Also, historically, mental health providers have not actively sought ways to reach these populations and/or have not treated them in culturally appropriate ways. Fortunately, these undesirable patterns are changing, as mental health practitioners become more aware of ways to engage older adults and people from racial and ethnic minorities and as the pool of persons who can work with these populations increases.

We also discuss how the dimensions of the STS model can be applied to older adults and people from racial and ethnic minorities and which instruments are suitable assessment tools of these dimensions. The appropriate assessment of personality in these special populations cannot be accomplished simply by issuing a list of culturally sensitive instruments. Nor can this issue be resolved by cataloguing a series of abnormal behaviors that clinicians should interpret in a culturally sensitive and nonpathological manner. Moreover, communication between clinicians and scholars would be further complicated by a proliferation of age- or culture-specific instruments.

In this chapter, we have made specific recommendations regarding personality assessment of special populations based on the STS model; however, it is important to highlight issues that cut across all the suggestions discussed: assessor bias, education and training for working with diverse populations, and a better understanding of the role of moderator variables such as age and socioeconomic status (Gray-Little, 1995). Despite the frequent association between psychopathology and socioeconomic status, very little attention has been given to understanding the relation. Thus we appear to be culturally sensitive when statements are made that the differences between groups are due to socioeconomic status instead of race; yet we are no closer to understanding the relation between personality and racial and ethnic differences. Building on the work of Beutler and Clarkin (1990), we suggest that researchers and clinicians must be willing to learn new skills and ways of thinking, such that each person is treated as an individual rather than on the basis of age or racial stereotypes.

12

Integrating and Applying Assessment Information
DECISION MAKING, PATIENT FEEDBACK, AND CONSULTATION

Richard W. Lewak and R. Sean Hogan

The psychological assessment of personality and psychopathology began on a large scale during World War I with the goal of screening out psychologically disturbed conscripts. Though heavily utilized, the early rationally and intuitively developed assessment instruments were quickly shown to be invalid (Greene, 2000). In response, psychologists in the 1940s and 1950s relied heavily on empirical, atheoretical methods to develop assessment instruments (Friedman, Lewak, Nichols, & Webb, 2001). Vigilant against the intrusion of tester bias, psychologists developed a medical, objective, and scientific approach to psychological assessment. Consequently, the language of psychological reports, reflecting this new paradigm, became psychometric, statistical, objective, distant, and unilateral (Fisher, 1994). Psychiatrists requested psychological testing without consultation with psychologists, psychologists selected tests and wrote reports without consulting with psychiatrists, and no one consulted with the patients. In fact, test results were rarely shared with patients, and reports tended to by highly technical, often statistical, and almost always so judgmental that they were antithetical to therapeutic alliance building (e.g., "Mrs. F. tests as passive–aggressive, dependent, and narcissistic with paranoid traits").

This empirical, objective, and statistical approach to assessment was a clear improvement over the rational intuitive approach, though it clearly had undesirable consequences and, even early on, critics. They held that empiricism had gone too far, losing the uniqueness of the individual in the pursuit of the rigorous scientific method. Fisher (1994), for example, had suggested in the 1970s that patients should become more involved in the assessment process, discussing the purpose of their psychological assessment with the testing psychologist. Timothy Leary (1957) suggested that the patient's own viewpoint about his or her psychological condition could add incremental validity. Iconoclastically, he even suggested that the assessment process should aim to make patients feel "wiser and good" about themselves. The early critics, however, had little effect on the reigning paradigm of pure scientific objectivity.

Over the past 15 years, a more integrated (Beutler & Berren, 1995), collaborative (Finn & Tonsanger, 1992), and feedback-oriented (Lewak, Marks, & Nelson, 1991) approach to assessment and treatment planning has developed. This new approach was partly in response to changing views on the purpose of psychological assessment and therapist–patient interactions, and partly in response to changes in consumer laws. Still grounded in empiricism, this approach seeks to provide a more complete, integrated, and humanistic assessment of the individual. This new paradigm reflects a number of converging issues. For example, freedom of information legislation now makes it far more likely that patients will gain access to their records. The psychologist's code of ethics reflects this requirement and suggests that psychologists provide some feedback to patients as part of the assessment procedure (American Psychological Association, 1992). Reports written in the traditional style increase the chance of patients feeling judged or even attacked and criticized, with possible legal ramifications and potential harm to the public standing of psychologists.

Managed care also has provided an impetus to the acceptance of this new paradigm. As cost represents an increasingly important variable in the mental health equation, the efficacy of assessment must be unquestionable (see Groth-Marnat, 1999a). Reports that are accurate but balanced, reflecting strengths as well as vulnerabilities, and that provide concrete therapeutic strategies that are shared with patients are more likely to be accepted by patients. Assessment reports that patients and referral sources find useful will lead to greater demand and the greater likelihood that the cost of assessment will be born by managed care. Integrative assessment clearly reflects the new paradigm in assessment psychology by showing, for example, how a patient's current defenses are understandably linked to early painful experiences, describing patient strengths as well as vulnerabilities, and articulating practical therapeutic strategies. It incorporates the collaborative approach developed by Fisher (1994) and Finn and Tonsager (1992) and the feedback approach developed by Lewak and colleagues (1991) in providing a more thorough, balanced, and therapeutically useful assessment.

Though this approach to assessment has been shown to be therapeutically useful without a loss of validity, few books provide the language and constructs of the new approach (see Finn & Tonsager, 1992; Lewak et al., 1991). Too often psychologists present results of a psychological assessment in a way that leaves a fractionated "part–object" view of the testee (Ganellen, 1996). The rote reporting of results from each of the tests, often without integrating contradictions or making the test results relevant to the individual, has a tendency to not only confuse the reader, but also to a distorted impression of the patient (Fisher, 1994).

Part of the problem may be due to the way that assessment psychologists are trained. Many doctoral programs specialize in one particular test over other tests, so that the programs become associated with specialists in one particular area of assessment (e.g., the University of Minnesota emphasizes the Minnesota Multiphasic Personality Inventory; MMPI). Consequently, many psychologists lack the integrative skills, particularly when administering a battery of tests. The problem is complicated further by the fact that integrating such a wide array of data in a clear and consistent manner is a challenging exercise. Integrated assessment can be difficult for graduate psychology students to learn, partly because they often lack the clinical expertise and judgment necessary to make the inferences required to integrate data from several tests with history and the presenting problem. Unfortunately, this problem is also compounded by the fact that there is a lack of research in the art of test integration. Ganellen (1996) highlighted this lack of research focus by pointing out that out of 16,000 books and articles published since 1947 on two of the most commonly used assessment instruments, the Rorschach and MMPI, fewer than 50 studies examined the relation between the two tests, less than one-third of a percent of the total. Little wonder that psychologists are often not well prepared to integrate test data.

Even when psychologists are well versed in a number of tests, they often have a tendency to present the results in a piecemeal manner using global, general terms. They may be unprepared or feel overwhelmed by the task, or they may feel that they are "not allowed" to integrate test results with the collateral and feedback data as a basis for generating inferences about the particular patient. To deal with data overload, many psychologists, when using the MMPI-2, for example, copy the descriptors associated with a particular scale elevation or code type without reconciling any discrepancies or generating higher-order hypotheses about a patient. For example, a psychological report might state: "Mrs. Smith scored highly on scale 4 on the MMPI-2, suggesting alienation, distrust, and a rebelliousness toward authority. She also scored highly on scale 7 of the MMPI-2, which measures conformity, anxiety, guilt, and self-doubt." These statements initially appear contradictory, yet both can be true. The higher-order integration in this case is not made: namely, that it is probable that Mrs. Smith, when anxious, guilty, and self-doubting, tends to act out as a way of relieving anxiety and stress, and then experiences guilt and remorse without any resulting behavior change.

The purpose of this book is to provide a conceptual framework and the "nuts and bolts" of how to conduct an integrated assessment. This chapter addresses how to apply the assessment information by first integrating it, and then using the integrated data to provide feedback to the patient or referral source. Guidelines are provided on how to generate higher-order inferences from the assessment and historical and feedback data, with the aim of recommending the most efficient therapeutic strategies and collaborative help to the referral source.

BENEFITS OF INTEGRATIVE ASSESSMENT

Assessment data that are thoroughly integrated provide a more relevant appraisal of the individual and thus generate feedback that is more applicable to the goal of achieving therapeutic change and answering the referral question. In contrast, the traditional rote style of reporting assessment results may leave the reader confused as to which symptoms to target with the greatest overall therapeutic efficiency. In a managed care environment, effective, short-term psychotherapy is often required, so it is critical to understand which set of symptoms could best be targeted for maximum therapeutic benefit. Using the above example of Mrs. Smith to show how therapy can be more effectively linked to the assessment data, its aim would be to teach her to recognize when stress was building and which particular stressors were most anxiety provoking to her. The next step would be to teach her how to recognize the signs of escalating anxiety, and with it, guilt and self-doubt, leading to acting-out behaviors, so that she could identify alternative coping mechanisms. In this example, an efficient therapeutic strategy linked to her assessment results would entail teaching Mrs. Smith how to prevent the buildup of anxiety by anticipating it. In addition, helping her understand how she might have developed impulsive tension-reducing defenses as a way of dealing with stress, perhaps because as a child her caretakers were unreliable or absent, could improve her self-esteem and reduce her guilt, which might aid in the development of more mature defenses.

Integrative assessment is thus likely to help the referral source provide the patient with better self-understanding and therefore better self-esteem, and with it, more trust in the assessment process and psychotherapy. Too often, patients have felt criticized or judged by the feedback from the assessment data. It is difficult for a patient to feel understood and supported if he or she is called "manipulative, dependent, and passive–aggressive." On the other hand, telling the patient that he or she "has difficulty trusting others and consequently may feel a need to manipulate in order to get needs met," for example, is more likely to be accepted, particularly if this feedback is integrated in a manner that reveals how his or her early childhood conditioning experiences have precipitated such distrust. This kind of integrated client-oriented interpretation, when shared with patients, is more likely to make them feel validated, more completely understood, and therefore, potentially more invested in therapeutic change.

TEST INTEGRATION

Once tests have been administered, scored, and the results determined to be valid, the complex work of psychological integration begins. Accurate, relevant integration is a crucial prerequisite to providing useful client feedback and consulting with the referral source. However, integration can be daunting, as information from just one test—for example, the MMPI-2—can appear to be contradictory. Ten clinical scales covary against the backdrop of numerous other subscales and content scales, sometimes revealing divergent data. An individual tested using the MMPI-2 can obtain a clinical profile suggesting an absence of depression, with an average score on scale 2 (Depression), yet obtain an elevated Depression Content scale that suggests overt admission of depression. This kind of within-test contradiction is difficult to resolve, and between-test contradictions can be even more problematic. It is hard for a clinician to have interpretive confidence when the MMPI-2 data suggests the use of histrionic defenses (e.g., repression and denial) by an elevation on scale 3 (Hysteria), but the Rorschach reveals a positive Depression Index (DEPI), suggesting pessimism, guilt, and self-deprecatory attitudes (Exner, 2002). Too often, psychologists are unable to integrate such disparate data, so they tend to go with their initial or primary clinical impression and fit the data around their preconceived clinical construct.

Test integration, although more difficult, is more efficient and clinically useful. The integrative process involves examining discriminant and incremental data generated from a particular test and from different tests, and combining them with history, clinical, and feedback data. Once these data have been assimilated and refined, hypotheses are then generated about possible etiology, such as early childhood conditioning experiences, significant traumas, and other reasons why the patient is vulnerable to certain precipitating circumstances. How can this process of integration be done most efficiently?

STEPS IN TEST INTEGRATION

We have identified five steps by which clinicians can effectively integrate data from multiple tests to formulate a comprehensive assessment report that provides the kind of clinical information that leads to treatment interventions and patient participation:

1. Generating preliminary anchor hypotheses.
2. Refining the hypotheses.
3. Embellishing the anchor hypotheses.
4. Integrating history and assessment data.
5. Preparing feedback for the patient.

Generating Preliminary Anchor Hypotheses

We suggest that psychologists skilled in any well-validated and accepted personality test use the data from that test to create an "anchor" or "backdrop" hypotheses about the patient. These hypotheses form the foundation upon which the rest of the personality assessment description will be built. We feel that the MMPI-2 codetype can form an ideal anchor or backdrop for the preliminary hypotheses about the patient. Our preference for the MMPI-2 as the primary anchor stems from three facts: (1) It is the most widely used and researched objective personality inventory in the world, (2) its codetype data is readily summarized in interpretive manuals into concrete, easy-to-grasp personality constructs that include suggestions for etiology and treatment (e.g., Friedman et al., 2001; Greene, 2000; Lewak et al., 1991), and (3) its validity measures are considered superior to those of other personality tests (Lewak & Hogan, 2001; Pope, Butcher, & Seelen, 1993). Data from other tests can then flush out, enrich, and expand on the basic codetype data. For example, an MMPI-2 "2/7 codetype" predicts an anxious, agitated, guilt-prone depression in a neurotic individual who does not act out. Additional scales on the MMPI-2 may also be elevated, perhaps refining the way the anxious depression will be manifested.

It should be noted that other psychologists might prefer another instrument, such as the Rorschach, Millon Clinical Multiaxial Inventory–III (MCMI-III), California Psychological Inventory (CPI), Psychological Assessment Inventory (PAI), and so on, as their anchor test. Regardless of which instrument is the starting or anchor point, the initial hypothesis-building stage means that secondary and supplementary scale elevations are temporarily put aside while the assessment psychologist works with the preliminary hypothesis (e.g., of an anxious, agitated depression).

Examining data from the other tests should generate further preliminary hypotheses. Using the above example of the MMPI-2 2/7code type as the anchor, the assessing psychologist would then look to see if the Rorschach also suggests anxiety, depression, and guilt. Is there evidence of anxiety and depression on the PAI, MCMI-III, Thematic Apperception Test (TAT), or some other measure of personality? What other attributes can be added to the basic anchor of the 2/7 code type from the other test data? At this stage, the clinician should avoid a theoretical or clinically based interpretation about the individual.

This initial hypothesis-generating stage should be data driven. For example, in the 2/7 code type case, the clinician may assume that an anxious depression is clearly evident. Questions about what precipitated it and why the individual may be vulnerable to depression, anxiety, guilt, as well as other deeper questions, should be answered later in the integrative process. These questions are highly relevant, not only to the creation of a clear understanding of the patient, but also to highlight the therapeutic strategies that would be most helpful. However, the initial aim is to create a "big picture" of the individual while systematically integrating the test data.

In this phase, it is crucial that the assessing psychologist avoid the "confirmatory bias" (Ganellen, 1996; Haverkamp, 1993), which is the tendency for the clinician to form a superficial opinion about the patient and then to look for confirmation of the bias in the data. Unfortunately, testing data are plentiful and complex enough that this bias readily avails itself to a data-overloaded clinician. Students in psychology typically make this confirmatory bias error, often rushing to diagnose a patient before they have fully examined all of the data.

To summarize the procedures for this first step of data integration:

1. Collect and tabulate the test data. Use one test to generate an anchor or backdrop hypothesis for the rest of the data. We recommend the MMPI-2 be used to create the anchor hypothesis because of its robust validity scales and because the code-type information is readily summarized into a concrete, easy-to-grasp personality construct. The code type defines the basic description of the individual. For example, the 2/7 code type can be seen as an "anxious depression," the "2/4" as a "trapped depression," the "2/3" as a "somatizing, smiling depression," and so on.
2. Add the incremental, convergent, and discriminant data from other tests administered to build a fuller beginning picture of the patient.
3. Avoid the confirmatory bias trap. Do not be more open or closed to selective evidence of a particular diagnostic hunch.

Refining the Hypotheses

In the second stage of test integration, clinicians should begin to refine their hypotheses by incorporating the primary data from the other tests. Points of agreement within the results add incremental validity to the working hypotheses about the individual, whereas data that seem to disagree with the anchor hypothesis call upon the clinician to use his or her clinical skills to refine the original anchor hypothesis. For example, an individual in a child custody evaluation obtained a somewhat elevated MMPI-2 L (Lie) scale score (T = 63), and a moderate elevation on scale 6 (Paranoia) (T = 64). The anchor hypothesis would describe a somewhat rigid, naive individual who is overly sensitive to criticism and possibly exhibiting paranoid traits. The suggestions of paranoia are strengthened by elevations on the scales that indicate paranoia on both the MCMI-III and the PAI. However, a closer look at the Paranoia subscales on the MMPI-2 reveals low scores on Pa 1 (Persecutory Ideas) and Pa 2 (Poignancy) but a significant elevation on Pa 3 (Naiveté), suggesting less paranoia, while confirming a rigidity of values, self-righteousness, and a tendency to be punitive and unforgiving. In the clinical presentation, the individual does not exhibit paranoid traits, and none of his MMPI-2 critical items suggests paranoia. The Rorschach and TAT also do not reveal paranoid ideation. The individual's clinical presentation suggests a somewhat rigid individual, overly sensitive to criticism, whose history reveals that both parents tended to be critical, somewhat demanding and punitive.

The assessing psychologist's clinical skills are then utilized to help him or her modify the initial anchor hypothesis of paranoia. It is well known that an individual with a paranoid personality can manifest paranoia as a rigidity of values and a hypersensitivity to criticism, without florid paranoid ideation (Shapiro, 1976). In such a manner, the working hypothesis about an individual is refined based on within-test data, between-test data, and history, using clinical skills. This integrative process is particularly relevant in the psychotherapeutic recommendations, because suggestions of paranoia in the report, without alerting the referring colleague to the additional finding that the individual's paranoid personality structure is egosyntonic, could lead to ineffective therapeutic strategies. In this particular example, rather than focus on the treatment of paranoid ideation, the psychotherapy recommendations should focus on helping the patient become less self-critical and therefore, over time, less critical of others.

In general, interpretive confidence grows when different tests converge on the same hypotheses. When test data seem to disagree, however, the clinician should use his or her clinical skills to blend the contradictions rather than dismissing one of the findings. For example, predictions made on the basis of one test, suggestive of hypomanic traits and excessive energy, can be refined on the basis of other assessment data that suggest low energy and depression. Using clinical judgment, the assessor can blend the data into an interpretation of moodiness, tension, and irritability, with a possible vulnerability to cyclothymic episodes. Using another example, let's say that assessment data from one test suggest that an individual is suffering from a severe depression, whereas another test identifies histrionic features as the prominent finding. The psychologist then blends these clinical data into a formulation that suggests the presence of a "smiling depression," with the histrionic defenses operating to deny the depression, leading to numerous somatic symptoms and a bland, conforming presentation. In a similar manner, one test may suggest acting out and narcissism, whereas another test suggests strong needs for approval, leading to a prediction of a role-playing, subtly manipulative and passive–aggressive individual whose acting out is shaped by the need for social approval. In this manner, the assessing psychologist begins to refine the initial hypotheses by using clinical experience and judgment to integrate both the convergent and divergent data from the tests administered.

Embellishing the Anchor Hypothesis

Once the anchor hypothesis has been refined with the data from the other tests, the assessing psychologist should continue to further enrich the personality picture by examining the secondary scales, subscales, and various indices of the tests administered. Ideally, the data from the additional scales and subscales will confirm the anchor hypothesis—though the clinician must continue to avoid the confirmatory bias mentioned earlier. In most cases, subscale and secondary data will change the description of how a particular attribute is manifested, rather than changing the basic assumptions about the individual. For example, a personality picture suggesting an anxious, depressed, ruminative, guilt-prone individual may change slightly when subscale data are added that suggest a narcissistic, dependent, and manipulative style. This new data would have to be articulated against the backdrop of the anxiety, depression, and guilt. Blended together, using clinical experience and judgment, the picture forms of an individual who deals with anxiety by eliciting caretaking behavior through guilt inducement and passive dependency. The narcissism and manipulativeness are masked by a presentation of self-effacing guilt with a tendency to undermine others' anger by an exaggerated self-criticism. This level of integrative step is often quite difficult because it involves using advanced theoretical and clinical skills to blend data in the process of further elucidating the backdrop hypothesis.

Integrating History and Assessment Data

At this stage, the assessing psychologist has generated preliminary hypotheses about the individual that have been somewhat refined and embellished by data from subscales and other tests. Once the first three steps of integration have been completed, the psychologist usually is prepared to develop a hypothesis as to possible etiology, such as any early childhood conditioning experiences that may be associated with the interpreted assessment data. It is useful to think of the history-taking portion of the assessment process as a chance to let patients "tell their story." In addition, this aspect presents another opportunity to collect key data that can assist in further higher-order refinements of the backdrop hypothesis.

Few psychologists, regardless of their orientation, would dispute the importance of early childhood experiences in the development of personality style, defensive behaviors, and vulnerabilities to the restimulating effects of adult traumas that are similar to past traumas. A person's psychological test results provide an X-ray, so to speak, of his or her current personality organization that can provide clues to the underlying etiological dynamics (Caldwell, 2001; Lewak et al., 1991). The history taking provides the opportunity to look for possible conditioning events or traumatic experiences that might explain the assessment results. For example, the early loss of a parent through death, emotional abandonment, or neglect; the loss of a sense of security or self-esteem through humiliating or denigrating peer experiences; or the loss of basic trust because of an absent, addicted, or sexually abusive parent—all constitute severe trauma. Clinically, we understand that any kind of early traumatic loss or experience tends to make individuals more vulnerable, as adults, when exposed to loss or other events that trigger the emotional "scar tissue" related to the early trauma. It is also understood that frightening events, without a concomitant, soothing experience, can leave a child vulnerable to later experiences of anxiety and emotional insecurity. Being hated or disliked by one's parents, peers, or siblings, for example, or being born with eccentricities or deformities that leave one open to humiliation and ridicule can also be difficult to navigate psychologically in childhood, resulting in psychological "scar tissue" in adulthood.

The history-taking process also involves paying attention to the individual's strengths, noting successful adaptations throughout the life cycle. The assessing psychologist should pay particular attention to self-esteem–enhancing events and successful adaptations in dealing with disruptions and ego blows. Noting positive qualities, strengths, and adaptive abilities is generally not part of interpretive materials, as the majority of assessment training and literature focuses on the pathological interpretation of test results. This problem can be partially addressed by adding tests such as the California Psychological Inventory to the battery, which focuses on adaptive strengths as well as pathology (Consulting Psychologists Press, 1995). There is some literature addressing this issue with the MMPI (see Finn, 1996a; Kunce & Anderson, 1976); in addition, Lewak and colleagues (1991) provide both positive and negative descriptors for the MMPI-2 clinical scale and common code-type constructs, as well as feedback guidelines, etiological hypotheses, and treatment recommendations.

In Lewak and colleagues' (1991) MMPI-2 feedback approach, diagnostic constructs such as depression, hypochondriasis, hysteria, paranoia, hypomania, and so on, are understood using a fear-avoidance paradigm.

This hypothetical etiological paradigm is illustrated in Caldwell (2001), where psychopathology, as revealed by the eight clinical scales (1–4, 6–9) of the MMPI-2, is understood as reflecting an adaptive, fear-avoidance response to certain classes of traumatic events. For example, depression can be seen as an adaptive response to the experience of profound loss. One adaptive way of dealing with loss is to stop wanting, to shut down hope, and to become preoccupied with the avoidance of future loss. In that way, the possibility of further loss is minimized. Pessimism, negativity, and seeing the glass as "half empty" also could be seen as adaptive responses to the avoidance of further loss. Hysteria, with its emphasis on a positive social presentation and needs for approval and validation, could reflect an adaptive response to the fear of emotional pain. Accordingly, the person's need to deny negative reality, with a concomitant need for approval and reassurance, would make sense in the context of having been flooded with emotional pain. Similarly, individuals who exhibit paranoid traits may have experienced episodes of criticism, judgments, or even physical attack that threatened their personal safety. Becoming vigilant, constantly scanning the environment for danger, and inhibiting the expression of wants would make sense in the context of protecting oneself against the possibility of further attack or criticism. Caldwell hypothesized that each of the primary clinical scales of the MMPI-2, for example, can be understood as reflecting adaptive responses to different kinds of trauma (see Table 12.1).

We have found this fear-avoidance paradigm to be useful as a roadmap for the history-taking segment of the assessment, as most of the other tests of personality and psychopathology use the same diagnostic constructs as the MMPI-2. This fear-avoidance paradigm potentially facilitates a more useful history-taking process by alerting the assessing psychologist to possible conditioning experiences that would make more sense of the data and of the individual being tested. This kind of integrative overview should lead to a more empathic yet empirically grounded and sophisticated understanding of the patient. If the assessment data suggest severe depression and low self-esteem, for example, the psychologist should look for evidence in the history of ego-damaging loss. Did the patient experience a profound sense of loss due to a parental death? Or did the sense of loss arise because the patient felt "lost in the shuffle" as the one of many children in a poor family with an alcoholic father? Could the patient have felt emotionally abandoned by one parent and abused by another? Could there have been a somewhat unremarkable history, without obvious severe losses, but rather a continuous series of small blows to the individual's self-esteem or sense of security? The test data reveal a picture of the individual's current psychological state, while the history should explain how that state was created.

Our theoretical perspective is that psychopathology can be best understood as an adaptive response to events that precipitated it. There are empirical data to support such a perspective. For example, 60% of the adoles-

TABLE 12.1. MMPI-2 Scales and Associated Fears, Conditioning Experiences, and Defensive Responses

Scale	Fear	Possible conditioning experience	Defensive response
1	Death, physical attack, illness, or pain	Illness in patient or caretakers	Maintaining physical integrity by overprotecting the body
2	Irretrievable and significant loss	Early losses, deaths, severe setbacks perceived as catastrophic losses	Blocking wanting or needing in order to avoid further loss
3	Emotional pain	Emotionally traumatic events to which the patient responded by denial and shifting the focus of attention	Positivizing unpleasant experiences by selectively blocking inputs (denial, numbness)
4	Rejection, being unwanted or abandoned	Childhood abandonment, parental neglect, narcissistic parents	"Numbing out" emotional responding; not allowing oneself to get emotionally involved to prevent letdown
5	Trait scale: no associated fear		
6	Humiliation, being criticized, evaluated	Critical, judgmental, punitive, threatening, or attacking experiences	Maintaining constant vigilance against attack
7	Shock, unexpected events	Unexpected, frightening events, teasing, unexpected losses, or catastrophes	Thinking ahead and worrying to anticipate onset of shock
8	Hostility, being disliked or despised by those on whom one depends	Hatred, dislike, cruel abuse or neglect	"Shutting down" cognitive processing to avoid unbearable reality
9	Deprivation or failure	Poverty, deprivation, consistently motivating caretakers	Increasing activity level in an attempt to maintain reward schedule
0	Trait scale: no associated fear		

cents in the Marks, Seeman, and Haller (1974) criterion sample who were elevated on scales 6 and 8 of the MMPI (using adolescent norms) experienced a history of "severe thrashings" by their parents. This data suggest a consistent conditioning experience for the "6/8 code type." It is reasonable to hypothesize that a self-protected, distanced, and alienated stance toward others (the essence of the 6/8 code type) makes sense as an adaptive response to such harsh conditions. Furthermore, Marks and colleagues reported that 60% of their adult "3/2 code types" experienced the death of a parent in childhood. The majority of these individuals reported experiencing a secure and loving bond with the lost parent. The development of hysterical defenses such as denial, repression and positivizing, as reflected in the 3/2 code type, would make sense in the context of protecting against the experience of severe loss. Using the constructs outlined in Table 12.1, the assessor can be alerted to look for the anticipated fears, conditioning experiences, and defensive responses that often correlate with the diagnostic constructs represented by the eight major clinical scales of the MMPI-2. The above example illustrates this point, for once a patient has been assessed as having depressive tendencies or paranoid traits, regardless of which tests were used, the constructs outlined in Table 12.1, and further discussed in Lewak and colleagues (1991) and Caldwell (2001), can be applied to facilitate the history-taking and eventual feedback sessions in a more pointed, empathic, and potentially therapeutic manner.

Preparing the Patient for Feedback

Equipped with a history and the integrated assessment results, the psychologist can prepare to conduct a feedback session in order to validate the test results and collaborate with the patient to develop a richer and fuller understanding of his or her personality makeup. Finn (1996a) suggests that the assessment and feedback process can be used as a therapeutic intervention. Alternatively, the assessing psychologist may be preparing a report for, or directly coaching, the referral source on how to give the feedback to the patient, using the principals described below. The purpose of feedback is to validate the patient's psychological experiences, symptoms, behaviors, fears, and anxieties with the objective of determining a collaborative therapeutic strategy.

It is important to understand that an assessment is generally an anxiety-producing experience for most people. It involves the discussion of intensely personal information and usually is somewhat mysterious to the patient, who may fear the vulnerability of feeling somewhat "exposed" in the process. Sometimes people ascribe erroneous meaning to certain questions and procedures involved in an assessment. Accurate and more useful information, along with patient cooperation, is most likely obtained when a patient feels engaged in the process as a collaborator whose ideas and cooperation are taken seriously (Finn, 1996a).

To build the patient's trust and minimize resistance, it is recommended that the assessing psychologist frame the feedback in as positive a light as possible. However, this does not mean "sugar coating" the findings. Rather, the assessor should look for ways in which patients' behaviors can be understood as adaptive, given the conditioning experiences that elicited their defensive and maladaptive behaviors (see Lewak et al., 1991). The essence of the feedback is to reframe, as much as possible, patients' experiences so that they can view themselves and their "problems" in a more positive light. However, in some cases, reframing may not be appropriate. For example, it is important to help acting-out, antisocial, or narcissistic individuals understand how their manipulative or self-centered behaviors are maladaptive—though, even in these cases, it is possible to reframe their behaviors, pointing out how, at one time, these behaviors may have been adaptive, given their experiences. For example, the feedback for a psychopathic individual might proceed as follows:

> "Your profile suggests that you have difficulty trusting others and that you see the world as a 'dog eat dog' place, where you need to have power and control in order to feel good. Because you see the world in such terms, it is easy for you to justify manipulating others and 'getting one up on them,' After all, you feel that others would do the same to you if they could."

In this case, the assessment feedback, although not positive, is framed within the perspective of how it was once adaptive, and therefore may be more readily accepted by the patient.

Providing feedback in an empathic way leads into the topic of therapeutic strategies and behavioral changes that could be more adaptive. Using the example of the psychopath, the assessing psychologist could point out how the individual's tendency to manipulate people leads to others distrusting them and wanting to take advantage of them in a "tit for tat" process. The assessor could then wonder about the kinds of events that could have created the patient's cynical view of the world.

Essentially, the purpose of the feedback is sevenfold:

1. Verify the general accuracy of the test results.
2. Hone, refine, and individualize the results to make them fit the individual's setting, socioeconomic status, and circumstances (e.g., an educated professional with psychopathic traits is likely to present differently and experience different problems from a less educated individual with similar testing results).
3. Validate the patient's experiences, symptoms, and issues against the

backdrop of his or her conditioning experiences and precipitating circumstances.

4. Help the patient feel better by making sense of the symptoms and behaviors in relation to his or her past experiences and recent precipitating circumstances.
5. Collaborate with the patient in creating therapeutic goals that build on his or her strengths.
6. Provide tangible symptom relief and suggestions for ongoing self-help.
7. Help the patient identify potentially stressful situations, given his or her psychological "scar tissue," and develop new, more adaptive coping strategies.

HOW TO CONDUCT A FEEDBACK SESSION

Building Rapport

Rapport building begins prior to an assessment and is recommended to ensure accurate test results. The process of obtaining informed consent offers an initial opportunity to facilitate rapport building, as the patient is informed of the purpose of the testing, how the results will be used, who will have access to the results, and whether or not he or she will have an opportunity to ask questions or receive feedback regarding the results. Done well, this segment can lay the foundation for a more collaborative assessment process, in which the patient is engaged as an active participant in the testing. Finn (1996a) suggests that the assessor and patient meet prior to the assessment process for the purpose of building rapport. He recommends discussing any questions the patient would like answered about the assessment process in order to engage him or her in a more therapeutic and collaborative endeavor. Asking patients questions can be helpful, he notes, such as: "What would you like to learn about yourself from this assessment?" Patient responses to this question vary. Some have a specific complaint, such as, "My doctor thinks I'm depressed, but I'm not sure and I'd like to know"; or, "I'm always tense and worried and I don't know why I can't relax." Others might say something more global, to the effect of, "I want to know more about myself, my vulnerabilities, strengths, and areas that I could work on." Finn recommends engaging the patient in this type of rapport building to utilize the assessment process as a therapeutic intervention.

The patient's questions can help the assessor create a more useful assessment report and recommend more pertinent therapeutic strategies. Typically, the assessment question is asked by the referral source. Sometimes the referral questions are vague, asking for an assessment to "get to know the patient." In other cases, they are more specific, for example, asking about the patient's ability to deal with anger, vulnerability to becoming violent under stress, or suicide potential. Other referral questions may revolve around child custody issues or forensic defense or prosecution matters. In these cases, the potential use of feedback and establishment of a collaborative process is likely to be considerably different. Nevertheless, the same principles apply. For example, in forensic settings, giving attention to rapport building and providing informed consent can increase patient cooperation and the likelihood of getting more accurate and useful data.

The process of giving feedback in order to understand patients better is also applicable when doing integrative assessments, even if the results do not focus as much on therapeutic issues and clinical understanding. The following section focuses on the use of feedback to gain a deeper understanding and the development of more effective therapeutic strategies for dealing with difficult patients. The referral question and presenting problem are relevant for the feedback process, because the assessing psychologist needs to be able to frame the results around a specific purpose—usually to help the patient with growth strategies or the referring source with therapeutic or other recommendations. We discuss issues about specific referral questions later in the chapter.

Beginning Feedback and Addressing Test-Taking Attitudes

When patients first sit down for a feedback session, it is useful to ask them if they feel comfortable with the feedback process, or if they are anxious or apprehensive about it. Inquiries about what could be the "worst case scenario" in the feedback session could help them verbalize any fears and anxieties about how the assessment results might define them in a negative way. This opportunity is particularly important when giving feedback in child custody or work-related situations. Although it is not possible (or desirable) to reassure patients that test results will be benign, it is useful to reassure them that the results will be discussed with them and that they will be able to respond to the clinician's feedback. This assurance will help them feel that they are part of a collaborative process.

Explain that they are going to receive feedback about many aspects of their behavior, emotions, and functioning, and that, in some cases, this feedback may be generally accurate, even though it might overemphasize a particular aspect, whereas in other cases, it might miss the mark completely. Ask them to indicate when the feedback "hits the mark" and when it feels inaccurate. Clearly, patients will not readily accept all of the feedback. However, we have found that most people will accept descriptions of even severe psychopathology if they are phrased in a generally positive or adaptive manner. For example, using the fear-avoidance paradigm explained above, the paranoid patient could be told:

"Your psychological testing suggests that you are experiencing a great

> deal of fear and anxiety around the possibility of being criticized, judged, or even attacked. You may feel so much anxiety and fear that it is hard for you to know whom you can trust. You may find times when your ability to perceive who is your friend or enemy is fairly accurate, but at other times, you may be so fearful that you misjudge people as your enemies when, in fact, they are not."

Worded in this manner, the feedback is more likely to be accepted by the patient. However, if data about a particular set of personality attributes are irrefutable but the patient argues about the data's application to him or her, the assessing psychologist needs to find ways to articulate the psychopathology in less judgmental terms to which the patient can relate.

Some psychologists are comfortable showing patients the various graphs from different assessment instruments, such as the MMPI-2, the PAI, the CPI, and so on. If an assessor is willing to do so, many patients feel more secure knowing that the data are coming from objective, scientific instruments. For example, using the MMPI-2, the clinician might tell the patient: "You answered many questions, some of which you may have thought were unusual. We score your answers on various dimensions of personality," pointing to the 10 clinical scales of the MMPI-2. The assessor then points to the line at T = 50 and says: "Scores around this line are more or less in the average range. The higher you go on any of these dimensions of personality (*pointing to each of the clinical scales*), the stronger the feelings, attributes, or pain you are experiencing." Then, pointing to the validity scales at the left-hand side of the MMPI-2 graph, the assessor says: "These scales tell me about the way you answered the test. Were you open, candid, honest? Or perhaps you felt so badly that you even exaggerated how you felt?" Alternatively, "Did you approach the test with somewhat of a 'stiff upper lip,' tending to minimize your painful feelings and disturbing symptoms?"

In situations where the validity scales of the different tests suggest an exaggeration of symptoms, the assessor might state:

> "The way you answered the test suggests you may have gone out of your way to let me know how uncomfortable you are right now, perhaps even panicked about your psychological condition, and wanting to make sure that you let me know how badly you are feeling. Perhaps you wanted me to know how knocked off balance you feel, and the results suggest that, in this process, you might have overdone it."

In cases where the validity scales suggest a constricted, defensive approach, the therapist might say:

> "You approached the testing in a somewhat cautious way, perhaps fearful of being judged or criticized, or perhaps fearful that the test results were going to be used against you. You tended to put your best foot for-

ward, going out of your way to let me know that you are a person of high moral fiber and above reproach. You have managed to convey your need to be seen that way, but unfortunately, I have not been able to get to know you as thoroughly as I would like to."

The assessor then would discuss with the patient some of the reasons for his or her guardedness.

During this part of the feedback process, the assessor should be noting therapeutic strategies tied to the validated feedback. Test-taking attitude can obviously have therapeutic implications. For example, when patients exaggerate their symptomatology, and that tendency is confirmed during the feedback process, therapeutic strategies would focus on ways to help the patient feel more relaxed and less panicked—and, therefore, have less need to exaggerate. For individuals who are constricted and defensive in their test-taking attitude, one therapeutic strategy could be to help them learn to recognize and label their emotional experiences. For example, Gestalt techniques might be used to teach them how to amplify their feelings and become more comfortable with emotional experiences, in general.

The Three Levels of Personality Feedback

Giving feedback to people about their test results is an anxiety-producing process, both for the assessor and the assessee. Most textbook assessment results are written in negative language that is not conducive to building rapport. Moreover, patients are often instinctively fearful of being judged during the assessment process. Consequently, feedback may elicit resistance, especially if the assessor begins to use judgmental language or if the patient begins to feel labeled. Many people, however, can feel validated by the assessment results, often expressing a sense of relief that somebody knows how they feel and that there may be some relief for their symptoms (Finn, 1996a; Finn & Tonsager, 1992; Lewak et al., 1991).

To avoid resistance, we recommend that feedback about personality issues be organized into three hierarchical levels. In the first level, feedback should be given that validates the patient's existential experience. For example, with patients whose results indicate that they are depressed and anxious, the assessor might state something like the following: "Your testing suggests that currently, you're not as happy as you would like to be. Much of the time you probably feel a sense of apprehension, perhaps even a sense of constant anxiety, and little seems to give you pleasure. You may find yourself often worrying, with a nagging sense that something bad is about to happen. Making decisions, concentrating, thinking clearly, and generally feeling efficient and enjoying life seem to be particularly hard for you at this time. You may find yourself having difficulty sleeping, relaxing, and allowing yourself to be hopeful about the future." For people with depression, this level of information is typically conscious and often these patients express relief that their symptoms have a label and an explanation. Some patients' symptoms have become ego-syntonic, so they may express surprise that their symptoms are "unusual." Whatever the particulars, feedback at this level of experience is usually felt as validating, and people often express gratitude that their internal experiences are readily accessible through the assessment process.

At this first level of feedback, there is usually little resistance, particularly if the feedback is given in an empathic, nurturing, and validating way. If the patient does begin to resist the feedback, rather than disagree or argue with him or her, we suggest that the assessor "go with the resistance." For example, a person whose results reveal a paranoid personality structure could be told: "Your profile suggests that right now you're feeling somewhat vulnerable to being criticized, judged or even perhaps attacked. You may find yourself on edge, somewhat suspicious of other people's motives, because you don't know who to trust." If the patient resists at this point, stating something like "I don't experience those feelings at all," the assessor could use the denial as an opportunity to initiate a discussion about issues of trust, sensitivity to criticism, and the individual's experience of feeling unsafe around others. Patients' resistances provide opportunities to hone and refine the integrative process. Assessment reports should articulate not only how patients may be feeling and what kinds of symptoms and behaviors they are experiencing, but also their existential experience of others. Obtaining this information directly from patients can be an important aspect of the refining and integrating process.

The second level of feedback involves discussing with patients how their symptoms, behaviors, and existential experience may affect how others consequently respond to them. This level of feedback can sometimes lead to resistance because patients may have less insight about how they affect others than they have about their own internal experiences. However, if the assessing psychologist is mindful of not judging or blaming patients, but rather strives to reveal to them how their understandable defensive behaviors may be misinterpreted by others, then the feedback can proceed with minimal resistance. For example, with patients who are depressed, the feedback might state:

> "Others may see your tendency to see the glass as 'half empty' and label it as negative, rather than realizing that you are sensitive to loss and therefore uncomfortable 'counting your chickens before they hatch.' They may become irritated and judge you as unreasonably pessimistic. People may also become irritated because you don't have as much energy and optimism as perhaps they would like you to have. Those closest to you may become angry with you because you seem to have difficulty making decisions and have problems remembering important events."

This deeper level of feedback involves helping patients see how their symptoms and behaviors may be affecting others. Ideally, at this level, insights are created in which they are able to link their symptoms and behaviors into a psychological construct such as depression or anxiety, and also begin to understand how others may see them in return.

Resistance at this level of feedback should, once again, provide an opportunity for dialogue. If a patient begins to resist the interpretation of how others might see him or her, use it as an opportunity to ask questions such as: "Tell me, what is your experience of how others see you?" or, "Do others become angry with you when you behave in this way?" The assessor should exert ongoing effort to clarify the assessment data and integrate any new information at each level of feedback, in order to develop a more complete, accurate, and useful understanding of the patient.

The third level of feedback incorporates the first two levels and adds an integrative process. At this level, the assessor describes how patients' emotions, behaviors, and defenses make sense, given their past conditioning experiences and the precipitating circumstances, which were particularly painful because they restimulated past "psychological scar tissue." The aim here is to help patients realize that they are a product of both positive and negative experiences and that their maladaptive behaviors may have become adaptive at some point in their history. It is at this level that the patient and the assessor collaborate in developing an understanding of what types of events might be particularly disturbing, how to anticipate these situations, and what kind of therapeutic strategies would be most useful. Any continuing resistance provides an opportunity for more dialogue, which itself further refines the assessment and feedback data.

For example, let's imagine a depressed patient responding well to feedback about how she was currently feeling and agreeing about, and elaborating on, how a precipitating circumstance of threat of loss elicited a recurrence of depressive symptomatology. During her history-taking and feedback session, she might have even developed insight into how her early childhood losses created psychological scar tissue, making her vulnerable to the restimulating effects of adult losses. However, she may clarify interpretation further by stating something to the effect of: "But I've had a number of setbacks in my life, to which I didn't respond with depression. For example, when my dog died, I didn't get depressed, and a few years later, when my good friend died in a car accident, I did all right. If I have this 'scar tissue' around loss, why didn't I get depressed during these events?" This question provides an opportunity for dialogue and a refining of the feedback results. Collaborating with the patient about why particular events are unsettling and why others are not can lead to useful interpretation of the assessment data.

Alternatively, this dialogue may also provide an opportunity to focus on the patient's strengths and positive adaptive qualities. As noted previously, the assessment of positive traits and adaptive qualities is generally lacking in psychological texts and interpretive manuals, and therefore discussion of it is often lacking in assessment feedback and reports. However, data regarding adaptive and positive traits and qualities should be an essential element in any well-integrated understanding of patients. Furthermore, feedback about a patient's strengths is nearly always appreciated and can boost rapport, decrease resistance, and facilitate a more comprehensive and therapeutic understanding. Table 12.2 provides a summary of the basic principles involved in collaborative feedback.

Collaborating on Treatment Goals

Irrespective of the reason for the assessment, we would suggest that some discussion of treatment goals or strategies for change is an important component of the feedback process. Even when working in forensic settings, it is often desirable to give a patient some strategies for personal enhancement and growth. In a similar manner, even forensic evaluations that are not treatment-related could include a discussion of what type of therapy or treatment could be useful, given the patient's various issues. Treatment goals and recommendations should proceed logically from the patient's presenting problem, related symptoms, distress level, general level of impairment, as well as his or her past psychological scar tissue and coping patterns. Treatment goals should correspond to the three feedback levels outlined above. In the first level of feedback, the patient's symptoms and existential experience are described and validated. These usually involve some experience of anxiety, fear, stress, and general distress. The initial aim of treatment should be immediate implementation of symptom alleviation strategies; these may involve medication and/or hospitalization in more severe cases of psychopathology. In less severe cases, the development of coping strategies may be the focus (e.g., for anxiety attacks, severe bouts of depression, or intense suicidal ideation, etc.). Usually a combination of medication and practical symptom alleviation strategies is this first level of the feedback process.

The second level of the feedback process involves helping the patient achieve insight into how his or her behaviors and symptoms may affect others; that is, identifying how he or she attempts to influence others to act in ways that fulfill his or her needs. Learning various methods such as active listening, requesting feedback from others, or developing empathy through the use of Gestalt techniques could help the patient develop better awareness of his or her effect on others.

The third level of feedback involves "putting the story together," describing how the patient's childhood experiences may have led him or her to develop particular sensitivities around certain events that restimulate the psychological scar tissue. Once patients who are prone to depression, humiliation issues, or to low self-esteem, for example, understand that they are particularly sensitive to loss issues, they can then develop, with the aid of the therapist, strategies for anticipating what events are likely to knock

TABLE 12.2. Basic Principles of Collaborative Feedback

Therapist objective	Action taken	Patient experience
Verify general accuracy of test results. Validate patient's experience.	"Big picture" feedback based on test summary.	Patient feels validated regarding current feelings, fears, anxieties, and conscious experiences.
Hone, refine, and enrich the anchor hypothesis through the feedback process.	Use the individual scale data and add to anchor hypothesis. Provide feedback.	Patient begins to explore deeper feelings, linking feelings and behaviors in new ways, recognizing the effect he or she has on others; adds labels and explanations to previously inchoate experiences (e.g., "Now I realize why I wake at 2:00 A.M. and feel anxious all the time").
Individualize nomothetic test data—how do the data apply to this person?	Ask questions to refine how patient experiences particular symptoms, etc.	Patient feels part of the assessment process, exploring how he or she experiences a particular symptom cluster: • what fits well, what fits less well • feedback about the feedback
Verify psychological scar tissue–conditioning experiences.	Combine history with assessment data into feedback.	Patient feels a deeper sense of validation by linking past conditioning experiences and painful events with the development of understandable but currently nonadaptive defenses (e.g., depression as defense against further loss).
Verify how precipitating events are linked to past psychological scar tissue and arrive at collaborative agreement.	Combine history, assessment data, and precipitating events into feedback.	Patient develops higher-order understanding of why and how precipitating events restimulated past scar tissue and begins to develop new coping strategies. Patient feels relief and is less self-negating because his or her defenses now make "sense."
Explain how precipitating events restimulate past scar tissue, leading to increased defensive behavior.	Link assessment, historical precipitating events, and clinical data.	Patient feels self-empathy, relief, understood, less self-negating. Patient sees defenses as understandable and begins to realize they can be changed.
Collaboratively strive for three stages of therapy: 1. Symptom alleviation via medication, relaxation. 2. Learning to anticipate scar tissue-restimulating events and developing new coping strategies. 3. Dealing with past unresolved issues (e.g., unfinished mourning), learning self-efficacy, self-esteem, and healing past psychological scar tissue.	1. Refer for medications, if needed. 2. Create behavioral strategies (e.g., relaxation, thought stopping). 3. Recommend deep, reparenting-style therapies.	Patient gains immediate techniques for symptom relief. Patient learns to anticipate what events can "knock him or her off balance" (e.g., for people with depression, any situation involving loss). Patient creates a more mature and differentiated ego. Patient creates a more integrated personality organization; life becomes more enjoyable and adaptive.

377

them off balance and what kinds of new coping strategies will be most useful in these circumstances. Each level of feedback should lead logically to
therapeutic strategies involving data generated during that level of assessment.

FEEDBACK AND THERAPEUTIC STRATEGIES USING THE STS MODEL

The Systematic Treatment Selection (STS) model (Beutler & Harwood,
2000) has been an underlying theme throughout this book. Each component of the model can be used to frame feedback for patients, including
what kind of language to use and what kind of therapeutic strategies are
logically linked to the various components. The following section includes
recommendations for giving assessment feedback to patients around the
various STS themes. These types of feedback statements can be shared with
the referral source in the discussion of treatment recommendations.

Functional Impairment/Severity

Often, functional impairment is associated with severe psychopathology,
such as psychotic, bizarre, and idiosyncratic thinking as well as hostile acting-out behaviors. However, functional impairment is often heightened by
the presence of substance abuse, organic medical conditions, low intelligence, and/or lack of social and financial support. Although some prediction can be made about the severity of functional impairment on the basis
of assessment data, typically a clinical history, interview, and collateral data
are needed to identify the degree of impairment. Treatment of people who
are functionally impaired due to psychotic or schizoid disorders typically
would not include insight therapy, as this format could exert a disorganizing effect on the individual. More appropriate treatment modalities in these
cases might include helping the individual find a social support system,
such as a day treatment program or hospitalization, and certainly a referral
for medication. Participating in social skill-building groups and learning
self-care behaviors also may be useful for these patients.

Giving feedback to people who are severely functionally impaired is
often difficult. Assuming valid test results, feedback should be empathic,
validating, nurturing, and supportive. Deep and dynamic interpretations
are usually not as relevant to these individuals, who may be barely able to
"put one foot in front of the other," psychologically. However, it would be
appropriate to validate the individual's experiences of anxiety, fear, and
difficulty in thinking clearly and navigating ordinary life experiences.
Typically these individuals are grateful when their experience of isolation,

inability to cope, and cognitive disorganization is verbalized and labeled, without judgment, during the feedback process. For example:

> "Your results suggest that the world is a pretty frightening place for you right now. You might often feel bombarded by thoughts and feelings that you do not feel you have control over. At times you may find yourself hearing voices or seeing things that you are not sure are really there, or experiencing emotions that feel like they are invading you against your will. You may find yourself experiencing periods where emotions that feel almost alien overwhelm you, and you can't seem to control them. At these times, you may experience a sense of panic and dread because you are unable to think clearly and organize your life in ways you want. Though it may be frightening to trust this process and frightening to trust your therapist, people with similar feelings have experienced significant improvement with the right kind of therapy. There are medications that can help take away the 'noise' in your head and the constant sense of anxiety and dread that you appear to be experiencing. It is going to take some time to learn to trust your therapist. At first, your treatment may involve helping you organize your life so that you feel more effective and in control."

A sympathetic, nurturing, and reparenting therapeutic style is generally appropriate for individuals with this kind of severe impairment.

Social Support

The ability to participate in a community and its social support systems can be an important means of enhancing ego strength. Stress is more readily managed in the context of a supportive social milieu. Individuals who experience severe functional impairment and limited coping ability exhibit more psychological disorganization when they are isolated, without a social support system. On the other hand, individuals who have the opportunity and ability to participate in a caring social support system tend to benefit from the enhanced reality testing and positive self-esteem that result from belonging to a group. Individuals whose impairment is aggravated by extreme introversion or negative self-esteem would likely have more difficulty participating in a supportive social network. When giving feedback to individuals who lack social support and the skills to create it, the therapist could say:

> "Your results suggest that you have a tendency to withdraw from others and fear social contact. Perhaps you are afraid that you will be rejected and humiliated. Your natural shyness may be aggravated by low self-esteem and the tendency to feel that others are looking at you critically and disliking you. You could be helped by recognizing some of your

strengths and learning to relate better with others, perhaps in a support group, so that you can learn about how others perceive you, rather than assuming that you are disliked and going to be rejected."

When giving feedback to an individual who, despite severe psychopathology, appears to manifest some positive social skills and a functional social support system, the therapist could state:

"In spite of how badly you have been feeling, you appear to have a number of positive strengths. You like people and enjoy being around them, and you seem to be able to reach out to others and benefit from their emotional support and help. In spite of feeling badly, you allow yourself to feel that others can care for you, so that you are able to turn to them during difficult times."

Problem Complexity/Chronicity

Dealing with problem complexity in the assessment data involves examining the different types of psychopathology that are evident. For example, individuals who score highly on many scales of the MMPI-2, MCMI-III, or the PAI, etc., would likely present numerous and sometimes contradictory symptoms and complex defensive patterns. Problem complexity is increased by physical illnesses, psychosocial stress, organic brain impairment, and substance abuse. Typically, the more areas of concern revealed by the various personality measures, the more complex the problem. People with simple reactive depressions, for example, would tend to show elevations on one or two measures of disturbance, whereas people with borderline disorders would tend to have elevated scores on many of the measures of psychopathology across all the tests administered.

When giving feedback to the patients about the complexity of their problems, the assessor might state:

"Your testing suggests that you are struggling with a number of complex issues and feelings. You may find yourself becoming quite confused as to exactly what you are feeling and what kinds of situations elicit different feelings. You may find yourself experiencing confusing and mixed emotions that make it difficult for you to fully comprehend what is troubling you and what is so upsetting. These mixed and confusing emotions make it more difficult for you to find ways to cope, solve your problems, think clearly, and enjoy life. At times, you may find yourself acting in ways that are self-destructive, giving up even as you're getting ahead, and hurting people you love."

The more complex individuals' problems become, the more difficulty they have understanding their own personal reactions. Therapeutically, they need to learn how to identify and label appropriately their various conflicting emotions, fears, and anxieties, so that they can comprehend them in order to develop more mature coping strategies. Typically, therapy for people with complex problems runs a longer course and involves several different types of interventions and techniques.

Usually complex problems are associated with greater chronicity. The degree of chronicity can be inferred from the length and severity of the disturbance and the presence or absence of ego strength and coping abilities. Degree of chronicity is best determined from a thorough history, as it is hard to extrapolate solely from assessment data; severity of disturbance, as evidenced on assessment data, is not always well correlated with chronicity. For example, an individual producing test data that appear to indicate a chronic condition, such as a borderline personality disorder, may not have borderline traits or features. Given (1) long-term, stable, psychological adjustment with good work and family relationships, and (2) a recent, severe precipitating circumstance, the assessment data suggestive of a borderline personality would rather reflect a severe reactive condition. In general, if the history reveals a generally healthy, stable long-term adjustment and the absence of childhood conditioning experiences that would be anticipated to explain current symptoms, and a recent catastrophic precipitating circumstance has occurred, then it could be concluded that the assessment data reflect an acute, rather than a chronic, condition.

When giving feedback to individuals who have a true chronic condition, it would be important to discuss how frustrating it must be for them to have experienced long periods of inefficiency, impaired relationships, discomfort, or anxiety, along with the discouragement, apathy, and cynicism that often accompany chronic conditions. These conditions usually require long periods of psychotherapy involving warm, "motherly-type" reparenting therapists to heal deep-seated early traumas or issues that have remained unresolved. Chronically impaired individuals who have low ego strength and limited coping resources usually benefit from support groups and practical psychotherapies that help them develop everyday coping skills. As noted, insight therapies are typically contraindicated for more severely impaired patients, because the therapies tend to be psychologically disorganizing. However, as we will see below, chronically impaired individuals who are "internalizers" with a tendency to use intellectual defenses in the face of stress (Beutler et al., 2000) may benefit from insight therapy in spite of long-term psychological disorganization, whereas chronic patients who tend to be "externalizers" may be more vulnerable to psychological disorganization and therefore not as likely to benefit from insight therapy.

Coping Style

Coping style is readily inferred from the assessment results. Many personality instruments identify typically used defenses, coping strategies, and levels of ego strength. Coping styles involve a hierarchy of defenses, from very mature to less mature and maladaptive. Within the STS model, coping styles are classified along a continuum ranging from internalizers at one end to externalizers at the other end (Beutler et al., 2000). Defenses along this internal-versus-external dimension range from adaptive to maladaptive. *Internalizers*, for example, tend to use intellectual defenses and feel guilt, anxiety, self-doubt, and have low self-esteem. They typically inhibit aggressive impulses and tend to be intropunitive. Passivity, low self-esteem, anxiety, guilt, difficulties with decision making, and strong needs for reassurance are common descriptors for individuals with this coping style. In contrast, individuals who are *externalizers* tend to attribute their problems to sources outside themselves (i.e., to other people or difficult situations) and use projection, denial, and externalization as primary defenses. They are often extremely sensitive, may act out, and tend to blame others when stressed. Externalizers usually experience less subjective distress but more interpersonal conflicts.

Using the collaborative and integrative procedures outlined earlier, the purpose of psychotherapy would be to help individuals become more aware of their predominant coping style and to increase the effectiveness of their defenses. Specific feedback about coping ability and treatment strategies that would enhance it would depend on the individual's predominant coping style and current level of functioning. To an individual who tends to be an externalizer and shows little awareness of his or her defensive style, the following feedback might be appropriate:

> "Your test results suggest that, when stressed, you have a tendency to want to move into battle mode, ready to fight and resist what you see as others' unreasonable attempts to control and manipulate you. You may find that most stressful situations leave you feeling angry, as if others have victimized you. You do not tend to think about how you might have contributed to these difficulties, perhaps because it would be too painful or because you grew up with a critical, judgmental parent. When stressed, you may find yourself doing impulsive things to feel better—things that sometimes backfire and work against you. At other times, you may find yourself getting into conflicts with others, unsure how the conflict began, because you see yourself as trying to do the right thing and protect yourself."

Treatment modalities for externalizers would help them become more aware of their subjective distress through the use of insight and Gestalt techniques, instead of immediately externalizing it, so that it could be processed in a more adaptive manner.

To individuals who tend to internalize as a way of coping, such as anxious and depressed persons with low self-esteem and guilt, the following feedback may be appropriate:

> "One of the ways you cope with stress is to withdraw, to become quiet and refuse to allow yourself to communicate with others. When things go wrong you are quick to feel guilty, to blame and 'kick yourself,' and to feel that you are not lovable. You may find yourself so anxious and tense about things going wrong that you are always 'observing,' as if you are watching yourself in a movie, unable to relax, let down your guard, and 'switch off' your mind. You may be constantly wondering what could go wrong next, so that you frequently feel a sense of anxiety and apprehension. People with your coping style can get better if they learn to recognize that not all things that go wrong are their fault. It will be important to work on seeing reality more clearly so that you are not constantly judging yourself negatively and focusing on all of your negatives, rather than seeing things in a more balanced way. Treatment may involve teaching you to recognize when you are beating yourself up and how to shut off those thoughts and see things more realistically."

Treatment for internalizers should focus on building self-esteem, reducing guilt, controlling anxiety, and developing a more realistic self-appraisal. Treatment strategies for both internalizers and externalizers typically utilize insight therapy to identify the predominant style of coping, along with a variety of treatment modalities that foster the development of more adaptive defenses.

Given that there are numerous coping styles and strategies, some of which are more adaptive than others, treatment duration and complexity will depend on how adaptive an individual's defenses are; still, more mature and effective defenses are always possible. Some individuals oscillate between externalizing and internalizing coping styles when subjected to stress: At times they feel guilty, overwhelmed, ruminative, and self-doubting, but as stress builds, they tend to act out and blame others for their difficulties. They then seek reassurance and support from others but do not trust it if they receive it. Various treatment strategies would attempt to increase the effectiveness of defenses through a combination of insight, psychoeducation, and the teaching of practical coping skills, as needed.

Reactance/Resistance

If an individual feels threatened by information, he or she tends to resist its impact. One aim of the assessment and feedback process is to identify a person's typical resistances. Each personality type will have a tendency to resist certain kinds of information more readily. For example, patients with paranoia usually resist information they perceive as critical or judgmental, whereas patients with depression tend to resist attempts to help them view life in a more balanced or positive, rather than negative, manner. Patients with depression also tend to resist the notion that they can feel more hopeful and that optimism might produce greater happiness. Similarly, anxious individuals become increasingly resistant and anxious if they feel they are being disapproved of or when pushed toward behavioral change. Individuals with hypochondriacal tendencies generally resist the notion that stress increases their physical symptoms, whereas people with narcissistic tendencies generally feel wounded by what they perceive as criticism. On the other hand, there are individuals who are defensive and angry that consistently resist others as a result of their personality and defensive makeup. For example, people with compulsive disorders, passive–aggressive tendencies, and those who fear being controlled often resist therapeutic change. Patients with compulsive disorders generally worry that something has been missed in the treatment procedures, whereas those with narcissistic and paranoid features often report that the therapist does not fully understand them and therefore the insights and therapeutic strategies do not apply.

In our earlier discussion of the feedback process, we outlined how resistance can add value to the assessment. Noting the point at which the patient resists the feedback and then allowing the patient to redefine how the assessment information applies to him or her can result in a more accurate assessment. For example, when giving feedback around an issue with an individual who tends toward depression, the assessor might say:

> "People with your profile tend to be fearful of feeling hopeful and optimistic in case they are let down or their worst fear comes true when they are least prepared for it. You may find yourself resisting my attempts to help you become more hopeful and optimistic. In fact, you may find yourself dismissing these attempts to make you see things in a more balanced way as naïve and unrealistic. You may feel that staying negative and prepared for loss is more realistic than being positive or optimistic. You are likely to benefit from treatment that helps you see the world in a more balanced way. Learning to stop your negative thoughts and learning to see yourself more realistically would be a good beginning."

Identifying the typical resistances associated with the individual's personality or psychopathology is a crucial element of the assessment process, and it is important to understand that some individuals have a resisting personality style (e.g., people with passive–aggressive personalities). Resistance issues should be incorporated in the treatment suggestions and strategies. Individuals who exhibit high levels of resistance tend to benefit from paradoxical and nondirective therapies, whereas individuals who are passive and less resistant generally benefit from more directive, coaching, and in-structive-type therapies.

Subjective Distress

A proportion of all assessment data is face valid. These face-valid data, when endorsed, allow the patient an opportunity to dialogue with the as-sessor about his or her level of intensity, and severity, of distress. On the MMPI-2, for example, the face-valid data comes in the form of critical items and content scales, a high endorsement of which suggests a self-report of severe concerns or disturbance. The validity scales also provide good measures of distress. An individual endorsing a high number of un-usual or pathological items and reporting few, if any, defenses is claiming severe distress, whether veridically or for secondary gain. A patient's level of distress also can be inferred from less face-valid assessment data that measures ego strength and coping ability. When giving feedback to individ-uals about their level of distress, the assessment psychologist might say:

> "Your profile shows that you are currently experiencing a great deal of unhappiness, distress, fear, confusion, or even panic. You seem to be ex-periencing many different symptoms, some of which may be disorga-nizing and even frightening. You may find yourself having difficulty coping, so that even ordinary tasks can feel unbearable."

On the other hand, an individual who endorses little distress and dysfunc-tion may respond to feedback such as:

> "Your testing suggests that you currently feel little distress or unhappi-ness and that you generally feel balanced and resilient, so little knocks you off balance. People with your kind of test results rarely cry over spilled milk, rarely look backward, and rarely doubt themselves."

The level of currently experienced distress is linked to selection and ef-ficacy of therapeutic strategies. At very high levels, distress can interfere with a patient's ability to benefit from treatment. The greater the distress, the more the need for immediate, practical solutions that lower distress lev-els. In many cases, particularly the more severe ones, these solutions would include medication, crisis intervention measures, and the type of therapeu-tic techniques used to lower distress levels in a relatively short period of time (e.g., thought stopping, relaxation training, and cognitive restructur-ing). Additional therapeutic interventions might include referral to support groups, recommendations for making behavioral changes around sleep, diet, and exercise, and (in some cases) teaching self-soothing behaviors.

Though psychologically uncomfortable, moderate levels of distress can be associated with strong motivation for change. Positively reframed feedback to acutely distressed or anxious individuals who are still motivated to change might state:

> "Your results suggest that you are currently experiencing severe discomfort, anxiety, and distress. You may even be frightened by some of your symptoms. Typically, individuals who are experiencing as much discomfort as you can get significantly better with the right kind of treatment, and they are often highly motivated to follow treatment recommendations."

In some cases, chronically distressed individuals become apathetic and resigned to low levels of emotional experience. When apathy is predominant, feedback might state:

> "Your profile suggests that you have been feeling unhappy and distressed for a long period of time, and you appear to have given up hope that things can get much better. Research has shown that people who are as distressed as you can use their distress to help them work toward and develop change."

This feedback could then lead to a discussion of past therapeutic attempts and the reasons for the individual's loss of hope.

Individuals who are referred for assessment and show an absence of distress are usually either highly defensive or emotionally shut down and unaware of their feelings, or they are actually healthy and symptom-free. Therapeutic strategies for highly defensive people would involve helping them engage their feelings and unblock the emotional shutdown. One appropriate strategy would be to use insight therapies together with Gestalt techniques to get them to "loosen up" their overcontrol.

WORKING WITH THE REFERRAL SOURCE

Informed Consent

Prior to conducting an assessment, the psychologist should clarify the referral questions as well as who will pay for the assessment and who will have access to the results. Sometimes assessments are requested without it being clear to the patient that he or she is responsible for paying the fees. Some patients assume that their insurance will pay for the assessment, when, in fact, it may not. In other cases, attorneys refer patients for an assessment without clarifying to the client that he or she is responsible for paying assessment fees. Clarifying the fee structure, the timeline for reports, and the format of the assessment reports are important components of the informed consent.

A second important component in establishing informed consent is to clarify with the referral source and patient who will have access to the test results. Although the assessing psychologist cannot control how the assessment results will be used over a long period of time, he or she should consider the possible uses of the results. For example, a colleague was retained as an expert witness in a criminal case. As part of the defense strategy, a psychological evaluation was conducted on the defendant. As part of his assessment report, the psychologist wrote that the defendant had answered a number of "Lie scale" items. Although this was a literally true statement, the relatively large number of "Lie scale" items on the defendant's MMPI-2 was consistent with the profile of a somewhat naive, rigid, and unsophisticated individual. In the context of the assessment, the elevated Lie scale did not invalidate the results. However, during cross-examination, the district attorney selectively plucked various statements from the report, giving the jury the impression that the defendant was a "liar." Had the assessing psychologist been mindful of how every sentence in the assessment report could be used in a hostile cross-examination, the inaccurate representation of the defendant could have been avoided. Knowing who will have access to the test results can mitigate these kinds of problems.

Psychological reports should be written veridically, but the language should be modified to reflect who has access to the reports. A report written in overly technical language may be rejected by a psychotherapy patient, whereas a report written in too colloquial a language for a civil litigation might be rejected as unscientific by a judge. Writing the report to fit the setting and the target audience is an important part of the assessment process.

A third issue that can be addressed while establishing informed consent is to determine the patient's expectations and needs relative to the assessment process. Doing so can facilitate patient cooperation and potentially lead to a more therapeutic outcome (Finn, 1996a). The assessing psychologist may want to ask the patient what he or she wants to learn from results. The assessor also may want to ascertain the patient's attitudes toward the testing procedure. Does he or she have cultural, linguistic, or other issues that might hamper the assessment process? Has the individual had any negative experiences with assessment in the past, of which the assessing psychologist needs to be aware in order to allay his or her fears prior to the current assessment? All of these issues should be addressed with the client prior to the testing procedure.

Clarifying the Referral Question

Often, a referring colleague or agency requests an assessment to answer a number of referral questions. Sometimes these questions are vague or global. For example, the referral source may request a general evaluation to "get to know the patient better." At other times, the purpose may be more specific, such as asking for help with diagnosis, therapeutic strategies, aid in understanding a patient's resistance in therapy, or help in dealing with transference and countertransference issues. Referral questions are important because they provide a focus for the organization and analysis of the myriad of data generated during an assessment. The assessment report will have a different focus depending on whether it is written, for example, as a part of a child custody evaluation, part of a therapeutic assessment, or as part of a criminal defense or prosecution assessment.

In some cases, the referral question is not completely articulated by the referring colleague. For example, let's say a neurologist requests a personality evaluation for a college student who is experiencing academic difficulties. The referrer asks for aid in determining whether the students' learning problems are the result of psychological difficulties or a learning disability. Assessing only the personality and cognitive issues, however, would fail to address deeper issues such as familial relationships, interpersonal dynamics, and perhaps cultural or socioeconomic issues. Another example: A colleague conducting a child custody evaluation asks for independent evaluations to determine each ex-spouse's ability to parent effectively. However, during further discussions, the referral source verbalizes difficulties he or she has in working with one or both of the parents and states that he or she needs help with transference–countertransference dynamics.

When possible, it is important to talk to the referral source whenever a request for an evaluation is made, since the referral issues, both explicit and implicit, can be better identified through an interactive discussion. Sometimes the referring colleague has developed an impression of his or her patient but doubts this impression because of contradictory findings. Obtaining the referring colleague's clinical impression of the patient and discussing any diagnostic dilemmas with him or her can hone the referral question. For example: An individual appears manic during the initial intake, and the referring colleague asks for an assessment to confirm his or her impression of a manic disorder. However, the assessment data reveal that the individual is really anxious and agitated. It would be important to discuss in the assessment report how this individual may appear manic, but that his or her high energy and agitation is a manifestation of anxiety rather than an underlying mood disorder. In this way, anyone reading the report can be alerted to the fact that the testee can appear manic but is actually agitated and depressed.

It is also useful to call a referring colleague once the testing psychologist has gathered preliminary results. Discussing these results with the referral source can help in refining the assessment prior to beginning the writing of the report. In rare cases, the referring colleague may resist accepting some of the test results, perhaps feeling that they are too disparate from his or her initial clinical impression. Understanding how the referring colleague views the patient and helping him or her see the patient from the perspective of the test results is an important part of the assessment process.

As part of refining the referral question, it is sometimes important to let the referring colleague know which questions the assessment results can answer. At times, referrals include a number of diverse questions, some of which the assessing psychologist will not be able to answer. Discussing the questions that fall outside the assessment's purview and clarifying priorities then would be necessary.

Referral Source Collaboration Using the STS Model

The results of the assessment are typically shared in a written report that is mailed to the referring colleague. Earlier in this chapter, we recommended contacting the referring colleague directly in order to clarify the referral questions, so that the assessment report answers the questions as clearly as possible. We also recommend contacting the referring colleague directly in order to give a verbal summary of the findings. This discussion promotes professional collaboration regarding the patient and sets the stage for follow-up contacts to determine the usefulness of the assessment and to clarify further any remaining questions the referral source may have. Throughout this chapter the STS dimensions have been articulated as a basis for assessment integration and report writing. Though each of the dimensions is explicated in the body of the assessment report, further collaboration with the referring colleague may be needed around these dimensions. The following sections offer suggestions for discussing STS dimensions with the referral source.

Functional Impairment

The assessing psychologist will have appraised the level and severity of functional impairment. Sometimes referral sources are unaware of the depth of psychological disorganization or dysfunction from their initial consultation. It would be important to alert them to any "red flags" in the patient's results, particularly if the results suggest the possibility that a patient may need hospitalization or be disabled by his or her problems. For example, a woman who had experienced severe sexual and emotional abuse in childhood may evidence, in the assessment results, a tendency to become temporarily psychotic when past abuse issues are stimulated. In another situation, an individual may be vulnerable to psychotic episodes when he or she feels threatened in social situations. It would be important to alert the referral source regarding these patient vulnerabilities and provide ongoing consultation should psychotic disorganization occur during treatment. Functional impairment can also occur when a patient's coping mechanisms become so overwhelmed by stress that he or she cannot work or manage the requirements of daily life. In these cases, the assessor would need to discuss with the referring colleague how to help the patient manage the stress and booster his or her coping abilities.

Level of Social Support

It is important to help the referral source understand the relationship between social support and ego strength. The assessing psychologist would want to explain how the patient's stress is better managed in the context of a supportive social milieu. The assessor would want to discuss the patient's social strengths and weaknesses to help the referral source decide whether or not the results suggest the need for therapeutic interventions to improve social support, such as family therapy, social skills training, or referral to a support group. It would also be important to alert the referral source to any significant interpersonal problems that the patient may have, so that the issues can be addressed in therapy in order to maximize the potential for social support.

Problem Complexity/Chronicity

Patients with complex, chronic problems, whether moderate or severe, tend to resist treatment. Alerting the referring colleague that the patient is presenting with what appear to be chronic problems might be helpful in precluding the disappointment and frustration that can interfere with treatment. It is important to discuss with the referring colleague which of the patient's problems are most amenable to treatment in the initial phases of therapy, and which issues are likely to be more resistant and require long-term therapy.

Clarifying diagnostic dilemmas is important, for example, when the presenting problem and initial data appear to indicate the presence of a borderline personality disorder, whereas the assessment process clarifies that the patient is actually experiencing a severe acute crisis that has led to the appearance of a more severe and longstanding disorder. In this case, the referring colleague would be directed to focus more on crisis management and the treatment of issues related to acute trauma, rather than planning long-term treatment strategies. In contrast, when discussing a patient whose results indicate a chronic disorder, such as the initial phase of schizophrenia or a schizoid adjustment to a history of neglect and cruelty, the assessing psychologist would direct the referring colleague to plan long-term treatment strategies that would be appropriate for the patient's diagnosis.

Coping Style

When discussing a patient whose results indicate an internalizing coping style, the assessor might say:

"Internalizers tend to be intropunitive, using intellectual defenses, and they often feel guilt, anxiety, self-doubt, and have low self-esteem. They typically inhibit aggressive impulses, are passive, have difficulties with decision making, and have strong needs for reassurance. It will be important to help the patient develop a more realistic perspective so that he or she is not constantly focusing on negatives but seeing things in a more balanced way. Treatment may involve teaching him or her to shut off negative thoughts and see things more realistically."

When discussing an externalizing patient, the assessor might tell the referring colleague the following:

"The patient is an externalizer and will tend to see his or her problems as due to other people and difficult situations. He or she uses projection, denial, and externalization as primary defenses. He or she is likely sensitive to a paranoid degree, tends to blame others when stressed, and may act out, particularly when anger builds. He or she probably experiences less subjective distress than others and may lack the insight and motivation necessary to change. However, he or she is likely to experience interpersonal conflicts and may be able to focus on this issue in treatment. Help him or her become more aware of his or her subjective distress, instead of externalizing it, so that it can be processed and extinguished."

Reactance/Resistance

Understanding the level of a patient's resistance can be crucial for therapists deciding on how best to develop a treatment program. If a referral source is alerted that a patient is highly resistant, he or she can prepare themselves in such a way as to hopefully avoid developing a negative countertransference. Patient resistance might even be reframed as fulfilling crucial client needs for control, independence, identity, and competence. Therapists who appreciate this perspective are more likely to acknowledge that resistance may be important to the client rather than interpreting it as undermining the therapist's sense of competence. Once the therapist is internally prepared, he or she can carefully consider which techniques would be likely to optimize outcome. As discussed in Chapter 3, nondirective approaches, in which the client is given extensive choice about what he or she perceives to be helpful and what he or she may or may not be willing to do, may be the optimal direction. Resistance could be reduced by providing a nonauthoritarian and collaborative environment. Such a setting would meet the client's need for control yet also optimize the working relationship and thereby increase the chance for therapeutic change. In addition, paradoxical suggestions might be effective, since the patient could assert his or her control by changing in a direction that he or she chooses (but may be contrary to the therapist's explicit suggestions). Knowing that a client is resistant may also help decision makers match the patient with a therapist who would be more likely to work with him or her in an optimal manner (i.e., one that is more collaborative and egalitarian).

Level of Subjective Distress

As noted, patients who feel highly distressed may be motivated for therapeutic change or, if the distress is extremely high, may feel hopeless and defeated by the severity of their symptoms. Alerting the referral source verbally (and with follow-up consultation) to the patient's distress level could help him or her choose more appropriate therapeutic strategies. For example, when discussing a severely anxious and distressed individual, the assessing psychologist might state:

> "The client is extremely distressed by their current difficulties. Initially, this individual will probably need extensive 'hand holding' and reassurance that he or she is going to get better. The high level of distress should help motivate the patient to change, but he or she may initially need medication and crisis management, as well as the use of therapeutic techniques that assist with stress reduction. Although crying out for help, he or she may also be resistant to psychotherapy. For example, he or she may complain of a list of symptoms and concerns, yet when you try to work with him or her, will tell you how he or she has tried all of your therapeutic interventions and nothing has worked. If this kind of response occurs, it would be important to remain patient with this individual, and it would help to empathize with how hopeless and trapped he or she is feeling."

When the assessment results suggest a lack of motivational distress, the assessor might tell the colleague:

> "This individual does not appear to be experiencing any real distress, but he may be motivated to change if you can help him understand how it could improve any problem situations he may be involved in."

Regarding patients with acting-out, psychopathic defensive styles, for example, the assessing psychologist might tell the colleague:

> "Help the patient to understand how his or her high energy, difficulties with trust, and rebelliousness to authority can lead him or her to make impulsive and hasty decisions that are not thought through. This kind of individual may only be motivated to change if he or she can be shown how change can make him or her less likely to get into trouble and therefore potentially more successful in some aspect of his or her life."

It is important to help the referral source understand how the level of an individual's distress and coping style impacts the potential motivation for treatment and change.

CASE EXAMPLE

The case used throughout this book as an example is detailed in Chapter 3. In brief, a 22-year-old female presents with the chief complaint of panic attacks and a fear of social situations. She reports a disturbing history of physical and sexual abuse, emotional instability, self-defeating behaviors, and depression. Problems with promiscuity, drug use, identity confusion and a tendency to gravitate toward older married men were identified. How would the assessor give her feedback using the integrative model?

Validity/Test-Taking Attitude Issues

"Your results suggest that you answered the test questions openly and honestly and were willing to tell me about your feelings. You reported that you are a person who tries hard to do the right thing, that your values and morals are important to you. You currently are feeling knocked off balance and, at times, overwhelmed by your psychological difficulties. You may have gone out of your way to let me know how badly you are feeling, perhaps because you want some immediate help. You may find yourself at times immobilized by your difficulties so that you feel unable to function in ordinary daily situations. This might be quite frightening to you. The way you approached the test suggests that you may want help for your condition."

Symptoms and Personality Traits

"Your results further suggest that right now you are feeling very sad, pessimistic, and blue. You also appear to be feeling trapped. You are extremely sensitive, easily hurt, and feel vulnerable to being criticized, judged, disliked, or treated unfairly. You may be experiencing a great deal of stress and tension in addition to headaches, stomachaches, low back pain, and vague and shifting physical symptoms. These symptoms may be quite frightening to you and may make you feel that there is something hopelessly wrong with you.

"You test as somewhat shy and a little uncomfortable in new social situations. You are probably feeling fearful around others, wondering whom you can trust and with whom you can open up and get close to. You appear to be afraid of being abandoned emotionally. Becoming close to others and wanting their love and approval is important to you, and you long to connect with others and gain their emotional support. However, much of the time you feel a sense of dread because you anticipate being judged and hated by those with whom you would like to be close.

"Making decisions, thinking clearly, and getting things done seems particularly difficult for you at the present time. You may find yourself constantly on edge, obsessing about what could possibly go wrong next. Your test results suggest that you are having some difficulties with sleep, decision making, and 'getting going.' They also suggest that you cry easily, feel useless, and experience life as a strain much of the time. You even may have felt so hopeless that you've tried to kill yourself and, perhaps, you may be thinking about that even now. It's hard for you to concentrate, to keep your mind on any task or job for long, and to ever feel really happy or content. You tend to be your own worst critic, quick to judge and criticize yourself at the slightest mistake. At times you seem to blame yourself and feel worthless, useless, and unlovable. At other times you may find yourself brooding about how others have treated you badly, believing that, had others treated you better, things would have worked out better.

"When stress builds, it appears that you impulsively try to feel better, sometimes by using drugs or alcohol or making impulsive decisions. You are likely to gravitate toward relationships wherein someone will take care of you. However, while needing the support and validation, you find yourself doubting others, pushing them away, and yet constantly feeling insecure, believing that they don't love you enough in return. At times, you may terminate a relationship impulsively because you feel so insecure, hurt, or unloved, and then feel panicked because you feel so alone. Always anxious and on edge, your whole body likely takes the strain so that you are constantly feeling some physical symptoms of stress. At times, you may withdraw from others, becoming quiet and feeling hurt. At other times, you may become quite angry, feeling that you have to tell off people. Consequently, others may see you as somewhat moody and hard to understand, because they don't see how sensitive you are and how easily you are hurt by criticism and rejection. Being perceived in this way may be why you tend to take a long time to warm up to others, why you keep a wary distance from them until they prove themselves. When stressed, your profile suggests that you may become quite confused, almost as if you feel a sense of internal panic. At these times it may be hard to communicate with people."

Background/Etiology

"People similar to you tend to have grown up in environments where their parents were cold, distant, perhaps even critical, hostile, and, at times, cruel. Consequently, you may now find yourself feeling very insecure, unlovable, and unworthy. You may also feel constantly on edge, as if anticipating criticism and judgment, perhaps because of the way you felt as a child. You may have felt that it was useless to argue against what you perceived as criticism, unfair judgments, and rejections, so you may have learned the habit of withdrawing, staying quiet, and protecting yourself. At other times, when you felt outraged at some particularly painful unfairness, you may have become very angry, obstinate, stood your ground, and even become violent. If so, that is why you may have difficulty trusting others now and are fearful of opening up. You may feel that you cannot negotiate your wants successfully. Consequently, you may oscillate between periods of angry silence and periods of outrage and anger. Because you feel defeated and hopeless, you may also do things impulsively that are self-destructive but temporarily make you feel better."

Treatment Suggestion

Here are some suggestions that may help:

"1. Your results suggest that although your problems are complex, they can be resolved with the right kind of treatment. You appear to be suffering from depression and anxiety, and with these, come a number of different symptoms. For example, when you are depressed, it is easy to take things personally, to feel that others do not like you, and to feel criticized. People with your kind of depression often experience periods of anxiety and stress, and that is why you sometimes do things impulsively to reduce the stress but that may get you into trouble. Though it may seem confusing to you, your test results show that your problems are not as complex as you might think. Your therapist may want to recommend some medication to help you feel less depressed, sleep better, think more clearly and efficiently, and concentrate and remember things.

"2. Work with your therapist on understanding how you often felt criticized, judged, unfairly treated, and rejected as a child. Try to identify specific situations growing up when you felt particularly hurt and wounded and examine how you felt at the time. It will be important to try to have some empathy for yourself as a child, so that you can understand why you developed some of your behaviors as a way of coping. At times, you tend to cope with stress by blaming yourself and feeling defective, damaged, and unlovable. You have a tendency to internalize, to go inside, beat yourself up, and withdraw from the world. At other times, you seem to have an externalizing way of coping, tending to see your situation as due to other people and the ways they have mistreated you. At these times, you may act out your stress and do impulsive things that can backfire and get you into trouble. You would benefit from treatment that would help you not be so self-critical and withdrawn from others. Treatment could also help you learn to restrain the impulse to act out your stress and to get less angry and blame others less often.

"3. Most of us have a number of different ways of coping with life when it becomes stressful. Some people tend to express their stress by lashing out, whereas others deal with stress by blaming themselves and being self-critical. Your results suggest that sometimes you cope with stress by turning inward and feeling inadequate, easily hurt, and wounded, and then you withdraw. At other times when you feel hurt and tension builds, you might lash out at others. Try not to wait until you are deeply wounded before you confront people. Try to recognize what you are feeling, perhaps paying attention to what is going on inside you when you find yourself withdrawing from others. Whenever you find yourself criticizing or judging yourself, try to be more balanced. For example, make a list of your positive qualities whenever you find yourself focusing on all your negative ones.

"4. Whenever you are very anxious, tense, and edgy, develop ways to relax and deal with the stress so that you don't act out in self-defeating or self-destructive ways. Learn how to relax by deep breathing, exercising, and thinking positive thoughts, so that you can avoid those high levels of stress and tension that push you to do impulsive things.

"5. Work on improving your self-esteem by behaving in ways that you respect and like, and use self-affirmations so that you are not so quick to belittle yourself."

SUMMARY

We have attempted to outline the basic elements of integrative assessment, which involves a deeper level of psychological evaluation than merely reporting the results of test scores. Historically, the rote reporting of results, the use of judgmental, nonempathic language, and the strict adherence to empiricism have tended to leave a fractionated, part–object view of the individual tested. Integrative assessment fosters a more comprehensive and user-friendly assessment process. It involves taking a thorough history in order to develop an understanding of how an individual's current psychological makeup, coping style, and vulnerability to certain precipitating events are the product of possible early childhood psychological scar tissue. Integrative assessment involves blending assessment data with childhood conditioning experiences, clinical presentation, and precipitating circumstances into a rich description of the individual that is refined and honed through the feedback process. In collaboration with the patient and the referral source, treatment strategies can then be articulated that are tied to the individual's strengths, vulnerabilities, past history, personality structure, and coping style. The potential result is a more effective outcome for the patient. The objectives and recommended methods for integration and application of assessment results are outlined in Table 12.3.

TABLE 12.3. The Objectives and Recommended Methods for Test Integration and Application of Results

Objective	Method
Obtain valid test results.	Administer tests under appropriate conditions and with clear test instructions. Discuss assessment purpose, feedback procedure, and confidentiality issues. Work through any pretest anxieties, fears, and past bad assessment experiences.
Generate initial "big picture" anchor hypothesis (e.g., the client has a depression/acting out/personality disorder profile).	Based on expertise, choose one test as the basis for initial hypothesis.
Confirm, expand, and hone the original anchor hypothesis.	Examine the other tests for confirmation and modify/expand the original hypothesis accordingly.
Add nuance to the anchor hypothesis (e.g., what is the *nature* of the depression: somatizing, self-defeating, withdrawing, or anxious?).	Examine the individual scales and indices of the various tests. Identify and resolve any contradictions. Continue to enrich the original hypothesis. Use clinical skills at the intersection of contradictory scale information (e.g., one scale suggests acting out, whereas another suggests depression).
Create a rich, insightful description of the individual.	Examine the various subscales on the different tests administered. At this point, data should confirm or enrich the refined anchor hypothesis rather than change it significantly.
Create a picture of a real person whose behavior and symptoms have meaning in the context of his or her history and precipitating circumstances.	Obtain a history using the assessment data as a road map for possible conditioning experiences (e.g., depression profile suggests early childhood and/or recent losses; personality disorder profile suggests parental absence, neglect, etc.).
Obtain a collaborative understanding of how assessment data, precipitating circumstances, and childhood conditioning experiences fit together.	Provide feedback to patient of assessment results and history, showing how current symptoms/behaviors make sense, given the precipitating circumstances and childhood conditioning experiences that may have left psychological scar tissue.
Generate collaborative therapeutic strategies that are logically linked to symptoms and behaviors and based on strengths, psychological scar tissue, and precipitating circumstances.	During feedback, collaborate with patient to generate therapeutic strategies that would validate current fears/anxieties/symptoms and provide ongoing self-help strategies. Obtain feedback from the patient about the feedback accuracy.
Provide feedback to referral sources, discuss dilemmas or questions, and get feedback from referral sources about usefulness of assessment.	Write an empirically based report in nonjudgmental, nonjargon language describing the individual's etiology, therapeutic strategies linked to his or her scar tissue, and strengths. Provide referral source with opportunity to comment on accuracy of assessment. Resolve referral source questions and/or dilemmas.
Provide ongoing consultation for referral source.	Anticipate in the report resistance, transference, and countertransference issues. Contact the referral source at 3- and 6-month intervals to discuss progress and resolution of these issues.

13

The Integrated Psychological Report

Steven Kvaal, James Choca, and Gary Groth-Marnat

As the profession of clinical psychology has matured and expanded its scope, the issues relevant to psychological report writing have become more varied and complicated. Theoretical orientations have multiplied, and the variety of case conceptualizations and the psychological vocabularies used to describe them has increased. The types of referral questions and professionals exchanging information are more diverse. Given this diversity, it is essential to develop an integrated report-writing style that is tailored to the specific needs of both the referral setting and the client context. In addition, because the psychological report is often the only product of psychological practice that others see, and because it is likely to have significant consequences for the examinee, reports must be readable and meaningful. This chapter is designed to help students and practicing psychologists evaluate and improve their reports.

In pursuit of these goals, we review the research on report writing and general practice issues and discuss the suggested components of a typical psychological report. Finally, the major points are demonstrated in samples of actual reports.

RESEARCH AND PRACTICAL CONSIDERATIONS

There has been a paucity of research on psychological report writing (Reynolds, Mair, & Fischer, 1995). This lack of interest is unfortunate, given that the report is the final product of assessment and is typically the only component of the assessment process with which the consumer is familiar. Research in which consumers (i.e., psychiatrists, neurologists, attorneys) have rated the value of reports indicates that they are perceived as well organized and useful (Finn, Moes, & Kaplan, 2001)

Despite this generally favorable impression, there are also a number of ways in which reports might be improved. A review of research on the most frequent criticisms of psychological reports indicates that reports are often difficult for clients to read (Harvey, 1997), include difficult-to-understand technical terms not commonly shared across professions (e.g., Rucker, 1967; Weiner, 1985), do not provide explicit, useful recommendations (Finn et al., 2001; Tallent & Reiss, 1959a, 1959b), and do not provide enough of the data on which inferences and judgments are based (Garfield, Heine, & Leventhal, 1954; Mussman, 1964). Research also has shown that reports were more likely to be actually used when referral sources were asked to make *specific* information requests along with the general referral (Affleck & Strider, 1971; Armengol, 2001).

The above research suggests that reports can be improved by:

- Clearly stating the purpose of the report
- Using vocabulary that is understood by the referral source and other consumers of the report (including the person who has been evaluated)
- Writing in a readable and well-organized manner
- Addressing the referral question as specifically and explicitly as possible, in both case conceptualizations and recommendations
- Providing examples of the behavior or other data on which inferences and judgments are based.

These issues are addressed in detail below, organized according to their relevance to different components of the psychological report.

Clarifying the Referral Question

In 1971, Hartlage and Merck stated, "[Psychologists ought] to evaluate their own reports in terms of what these reports contribute to the operation of their unique settings, rather than to continue to grind out reports with good theoretical consistency but little decisional value" (p. 460). This point is still relevant to today's practitioners. *Decisional value* refers to the extent to which a report provides information that is useful in making site- and client-specific clinical decisions. Hartlage and Merk's injunction implies the need for relatively less emphasis on extended theoretical case conceptualizations and greater emphasis on recommendations than has often been the case.

Prior to starting an evaluation, the diagnostician should work closely with the client and the referral source to clarify the referral question and decisional needs (Armengol, 2001). The psychologist conducting the assessment and the referral source share the responsibility for clarifying the referral question(s). An example of a poorly worded referral question was provided by a colleague who was asked by a referral source, "Does this patient have personality dynamics?" Clarifying the referral question frequently requires additional contact with the referral source. It is our experience that much useful information can be obtained from direct personal contact that might not be available in written communication, due to a referral source's reluctance to commit speculations to paper or due to time constraints.

After repeated experiences with a referral source, one may develop a better understanding of the source's idiosyncratic vocabularies and unstated needs. For example, the psychology staff in one hospital eventually learned that the most appropriate issue for chronic pain patients referred from one particular unit for "biofeedback evaluation" was whether the patient had a personality disorder. In these cases, biofeedback was rarely an appropriate treatment recommendation. During the course of consulting with the referral source or during the client's evaluation, if the assessor discovers that the initial referral question is not the most important or appropriate issue, he or she should exercise professional judgment and address the more relevant issue. At the same time, the referral source should be provided with a clear rationale for the change of issues.

> *Example of nonspecific referral*: Mr. X. was referred for a psychological assessment by his doctor.

> *Example of more adequate referral*: Mr. X. was referred for a psychological evaluation by his physician in order to assess the influence of depression, or possible dementia, on his difficulty making decisions, his poor memory, and his persistent fatigue.

Managing Differing Agendas

Given the proliferation of referral sources and referral questions, we can no longer assume that there is a simple relationship between the assessing psychologist, the patient, and assessment report (Armengol, 2001). The subject of the psychological evaluation, the "patient," is often different from the primary recipient of the report, the referral source or client. In some cases, there may be multiple clients, all with objectives that differ from the patient's. The ostensible purpose of a report may also differ from either the referral sources' or the patients' unspoken "hidden agendas," such as supporting a particular point of view in a conflict between treatment providers. This discrepancy is especially likely in workers compensation evaluations, assessment of candidates for organ transplantation, due process assessment of a child with learning and behavior problems, probation hearing evaluations, or reports requested as "second opinions." Both clients and agendas can be relatively briefly identified in the initial statement of the referral question.

> *Example*: John Doe was referred by his insurance company to assess the presence and extent of disability, as well as to evaluate the appropriateness of vocational retraining.

> *Example*: Mrs. X. was referred by the transplantation review board for evaluation of psychological factors that may affect her ability to consent to, and benefit from, a liver transplant.

One of the most critical issues raised by multiple-purpose evaluations is confidentiality. The relevance of specific details and the potential for embarrassment and invasion of privacy vary according to the referral question, the referral source, and the purpose of the report. Consequently, it is important that a patient's consent be obtained, based upon adequate information about the purpose of a report and the intended recipients. Report writers also should be mindful that, in most cases, the examinee will have access to the report. Writers should thus strive to present information in as nonstigmatizing, nonjudgmental manner as possible. At the same time, writers need to be concerned with not compromising their clinical judgment by neglecting information that may be uncomfortable for an examinee to read. A useful strategy in this regard is to provide descriptions of clients' strengths as well as their weaknesses.

The competing concerns noted above often can be balanced by giving attention to the way ideas are worded. Terms can be selected that do not imply disparagement and that are potentially less difficult for the examinee to accept. Careful choice of words also can be used to reveal a problem that may not be relevant to the current referral question, and that may have a high potential for embarrassment, but that may need to be raised. For example, phrases and terms such as "problems in the family of origin" or "early trauma" may be used, respectively, in lieu of details about a father's alcoholism or an incident of abuse. Important issues should not be minimized just because they are uncomfortable, but, considering the issue of confidentiality, the writer should make sure that all details are relevant to the specific issue in question.

Documentation versus Conceptualization

The report of a psychological evaluation is different from a documentation of an examinee's concerns, although the two are not mutually exclusive. Studies dealing with the usefulness of psychological reports have typically ranked recommendations and treatment plans highest in importance, and written documentation lowest (Reynolds et al., 1995; Siegel & Fischer, 1981). Despite this importance, recommendations are frequently considered to be one of the weakest areas of a report (Finn et al., 2001).

Documentation assumes more relative importance in legal and forensic cases, where it is crucial to include all the data on which inferences are based, including specific quotes and identification of the source of each piece of information (Derby, 2001; Hoffman, 1986). Direct quotation is also appropriate in other circumstances where it is necessary to convey specific information, such as the characterization of an unusual thought disorder or the documentation of suicidal and homicidal ideation. However, our experience in helping students with their reports is that, perhaps because of uncertainty about their professional judgment, they typically err on the side of providing excessive circumstantial detail at the expense of explicit statements of the summary judgments they are being asked to provide.

It is generally felt that, although the report typically should go beyond the answer to the referral question, the diagnostician can choose the areas to be discussed in more detail and does not need to include absolutely all the information that was gathered about the examinee. By making the psychologist's professional judgment as explicit as possible throughout the report, the differences between "raw data" and inference can be made clear, and "biases" in the selection of material can be made as transparent as possible.

Structuring the Narrative

Good psychological report writers aspire to make their reports as readable as possible. To achieve this goal, the report should flow smoothly. Paragraphs should be organized by themes, with each paragraph developing one theme, or part of a theme, in a coherent manner. An introductory sentence or two should describe the overall theme and include an assessment of the severity of the issue. This format is compatible with Ownby's (1997) recommendation that paragraphs include a topic sentence that introduces a construct (such as *intelligence*), followed by relevant data and an evaluation.

> *Example*: Mr. Smith's intellectual abilities are in the average range. All of the global scores obtained with the WAIS-III were in that range. Judging from the subtest scores, all of the specific abilities examined

were in or about that range, and there were no indications of significant cognitive deficits.

Important issues should be readily identified, not "buried" within the body of an extensive report. For example, suicidal or homicidal ideation should be placed prominently in the report, and both should be addressed clearly in the summary and recommendation sections.

Organizing themes can include *diagnoses* (e.g., depression) or *symptom clusters* (e.g., reexperiencing symptoms in PTSD), *interpersonal style or conflicts* (e.g., externalizing blame, withdrawal), *functional domains* (e.g., intelligence, emotional expression), or more *specific issues* such as the ability to provide informed consent. It is important to address predisposing, precipitating, maintaining, and exacerbating factors, although these may be more appropriately reviewed in the concluding sections of the report, where they can be linked to specific recommendations.

In order to develop treatment plans that are likely to improve treatment outcome, it is important to be guided by relevant empirical literature (see Chapter 3). For reports that focus on treatment planning, some domains are more important than others (Armengol, Moes, Penney, & Sapienza, 2001; Beutler, Clarkin, & Bongar, 2000). For example, internalizing clients are more likely to respond well to insight-oriented interventions that increase their awareness. In contrast, externalizing clients do not respond as well to introspective approaches but do best with specific, concrete strategies for developing behavioral change.

> *Example*: The statement "Mr. X. reports a longstanding history of aggression," followed by details of his history, identifies the chronic nature of the problem. A subsequent paragraph's introduction, "Mr. X.'s case is complicated by a 10-year history of alcohol abuse that appears to have exacerbated his aggressiveness," draws attention to comorbid influences on the presenting complaint.

Readability of Reports

Reports are usually the most tangible part of the assessing psychologist's work. The appearance and style of the report, especially its adherence to basic rules of grammar and stylistic conventions, may have a bearing on the recipient's view of the psychologist, the psychologist's professionalism, and the validity of the information in the report. When in doubt about psychology-specific composition issues, refer to the American Psychological Association's *Publication Manual* (2001), which includes a concise summary of general grammar and style. For a broader review of grammar and style, with special attention to typical problems when English is a second language, see Hacker (1999).

The readability of a psychological report has new relevance, because—as a result of current ethical, professional, and legal guidelines—the subject of a report is quite likely to obtain and read the report. Unfortunately, psychologists have a natural tendency to write technical reports that are not easily understood by patients (Harvey, 1997). Readability can be enhanced by using shorter sentences, translating psychological concepts into everyday language, reducing the use of acronyms, and increasing the use of subheadings. Feedback from peers and consumers also can be helpful in making reports more readable.

Conveying the Level of Certainty

As diagnosticians, we need to trust our findings, but we also need to be mindful of the limitations of our data. Some of our findings are so trustworthy that we can predict, with a 95% level of confidence, what the finding is likely to be if the test were to be taken again. Some of the tests in our armamentarium, however, do not enjoy that kind of reliability. Moreover, some interpretations may be directly derived from test data, whereas other conclusions may rely on a number of assumptions and be much more speculative. For instance, when we discuss the limited abilities of an individual with an intelligence quotient of 65, we can be fairly certain of the functions that the person may be able to perform and those that are beyond his or her capacity. Our findings, on the other hand, may not allow the same level of certainty about the behavior of a person with a moderately high score on a dependency scale. Worse yet, if we were to discuss etiological issues, such as why the person has a narcissistic personality style, our contentions would be even more speculative.

Because of the potential benefits of speculative material, such discussion should not be discouraged. However, a good report should distinguish between valid assertions based directly on reliable data and more speculative interpretations associated with a less solid foundation. The level of certainty can be conveyed to the reader through the use of appropriate phrasing. Statements to the effect that an individual *may* demonstrate a particular characteristic, or *is similar* to people who have a particular attribute, can convey an appropriate level of uncertainty. A statement such as *one possible way of looking at Mr. Smith* expresses an even more tentative contention.

Disposition

The APA ethical code states, "Psychologists strive to benefit those with whom they work and take care to do no harm. . . . Because psychologists' scientific and professional judgments and actions may affect the lives of others, they are alert to and guard against personal, financial, social, organizational, or political factors that might lead to misuse of their influence" (American Psychological Association, 2002, p. 1062).

The sometimes divergent or hidden agendas of examinees have implications for the use of a report as well as for its content. Psychologists should assume some responsibility for the appropriate use of their work and not assume the process has been completed once they have submitted their report. For example, having evaluated a child for class placement and having made recommendations for managing a behavior problem, a psychologist may, following best ethical practice, contact the school to ascertain whether the report was received by the appropriate person, whether its conclusions and recommendations were understandable, and whether the recommendations were implemented. In our experience, many nonpsychologists welcome a more informal verbal exchange of information in addition to, or accompanying, the report itself. Verbal exchanges are often more likely to have an immediate impact, as the assessor cannot be certain when or how much of a written report will be read or by whom. The steps taken to ensure appropriate use of a report should be included in the report itself, when possible, or in a subsequent addendum.

> *Example*: The contents of this report were shared with Mrs. Z., who concurred with our recommendations and agreed to begin weekly sessions of individual psychotherapy with Dr. B.

> *Example*: Although Mrs. B. has expressed some suicidal ideation, she denies having a plan or intent. She has made a verbal agreement not to attempt to harm herself and to contact her psychologist, should she find herself considering such actions. Her suicidal ideation will be monitored by her therapist at weekly treatment sessions. She also has been referred to Dr. Z., a psychiatrist, for evaluation of the appropriateness of medication for her depression.

Length of the Report

The average psychological report is from five to seven single-spaced pages (Finn et al., 2001). This length is particularly likely for reports written in vocational, psychological, or educational settings. However, length can vary substantially. Psychological reports in many medical settings resemble those done by physicians, which are typically two to three pages long. In contrast, reports written for forensic settings are typically much longer, because of the need for detail, integration of information from a wider range of sources, substantiation of findings, and anticipation of counterarguments. A typical forensic report is 7 to 10 single-spaced pages, although some forensic reports can be as long as 20 pages.

THE USE OF COMPUTERS

Psychodiagnosticians typically use computers when writing reports. In addition to making report writing easier, computers store the report as a computer file, which makes it possible to move in the direction of a paperless office (Trudel & Taylor, 2001). Computer-based interpretations can utilize large data bases and generate numerous possible interpretations. Scoring and interpretive programs are available for most of the major psychological tests. A software program is also available for the STS model, which assists with developing a treatment plan, provides examples of how techniques can be implemented, and helps with client monitoring and outcome assessment (Beutler & Williams, 1999).

Going beyond test-processing and word-processing tasks, computer technology has made it possible to function more effectively and accurately. For instance, diagnosticians typically find themselves repeating similar information in their reports. From the mental status examination to the explanation of a scale elevation to the description of a particular profile of abilities in an intelligence test, different reports may contain very similar narrative segments. The assessor can compose the description of a mental status examination that covers all of the areas of the typical examination and describes all of the functions as intact. When this narrative is imported into the record of a person who is left-handed, has trouble paying attention, or is delusional, those elements of the narrative can then be changed to reflect the actual findings for the particular case.

In addition to such "fill-in-the-blanks" segments, clinicians can develop coding and index systems to increase their efficiency and accuracy. Readers may be familiar with the coding systems developed for the MMPI or the MCMI (Butcher, Dahlstrom, Graham, Tellegen, & Kaemmer, 1989; Millon, Davis, & Millon, 1997). Coding reports, and keeping a directory of the codes with the file names where the report is to be found, allows clinicians to borrow relevant portions of previously written reports. In specialty settings (e.g., a pain clinic, an elementary school) there may be a very finite number of different syndromes (e.g., different learning disabilities) that are seen on a regular basis. In those cases, it is more efficient to have a collection of narratives that can be imported into a report, as needed.

Even in a general psychiatric clinic, there may be occasional patients who resemble each other. To take advantage of previous reports, clinicians can create a computerized index file containing patients they have seen. In addition to the date and file name, this index file may contain the DSM-IV diagnoses and a summary of the case, perhaps taken from the report itself. When a new patient is tested, this index file can be searched for previous reports that may have reusable parts. In that manner, the diagnostician can obtain ready-made segments, such as a description of a depressed state, or how a schizotypal personality disorder has contributed to the development of a psychotic disorder.

However, when using computer-based or previously written interpretations, clinicians need to exercise a number of cautions. Although many of the computer-based narrative interpretations may be quite accurate, many other such interpretations will be incorrect. This possibility means that clinicians need to sift carefully through the narrative interpretations to differentiate between the accurate and inaccurate descriptions of the client. Even when the interpretations are considered to be accurate, they may not be necessarily relevant enough to include in the report, given the referral question. In addition, clinicians using segments of previously written reports must ensure that names or inapplicable details from one patient are not erroneously inserted into the report of another person. Using such a system makes it imperative that the psychologist read every report carefully, from beginning to end, including headers and footers, prior to dissemination.

COMPONENTS OF THE PSYCHOLOGICAL REPORT

There is no agreed-upon structure for a psychological report. Reports can be highly structured around specific headings and subheadings or presented in a letter format. Test scores can be presented in the body of a report, included as an appendix, or not reported at all. For more extended reviews of research and alternatives to report-writing styles, the reader is referred to Groth-Marnat (1999, 2000, in press-b), Ownby (1997), Reynolds and colleagues (1995), Tallent (1993), Wolber and Carne (1993), or Zukerman (2000). However, these options are not meant to paralyze writers and readers of mental health records but, instead, to promote diversity and thoughtfulness. The following section provides a review of components found in most psychological reports.

Reason for Referral

A psychological report typically starts with a section that includes the patient's name and demographic information such as age, ethnicity, and marital status. Location may be pertinent, particularly if the assessor's practice serves a broad geographical area. The inclusion of demographic information helps identify the patient and provides base-rate information that may be relevant for differential diagnoses. The name of the referral source and the relationship of this person to the patient are often important, as are the referral question and the purpose of the report.

A recommended way to begin a report is to include a brief sentence orienting the reader to the client. For example: "Mr. X. is a 35-year-old white divorced male who is experiencing depression and anxiety." This overview is followed by a statement of the referral question—for example: "The evaluation was requested in order to determine the extent of his depression and anxiety, to develop a formal diagnosis, to assess the presence of suicidal ideation, to identify his relevant resources and strengths, and to provide recommendations for treatment." The advantage of listing all referral questions is to allow easy reference to them at the end of the report, in the summary and recommendations sections. Often this listing can be done by numbering or bulleting each of the points. This reiteration is particularly important because some time-conscious professionals may read *only* the "Reason for Referral" and the "Summary" and "Recommendations" sections, neglecting the body of the report.

Procedures

A section listing the procedures comprising the evaluation is typically included in forensic cases. The listing of procedures begins with the clinical interview held with the patient and other informants. Informants are identified by name and by their relationship to the patient. Other sources of information may include medical or other records referred to in the report. These sources should be listed with the authors and the dates of the reports. Psychological tests should be noted, with abbreviations in parentheses; abbreviations can be used thereafter in the body of the report. It also can be useful to include the dates the tests were given as well as the total face-to-face time spent with the client.

Presenting Complaint

This section of the report includes a description of the presenting problems. Some psychologists prefer to include the history of the problem in a separate section; others include it in this section, along with the description of the problem in its current state. Given that patients typically have been experiencing distress for some time before their evaluation, this section also should address the question of why the patient was referred for, or is seeking, treatment at this particular time (Budman & Gurman, 1988), if the issue was not already addressed as part of the referral problem.

It is important to identify explicitly any discrepancies in information provided by the different sources. For example, if a man describes a supportive marital relationship whereas his spouse reports that she is considering divorce, such a discrepancy obviously should be noted. Noting such discrepancies is often an issue in conditions where denial or minimization is common, as is the case with patients who have substance abuse problems or those complaining of somatic symptoms.

Psychosocial History

The psychosocial history should be organized by themes, such as the character of interpersonal relationships or predominant issues in the patient's work or educational history. Typical components include previous psychological problems and treatment outcomes, medical history, family background, social relationships, educational history, and occupational history (see Chapter 4). It is important to tailor the psychosocial history to the referral question. For example, if the referral is for vocational assessment, the history sections should focus on the client's past work history, aspirations, goals, and interests. It may not be appropriate to focus on such factors as problematic family relations or personal difficulties, unless these are directly related to the client's vocational options.

Behavioral Observations and Mental Status Examination

Behavioral observations are a critical component of every report. Observations of patients during the assessment process provide additional data on which to base evaluations and diagnosis—data that is often more valid than the patient's self-report (e.g., Mazure, Nelson, & Price, 1986). Observations may shed a new light on other sources of data, perhaps allowing a different interpretation of a statement made by the examinee than the statement otherwise would have merited. It is imperative to note if there is evidence of disorientation, disorganization of behavior or thought processes, or lack of cooperation. Other influences that may compromise the accuracy of the data, such as limited command of the English language or medication that may impair attention and concentration, also should be noted. Behavioral observations should be worded as concretely as possible; inferences based on observations are more appropriate in the section on the presenting problem and especially the discussion/interpretation and impressions sections. For example, instead of stating that a client appeared *depressed*, it is preferable to describe behaviors from several domains that are consistent with depression (i.e., "There was evidence of psychomotor retardation in the client's slow speech and long latencies; his affect was flat and unvarying").

One exception to this recommendation occurs when a more comprehensive Mental Status Exam (MSE) is a component of the report. An MSE is typically based primarily on the client's behavior combined with conclusions related to this behavior (see Zukerman, 2000, pp. 26–43). For example, a clinician may observe aspects of a patient's behavior and conclude that the person is oriented or has good insight into his or her behavior. Recommended components of mental status reports include:

- Orientation (to time, place, person)
- Appearance
- Attitude toward the evaluation process
- Verbalizations (articulation, rate, volume)
- Psychomotor activity
- Affect (character, stability, range, appropriateness to content)
- Thought processes and contents
- Insight and judgment

A further exception to the mere description of behavior occurs when clinicians make inferences regarding the validity of the assessment procedures. Because these inferences are often based on behavioral observations (e.g., degree of motivation, fatigue, accuracy as a historian), this part of the assessment is traditionally included at the end of the behavioral observations section. A representative statement might be: "Given the patient's high level of motivation and the validity indicators on the MMPI-2, the assessment results appear to be an accurate assessment of his current level of functioning." If, on the other hand, the results seem to be compromised in some ways, then this section is often a good place to discuss this issue.

Results

The results section lists the scores on the various tests. This listing can either be presented as text in the body of the report itself or in a table format. Some tests, such as the MMPI-2, MCMI-III, and intelligence tests, have scores that are easily presented in a table as part of the report. When appropriate, the norms on which comparisons are based should be indicated (i.e., whether a patient's scores are being compared with a general sample or with smaller samples based on age, gender, education, etc.). Some test results, such as narratives from the Thematic Apperception Test or human figure drawings, tend to be more difficult to include. Typically they are summarized; for example: "TAT stories were characterized by strong needs for achievement and affiliation, but these two needs were frequently in conflict with one another."

It should be noted that many psychological reports do not include a listing of test scores. When any scores are included, they tend to be only the more salient scores, and they are imbedded in the narrative. The rationale for this practice is that, because many or most readers are not trained to interpret scores properly, inclusion of any or all scores opens the door to misinterpretations. Moreover, including test scores requires additional explanations that may not be necessary otherwise. For instance, if a clinician, for good cause, decides to disregard a high or low score, and if all scores are presented in the report, he or she may be required to explain why the particular score was not included in the narrative.

In contrast to the above view, other psychologists argue for the inclusion of scores (see Pieniadz & Kelland, 2001). One clear argument in favor of this position is that the standard of care in many other health fields calls for the inclusion of test results, even though there may be a risk that the scores may be misinterpreted. For example, every medical record contains all of the patient's laboratory test values, even though such values need to be interpreted by a qualified professional. In fact, one of the advantages of presenting scores is that it makes our work appear more legitimate and data-based. Moreover, as other professionals gain access to scores from our testing instruments, they become more knowledgeable about psychological testing per se, and may be more likely to request our work in the future. When the reader is another psychologist, the inclusion of the scores adds a depth of understanding that could not otherwise be achieved. Finally, the inclusion of test scores in table form allows for a more flowing narrative, because the writer no longer has to be concerned about presenting the salient scores as the issues presented by the case are discussed. A related issue is whether to discuss statistical findings, such as confidence levels. A suggestion that may help reduce statistical confusion is to indicate the degree of elevation (such as "very high," high," "average," etc.) when including test scores. In addition, standard scores that are easily understood by a wide range of readers (e.g., percentiles) are preferred over more obscure scores (e.g., base rates; Finn et al., 2001).

Another area characterized by a wide range of variation involves the inclusion of data to support specific inferences and judgments in the narrative. Some psychologists favor making declarative statements in their interpretation and summary sections. Such statements are typically the end result of integrating a wide number of converging sources of information about the client. Such integrations might involve ignoring a score elevation if other sources of information (behavioral observations or medical history) do not support the conclusions typically suggested by the high score. Detailing the clinician's reasoning processes may result in an overly tedious report. However, in the absence of supportive data the reader must make a leap of faith regarding the clinician's inferences. We favor the middle ground of providing enough foundation to inform the reader of the basis of our conclusions, while not burdening the narrative with excessive justification. Consider, for instance, the following text:

> "Mr. Fernández's unusual responses to a series of ambiguous inkblots (Rorschach inkblot test) indicate that he is having difficulties with his contact with reality. Behavioral observations and past history also reveal ideas that are peculiar or delusional. During the interview, he sometimes began with a notion that was indisputably real, but then he inserted other thoughts that were not logical or connected."

In this example, the reader is informed that conclusions are based on the Rorschach and confirmed by history and behavioral observations. However, the narrative is not burdened with the details of Rorschach markers that indicate the lack of contact with reality.

Discussion/Interpretation and Impressions

The section dealing with the clinician's interpretations is typically the most difficult part of the report. A valuable source of options for accurate and effective descriptions and phrasing is Zuckerman's (2000) *Clinician's Thesaurus: The Guidebook for Writing Psychological Reports*. This section, and the summary and recommendation section, are the most meaningful and useful parts of the report. They are also the portions of the report that provide the most opportunity for the writer's creativity. These sections provide answers to specific referral questions while enhancing the reader's understanding of the patient as a whole.

A good discussion section is not unlike a piece of literature, wherein a character is developed or a mystery is solved. It should focus on the examinee, only using data as the pillars supporting the narrative. If test results are referred to in this section, it is preferable to use descriptive phrases ("very high," "average," etc.) rather than scores. The goal is to review the relevant aspects of the examinee in a way that makes him or her "come alive." The narrative should balance idiographic and nomothetic approaches by showing the individual in his or her uniqueness, while identifying the elements that he or she has in common with others. The narrative also should address any relevant concurrent or future behaviors that can be predicted on the basis of empirical research.

Most discussion sections follow one of a finite number of organizational schemes—just as, even in the creative world of literature, recurrent story progressions are commonly used (see May, 1980). Five of these narrative schemes are discussed: (1) the review of functions, (2) the developmental issues, (3) the personality, (4) the diagnostic issues, and (5) the review of test results (Choca & Van Denburg, 1996).

The *review of functions* scheme organizes the narrative through a sequential description of the psychological functions deemed important. The writer's theoretical orientation may guide the choice of the salient functions to be covered and the progression from one theory-based construct to the next. Using a review of functions scheme, an intellectual evaluation may start with a discussion of the patient's global abilities, proceed to review the individual's mental control and flexibility, and eventually address abstract capacity, verbal capacity, visuospatial capacity, and so on (see Groth-Marnat, 2000). Often it is important to consider a patient's relative cognitive strengths and weaknesses. For example, a patient may have a fairly high level of general intelligence but considerable difficulties with memory. Memory difficulties can be further divided into subcomponents, such as auditory–verbal versus visual memory. Often it is important to describe the cause of memory and other cognitive difficulties, if known (e.g., exposure to neurotoxic substances, head injury, Alzheimer's disease, etc.). A frequent problem with descriptions of intellectual abilities is the use of technical language (e.g., "The patient shows difficulties with visual sequencing"). Although this specificity of language can be useful when communicating with a knowledgeable professional, it runs the risk of making the report difficult to read for others. Technical terms or implications for daily functioning can usually be translated into everyday language (e.g., "The client is likely to have difficulty reading and following directions on street maps").

There is a potentially wide array of functioning issues to address in a personality report. Three of the most important are the client's cognitive, emotional, and interpersonal–intrapersonal functions. In addition to the information offered by an intelligence test, cognitive functions also include level of insight, degree of conventionality, ability to solve practical, everyday problems, intellectual efficiency, and ability to deal effectively with emotions (i.e., emotional intelligence).

Emotional functioning is often divided into mood and affect. *Mood* refers to the subjective emotional experience of the client and may include long-term features that characterize his or her personality (i.e., trait features) as well as more temporary fluctuation (i.e., state features). Mood ranges on a continuum from euphoria to dysphoria. It is often useful to discuss where on this continuum the client typically functions as well as how changeable his or her mood is (i.e., range and lability). Whereas mood refers to the person's own experience, *affect* refers to those responses to the environment that are observable. One of the most important clinical dimensions of affect is the degree to which the affect is appropriate to the situation. Some clients are highly reactive to, and unstable in, even minimally stressful situations. Thus their problem-solving skills and behavioral repertoire may deteriorate quite easily. In contrast, other persons are fairly resistant to stressors. The discussion of emotional functioning should clearly establish whether or not a client has features relevant to the diagnosis of a thought disorder (e.g., flat affect) or a mood disorder (e.g., unstable moods, predominantly dysphoric).

In terms of the interpersonal style, the two basic relational continua include (1) the extent to which a client expresses loving versus hostile patterns (the love–hate dimension), and (2) the extent to which a client expresses dominant versus submissive patterns (the dominant–submissive dimension). Many of the measures described previously in this volume address these dimensions. For example, the CPI assesses such qualities as degree of responsibility, control over behavior, and the extent to which a client feels a sense of belonging to, and empathy with, his or her community. The MCMI-III describes many personality patterns of interpersonal behavior, such as the active, engaged patterns of histrionic styles or the removed, distant patterns of schizoid styles. Descriptions of interpersonal functioning also may address the client's style of coping with interpersonal conflict. For example, some clients become actively engaged in problem solving when in conflict with others, whereas others become highly suspicious, defensive, and hostile, thereby creating interpersonal distance that may further aggravate conflicts and alienate sources of potential support.

In addition to describing interpersonal patterns, it is often important to elaborate on internal processes (i.e., intrapersonal style). For example, some patients are pessimistic and self-critical, whereas others are optimistic and actively work to enhance their self-esteem. Some clients have internalized a view of themselves as helpless and needing others to take care of them; others see themselves as extremely independent and autonomous.

One strategy for organizing results around functions and domains is to use a grid (see Beutler, 1995; Groth-Marnat, 1999), with the domains/functions (intellect, coping style, contact with reality, etc.) listed on the left side as row heads. For example, if a referral source wanted information on treatment planning, relevant domains would include the client's coping style, level of social support, and resistance level. The sources of data (history, behavioral observations, MMPI-2, CPI, etc.) can be listed as column heads at the top of the grid. Relevant information can be entered into the body of the grid based on the domain and information source. When it comes time to write the report, clinicians can then develop descriptive paragraphs based on the information within the grid, organized by the various domains and functions. For example, a review of Tables 13.1 and 13.2 indicates that the client had a number of characteristics consistent with a compulsive personality. The boxes within the grid provide information supportive of this inference, including an emphasis on detail and duty, and a disdain for others.

Using the domains/functions format has the advantage that it can be fairly easily organized (especially by using the grids shown in these two tables) and usually does a good job of answering the referral question. However, this format may not do an optimal job of developing a coherent narrative of the person or fully describing the "feel" of who he or she is as an individual. The next three schemes are harder to mold into an adequate report, but they have the potential of making the discussion more interesting and preserving the integrity of the individual. With these schemes, the narrative then becomes more like a story or an argument for a particular point of view, and the order of the elements is dictated by the theme being developed. Because each paragraph advances the theme, there is more cohesion in the discussion than occurs through the sequential listing of the different functions that comprise the individual.

Using the *developmental* scheme, the writer describes the influences experienced by the patient throughout the years, and the way that he or she reacted at different stages in life. Consider, for instance, the task of writing the discussion section for a report on Melvin Udall, the main character in the movie *As Good as It Gets*. The writer might start by discussing the effects of Melvin's overly strict father, who rapped him on the hands with a ruler whenever he made a mistake. Perhaps the mother could be described as distant and unavailable. This type of upbringing may be said to have left Melvin apprehensive about venturing out, because it created a great deal of fear about making mistakes. At this point, the patient's personality attributes could be detailed. Those traits, in turn, could be seen as resulting in an angry demeanor and a self-defeating, constricted, and unfulfilling life, in spite of Melvin's talents and vocational success. (We use this fictional character and this scheme as the patient in one of the sample reports at the end of the chapter.)

The *personality* scheme starts with a description of the patient's basic personality style, followed by a review of the life situation that the patient is facing and the interplay between the personality style and the environmental forces. In his story *The Overcoat*, Gogol describes the compulsive personality of the protagonist, a scribe who practices writing different letter fonts for recreation. After having presented this rigid and overly formal individual, Gogol introduces the situation his protagonist faces when he is in dire need of a new overcoat. The story goes on to detail the sacrifices this scribe makes in order to afford the new coat. When the coat is stolen the first time it is worn, the psychotic break that follows comes as no surprise. A report based on the personality scheme format also may isolate and develop those aspects that are particularly important to the narrative, given the referral question. For example, if the referral question emphasized treatment recommendations, the narrative could focus on the relationship of personality factors to the variables of the STS model, such that separate paragraphs could be devoted to problem severity, problem complexity, motivational distress, coping style, resistance potential, and level of social support.

Using the *differential diagnostic* scheme, the test and interview information could be presented under the rubric of a differential diagnosis debate. The report would explore the diagnostic issues that the patient presents and how the history and the test data can be used to clarify those issues. In Ken Kesey's masterpiece *One Flew Over the Cuckoo's Nest*, the author raises the issue of whether the main character, R. P. McMurphy, suffers from a psychiatric disorder. A report about this individual might start by posing the diagnostic uncertainty and then explore the data supporting one side or the other. The assessment might show, for instance, signs of a borderline personality disorder with antisocial elements. On the other hand, psychological data also might show that the patient was in good contact with reality, was not depressed or manic, and was not burdened by anxieties or apprehensions.

We strongly discourage organizing the discussion section as a *review of test results*. In this scheme, results are organized by the tests administered, and the inferences derived from the data are addressed within the discussion of each particular test. In a neuropsychological battery, for instance, a report might start with a discussion of scores from the Wechsler Adult Intelligence Scale (WAIS-III), followed by the findings from the next instrument in the battery. This test-by-test approach is undesirable for several reasons. First, it tends to bore the reader with the somewhat tiresome recounting of findings from each of the particular instruments, regardless of the relevance to the referral issues. Indeed, referral sources are much less interested in test scores than in the meaning of the overall assessment. The test-by-test scheme deemphasizes the most interesting and important element of our work: the examinee. It presents the person as a series of test scores rather than as a living, struggling, functioning human. In addition, it is a mechanical and fragmented format and does not utilize the clinician's ability to integrate information into a coherent description based on multiple sources of information. It is exactly this integrating function of the clinician that makes the information most meaningful and relevant to the referral source and the client.

Diagnostic Impressions

Many referral sources request DSM-IV diagnoses, and such diagnoses are typically required for billing purposes. However, there is accumulating evidence of (1) the limited predictive validity of such categorical diagnoses (Beutler & Malik, 2002b; Carson, 1997; Groth-Marnat, Roberts, & Beutler, 2001; Houts, 2002), and (2) the presence of clinically significant psychosocial impairment in subclinical cases. This means that it is important that the discussion section of the report provide sufficient elaboration of the particulars of each case as well as a clear rationale for the relevance of diagnosis.

Summary and Recommendations

The value of a psychological report rests, in large part, on the summary and recommendations generated by the evaluation. As was suggested previously, an effective way of organizing the summary is to address each of the referral questions in a brief, succinct manner. Bulleting or numbering each recommendation makes the information easy to locate.

Recommendations need to take into account the client's strengths, interests, and resources, as well as the problems uncovered by the evaluation (see Egan, 2002, for a discussion of the importance of these factors in therapy). Research and clinical experience suggest that recommendations are most effective when they are as concrete as possible (Armengol et al., 2001). Higher-order constructs should serve an intermediary function between the presenting problems and the recommendations. For example, cognitive therapy might be recommended to address *depressogenic cognitions*, the hypothesized mediating construct between a patient's chronic health condition and his or her depressed mood and fatigue; however, examples should be given of the client's specific problematic cognitions in order to particularlize the recommendation and improve its understandability to a more general audience. Each recommendation should be linked explicitly with the critical themes or problems identified in the body of the report as well as the referral questions (Armengol et al., 2001)

> *Example of nonspecific recommendation*: I recommend that Mr. Jones undertake a course of cognitive therapy.

> *Example of specific recommendation, linked with presenting problems*: I recommend that Mr. Jones receive a course of cognitive therapy to address the depressogenic cognitions noted above. These cognitions about himself and his work performance are likely contributing to his current complaint of little motivation and sense of futility.

Good recommendations are also typically geared to the expertise and interests of the referral source. It is usually inappropriate, for instance, to tell a psychiatrist what medication to use, or a speech pathologist which articulation problem needs to be treated. However, patients can be tactfully referred to an appropriate provider for an evaluation of the appropriateness of medication for symptoms or disorders identified in the report.

The degree of detail in each recommendation will depend on the client and purpose of the report. For example, workers compensation carriers typically want to know not only whether to treat or not but the modality of therapy (e.g., individual, group), the number of sessions, their frequency, and the expected duration. In order to maximize outcomes and increase the rate of improvement, managed care organizations are increasingly expecting such recommendations to be based on empirical research. The STS variables detailed in Chapter 3 and discussed throughout this volume provide such a basis. Given the limited predictive validity of many diagnoses, tailoring treatment according to these variables, rather than to diagnoses per se, is more likely to enhance response to treatment.

EXAMPLES OF CASE REPORTS

Case 1

The following evaluation was based on information derived from viewing the film *As Good as It Gets*. The main character, Melvin Udall, demonstrates many of the classic features that characterize an obsessive–compulsive disorder, with corresponding features of a compulsive personality. The "test results" were developed from inferences made of the client's history and behavioral observations. Note that the Emotional Assessment System is not described in this book, but the central domains that are being assessed should be relatively familiar to readers. In contrast, the MCMI-III is thoroughly covered in Chapter 7. The report is organized according to the standard structure used in most reports. However, the discussion section is an example of using a developmental narrative to best summarize and understand the central features of the person. Note that the organization of the different features of the case is summarized by using the grid described previously (see Table 13.1). The recommendations also focus on understanding the challenges, issues, and techniques of therapy that would be most relevant for the "patient."

Identifying Information

Name: Melvin Udall
Sex: Male
Date of birth: 5/22/51
Date of evaluation: 8/12/01
Referring clinician: Robert Newhart, MD
Ethnicity: European American

Reason for Referral

Mr. Udall is a 50-year-old white single male who was referred for a psychological evaluation regarding his obsessions, compulsions, and interpersonal problems. The patient had not been making much progress in the treatment he had been receiving from his psychiatrist, Dr. Robert Newhart, and had been noncompliant with his medication. Testing was requested in order to determine his personality structure, the role that characterological factors may be playing in his lack of progress, and to provide suggestions for treatment.

Presenting Complaints

Mr. Udall has a compulsion to check repeatedly the multiple locks on his front door. In addition, he hops around on sidewalks to avoid stepping on any cracks. He feels this habit results from an irrational superstition in which he claims he does not believe. Nevertheless, he feels so uncomfortable when he steps on the cracks that he believes he is incapable of behaving in any other way. Furthermore, Mr. Udall has a fear of germs. In addition to practicing cleanliness to an excessive degree, he takes his own napkin and eating utensils to restaurants so as not to touch their utensils.

   Mr. Udall is aware that his behavior aversely affects his interactions

TABLE 13.1. Mapping Information from Different Sources into a Narrative: Case 1

	History	Observations	EAS	MCMI-III
Intellect	Good student	Excellent vocabulary, good ability to express self.	Not applicable.	Not applicable.
Childhood antecedents	Father characterized as a strict man who punished for minor mistakes. Mother was distant and ineffective.	Not applicable.	Not applicable.	Not applicable.
Compulsive personality		Compulsive characteristics.	Elevation of the Compulsive scale, indicating overly disciplined and meticulous personality traits.	Elevation of the Compulsive scale, indicating overly disciplined and meticulous personality traits.
Narcissistic element		Mild grandiosity, inclined to treat others with disdain.	Elevation of the Narcissistic scale, indicating an inflated self-image.	Elevation of the Narcissistic scale, indicating an inflated self-image.
Schizotypal element	Has no relationships.	Is peculiar.	Subclinical elevation of the Schizotypal scale, suggesting a tendency toward peculiar habits.	Elevation of the Schizotypal scale, indicating interpersonal isolation and a tendency toward peculiar habits.
Resentment and anger		Is typically sarcastic and insulting.	Elevation of the Anger scale indicates a tendency toward verbally expressed anger.	Elevation of the Negativistic scale indicates a tendency toward resentment.
Obsessive–compulsive disorder	Detail symptoms.	Fear of germs, avoids stepping on sidewalk cracks, must lock and unlock door several times.	Elevation of the Anxiety scale, indicating a high level of tension.	Elevation of the Anxiety scale, indicating a high level of tension.
Good contact with reality	No psychotic symptoms.	No psychotic symptoms.	No elevation in Thought Disorder scale.	No elevation in Thought Disorder scale.
No other psychopathology	No other complaints.	No other symptoms.	No other elevations.	No other elevations.

419

with others across a range of personal and work relationships. He constantly insults and mistreats people verbally. Although he professes not to care about the opinions of others, he is painfully aware that this mode of operation makes him function very poorly whenever he has to deal with others. However, he again feels so uncomfortable when he tries to behave in any other manner that he immediately reverts to his usual mode.

Procedures

Clinical interview with Mr. Udall; Emotional Assessment System (EAS); Millon Clinical Multiaxial Inventory–III (MCMI-III); Rorschach.

Background Information

Psychiatric History. Mr. Udall has been in individual psychodynamic psychotherapy on an intermittent basis for much of his adult life. This therapy has apparently had a limited effect on his actual behavior and social impairments, but it allows him to feel better. Currently, he is refusing to take medication (clomipramine) that would potentially relieve the compulsive behavior. [Note that in reporting medications, the convention is to capitalize letters for product/brand names (e.g., Anafranil) and use lowercase for generic, chemical names (e.g., clomipramine).]

Medical History. The patient has never had any major medical problems or injuries. He was considered to be in good physical health at the time of the testing.

Social History. Mr. Udall has a history of problematic, unsupportive relationships with both of his parents, who are deceased. He was born and raised in New York City. He recalls that his father was a "strict" man who was quick with corporal punishment. The patient remembers times when, as a child, his father would rap his hand with a ruler for seemingly minor mistakes. He recalls that his mother, on the other hand, was distant and ineffective, too involved in herself to have much of a meaningful interaction with her son.

Mr. Udall has not developed any supportive relationships in his adult life. He has many acquaintances but no real friendships. He prefers to spend his time in his condominium, watching television or reading and writing novels. He made some attempts at dating during his early 20s, but these attempts did not go well, and he abandoned this effort altogether. He sees himself as heterosexual but is not sexually active.

Educational History. Mr. Udall has a bachelor's degree in literature.

By his report, he was a better-than-average student for most of his academic career.

Occupational History. In spite of his psychological symptoms, the patient has maintained a functional work life, earning his living as a writer. During recent years he has been writing romance novels that have been extremely successful. As a result of that success, he has become reasonably wealthy.

Behavioral Observations and Mental Status Examination

Mr. Udall appeared for the assessment procedure slightly early. He was neatly dressed and was cooperative throughout the evaluation. However, he took an unusually long time to complete his responses. For example, he carefully considered each response on the Rorschach and provided a large number of overall responses. In addition, the history he provided was extremely detailed. At various times during the procedure, he made statements such as "Are you happy with that answer?" or "I'm not sure what you'll make of that, but I don't really care anyway."

Throughout the examination, the patient was alert, oriented to time and place, and verbally coherent. Speech, language, calculations, construction ability, abstractions, and memory were all intact. His thought process was orderly and effective. His thought content, however, showed a preoccupation with obsessions. Maladaptive compulsive behaviors were present. His affective response was appropriate to the content of the conversation. His mood was within normal limits, and he demonstrated a good range of emotions. No suicidal or homicidal ideation was verbalized. His psychomotor activity and anxiety levels were within the normal range during the course of both interview and testing. Given his mental status, behavioral observations, and the pattern of test responses, the results appear to be an accurate assessment of his current level of functioning.

Test Results

EAS	*T*-score	High/very high scores
Tier A: Validity Indicators		
Aa Attention	46	
Ac Comprehension	42	
Ad Disclosure	32	
Ai Inconsistency	55	

EAS	T-score	High/very high scores
Tier B: Basic Scales—Personality		
B01 Introversive–Schizoid	76	High
B02 Avoidant	49	
B03 Cooperative–Dependent	30	
B04 Dramatic–Histrionic	37	
B05 Self-assured–Narcissistic	75	High
B06 Competitive–Antisocial	51	
B07 Disciplined–Compulsive	84	Very high
B08 Schizotypal	65	
B09 Borderline	43	
Tier B: Basic Scales—Mood		
B10 Anxiety–Anxiety Disturbance	75	High
B11 Anger–Explosive Disturbance	70	High
B12 Pessimism–Depression	48	
B13 Optimism–Mania	39	
Tier B: Basic Scales—Pathological Defenses		
B14 Somatic Concerns	53	
B15 Eating Disturbance	40	
B16 Substance Abuse	43	
B17 Distrust–Paranoia	52	
B18 Thought Disturbance	49	
Tier B: Environmental		
B19 Current Stress	44	
B20 Posttraumatic Stress	56	
Tier B: Level of Functioning		
B21 Global Functioning	54	

MCMI-III	Elevations	High/very high scores
Disclosure	75	
Desirability	80	High
Debasement	65	
Schizoid	78	High
Avoidant	83	High
Depressive	65	
Dependent	58	

MCMI-III	Elevations	High/very high scores
Histrionic	53	
Narcissistic	81	High
Antisocial	65	
Aggressive (Sadistic)	74	
Compulsive	90	Very High
Negativistic	77	High
Masochistic	53	
Schizotypal	78	High
Borderline	63	
Paranoid	65	
Anxiety Disorder	80	High
Somatoform Disorder	52	
Bipolar Manic Disorder	57	
Dysthymic Disorder	60	
Alcohol Dependence	63	
Drug Dependence	60	
Posttraumatic Stress	60	
Thought Disorder	54	
Major Depression	65	
Delusional Disorder	66	

Discussion

The mental status examination gave no indications of cognitive or memory deficits. The impression was of an individual with above-average general abilities and with outstanding verbal skills.

According to Mr. Udall's recollections, his father was a strict and fairly unfeeling individual who was never pleased with him. Mr. Udall remembers times when his father would hit him on his hands with a ruler for making a seemingly minor mistake. The patient described his mother as distant and unavailable. At least from his point of view, it seemed that the best the young Mr. Udall could do was to avoid making mistakes in order to evade punishment. Although he was expected to work hard for his achievements and to excel, the emphasis remained on avoiding the mistakes that would bring down the wrath of authority figures, predominantly his father.

It is easy to visualize how such upbringing may have produced the kind of compulsive personality with narcissistic and schizotypal elements that was indicated by Mr. Udall's self-report inventories. The findings suggested that he is the type of individual who is orderly and plans for the future. He believes in discipline and self-restraint, especially regarding expressions of warmth and closeness to others. Mr. Udall tends to be somewhat proper and formal. He is usually conscientious, well prepared, efficient, dependable, industrious, and persistent. Others are likely to see him as perfectionistic, rigid, and picayune.

Because the patient tends to have a grandiose self-image and to see other people as his inferiors, an egotistical and conceited flavor tends to permeate his relationships. Results indicated that Mr. Udall would like to experience affection and appreciation from others, but people present a problem for him. Relating to others carries the risk of rejection and makes him feel vulnerable. He avoids close relationships and relates in a cold and distant manner in order to minimize his feeling of vulnerability. Thus the patient prefers a life of isolation, with very few relationships. At the time of the testing, there was no one in his life to whom he felt close.

In addition to Mr. Udall's isolation, the testing indicated that he is somewhat eccentric and has some habits others may find peculiar. At times he can appear anxious and apprehensive or may demonstrate a flattening of affect. Finally, Mr. Udall may have feelings of depersonalization, emptiness, or meaninglessness.

One way of looking at Mr. Udall's problems is to consider that he entered adulthood with a flawed personality that significantly encumbered his development. Although he was able to succeed in college, his tendency toward awkward, insensitive, and abrasive behavior precluded the establishment of supportive, mature, and reciprocal relationships outside of the home.

In some ways, his choice of careers was an excellent one. A writer can be an individual performer, a person who does not have to interact much with others. Moreover, writing allows him to use the frustration of his unfulfilled social and sexual needs to fuel the romantic fantasies that are the bases for his novels. On the other hand, Mr. Udall's choice of career has probably aggravated some of the pathological aspects of his personality. This career has allowed him to isolate himself and be disdainful of others without impairing his livelihood. His success at writing romantic novels, most typically read by women, is seen by him as further evidence that women are dim-witted, which encourages his self-defeating but protective withdrawal. In addition, his successes may have increased his arrogance and disdain for others.

As time has passed, Mr. Udall's symptoms and peculiarities have worsened. By the time of his testing, his compulsions were so pronounced that he had become increasingly dysfunctional. His preoccupation with cleanliness and avoiding germs, his need to check the locks on his front door, and his need to avoid stepping on cracks when he walked had reached levels of severity that made it very difficult for Mr. Udall even to venture out of his home. His constant sarcasm, possibly used as a defense against his feelings of inadequacy, had alienated all of the people around him. A possible interpretation of one aspect of his social behavior is that his need for mothering is extremely pressing. Indeed, when his surrogate mother—a waitress at the restaurant where he goes for his meals—is off work, he is unable to eat.

On the positive side, Mr. Udall is an extremely intelligent and gifted individual. He is insightful and interpersonally perceptive. In spite of his peculiarities, he has always remained in good contact with reality. In fact, outside of the obsessive–compulsive disorder, there is no history of any other clinical syndromes. He is capable of higher-order defenses, such as altruism. The latter could be used to help him fill his own unmet needs in ways that are helpful to society, in general, and to the people around him, in particular.

Variables relevant to treatment planning include Mr. Udall's functional impairment and the complex pattern of his difficulties. He needs to be in control of relationships and, as a result, is likely to resist direct forms of therapeutic intervention. For the most part, he uses an internalizing style of coping, in that he thinks through and develops a moderate level of insight into his behavior. At the same time, he is likely to externalize some of his anger through abrasive and sarcastic interactions. Due to the pattern of his symptoms and coping style, his social support is extremely limited.

Diagnostic Impressions

Axis I   Obsessive–compulsive disorder—300.3
Axis II   Compulsive personality disorder—301.4 with narcissistic and
            schizotypal elements
Axis III   No known medical problems contributing
Axis IV   External stress: None noted
Axis V   Level of functioning: Serious impairment of social functioning
            (GAF = 45)

Summary and Recommendations

The following summary and recommendations are particularly important, given the referral questions:

- Mr. Udall has a great deal of anger that he expresses in a self-defeating manner. He suffers from a compulsive personality disorder with narcissistic and schizotypal elements. In addition to having problems with anger and a personality disorder, he also fulfills the criteria for an obsessive–compulsive anxiety disorder. Psychological strengths include his considerable talent as a writer, his insight regarding his difficulties, and a level of discomfort that is sufficient to provide high motivation for change.
- Even though the client would like to have more meaningful relation-

ships with others, he feels that such relationships would be threatening, since they would demand more emotional involvement than he is willing to give. His withdrawal is also self-justified in that he feels disdainful of, and superior to, others. In order to protect himself from the dangers of relationships, he has become progressively more withdrawn. This style of coping has resulted in a worsening of his symptoms.

   • Mr. Udall would benefit from a period of psychotherapy. Given the personality described above, he may find it easier to establish a therapeutic alliance with a professional whose style is formal, proper, punctual, and predictable. Judging from the feelings Mr. Udall has expressed about women, it would probably be easier for him to establish a therapeutic alliance with a male. Given his use of intellectualization as a defense and his intellectual capacity, it would be useful to find a therapist the patient would consider intellectually capable. Keeping initial distance and allowing him to control significant parts of the session also would help him feel at ease. Explanations of the diagnosis, the nature of the "illness," and the expected course of treatment are likely to have particular appeal for Mr. Udall. The difficulty may be found in attempting to move him from a superficial therapeutic alliance to a more meaningful involvement in the relationship. Increasing social support beyond the therapy session would be an important goal but would likely encounter the same difficulties as working with him within the therapeutic session. Helping him explore the defenses he uses or enhancing his tolerance for control by others may also be difficult to accomplish. The important role his personality plays in the problems he has been experiencing, his lack of social support, his increasing functional impairment, and his maladaptive defensive/coping strategies suggest the need for commitment to a relatively lengthy course of treatment. Specific diagnostic-based techniques that are likely to be beneficial include thought stopping, disrupting the obsessive–compulsive patterns, and relaxation training. Positive client resources include high verbal skills and considerable insight into his difficulties. Consideration should be given to the use of medication to help the patient with his obsessive–compulsive symptoms. He would have to be convinced, however, of the benefit of this treatment.

Case 2

The second case is the sample case that is discussed throughout the book. Interpretations of R.W.'s individual test scores can be found in the chapters on the relevant tests (MMPI-2, MCMI-III, CPI, Rorschach), and the scores are summarized in Appendix A. In order to get a more complete picture of the case, as well as the individual contributions that each test can make, readers are encouraged to read each of the interpretations (at the end of the relevant test-oriented chapters). This report represents a summary of the key features of these interpretations as well as being an example of a complete report. The Discussion/Interpretation and Impressions section is organized according to various domains (cognition, mood/affect, interpersonal relations) rather than according to a developmental narrative (as in the previous sample case). Table 13.2 provides a grid of the various results, so that they can be easily summarized according to the chosen domains. The report also emphasizes treatment recommendations based on the STS variables.

Identifying Information

Name: R.W.
Sex: Female
Date of birth: 1/20/78
Date of evaluation: 2/28/01
Evaluated by: Dr. Jones
Referring clinician: Dr. Renney
Ethnicity: Mexican American

Referral Question

R.W. is a 22-year-old Mexican American female who is currently supported by her 42-year-old boyfriend of 6 years. Although she received her GED, the client is not currently employed or in school. She was referred for evaluation in order to clarify her diagnosis and assist in treatment planning.

Evaluation Procedures

February 20, 2001–February 27, 2001
Clinical interview
Wechsler Adult Intelligence Scale—Third Edition (WAIS-III)
Rorschach Inkblot Test
Minnesota Multiphasic Personality Inventory–2 (MMPI-2)

April 9, 2001–April 23, 2001
Minnesota Multiphasic Personality Inventory–2 (MMPI-2)
California Psychological Inventory (CPI)
Millon Clinical Multiaxial Inventory–III (MCMI-III)

Background Information

When she sought counseling in June 1 year ago, the client presented with panic attacks and social anxiety. Specifically, R. W. reported feeling scared to go outside the house. She reported that these attacks started when she was in high school and dating a softball coach from an adjoining high school. The client explained that people stared at her accusingly and disre-

TABLE 13.2. Mapping Information from Different Sources into a Narrative: Case 2

	History	Observations	WAIS-III	MMPI-2/MCMI-III	Rorschach
Cognition	Poor internal–external differention.	Coherent, articulate, unusual ideation.	Average range.	Possible thought disorder.	Incoherent, illogical, peculiar.
Mood/affect	Poor emotional control.			Depression, anxiety, anger.	Withdrawal from affect.
Interpersonal relations	Impaired, difficulty trusting.			Active ambivalence, rebelliousness.	Oppositional, misperceives others, introverted.
Coping style	Acting out, rejects external organization.	Fair amount of insight.		Externalizing.	Passive fantasy, magical thinking.
Resistance level	Moderate resistance.			Moderate resistance.	
Conflict areas	Authority, interpersonal relations, work.		Rebelliousness reduces potential.	Authority.	Limited coping, decompensates under stress, avoidance.
Motivational distress		Moderate distress.		Good level; motivated for change.	Low distress.
Social support	Possibly isolated.				Distrust.

428

spectfully for dating a married man, sometimes accusing her of breaking up his home. The two continue to date, and she continues to feel uncomfortable when in public. Since graduating from high school, however, she is less anxious and self-conscious. When surrounded by people, the client maintains that she continues to sense other people's rejection of her; she becomes afraid, and this fear keeps her from going places by herself. She reports that she can only go to public places if her boyfriend first accompanies her. The only course that helps her is physical activity and athletics. She views her athletic ability as a strength and wants to become a professional basketball player.

The client presents with a history of emotional changeability that she refers to as "highs and lows." For example, she responded to the following MMPI-2 questions (not actual MMPI-2 items) in the following manner:

Sometimes I feel as if my mind is going so fast I can't keep track of everything. (True)
At times my moods change extremely quickly. (True)
I often feel as if I am ready to fall apart. (True)

She describes a pattern of doing well, making mistakes, and then feeling depressed. The client reports that, until recently, she would find solace by going off by herself when she felt low. When she could get away from others, she would experience less fear and less concern about the consequences of her actions, at least temporarily. Frequently, the pattern of self-imposed isolation would be broken by episodes of acting out, either through promiscuous sexual behavior or through drug and alcohol use. After she returns from these periods of escape, she begins to feel very depressed and fearful. More recently, she has found it difficult to get away from people, experiencing tremendous feelings of anxiety and fear at the thought of going off by herself, even to the point of experiencing panic attacks when she gets ready to leave the house.

The client has reported to her current therapist that she feels very fragmented and conflicted, even describing three different people within herself: She describes W. as the older, mature person; T. as the angry, aggressive, and rebellious one who is younger and more immature; and B. as the baby who cries because her parents abandoned her and her stepfather sexually abused her. She is not sure if these personified conflicts represent real people inside of her or simply different sides of her own conflict, but she does hear internal voices from each, within her head.

Until the age of 10, the client reports living in a traditional home with her mother, father, two younger sisters, and an older brother. At this age, her parents divorced. For about a year, she and her siblings lived with her maternal grandmother. Then her mother remarried, and they lived with her mother and stepfather. She describes her stepfather as an authoritative

Mexican American male who had little regard for women. He began physically abusing her as part of routine discipline and, by the time she was 12, he was making many sexual approaches and comments to her. He tried to force himself on her on one occasion, but she repelled this advance and thereafter became very oppositional, opposing anything that her stepfather told her to do. He responded with more violence and frequently hit her so hard that she carried marks for days. At age 13, the client reports that her mother and stepfather got divorced and that her mother became very bitter and distant. She felt abandoned once again and maintains that she raised herself and her younger sisters.

The client's main source of social support is her boyfriend. At the time of the assessment, the client reports that he gives her stability and that she is comfortable with their relationship.

The results of this assessment should be interpreted with caution. The validity of the assessments is questionable, given the client's inconsistent response patterns and possible confusion. Additionally, the client's low educational level may have suppressed her performance on academic tasks.

Discussion/Interpretation and Impressions

The client obtained a Verbal IQ of 111, a Performance IQ of 90, and a Full Scale IQ of 102. Overall, this places her in the average range, or the 55th percentile, when compared with her age-related peers. Relative strengths include her understanding of spoken language and her good vocabulary. In contrast, relative weaknesses include inattention, poor concentration, and the slow pace at which she responded to tasks presented to her. This finding suggests that she might be somewhat slow and poorly motivated in day-to-day activities, such as getting started in the morning. In addition, her difficulties with attention suggest that she may forget relevant details, such as meetings that she was supposed to attend. She is also likely to find it difficult to stay focused on a task for any length of time. It is quite likely that her current level of distress is sufficiently high to reduce cognitive abilities that require attention, concentration, and a rapid response to tasks. In addition, poor education may have slightly suppressed her performance on the academic-based tasks of the assessment. For both these reasons, the IQs she obtained may be an underestimate of her optimal level of functioning.

During the interview, the client presented coherently and articulately. She indicated that her cognitive functioning was usually an area of strength. However, it appears that at the present time, the client is inefficiently using her cognitive processes in that she demonstrated a poor ability to distinguish between her external and internal experiences or to separate or integrate her perception of the world. There is evidence of unusual ideation, disorganization, and poor perceptual processes. In order to cope with these unhelpful states, she tries to confine her experiences to a relatively narrow range. She perceives events as occurring beyond her control and has a low tolerance to stress. Her disorganized thoughts and poor perceptual processes are sufficient to suggest an emerging formal thought disorder.

The client presents with moderate to high levels of depression and anxiety. Additionally, she presents with moderate levels of anger. She appears to underutilize her cognitive resources to control her emotions. This lack of emotional control seems to be pervasive, as the client has a history of acting out and reports feeling unable to control her temper. Under extreme stress her thoughts are likely to become progressively more confused, and her reality testing is likely to decrease.

R.W. demonstrates significantly impaired interpersonal functioning. Her pattern is characterized by active ambivalence. She presents with needs for dependency and approval, on the one hand, and independence and autonomy, on the other. However, her tendency toward self-reliance is likely more from a sense of alienation from others and rebelliousness than any great degree of self-confidence. She has a tendency to become isolated and uninvolved. She experiences anxiety in social situations and has difficulty trusting others. The client demonstrates an externalizing coping style. She reports a strong sense of rebelliousness toward both authority figures and social organizational structures, in general. This rebelliousness may be particularly salient in academic settings. The client has strong tendencies to act out. Her academic achievements may be far below her academic potential because her energy is directed more toward rejecting external organization than working within the limits imposed on her. However, she can also be self-reflective and self-critical. Specifically, she demonstrates a fair amount of insight into her rebelliousness and reports regret following her periods of acting out.

In addition to the above difficulties, there are a number of client strengths that could be utilized to enhance her self-esteem and as tools for therapy. Her level of insight and ability to articulate her feelings is good. In addition, her level of distress suggests that she will be motivated to change. Her unconventional orientation might be used to develop creative ways of perceiving her situation and creating change. In addition, her intellectual abilities are at least in the average range, which would enable her to understand the process of therapy (develop insights) and to obtain further education.

Diagnostic Impression

Based on the information gathered from the client and her present therapist, the following diagnostic impressions were indicated: There was a question raised about whether a dissociative identity disorder or bipolar disorder were present. At this time, there is little evidence of these disorders; rather, an emerging formal thought disorder is indicated.

Axis I   R/O emerging undifferentiated schizophrenic disorder
          in prodromal phase
          Social phobia—300.23
Axis II   Borderline personality
Axis III No diagnosis
Axis IV   Lack of extensive social support; alienated from family
Axis V   GAF = 35; highest past year = 35

Recommendations

The client is functioning with high levels of impairment. She reports moderate levels of subjective distress, mostly related to her fear of going outside. This fear constitutes a good motivational basis for counseling. She poses no risk to others and low-to-moderate risk to herself. She continues to be a good candidate for weekly outpatient psychotherapy. A psychiatric consultation for antipsychotic medication is strongly suggested.

The client presents an externalizing coping style, intruding on the environment, and forcing integration of different aspects. She does not accurately perceive her impact on people. The client also tends to be out of touch with her feelings, although she does have some degree of insight, at times. The tendency to become isolated and uninvolved indicates the potential value of group-oriented therapy, as this format may facilitate the development of social attachments.

R.W. seems to be person-specific in her resistance level. She has a tendency to be initially highly resistant, which is manifested by testing the limits and acting out defiantly. However, she seems to have developed a strong alliance with her therapist, with whom she has been in treatment for almost a year. A behaviorally focused therapy may be particularly useful. However, given her resistance, modifications may be necessary, such as giving her self-help manuals and making homework assignments flexible. Although R.W. has been in counseling for almost a year, it may be useful to discuss roles and expectations within the therapeutic relationship. This kind of discussion may be important in light of the client's resistance.

The overall prognosis for this patient is guarded, although she is sufficiently distressed to be motivated to change. She illustrates this motivation by participating actively in therapy. The probability of relapse is high, since many of her symptoms are pervasive and chronic. Work with family and social support systems may help to prevent relapses. The chronicity of the client's problems indicates a need for long-term intervention focusing on behavior management and skill building. Initial goals should include symptom removal, whereas long-term goals may include exploring cognitive schemas, relationship patterns, and her rejection of authority figures and any social demands.

SUMMARY

Psychologists must ensure that the professional judgments and recommendations they provide in their reports are based on current clinical science. In addition, because the consumers of psychological reports are more varied now than in the past, and because there may be multiple clients who have access to a report, including nonpsychologists, psychologists must take particular care to present information and conclusions without jargon and in a nonpejorative manner. Both research and clinical experience indicate that psychological reports are more likely to be used when they provide information that is relevant to the clinical concerns and questions that have motivated the referral. Such information should include not only diagnoses, which may be of limited predictive value, but characteristics of patient and problems that have more relevance to treatment planning (e.g., chronicity, comorbidity, resistance), as noted in more detail in other chapters of this volume.

We have described the standard components of psychological reports. However, there are many possible organizational schemes for the most integrative section of any report, the discussion section. These schemes include a review of functions, a description of the client's developmental progression, a description of the interplay between personality style and environment, discussion of differential diagnoses and, least favored because it is the least coherent and most fragmentary, a review of test results. The psychologist's responsibility does not end with submission of a report, but includes ensuring that recommendations are understood and relevant, and that the report is used appropriately in the best interests of all parties. Finally, we have provided two case reports to illustrate our main points.

Test Scores for Case Example R. W.

IDENTIFYING INFORMATION

Name: R.W.
Sex: Female
Date of birth: 1/20/78
Date of evaluation: 2/28/01
Referring clinician: Dr. Renny
Ethnicity: Mexican American

REFERRAL

R.W. is a 22-year-old, Mexican American female who is currently supported by her 42-year-old boyfriend of 6 years. Although she received her GED, the client is not currently employed or in school. She was referred for evaluation in order to clarify diagnosis and assist in treatment planning.

BACKGROUND

The client presented with panic attacks and social anxiety when she sought counseling 1 year ago. Specifically, the client reported feeling scared to go outside the house and experienced regular panic attacks when she attempted to do so. She reported that these attacks started when she was in high school dating a softball coach from another high school. Initially, the clientexplained, when people became aware of her relationship, they stared at her accusingly and disrespectfully. They made comments and derided her for dating a married man, and sometimes accused her openly of breaking up his home. She became very fearful of their disapproval and less and less involved in social groups. Over time, she developed a fear of going out. This fear was exaggerated, on several occasions, because of panic attacks that came on when she was in public places.

On one of these occasions, she fainted and had to leave a restaurant and go to an emergency room before she could start breathing again.

The two continue to date and she continues to feel uncomfortable when in public. Since graduating from high school, however, she is less anxious and self-conscious. When surrounded by people, the client maintains that she continues to sense other people's rejection of her; she becomes afraid and this keeps her from going places by herself. She reports that she can only go to public places if her boyfriend accompanies her first. The only thing that helps her is physical activity and she views her athletic ability as a strength and wants to become a professional basketball player.

The client presents with a history of emotional changeability that she refers to as "highs and lows." She describes a pattern of doing well, messing up, and then feeling depressed. The client reports that, until recently, when she felt low, she would find solace by going off by herself. When she could get away from others, she would experience less fear and less concern about the consequences of her actions, at least momentarily. Frequently, these periods of self-imposed isolation would be associated with episodes of acting out, either through promiscuous sexual behavior or through drug and alcohol use. After she returned from these periods of escape, she would begin to feel very depressed and fearful. More recently, she has found it difficult to get away from people, experiencing tremendous feelings of anxiety and fear at the thought of going off by herself, even to the point of panic attacks when she gets ready to leave.

The client has reported to her current therapist that she feels very fragmented and conflicted, even describing three different people within her. She describes W. as the older, mature person; T. as the angry, aggressive, and rebellious one who is younger and more immature; and B. as the baby who cries because her parents abandoned her and her stepfather sexually abused her. She isn't sure if these personified conflicts represent real people inside of her or simply different sides of her own conflict, but she does hear internal voices from each.

Her parents are divorced but until the age of 10, the client reports living in a traditional home with her mother, father, two younger sisters, and an older brother. For about a year after the divorce, she and her siblings lived with her maternal grandmother. Then her mother remarried and they lived with her mother and stepfather. She describes her stepfather as an authoritative, Mexican American male who had little regard for women. He began physically abusing her as part of routine discipline and by the age of 12, he was making many sexual approaches and comments to her. He tried to force himself on her on one occasion, but she repelled this advance and thereafter became very oppositional, going against anything that her stepfather told her to do. He responded with more violence and frequently hit her so hard that she carried marks for days. At age 13, the client reports that her mother and stepfather got divorced and that her mother became very bitter and distant. She felt abandoned once again and maintains that she raised herself and her younger sisters.

The client's main source of social support is her boyfriend. She has no contact with her family and has no friends. At the time of the assessment, the client reports that he gives her stability and she is comfortable with their relationship.

WAIS-III

IQ scores

Verbal IQ	111
Performance IQ	90
Full Scale IQ	102

Index scores

Verbal Comprehension Index	109
Perceptual Organization Index	109
Working Memory	86
Processing Speed	86

Subtest	Scaled score	Subtest	Scaled score
Vocabulary	13	Picture Arrangement	11
Similarities	11	Picture Completion	13
Information	11	Block Design	9
Comprehension	13	Matrix Reasoning	13
Arithmetic	8	Coding (Digit Symbol	8
Digit Span	8	Symbol Search	7
Letter–Number Sequencing	7	Object Assembly	(not given)

BAR-ON EMOTIONAL QUOTIENT INVENTORY
(EQ-i; SIMULATED SCORES BASED ON
HISTORY AND OTHER TEST RESULTS)

Total EQ = 85

Intrapersonal EQ = 80 (low)
    Emotional self-awareness   102 (average)
    Assertiveness   98 (average)
    Self regard   80 (low)
    Self actualization   81 (low)
    Independence   74 (very low)

Interpersonal EQ = 82 (low)
    Interpersonal relationship   84 (low)
    Social responsibility   86 (low)
    Empathy   95 (average)

Adaptability EQ = 83 (low)
    Problem solving   80 (low)
    Reality testing   78 (very low)
    Flexibility   86 (low)

Stress Management = 86 (low)
    Stress tolerance   76 (very low)
    Impulse control   91 (average)

General Mood = 86 (low)
    Happiness   87 (low)
    Optimism   85 (low)

MMPI-2 (SECOND ADMINISTRATION)

Validity scales		Supplementary scales	
VRIN	75	MAC-R	55
TRIN	50	APS	50
L	51	AAS	78
F	98	PK	70
K	28	OH	44
F(B)	74		
S (experimental)	33	Content scales	
		ANX	54
Clinical scales		FRS	51
1	53	OBS	64
2	67	DEP	64
3	43	HEA	53
4	65	BIZ	52
5	67	ANG	74
6	65	CYN	67
7	65	ASP	56
8	78	TPA	55
9	72	LSE	55
0	58	SOD	70
		FAM	82
		WRK	67
		TRT	54

MCMI-III

	BR	
Validity Scales		
Validity	0	
Disclosure	54	
Desirability	35	
Debasement	56	
Basic Personality Disorders		
Schizoid	78[a]	High
Avoidant	72	
Depressive	68	
Dependent	60	
Histrionic	60	
Narcissistic	98[c]	Extremely high
Antisocial	68	
Sadistic	64	
Compulsive	20	
Negativistic	79[a]	High
Self-defeating	86[b]	Very high
Severe Personality Disorders		
Schizotypal	63	
Borderline	84[a]	High
Paranoid	73	
Basic Clinical Syndromes		
Anxiety	75[a]	High
Somatoform	26	
Bipolar	72	
Dysthymia	47	
Alcohol Dependence	63	
Drug Dependence	64	
PTSD	60	
Severe Clinical Syndromes		
Thought Disorder	43	
Major Depression	38	
Delusional Disorder	65	

[a]75–84; [b]85–94; [c]95+.

CPI

Class I	T-scores	
Dominance	40	
Capacity for Status	34	Low
Sociability	33	Low
Social Presence	38	Low
Self-acceptance	46	
Independence	50	
Empathy	50	

Class II		
Responsibility	32	Low
Socialization	28	Very low
Self-control	32	Low
Good Impression	33	Low
Communality	44	
Well-being	37	
Tolerance	46	

Class III		
Achievement via Conformance	31	Low
Achievement via Independence	52	
Intellectual Efficiency	39	Low

Class IV		
Psychological Mindedness	48	
Flexibility	48	
Femininity–Masculinity	34	Low

RORSCHACH RESPONSES

Card I

2 sec/30 sec

1.   That's a frog with butterfly wings.
           (Q) Take your time and look some more. I'm sure you'll find something else
           too.
           That's all I see.
           ****Note: Defensive.

Inquiry
           There's the frog . . . there's the pinchers . . . there's the wings, like a
   butterfly. It's the whole thing. Those are the frog's eyebrows.
           (Q) I'm not sure I C it like you do.
           The whole thing. Shape of the whole thing.

Card II

1 sec/3 min

2.   It's a vagina that has blood coming out of it.
3.   It cb the face of a guy who has a beard who is sticking his tongue
   out. He cb 1 of those wolf people.
4.   Or it cb 2 wolves kissing w/ their noses . . . Eskimo kissing.
           I don't C anything else.

Inquiry
           This part are the lips of the vagina. . . . That's the blood coming out.
           (Q) What makes it ll blood?
           Red.

   With the man, here's his eyes and his tongue sticking out. . . . Here's his
   beard. . . . That's why I felt that he ll a wolfman, because most of his
   face is covered with hair.

           (Q) You also said that it could be two wolves kissing?
           Here's the wolves. Here's their ears & their noses and they're both kissing.
           (Q) Eskimo kissing?
           Rubbing their noses together.

Card III

9 sec/2 min

5.   The 1st thing that comes to mind is fallopian tubes.
6.   There's a butterfly in there.
7.   Here's a dove's head w/ the body of a seahorse.
8.   There's 2 people pouring tea. They cb guys because they have dicks
   coming, I's sorry, I should say penis. But they have high heels on so . . . they have
   bird necks, like ostriches . . . like elegant, from the 1920s or something.
9.   And somebody's muscular stomach. That's about it.
           That's about it.

Inquiry
           Oh, yeah. There's the . . . what are they called? Ovaries. The tubes come
   down.

Rt here. Just ll a butterfly.
This is the bird's head and the seahorse body.

This is the bird's neck. Here's his penis, his body around here. There's the teapot and they're both pouring tea.

The stomach is right here.
(Q) Muscular?
The way it ripples like muscles where it's lighter.

Card IV

10 sec/1 min

10.   This cb an android who is leaning back on the tree. It's like
someone lifted him up and put him on a tree, or he cb growing out of a
tree, like part of it.... His arms ll branches.

Inquiry
The android's here. Here are his big feet because he's leaning. This is the top of the tree. I thought he may be growing with the tree because he's connected.

Card V

2 sec/40 sec

11.   That is a butterfly.
12.   Or it could be a snail w/ wings.

Inquiry
The head, antenna, and wings.
(*Turns card around*) The other way, this is the snail's head because it ll a snail's antenna, with wings here.

Card VI

9 sec/2½ min

13.   That cb a violin or a guitar.
The top is like a butterfly but has whiskers like a cat . . . and what's going
through the butterfly ll a penis, & it cb attached to another
animal that's mouth is like pinchers, & he grabs the penis & the butterfly is
stuck. The animal doesn't have arms or legs, so it's stuck.

Inquiry
Rt here shaped like a butterfly, with whiskers on sides. This thing here is a
penis.
(Q) Another animal?
St down here. Ll it's gotten hold of them.

Card VII

7 sec/2 min

14.   That cb 2 little girls facing e.o., w/ ponytails up in the
air. The heads are facing e.o., but their bodies are facing the other way.
They are sitting on 2 Siamese cats who are connected at the butt. They don't
have a tail. They both have monkey mouths w/ the painting of a clown
mouth on it. Oh, one more thing. Their ponytails are the cat tails.

Inquiry

Those are the 2 cat tails. They are facing out. The butts are here.

Here are their hands. The pony tails are made of the cats' tails. They cut them off. The lips are sticking out like a monkey's.

(Q) What makes it ll the painting of a clown mouth on it?

Darker here at the tip, like it's painted over.

Card VIII

5 sec/3 min

15.   Hmmmm. . . . More color. . . . They cb 2 whales. One has the beak of a bird and the tail of a mouse. There's an alien creature connecting the 2 whales sucking the life from them. But they keep recreating themselves from the pink and orange blob. U C, the pink and orange are good and the torquoise is evil. So it's like a cycle that goes over & over again & never stops.

Inquiry

16.   The space thing is rt here. This is the evil. The whales are rt here. This guy's got a beak like a bird, and the other one's face ll a rat. Here's the bad sucking the good.

(Q) Show me where U C it.

(*points*) This is the good regenerating them. It just goes around in a circle.

Card IX

25 sec/2½ min

17.   Can I turn it around? This is an elephant w/ pink ears. He has a really tough backbone. He has legs. U can C all his insides but he has no feelings.

Inquiry

Here are the elephant's ears and head. Here are his legs. This is his core.

(Q) Show me where the legs are.

The legs are the orange part.

(Q) You said, "U can C all his insides but he as no feelings"?

I knew U were going to ask me that. This is about me that I say he can't feel. Looking at this card makes me feel down. You can't show feelings because someone could see. He's not equipped with emotions. This relates to me. I don't feel emotions and I don't feel that I should try to. This is the stuff I would talk with Renée about.

Card X

½ sec/1 min

18.   It ll fireworks are going off. There are fish everywhere. There are crabs, seahorses, & seaweed flying around like something blew it all up . . . but they are all connected.

Inquiry

(*Turns card upside down*) These are the fireworks. This is the seaweed. This yellow part are fish. These are the 2 crabs. The 2 seahorses are flying here.

(Q) This is all one scene?

Yeah. They're all connected. They are all touching.

SEQUENCE OF SCORES

Card	Resp. No	Location and DQ	Loc. No.	Determinant(s) and Form Quality	(2)	Content(s)	Pop	ZScore	Special Scores
I	1	Wo	1	F-		A		1.0	INC2
II	2	D+	6	FCu		Hd,Bl,Sx		3.0	MOR, PHR
	3	DdSo	99	Mp-		Hd		4.5	ALOG, PHR
	4	D+	6	FMao	2	A		3.0	COP, GHR
III	5	Do	1	Fu	2	An			
	6	Do	3	Fo		An			
	7	Do	2	Fu		A			INC2
	8	D+	1	Mao	2	H,Sx,Hh, Cg	P	3.0	INC2, DR, PHR
	9	Do	8	FV-		An			
IV	10	W+	1	Mp.FDo		(H),Bt	P	4.0	FAB2, ALOG, PHR
V	11	Wo	1	Fo		A	P	1.0	
	12	Wo	1	Fu		A		1.0	INC2
VI	13	Wo	1	Fu		Sc		2.5	
	14	W+	1	FMa-		A,Sx		2.5	INC2,FAB2, AG, PHR
VII	15	W+	1	Mp.FY-	2	H,A	P	2.5	INC2, FAB2, MOR, PHR
VIII	16	W+	1	Fma.C-	2	A,(A),Id		4.5	INC2, FAB2, AG, AB, PHR
IX	17	Wo	1	F-		A,An		5.5	FAB2, PER
X	18	W+	1	ma.FMau	2	Ex,A,Bt	P	5.5	FAB

SUMMARY OF APPROACH

I: W	VI: W.W
II: D.DdS.D	VII: W
III: D.D.D.D.D	VIII: W
IV: W	IX: W
V: W.W	X: W

STRUCTURAL SUMMARY

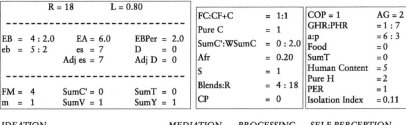

Location Features		
Zf	=	14
ZSum =		43.5
ZEst =		45.5
W	=	10
(Wv =		10)
D	=	7
W+D	=	17
Dd	=	1
S	=	1

Determinants		Contents		S-Constellations	
Blends	**Single**	H	= 2	☐ FV+VF+V+FD>2	
M.FD	M = 2	(H)	= 1	☐ Col-Shd Blends>0	
M.FY	FM = 2	Hd	= 2	☐ Ego <.31 or >.44	
FM.C	m = 0	(Hd)	= 0	☐ MOR>3	
m.FM	FC = 1	Hx	= 0	☐ Zd> ±3.5	
	CF = 0	A	= 10	☑ es>Ea	
	C = 0	(A)	= 1	☐ CF+C>FC	
	Cn = 0	Ad	= 0	☑ X+%<.70	
	FC' = 0	(Ad)	= 0	☐ S>3	
	C'F = 0	An	= 4	☐ P<3 or >8	
	C' = 0	Art	= 0	☐ Pure H<2	
	FT = 0	Ay	= 0	☐ R<17	
	TF = 0	Bl	= 1	2 Total	
	T = 0	Bt	= 2		

DQ		
		(FQ-)
+	= 8	(3)
o	= 10	(4)
v/+	= 0	(0)
v	= 0	(0)

		Special Scores	
		Lvl-1	Lvl-2
DV	= 0 x1		0 x2
INC	= 0 x2		7 x4
DR	= 1 x3		0 x6
FAB	= 1 x4		5 x7
ALOG	= 2 x5		
CON	= 0 x7		
	Raw Sum6 = 16		
	Wgtd Sum6 = 80		
AB	= 1	GHR =	1
AG	= 2	PHR =	7
COP	= 1	MOR =	2
CP	= 0	PER =	1
		PSV =	0

Determinants (continued):
FV = 1, VF = 0, V = 0, FY = 0, YF = 0, Y = 0, Fr = 0, rF = 0, FD = 0, F = 8, (2) = 6

Contents (continued):
Cg = 1, Cl = 0, Ex = 1, Fd = 0, Fi = 0, Ge = 0, Hh = 1, Ls = 0, Na = 0, Sc = 1, Sx = 3, Xy = 0, Idio = 1

Form Quality			
	FQx	MQual	W+D
+	= 0	0	0
o	= 5	2	5
u	= 6	0	6
-	= 7	2	6
none =	0	0	0

RATIOS, PERCENTAGES, AND DERIVATIONS

R = 18   L = 0.80

EB =	4 : 2.0	EA = 6.0	EBPer =	2.0
eb =	5 : 2	es = 7	D =	0
		Adj es = 7	Adj D =	0

FM =	4	SumC' = 0	SumT = 0
m =	1	SumV = 1	SumY = 1

FC:CF+C	=	1:1
Pure C	=	1
SumC':WSumC	=	0 : 2.0
Afr	=	0.20
S	=	1
Blends:R	=	4 : 18
CP	=	0

COP = 1		AG = 2
GHR:PHR		= 1 : 7
a:p		= 6 : 3
Food		= 0
SumT		= 0
Human Content		= 5
Pure H		= 2
PER		= 1
Isolation Index		= 0.11

IDEATION

a:p	= 6 : 3	Sum6	=	16
Ma:Mp	= 1 : 3	Lvl-2	=	12
2AB+(Art+Ay)	= 2	WSum6	=	80
MOR	= 2	M-	=	2
		M none	=	0

MEDIATION

XA%	= 0.61
WDA% =	0.65
X-%	= 0.39
S-	= 1
P	= 5
X+%	= 0.28
Xu%	= 0.33

PROCESSING

Zf	= 14
W:D:Dd =	10:7:1
W : M	= 10 : 4
Zd	= -2.0
PSV	= 0
DQ+	= 8
DQv	= 0

SELF-PERCEPTION

3r+(2)/R	= 0.33
Fr+rF	= 0
SumV	= 1
FD	= 1
An+Xy	= 4
MOR	= 2
H:(H)+Hd+(Hd)	= 2:3

PTI=5	☐ DEPI=3	☐ CDI=1	☐ S-CON=2	☐ HVI=No ☐ OBS=No

CONSTELLATIONS TABLE

S-Constellation (Suicide Potential)

☐ Positive if 8 or more conditions are true:
NOTE: Applicable only for subjects over 14 years old.

- ☐ FV+VF+V+FD [2] > 2
- ☐ Col-Shd Blends [0] > 0
- ☐ Ego [0.33] < .31 *or* > .44
- ☐ MOR [2] > 3
- ☐ Zd [-2.0] > ±3.5
- ☑ es [7] > EA [6.0]
- ☐ CF + C [1] > FC [1]
- ☑ X+% [0.28] < .70
- ☐ S [1] > 3
- ☐ P [5] < 3 or > 8
- ☐ Pure H [2] < 2
- ☐ R [18] < 17

2 Total

PTI (Perceptual-Thinking Index)

- ☑ (XA% [0.61] < 0.70) *and* (WDA% [0.65] < 0.75)
- ☑ X-% [0.39] > 0.29
- ☑ (Sum Level 2 Special Scores [12] > 2) *and* (FAB2 [5] > 0)
- ☑ ((R [18] < 17) *and* (WSum6 [80] > 12)) *or* ((R [18] > 16) *and* (WSum6 [80] > 17))
- ☑ (M- [2] > 1) *or* (X-% [0.39] > 0.40)

5 Total

DEPI (Depression Index)

☐ Positive if 5 or more conditions are true:

- ☑ (FV + VF + V [1] > 0) *or* (FD [1] > 2)
- ☐ (Col-Shd Blends [0] > 0) *or* (S [1] > 2)
- ☐ (3r + (2)/R [0.33] > 0.44 *and* Fr + rF [0] = 0) *or* (3r + (2)/R [0.33] < 0.33)
- ☑ (Afr [0.20] < 0.46) *or* (Blends [4] < 4)
- ☐ (SumShading [2] > FM + m [5]) *or* (SumC' [0] > 2)
- ☐ (MOR [2] > 2) *or* (2xAB + Art + Ay [2] > 3)
- ☑ (COP [1] < 2) *or* ([Bt+2xCl+Ge+Ls+2xNa]/R [0.11] > 0.24)

3 Total

CDI (Coping Deficit Index)

☐ Positive if 4 or more conditions are true:

- ☐ (EA [6.0] < 6) *or* (AdjD [0] < 0)
- ☐ (COP [1] < 2) *and* (AG [2] < 2)
- ☑ (Weighted Sum C [2.0] < 2.5) *or* (Afr [0.20] < 0.46)
- ☐ (Passive [3] > Active + 1 [7]) *or* (Pure H [2] < 2)
- ☐ (Sum T [0] > 1) *or* (Isolate/R [0.11] > 0.24) *or* (Food [0] > 0)

1 Total

HVI (Hypervigilance Index)

☐ Positive if condition 1 is true and at least 4 of the others are true:

- ☑ (1) FT + TF + T [0] = 0
- ☑ (2) Zf [14] > 12
- ☐ (3) Zd [-2.0] > +3.5
- ☐ (4) S [1] > 3
- ☐ (5) H + (H) + Hd + (Hd) [5] > 6
- ☐ (6) (H) + (A) + (Hd) + (Ad) [2] > 3
- ☐ (7) H + A : Hd + Ad [14:2] < 4 : 1
- ☐ (8) Cg [1] > 3

OBS (Obessive Style Index)

- ☐ (1) Dd [1] > 3
- ☑ (2) Zf [14] > 12
- ☐ (3) Zd [-2.0] > +3.0
- ☐ (4) Populars [5] > 7
- ☐ (5) FQ+ [0] > 1

☐ Positive if one or more is true:

- ☐ Conditions 1 to 5 are all true
- ☐ Two or more of 1 to 4 are true *and* FQ+ [0] > 3
- ☐ 3 or more of 1 to 5 are true *and* X+% [0.28] > 0.89
- ☐ FQ+ [0] > 3 *and* X+% [0.28] > 0.89

NOTE: '' indicates a cutoff that has been adjusted for age norms.*

Test Publishers/Distributors

AGS Publishing
4201 Woodland Road
Circle Pines, MN 55014-1796
800-328-2560
www.agsnet.com

List includes: Kaufman Assessment Battery for Children, Kaufman Adolescent and Adult Intelligence Test, Kaufman Brief Intelligence Test.

American Orthopsychiatric Association, Inc.
330 Seventh Avenue, 18th Floor
New York, NY 10001
212-564-5930
www.amerortho.org

List includes: Bender Visual Motor Gestalt Test.

Center for Behavioral Health Care Technologies, Inc.
3600 South Harbor Boulevard, #86
Oxnard, CA 93035
805-677-4501
cbhti.com
www.systematictreatmentselection.com

List includes: Systematic Treatment Selection software.

Consulting Psychologists Press
3803 East Bayshore Road
PO Box 10096
Palo Alto, CA 94303
800-624-1765
650-969-8901

www.cpp-db.com
www.SkillsOne.com

List includes: California Psychological Inventory, Fundamental Interpersonal Relations Orientation–B, Myers–Briggs Type Indicator, Strong Interest Inventory.

Jastak Associates, Inc.
PO Box 3410
15 Ashley Place, Suite 1A
Wilmington, DE 19804
800-221-WRAT

List includes: Wide Range Achievement Test

NCS Pearson
5605 Green Circle Drive
Minnetonka, MN 55343
800-627-7271
www.ncspearson.com/assessments

List includes: Bender Visual Motor Gestalt Test, Brief Symptom Inventory, Career Assessment Inventory, Children's Depression Inventory, Millon Adolescent Clinical Inventory, Millon Behavioral Health Inventory, Millon Clinical Multiaxial Inventory, Minnesota Multiphasic Personality Inventory, Rorschach, Symptom Checklist–90–R, Sixteen Personality Factor (16 PF), Taylor–Johnson Temperament Analysis, Thematic Apperception Test, Test of Memory Malingering.

Psychological Assessment Resources
16204 North Florida Avenue
Lutz, FL 33549
800-331-8378
www.parinc.com

List includes: Bar-On Emotional Quotient Inventory, Bender Visual Motor Gestalt Test, Hare Psychopathy Checklist—Revised, House–Tree–Person, Kaufman Adolescent and Adult Intelligence Test, NEO-PI-R, Personality Assessment Inventory, Personality Disorder Interview–IV, Rorschach, Self-Directed Search, Sentence Completion Series, State Trait Anger Expression Inventory, Taylor–Johnson Temperament Analysis, Test of Nonverbal Intelligence, Thematic Apperception Test, Wide Range Achievement Test.

Psychological Corporation
19500 Bulverde Road
San Antonio, TX 78259
800-872-1726
www.psychcorp.com

List includes: Beck Depression Inventory, California Verbal Learning Test, Wechsler Adult Intelligence Scale, Wechsler Individual Achievement Test, Wechsler Intelligence Scale for Children, Wechsler Preschool and Primary Scale for Children,

Wechsler Memory Scale, Wechsler Test of Adult Reading, Wide Range Test of Memory and Learning.

Riverside Publishing Company
425 Spring Lake Drive
Itasca, IL 60143-2079
800-323-9540
www.riverpub.com

List includes: Stanford–Binet

Western Psychological Services
12031 Wilshire Boulevard
Los Angeles, CA 90025-1251
800-648-8857
www.wpspublish.com

List includes: Bender Visual Motor Gestalt Test, Children's Depression Inventory, Draw-A-Person, Eating Disorders Inventory, House–Tree–Person, Human Figure Drawing Test, Family Apperception Test, Millon Index of Personality Styles, Personality Assessment Inventory, Psychopathy Checklist—Revised, Roberts Apperception Test, Rorschach, Sixteen PF (16 PF), Self-Directed Search, State–Trait Anger Expression Inventory, Thematic Apperception Test, Taylor–Johnson Temperament Analysis, Tell Me a Story, Wide Range Achievement Test.

STS Analysis

The clinician response-prompted STS version is designed for use by an evaluating clinician after having completed a semistructured diagnostic interview and a review of the patient's history. These tasks can be supplemented or replaced by entering the scores of formal psychological tests and questionnaires directly into STS. The STS system is intended to help the clinician organize the relevant information and develop a treatment plan, project the course of treatment, and identify potential problems and goals. The system also allows for periodic updating and tracking patient progress by comparing the patient's results with normative projections of patients who have similar personal characteristics and problem areas.

Interface with STS typically begins with a patient-initiated assessment. This onscreen assessment can be accomplished after the patient obtains a record number from a subscribing provider and accesses the Web-based self-report program. An alternative is to access the STS through the telephone, using the IVR-based option. This latter function is engaged by a phone call from a prospective patient to a toll-free number after first enrolling with a subscribing provider. Voice prompts guide the patient through an intake tree designed to gather relevant, treatment-specific information prior to clinician contact. Responses are made by pressing numbers on the touchtone phone—for example, "1" is "No," "2" is "Yes," "3" is "Repeat," "4" is "Go back one," and "5" is "Help." The rationale for this option is several-fold: convenience, time–cost savings (for patient, therapist, and managed care organization), and the provision of a mechanism dedicated to the assignment of the most effective therapist and therapy for the individual patient and his or her unique presenting problem(s). Regarding the informed assignment of therapists and therapy, the STS system employs an extensive database that includes objective therapist performance data and objective and subjective patient outcome data to render an individualized treatment plan, prognosis, and profile of treatment- and patient-specific evidence of therapist effectiveness. Through the use of this "evolving" and "learning" database, patients (and their problems) are matched with optimal therapists and therapies. The database evolves because it continually evaluates and stores patient, therapist, and therapy data in an effort to maximize the empirically established algorithmic-driven selection of empirically supported treatment and therapy guidelines. That is, based on empirically supported STS algorithms, continually updated (i.e., current) patient and therapist data are employed to facilitate the optimal selection of clinician, type of treatment, and therapeutic strategies.

Because the STS system—for both intake and update, by patient or clinician—is accessible via Web browser or telephone, convenience of access is one of its more attractive features. The STS web interactive system has many useful and convenient features to assist the clinician or clinic manager in evaluating, assigning, and tracking cases. For example, clinicians can log on to STS through their Web browser, allowing access to patient information from virtually any location that has Internet access. All STS functions and associated production are highly secure—that is, data are encrypted and only accessible to those with the designated credentials and prior/current authorization. Patient names connected with identifying information are never sent over the Internet or other public channels. Additionally, a clinician may access only data that are relevant to those patients under his or her care. Once the program is engaged, the clinician has access to the full array of information provided by the system (e.g., patient diagnostic information, graphic representations of predisposing patient qualities, normative data, appropriate treatment strategies, relevant/indicated empirically supported treatment "best practices," prognostic information, and treatment summaries, including specific patient change/growth trajectories).

The figures in the following pages represent specific STS browser windows. These windows normally appear in color on the computer monitor to direct the clinician through the process of evaluating a patient. The use of color and design is an important feature of the STS program because it enhances the information/interpretability of the diverse array of information provided by the program; for example, patient change trajectories (predicted, actual, and actuarial) and treatment-relevant predisposing patient characteristics are depicted in different colors; therapist profile information is provided in a similar manner.

The initial log-in screen for Web-enabled STS, accessible by patients, clinicians, or HMO/insurance users, is depicted in Figure C.1. The features to which each has access and rights are not only tailored for appropriateness, but specific, user-related features are also restricted or controlled accordingly.

Once the prospective user is logged into the system, the second STS screen provides a menu that allows either the clinical or administrative user to select from among a variety of program options. Both patients and clinicians may access STS over the Internet or via telephone. This accessibility allows the patient to provide a wealth of intake or follow-up information, easily and conveniently, and clinicians have the convenience of gathering information from any location that allows them access to an Internet-connected computer terminal, laptop, or palm.

The following short outline provides some basic information regarding the entry points for STS system users (clinical, patient, and administrative).

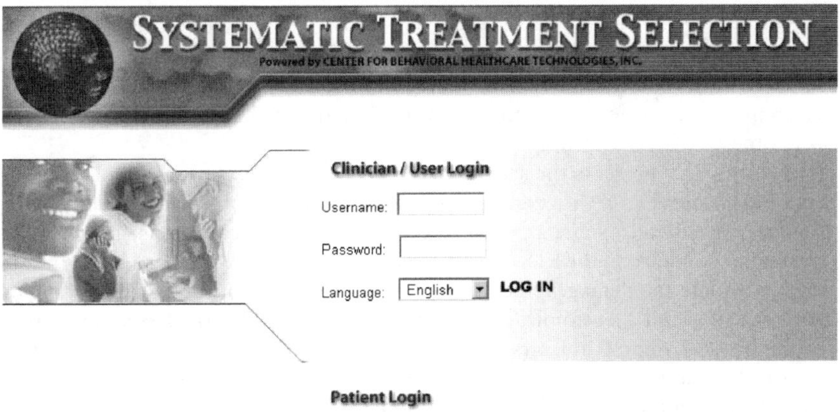

FIGURE C.1. Opening screen.

1. Intake (first time a patient has entered the system):
   a. May be completed by the clinician—after seeing the patient for the first time.
   b. May be completed by the patient—while viewing a screen accessed through an Internet Web browser, in the privacy of his or her home.
   c. May be completed by the patient—answering aural questions directly over the telephone by dialing an "800" number (if contact by telephone, then there is no computer screen).

2. Update or follow-up:
   a. Completed by the clinician—through his or her Web browser. Once the session update is completed, the claim form is automatically generated.
   b. Completed by the patient—while viewing a screen accessed through an Internet Web browser, in the privacy of his or her home.
   c. Completed by the patient—answering aural questions directly over the telephone by dialing an "800" number (if contact by telephone, then there is no computer screen).

3. Case management, clinical planning, and provider profiling function (used by HMO administration):
   a. The clinician/provider can access and monitor the progress of each of his or her patients.
   b. This option and the capabilities provided are subject to the security level granted to the user.
   c. Clinician/provider profiling menu option.

The system user can monitor general performance across the clinicians and providers who belong to the STS computer system. Performance is based on the symptomatic change of a single patient or several patients, and is associated with the specific STS dimensions of patient predisposing characteristics. It should be duly noted that "performance monitoring" is not relevant to therapist quality or experience but rather to the "chemistry" a therapist experiences with some patients, and not with others.

Figure C.2 represents the screen that appears once the clinician has logged in. This window provides a variety of menu options, from which the clinician can select to add a new patient, update a patient's record/file, or access a help program for the STS system. In addition, the STS computer program includes a standard intake information template and demographics profile (see Figure C.3). The intake/demographics screen can vary and is customizable to suit a wide variety of providers and payers.

Figure C.4 depicts the first of two "problem area checklists." This screen is shown to a clinician conducting a patient intake with the STS program. A patient who is completing a self-report responds to a separate generic list of questions. The information gathered from a clinical interview and a variety of self-report measures provide the relevant data for the problem area checklist.

Figure C.5 illustrates some of the typical types of STS questions that the clinician is requested to answer about the patient. In total, there are 164 questions, but the actual length varies as a function of the number of problems identified in the problem area checklist. In total, 31 subscales are available, representing various symptom clusters, coping styles, social and interpersonal adjustment levels, and treatment predic-

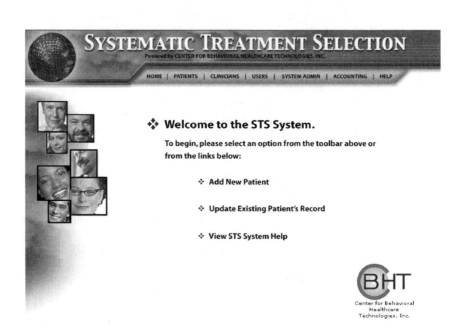

FIGURE C.2. Log-in screen.

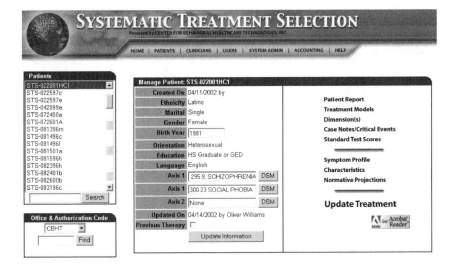

FIGURE C.3. Intake and demographic information.

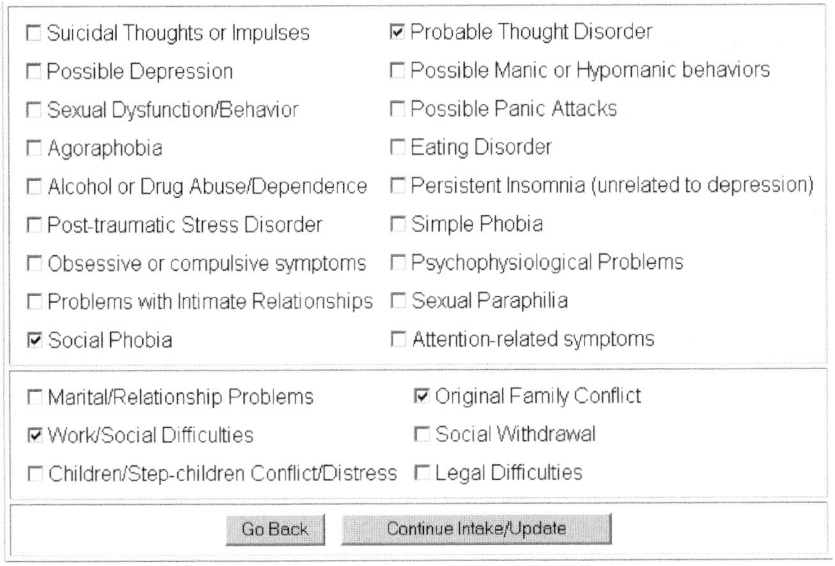

☐ Suicidal Thoughts or Impulses	☑ Probable Thought Disorder
☐ Possible Depression	☐ Possible Manic or Hypomanic behaviors
☐ Sexual Dysfunction/Behavior	☐ Possible Panic Attacks
☐ Agoraphobia	☐ Eating Disorder
☐ Alcohol or Drug Abuse/Dependence	☐ Persistent Insomnia (unrelated to depression)
☐ Post-traumatic Stress Disorder	☐ Simple Phobia
☐ Obsessive or compulsive symptoms	☐ Psychophysiological Problems
☐ Problems with Intimate Relationships	☐ Sexual Paraphilia
☑ Social Phobia	☐ Attention-related symptoms

☐ Marital/Relationship Problems	☑ Original Family Conflict
☑ Work/Social Difficulties	☐ Social Withdrawal
☐ Children/Step-children Conflict/Distress	☐ Legal Difficulties

Go Back	Continue Intake/Update

FIGURE C.4. STS problem area checklist.

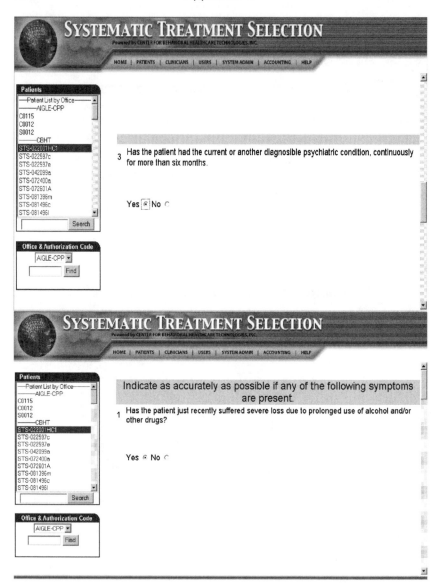

FIGURE C.5. Typical STS question screens.

tors. The usual length of time for a clinician to complete the response form is about 20 minutes. The length of time for patients is only slightly longer.

The STS question–response process actually flows through three "levels"; however, this progression is not typically apparent to the user. Each level builds upon the various predictive patient dimensions and adds precision to the definition of the treatments of choice. The progression begins with the most essential dimensions of problem severity, degree of risk, and general functionality through motivational distress (i.e., arousal), general well-being (i.e., general subjective distress and self-esteem), and continues through coping style and resistance/reactance. The clinician or patient (if answering over the phone via IVR or over the Internet via access to the STS program) may opt to stop at any place in the question series. Whenever the individual logs back in with a user name and password, the system automatically resumes assessment from the point at which he or she previously disengaged.

In order to further shorten clinician time investment, the STS allows the clinician to input scores from a variety of standard psychological tests, many of which have been described in the previous chapter (e.g., MMPI-2, MCMI, BDI, SCL-90-R, BDI, etc.). These scores replace the responses to a series of questions regarding coping style, resistance levels, impairment, and the like. When the clinician finishes the evaluation, a press of a button produces a narrative treatment planning report and a number of charts and graphs to assist him or her. After accessing the computer database for appropriate comparative norms, the following outputs are provided by the STS program (some representations of selected outputs are provided for illustrative purposes):

1. A complete STS online report with tailored treatment plan (Figure C.6).

2. A patient predisposing characteristics profile bar chart. The following (Figure C.7) is an example of one patient's predisposing characteristics profile, depicting all of the relevant STS treatment dimensions.

3. The next figure (Figure C.8) is an example of one patient's symptom profile bar chart, based on a limited number of assessments.

4. A line graph "predicting" the quantitative prognosis of the patient at intake is provided by the STS system. As treatment progresses, the patient's actual progress is included or tracked (Figure C.9). The intake assessment provides baseline information on patient level of impairment in various symptom areas (e.g., alcohol, depression, suicidality, anxiety, etc.), and general distress. The computer program also allows the clinician to enter case notes directly into a database and to supplement this narrative review of progress with an abbreviated follow-up evaluation of various problem areas and general distress. A graphic representation of progress is then provided, comparing the patient's progress to the initially projected rate of change. If the patient is progressing at the expected rate, the projected and obtained scores will converge. If the actual progress departs from the projected course, the chart is flagged for review. If obtained progress is slower than expected, the clinician is advised to review the patient's progress and to alter treatment. The following figure (Figure C.9) represents the perspective of well-being. The trajectories and normative cutoff lines are always color-coded in the user's browser for ease of interpretation.

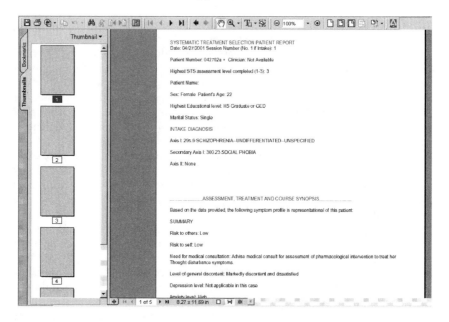

FIGURE C.6. STS online report.

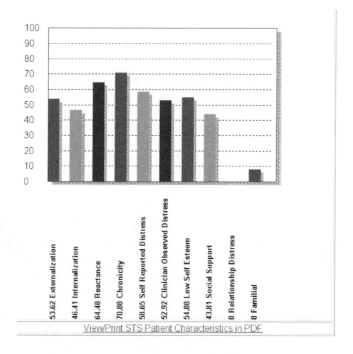

FIGURE C.7. Predisposing patient characteristics profile.

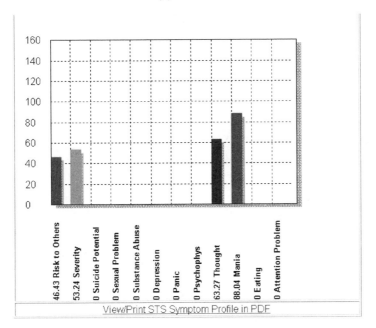

FIGURE C.8. Patient symptom profile.

5. A specific item-response review option (not shown) from each problem area and STS dimension is available for the clinician, should he or she wish to gather additional patient diagnostic/problem area information.

6. A clinician recommendation link (for patients and administrative users). The page containing the patient–clinician matching analysis (Figure C.10) provides clinician performance and experience data. This information allows for an informal selection of the best (most effective) therapist for any particular patient. The following figure is an example of the clinician recommendation function (Best Therapist Selection) from the STS system. STS automatically selects the best therapist for the particular patient in question, based on previous performance data from the expanding patient data pool. Matching algorithms search for a therapist (or any number of therapists specified) who has shown the best success with similar patients, based on all of the available data.

7. The STS system selects appropriate treatment manuals and standards of care from among an existing STS database. Figure C.11 represents this treatment manuals/standards of care option. Therapists are provided with a list of empirically supported treatments selected and matched specifically to the patient and his or her presenting problem(s). Clinicians may access the information on treatment manuals and standards by clicking on the "View Treatment Models" option in the Report Menu (see Figure C.11). By clicking one of the large buttons, the "standard of care" matched to this particular patient is readily viewable and printable.

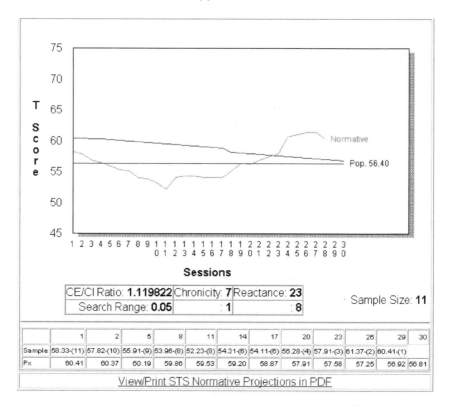

FIGURE C.9. Lack of well-being.

A demo illustrating the capability of the STS program is available to interested therapists. To access the demo program, therapists should utilize the following URL: *www.systematictreatmentselection.com*. All the user needs to do is follow the instructions provided for the demonstration procedure. If you choose to do so, you may complete an intake and two updates, as well as print relevant reports and a variety of other treatment-specific output materials.

CASE EXAMPLE: R.W.

The previous figures contain information on R.W., the individual whose description was provided in Chapter 2 and who is followed throughout this volume. R.W. is a 22-year-old, Mexican American woman. She has a history of panic attacks, associated with apparent agoraphobia, social phobias, and significant paranoid ideation. She carries a provisional diagnosis of undifferentiated schizophrenia (295.9) and social phobia (300.23). Her history suggests a good deal of social distrust and isola-

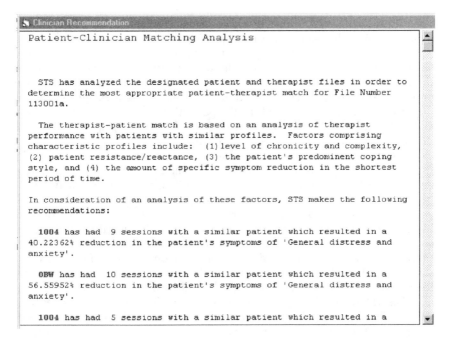

FIGURE C.10. Patient–clinician matching analysis.

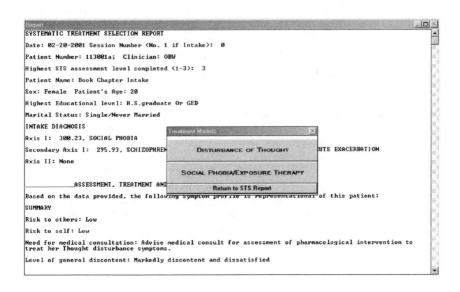

FIGURE C.11. Treatment manual option.

tion, largely the result of her having initiated a long-term but illicit relationship with a high school teacher while she was yet underage.

The clinician gathered background information on R.W., administered several assessment tools, and then collected the information and sat down at the computer to complete the clinician version of the STS treatment planning program. After completing the questions (see Figure C.5 for examples), the clinician may then choose to look at the patient's profile of symptoms (Figure C.8), which reveals significant elevations (over $T = 50$) of symptoms in the domains of thought disturbance and hypomania.

The treating clinician may choose to review the patient's status on the STS treatment planning dimensions (Figure C.7). The first two scales reveal a tendency toward externalizing over internalizing qualities. Thus she may be expected to have many external fears, to anticipate being harmed, and to be hypersensitive to others' opinions and criticisms. She also has a high level of trait-like resistance (called "reactance" in Figure C.7), indicating that she invests a good deal of energy in asserting her autonomy and may have problems with authorities and with any perceived loss of interpersonal control. Elevations also suggest that her problem is complex/chronic, that she experiences a moderate level of subjective distress, but that she has adequate social support.

The STS report (Figure C.6) suggests the need for long-term treatment, including the use of psychoactive medications designed to affect thought processes, and efforts to structure the patient's environment to reduce the degree of instability and variability of response. The externalizing patterns suggest the need to focus on discrete symptoms and to assume a concrete and structured approach to (1) acquire more effective thought and emotion management, (2) practice effective person skills, and (3) test out suspicions of others' motives and behaviors. The high levels of resistance suggest that self-directed treatments should be employed to supplement therapist activities and reduce the degree of confrontation. Self-help manuals focusing on impulse control, anxiety management, and cognitive skill building are recommended.

Once the therapist has gathered this information, he or she may want to turn to the projection of treatment course (depicted in Figure C.9). This figure shows that treatment is likely to be erratic (green lines), with ups and downs over a long period of time. Thus efforts directed toward increasing and/or maintaining the patient's stability, rather than making dramatic changes in functioning, become the primary focus.

Indeed, after a long course of treatment, slow progress is confirmed by periodic updates (red lines); this patient's course was somewhat more stable than predicted from a subgroup of similar patients in the normative samples. Thus, the clinician can feel comforted by observing that the treatment is associated with an improved course and increased stability in subjective feelings of well-being. Indeed, there may be some reduction of symptoms over time, returning the patient to the approximate mean of patients in the normative group.

References

Ackerman, M. J. (1999). *Essentials of forensic psychological assessment.* New York: Wiley.

Ackerman, P. L., & Heggestad, E. D. (1997). Intelligence, personality and interests: Evidence for overlapping traits. *Psychological Bulletin, 121,* 219–245.

Acklin, M. W., McDowell, C. J., II, Verschell, M. S., & Chan, D. (2000). Interobserver agreement, intraobserver reliability, and the Rorschach Comprehensive System. *Journal of Personality Assessment, 74,* 15–47.

Adams, S. H. (1994). Role of hostility in women's health during midlife: A longitudinal study. *Health Psychology, 13,* 488–495.

Affleck, D., & Strider, F. (1971). Contribution of psychological reports to patient management. *Journal of Consulting and Clinical Psychology, 53,* 790–802.

Agronick, G. S., & Duncan, L. E. (1998). Personality and social change: Individual differences, life path, and importance attributed to the women's movement. *Journal of Personality and Social Psychology, 74,* 1545–1555.

Alterman, A. J., McDermott, P. A., Cacciola, J. S., Rutherford, M. J., Boardman, C. R., McKay, J. R., & Cook, T. G. (1998). A typology of antisociality in methadone patients. *Journal of Abnormal Psychology, 107,* 412–422.

Amador, X. F., Friedman, J. H., Kasapis, C., Yale, S. A., Flaum, M., & Gorman, J. M. (1996). Suicidal behavior in schizophrenia and its relationship to awareness of illness. *American Journal of Psychiatry, 153,* 1185–1188.

Amchin, J. (1991). *Psychiatric diagnosis: A biopsychosocial approach using DSM-III-R.* Washington, DC: American Psychiatric Press.

American Psychiatric Association. (1968). *Diagnostic and statistical manual of mental disorders* (2nd ed.). Washington, DC: Author.

American Psychiatric Association. (1980). *Diagnostic and statistical manual of mental disorders* (3rd ed.). Washington, DC: Author.

American Psychiatric Association. (1987). *Diagnostic and statistical manual of mental disorders* (3rd ed., rev.). Washington, DC: Author.

American Psychiatric Association. (1991). *DSM-IV options book: Work in progress.* Washington, DC: Author.

American Psychiatric Association. (1994). *Diagnostic and statistical manual of mental disorders* (4th ed.). Washington, DC: Author.

American Psychiatric Association. (2000). *Diagnostic and statistical manual of mental disorders* (4th ed. text, rev.). Washington, DC: Author.

American Psychological Association. (1990). *APA guidelines for providers of psychological services to ethnic, linguistic, and culturally diverse populations.* Washington, DC: Author.

American Psychological Association. (1992). Ethical principals of psychologists and code of conduct. *American Psychologist, 47,* 1596–1611.

American Psychological Association. (1993). *Responsible test use: Case studies for assessing human behavior.* Washington, DC: Author.

American Psychological Association. (2001). *Publication manual* (5th ed.). Washington, DC: Author.

American Psychological Association. (2002). Ethical principles of psychologists and code of conduct. *American Psychologist, 57,* 1060–1073.

Anderson, T., & Strupp, H. H. (1996). The ecology of psychotherapy research. *Journal of Consulting and Clinical Psychology, 64,* 776–782.

Antonuccio, D. O., Danton, W. G., & DeNelsky, G. Y. (1995). Psychotherapy versus medication for depression: Challenging the conventional wisdom with data. *Professional Psychology: Research and Practice, 26,* 574–585.

Antony, M. M., Orsillo, S. M., & Roemer, L. (Eds.). (2001). *Practitioner's guide to empirically based measures of anxiety.* New York: Kluwer Academic/Plenum Press.

Apostal, R. A. (1971). Personality descriptions of mental health center patients for use as pre-therapy information. *Mental Hygiene, 55,* 119–120.

Archer, R. P. (1999). Introduction to a special section: Perspectives on the Rorschach. *Assessment, 6,* 307–310.

Archer, R. P., & Gordon, R. A. (1988). MMPI and Rorschach indices of schizophrenic and depressive diagnoses among adolescent inpatients. *Journal of Personality Assessment, 52,* 276–287.

Archer, R. P., & Krishnamurthy, R. (1993a). Combining the Rorschach and MMPI in the assessment of adolescents. *Journal of Personality Assessment, 60,* 132–140.

Archer, R. P., & Krishnamurthy, R. (1993b). A review of MMPI and Rorschach interrelationships in adult samples. *Journal of Personality Assessment, 61,* 277–293.

Archer, R. P., & Krishnamurthy, R. (1997). MMPI-A and Rorschach indices related to depression and conduct disorder: An evaluation of the incremental validity hypothesis. *Journal of Personality Assessment, 69,* 517–533.

Archer, R. P., & Newsom, C. R. (2000). Psychological test usage with adolescent clients: Survey update. *Assessment, 7,* 227–236.

Armengol, C. G. (2001). The referral process. In C. G. Armengol, E. Kaplan, & E. J. Moes (Eds.), *The consumer-oriented neuropsychological report* (pp. 47–60). Lutz, FL: Psychological Assessment Resources.

Armengol, C. G., Moes, E. J., Penney, D. L., & Sapienza, M. M. (2001). Writing client-centered recommendations. In C. G. Armengol, E. Kaplan, & E. J. Moes (Eds.), *The consumer-oriented neuropsychological report* (pp. 141–160). Lutz, FL: Psychological Assessment Resources.

Aronoff, G. M., & Evan, W. O. (1982). The prediction of treatment outcome at a multidisciplinary pain center. *Pain, 14*, 67–73.

Asaad, G. (2000). Somatization disorder. In M. Hersen & M. Biaggio (Ed.), *Effective brief therapies: A clinician's guide* (pp. 179–190). San Diego, CA: Academic Press.

Atkinson, D. R., Morten, G., & Sue, D. W. (1983). Proposed minority identity development model. In D. R. Atkinson, G. Morten, & D. W. Sue (Eds.), *Counseling American minorities: A cross-cultural perspective* (pp. 191–200). Dubuque, IA: William C. Brown.

Austin, E. J., Deary, I. J., & Gibson, G. J. (1997). Relationships between ability and personality: Three hypotheses tested. *Intelligence, 25*, 49–70.

Austin, E. J., Deary, I. J., Whiteman, M. C., Fowkes, F. G. R., Pedersen, N. L., Rabbitt, P., Bent, N., & McInnes, L. (2002). Relationships between ability and personality: Does intelligence contribute positively to personal and social adjustment? *Personality and Individual Differences, 32*, 1391–1411.

Austin, E. J., Hofer, S. M., Deary, I. J., & Eber, H. W. (2000) Interactions between intelligence and personality: Results from two large samples. *Personality and Individual Differences, 29*, 405–427.

Aylward, E., Walker, E., & Bettes, B. (1984). Intelligence in schizophrenia: A meta-analysis of the research. *Schizophrenia Bulletin, 10*, 430–459.

Baer, R. A., Wetter, M. W., & Berry, D. T. (1992). Detection of under-reporting of psychopathology on the MMPI: A meta-analysis. *Clinical Psychology Review, 12*, 509–525.

Bagby, R. M., Joffe, R. T., Parker, J. D. A., Kalemba, V., & Harkness, K. L. (1995). Major depression and the five-factor model. *Journal of Personality Disorders, 9*, 224–234.

Ball, J. D., Archer, R. P., Gordon, R. A., & French, J. (1991). Rorschach depression indices with children and adolescents: Concurrent validity findings. *Journal of Personality Assessment, 57*, 465–476.

Bar-On, R. (1997). *The Emotional Quotient Inventory (EQ-i): Technical manual.* Toronto: Multi-Health Systems.

Bar-On, R. (2000). Emotional and social intelligence: Insights from the Emotional Quotient Inventory. In R. Bar-On & J. D. A. Parker (Eds.), *The handbook of emotional intelligence: The theory and practice of development, evaluation, education, and application—at home, school, and in the workplace* (pp. 363–388). San Francisco: Jossey-Bass.

Bar-On, R. (2002). *Bar-On Emotional Quotient Inventory: Short (EQ-i:S): Technical manual.* Toronto: Multi-Health Systems.

Bar-On, R., & Parker, J. D. A. (Eds.). (2000). *The handbook of emotional intelligence: Theory and praxtice of development, evaulation, education, and application— at home, school, and in the workplace.* San Francisco: Jossey-Bass.

Barber, J. P., Crits-Christoph, P., & Luborsky, L. (1990). A guide to the CCRT standard categories and their classification. In L. Luborsky & P. Crits-Christoph (Eds.), *The core conflictual relationship theme* (pp. 35–49). New York: Basic Books.

Barber, J. P., Luborsky, L., Crits-Christoph, P., & Diguer, L. (1995). A comparison of core conflictual relationship themes before psychotherapy and during early sessions. *Journal of Consulting and Clinical Psychology, 63*, 145–148.

Barber, J. P., Luborsky, L., Gallop, R., Frank, A., Weiss, R. D., Thase, M. E., Connolly,

M. B., Gladis, M., Foltz, C., & Sigueland, S. (2001). Therapeutic alliance as a predictor of outcome and retention in the National Institute on Drug Abuse Collaborative Cocaine Treatment Study. *Journal of Consulting and Clinical Psychology, 69,* 119–124.

Bargh, J.A., & Chartrand, T.L. (1999). The unbearable automaticity of being. *American Psychologist, 54,* 462–479.

Barlow, D. H. (Ed.). (l985). *Clinical handbook of psychological disorders: A step-by-step treatment manual.* New York: Guilford Press.

Barlow, D. H., Gorman, J. M., Shear, M. K., & Woods, S. W. (2000). Cognitive-behavioral therapy, imipramine, or their combination for panic disorder: A randomized controlled trial. *Journal of the American Medical Association, 283,* 2529–2536.

Barrera, M. (1983). A method for the assessment of social support networks in community survey research. *Connections, 3,* 8–13.

Barrick, M. R., & Mount, M. K. (1991a). Autonomy as moderator of the relationship between the big five personality dimensions and job performance. *Journal of Applied Psychology, 78,* 111–118.

Barrick, M. R., & Mount, M. K. (1991b). The big-five personality dimensions and job performance: A meta-analysis. *Personnel Psychology, 44,* 1–26.

Barron, F. (1953). Some test correlates of response to psychotherapy. *Journal of Consulting Psychology, 17*(4), 235–241.

Bathurst, K., Gottfried, A. W., & Gottfried, A. E. (1997). Normative data for the MMPI-2 in child custody litigation. *Psychological Assessment, 9,* 205–211.

Beck, A. T., Steer, R. A., & Brown, G. K. (1996). *BDI-II manual.* San Antonio, TX: Psychological Corporation.

Beck, A. T., Ward, C. H., Mendelson, M., Mock, J., & Erbaugh, J. (1961). An inventory for measuring depression. *Archives of General Psychiatry, 4,* 53–56.

Beech, A., & Williams, L. (1997). Investigating cognitive processes in schizotypal personality and schizophrenia. In G. Matthews (Ed.), *Cognitive science perspectives on personality and emotion* (pp. 475–502). Amsterdam: Elsevier.

Bellak, L. (1947). *A guide to the interpretation of the Thematic Apperception Test.* New York: Psychological Corporation.

Bellak, L., & Bellak, S. (1949). *The Children's Apperception Test.* Larchmont, NY: C.P.S.

Bellak, L., & Bellak, S. (1973). *The Senior Apperception Technique.* Larchmont, NY: C.P.S.

Ben-Porath, Y. S., & Butcher, J. N. (1989a). The comparability of MMPI and MMPI-2 scales and profiles. *Psychological Assessment: A Journal of Consulting and Clinical Psychology, 1,* 345–347.

Ben-Porath, Y. S., & Butcher, J. N. (1989b). Psychometric stability of rewritten MMPI items. *Journal of Personality Assessment, 53,* 645–653.

Ben-Porath, Y. S., Butcher, J. N., & Graham, J. R. (1991). Contribution of the MMPI-2 content scales to the differential diagnosis of psychopathology. *Psychological Assessment, 3,* 634–640.

Ben-Porath, Y. S., McCulley, E., & Almagor, M. (1993). Incremental validity of the MMPI-2 content scales in the assessment of personality and psychopathology by self-report. *Journal of Personality Assessment, 61*(3), 557–575.

Ben-Porath, Y. S., & Tellegen, A. (1993). Continuity and changes in MMPI-2 validity indicators: Points of clarification. *MMPI-2 News and Profiles, 3,* 6–8.

Bender, L. (1938). *A visual motor gestalt test and its clinical uses. Research Monograph* (No. 3). New York: American Orthopsychiatric Association.

Bennett, B., Bryant, B., VandenBos, G., & Greenwood, A. (1990). *Professional liability and risk management.* Washington, DC: American Psychological Association.

Berger, K. S. (1994). *Late adulthood: Developing through the life span.* New York: Worth.

Bergner, M., Bobbitt, R. A., Carter, W. B., & Gilson, B. S. (1981). The Sickness Impact Profile: Development and final revision of a health status measure. *Medical Care, 19,* 787–788.

Berry, D. T., Baer, R. A., & Harris, M. J. (1991). Detection of malingering on the MMPI: A meta-analysis. *Clinical Psychology Review, 11,* 585–591.

Berry, D. T., Wetter, M. W., Baer, R. A., Larsen, L., Clark, C., & Monroe, K. (1992). MMPI-2 random responding indices: Validation using a self-report methodology. *Psychological Assessment, 4,* 340–345.

Berry, J. W., & Annis, R. C. (1974). Acculturative stress: The role of ecology, culture, and differentiation. *Journal of Cross Cultural Psychology, 5*(4), 382–406.

Betancourt, H., & Lopez, S. R. (1993). The study of culture, ethnicity, and race in American psychology. *American Psychologist, 48,* 629–637.

Beutler, L. E. (1983). *Eclectic psychotherapy: A systematic approach.* New York: Pergamon Press.

Beutler, L. E. (1995). Integrating and communicating findings. In L. E. Beutler & M. R. Berren (Eds.), *Integrative assessment of adult personality* (pp. 25–64). New York: Guilford Press.

Beutler, L. E. (2001). Comparisons among quality assurance systems: From outcome assessment to clinical utility. *Journal of Consulting and Clinical Psychology, 69,* 197–204.

Beutler, L. E., & Berren, M. R. (1995). *Integrative assessment of adult personality.* New York: Guilford Press.

Beutler, L. E., Brown, M. T., Crothers, L., Booker, K., & Seabrook, M. K. (1996). The dilemma of factitious demographic distinctions in psychological research. *Journal of Consulting and Clinical Psychology, 64,* 892–902.

Beutler, L. E., & Clarkin, J. F. (1990). *Systematic treatment selection: Toward targeted therapeutic interventions.* New York: Brunner/Mazel.

Beutler, L. E., Clarkin, J. F., & Bongar, B. (2000). *Guidelines for the systematic treatment of the depressed patient.* New York: Oxford University Press.

Beutler, L. E., Engle, D., Mohr, D., Daldrup, R. J., Bergan, J., Meredith, K., & Merry, W. (1991). Predictors of differential response to cognitive, experiential, and self-directed psychotherapeutic procedures. *Journal of Consulting and Clinical Psychology, 59,* 333–340.

Beutler, L. E., Goodrich, G., Fisher, D., & Williams, O. B. (1999). Use of psychological tests/instruments for treatment planning. In M. E. Maruish (Ed.), *The use of psychological tests for treatment planning and outcome assessment* (2nd ed., pp. 81–113). Hillsdale, NJ: Erlbaum.

Beutler, L. E., & Harwood, T. M. (1995). How to assess clients in treatment planning.

In J. N. Butcher (Ed.), *Clinical personality assessment* (pp. 59–77). New York: Oxford Univeristy Press.

Beutler, L. E., & Harwood, T. M. (2000). *Prescriptive psychotherapy: A practical guide to Systematic Treatment Selection.* New York: Oxford University Press.

Beutler, L. E., Harwood, T. M., Alimohamed, S., & Malik, M. (2002). Functional impairment and coping style. In J. Norcross (Ed), *Psychotherapy relationships that work: Therapist contributions and responsiveness to patient needs* (pp. 145–170). New York: Oxford University Press.

Beutler, L. E., Harwood, T. M., & Holaway, R. (2002). How to assess clients in pretreatment planning. In J. N. Butcher (Ed.), *Clinical personality assessment* (2nd ed., pp. 76–95). New York: Oxford University Press.

Beutler, L. E., Kim, E. J., Davison, E., Karno, M., & Fisher, D. (1996). Research contributions to improving managed health care outcomes. *Psychotherapy, 33,* 197–206.

Beutler, L. E., & Malik, M. L. (2002a). Diagnosis and treatment guidelines: The example of depression. In L. E. Beutler & M. L. Malik (Eds.), *Rethinking the DSM* (pp. 251–278). Washington, DC: American Psychological Association.

Beutler, L. E., & Malik, M. L. (Eds.). (2002b). *Rethinking the DSM: Psychological perspectives.* Washington, DC: American Psychological Association.

Beutler, L. E., Mohr, D. C., Grawe, K., Engle, D., & MacDonald, R. (1991). Looking for differential effects: Cross-cultural predictors of differential psychotherapy efficacy. *Journal of Psychotherapy Integration, 1,* 121–142.

Beutler, L. E., Moleiro, C., & Talebi, H. (2002). Resistance. In J. Norcross (Ed.), *Psychotherapy relationships that work: Therapist contributions and responsiveness to patient needs* (pp. 129–144). New York: Oxford University Press.

Beutler, L. E., Moleiro, C., Malik, M., & Harwood, T. M. (in press). A new twist on empirically supported treatments. *Revista Internacional de Psicologia Clínica y de la Salud.*

Beutler, L. E., Moleiro, C., Malik, M., Harwood, T. M., Romanelli, R., Gallagher-Thompson, D., & Thompson, L. (in press). A comparison of the Dodo, EST, and ATI factors among co-morbid stimulant dependent, depressed patients. *Clinical Psychology and Psychotherapy.*

Beutler, L. E., Storm, A., Kirkish, P., Scogin, F., & Gaines, J. A. (1985). Parameters in the prediction of police officer performance. *Professional Psychology: Research and Practice, 16,* 324–335.

Beutler, L. E., & Williams, O. B. (1999). *Systematic treatment selection (STS): A software package for treatment planning.* Ventura, CA: Center for Behavioral Health Technology.

Bickman, L., Karver, M. S., & Schut, L. J. A. (1997). Clinician reliability and accuracy in judging appropriate level of care. *Journal of Consulting and Clinical Psychology, 65,* 515–520.

Binstock, R. H. (1992). The oldest old and "intergenerational equity." In R. M. Suzman, D. P. Willis, & K. G. Manton (Eds.), *The oldest old* (pp. 394–417). New York: Oxford University Press.

Bjorkqvist, K., & Oesterman, K. (2000). Social intelligence - empathy = aggression? *Aggression and Violent Behavior, 5,* 191–200.

Blake, R. J., Potter, E. H., Jr., & Slimak, R. E. (1993). Validation of the structural scales of the CPI for predicting the performance of junior officers in the U.S. Coast Guard. *Journal of Business and Psychology, 7,* 431–448.

Blau, T. H. (1998). *The psychologist as expert witness* (2nd ed.). New York: Wiley.

Blieszner, R. (1995). Friendship processes and well-being in the later years of life: Implications for interventions. *Journal of Geriatric Psychiatry, 28,* 165–182.

Block, J. (1995). On the relation between IQ, impulsivity, and delinquency: Remarks on the Lynam, Moffitt, and Southamer-Loeber (1993) interpretation. *Journal of Abnormal Psychology, 104,* 395–398.

Bloom, R. W. (1993). Psychological assessment for security clearances, special access, and sensitive positions. *Military Medicine, 158,* 609–613.

Boccaccini, M. T., & Brodsky, S. L. (1999). Diagnostic test use by forensic psychologists in emotional injury cases. *Professional Psychology: Research and Practice, 31*(1), 251–259.

Bockian, N., Meager, S., & Millon, T. (2000). Assessing personality with the Millon Behavioral Health Inventory, the Millon Behavioral Medicine Diagnostic, and the Millon Clinical Multiaxial Inventory. In R. J. Gatchel & J. N. Weisberg (Eds.), *Personality characteristics of patients with pain* (pp. 61–88). Washington, DC: American Psychological Association.

Boone, D. E. (1994). Validity of the MMPI-2 Depression content scale with psychiatric inpatients. *Psychological Reports, 74*(1), 159–162.

Borum, R., & Grisso, T. (1995). Psychological test use in criminal forensic evaluations. *Professional Psychology: Research and Practice, 26,* 465–473.

Boscan, D. C., Penn, N. E., Vesasquez, R. J., Reimann, J., Gomez, N., Guzman, M., Moreno Berry, E., Diaz Infantes, L., Jaramillo, L. F., & Corrales de Romero, M. (2000). MMPI-2 profiles of Colombian, Mexican, and Venezuelan university students. *Psychological Reports, 87,* 107–110.

Boyd-Franklin, N. (1989). *Black families in therapy: A multisystems approach.* New York: Guilford Press.

Brand, C., Egan, V., & Deary, I. (1994). Intelligence, personality, and society: "Constructivist" versus "essentialist" possibilities. In D. K. Detterman (Ed.), *Current topics in human intelligence* (Vol. 4, pp. 29–42). Norwood, NJ: Ablex.

Brandwin, M. A., & Kewman, D. G. (1982). MMPI indicators of treatment response to spinal epidural stimulation in patient with chronic pain and patients with movement disorders. *Psychological Reports, 51,* 1059–1064.

Brems, C., & Lloyd, P. (1995). Validation of the MMPI-2 Low Self-Esteem Scale. *Journal of Personality Assessment, 65*(3), 550–556.

Brown, T. A., DiNardo, P. A., & Barlow, D. H. (1994). *Anxiety Disorders Interview Schedule for DSM-IV (ADIS-IV).* San Antonio, TX: Psychological Corporation.

Brtek, M. D., & Motowidlo, S. J. (2002). Effects of procedure and outcome accountability on interview validity. *Journal of Applied Psychology, 85,* 185–191.

Bryant, F. B., & Yarnold, P. R. (1990). The impact of Type A behaviour on subjective life quality: Bad for the heart, good for the soul? *Journal of Social Behaviour and Personality, 5,* 369–404.

Budman, S. H., & Gurman, A. S. (1988). *Theory and practice of brief therapy.* New York: Guilford Press.

Burger, G. K., Pickett, L., & Goldman, M. (1977). Second-order factors in the California Psychological Inventory. *Journal of Personality Assessment, 41,* 58–62.

Buros, O. K. (Ed.). (1978). *Eighth mental measurements yearbook.* Highland Park, NJ: Gryphon Press.

Butcher, J. N. (Ed.). (1972). *Objective personality assessment: Changing perspectives.* New York: Academic Press.

Butcher, J. N. (1985). Current developments in MMPI use: An international perspective. In J. N. Butcher & C. D. Spielberger (Eds.), *Advances in personality assessment* (Vol. 4, pp. 83–92). Hillsdale, NJ: Erlbaum.

Butcher, J. N. (1990). *Use of the MMPI-2 in treatment planning.* New York: Oxford University Press.

Butcher, J. N. (1993). *User's guide for the MMPI-2 Minnesota Report: Adult clinical system* (rev. ed.). Minneapolis, MN: National Computer Systems.

Butcher, J. N. (1996). *International adaptations of the MMPI-2: Research and clinical applications.* Minneapolis: University of Minnesota Press.

Butcher, J. N. (1998). *Butcher Treatment Planning Inventory.* San Antonio, TX: Psychological Corporation.

Butcher, J. N. (1999). *MMPI-2: A beginner's guide to the MMPI-2.* Washington, DC: American Psychological Association.

Butcher, J. N., Aldwin, C., Levenson, M., Ben-Porath, Y. S., Spiro, A., & Bosse, R. (1991). Personality and aging: A study of the MMPI-2 among elderly men. *Psychology of Aging, 6,* 361–370.

Butcher, J. N., Berah, E., Ellertsen, B., Miach, P., Lim, J., Nezami, E., Pancheri, P., Derksen, J., & Almagor, M. (1998). Objective personality assessment: Computer-based MMPI-2 interpretation in international clinical settings. In C. Belar (Ed.), *Comprehensive clinical psychology: Sociocultural and individual differences* (pp. 277–312). New York: Elsevier.

Butcher, J. N., Dahlstrom, W. G., Graham, J. R., & Tellegen, A. (1990, May). The MMPI-2 and Classic Coke. *APA Monitor,* p. 1.

Butcher, J. N., Dahlstrom, W. G., Graham, J. R., Tellegen, A. M., & Kaemmer, B. (1989). *Minnesota Multiphasic Personality Inventory–2 (MMPI-2): Manual for administration and scoring.* Minneapolis: University of Minnesota Press.

Butcher, J. N., Graham, J. R., Dahlstrom, W. G., & Bowman, E. (1990). The MMPI-2 with college students. *Journal of Personality Assessment, 54,* 1–15.

Butcher, J. N., Graham, J. R., Williams, C. L., & Ben-Porath, Y. S. (1990). *Development and use of the MMPI-2 content scales.* Minneapolis: University of Minnesota Press.

Butcher, J. N., Jeffrey, T., Cayton, T., Colligan, S., DeVore, J., & Minnegawa, R. (1990). A study of active duty military personnel with the MMPI-2. *Military Psychology, 2,* 47–61.

Butcher, J. N., & Owen, P. (1978). Survey of personality inventories: Recent research developments and contemporary issues. In B. Wolman (Ed.), *Handbook of clinical diagnosis.* New York: Plenum Press.

Butcher, J. N., & Pancheri, P. (1976). *Handbook of cross-national MMPI research.* Minneapolis: University of Minnesota Press.

Butcher, J. N., & Rouse, S. V. (1996). Personality: Individual differences and clinical assessment. *Annual Review of Psychology, 47,* 87–111.

Butcher, J. N., Rouse, S. V., & Perry, J. N. (2000). Empirical description of psychopathology in therapy clients: Correlates of MMPI-2 scales. In J. N. Butcher (Ed.),

Basic sources on the MMPI-2 (pp. 487–500). Minneapolis: University of Minnesota Press.

Butcher, J. N., & Williams, C. L. (2000). *Essentials of MMPI-2 and MMPI-A interpretation* (2nd ed., p. 494). Minneapolis: University of Minnesota Press.

Butcher, J. N., Williams, C.-L., Graham, J. R., Archer, R., Tellegen, A., Ben-Porath, Y. S., & Kaemmer, B. (1992). *MMPI-A: Manual for administration, scoring, and interpretation.* Minneapolis: University of Minnesota Press.

Byrne, R. W., & Whiten, A. (1997). Machiavellian intelligence. In A. Whiten & R. W. Byrne (Eds.), *Machiavellian Intelligence II: Extensions and evaluations* (pp. 1–23). Cambridge, UK: Cambridge University Press.

Caldwell, A. B. (2000). MMPI-2 data research file for clinical patients. In R. L. Greene (Ed.), *The MMPI-2: An interpretive manual* (2nd ed., p. 494). Boston: Allyn & Bacon.

Caldwell, A. B. (2001). What do the MMPI-2 scales really measure?: Some hypotheses. *Journal of Personality Assessment, 76,* 1–17.

Camara, W. J., Nathan, J. S., & Puente, A. E. (2000). Psychological test usage: Implications in professional psychology. *Professional Psychology: Research and Practice, 31,* 141–154.

Camara, W., Norton, J., & Puente, A. (2000). Psychological test usage: Implications in professional psychology. *Professional Psychology: Research and Practice, 31,* 141–154.

Campbell, D. P. (1995). The psychological test profile of brigadier generals: Warmongers or reluctant warriors? In D. Lubinski & R. V. Dawis (Eds.), *Assessing individual differences in human behavior: New concepts, methods, and findings* (pp. 145–175). Palo Alto, CA: Consulting Psychologists Press.

Carbone, E. G., Cigrang, J. A., Todd, S. L., & Fiedler, E. R. (1999). Predicting outcome of military basic training for individuals referred for psychological evaluation. *Journal of Personality Assessment, 72*(2), 256–265.

Carmelli, D., Swan, G. E., & Cardon, L. R. (1995). Genetic mediation in the relationship of education to cognitive function in older people. *Psychology and Aging, 10,* 48–53.

Carroll, J. B. (1993*). Human cognitive abilities: A survey of factor-analytic studies.* New York: Cambridge University Press.

Carson, R. C. (1997). Costly compromises: A critique of the diagnostic and statistical manual of mental disorders. In S. Fisher & R. P. Greenberg (Eds.), *From placebo to panacea: Putting psychiatric drugs to the test* (pp. 98–112). New York: Wiley.

Castonguay, L. G., Goldfried, M. R., Wiser, S., Raue, P. J., & Hayes, A. M. (1996). Predicting the effect of cognitive therapy for depression: A study of unique and common factors. *Journal of Consulting and Clinical Psychology, 64,* 497–504.

Cattell, R. B., Ever, H. W., & Tatsouka, M. M. (1970). *Handbook for the Sixteen Personality Factor Questionnaire.* Champaign, IL: Institute for Personality and Abilities Testing.

Chambless, D. L., & Ollendick, T. H. (2001). Empirically supported psychological interventions: Controversies and evidence. *Annual Review of Psychology, 52,* 685–716.

Cheeseman, J. (1996). *Population projections of the United States by age, sex, race, and Hispanic origin: 1995 to 2050* (U.S. Bureau of the Census, Current Population Reports, P25–1130). Washington, DC: U.S. Government Printing Office.

Cheung, F. M. (1985). Cross-cultural considerations for the translation and adaptation of the Chinese MMPI in Hong Kong. In J. N. Butcher & C. D. Spielberger (Eds.), *Advances in personality assessment* (Vol. 4, pp. 131–158) Hillsdale, NJ: Erlbaum.

Chiles, J. A., Lambert, M. J., & Hatch, A. L. (1999) The impact of psychological interventions on medical cost offset: A meta-analytic review. *Clinical Psychology: Science and practice, 6,* 204–220.

Choca, J. P., & Van Denburg, E. J. (1996). *Manual for clinical psychology trainees.* New York: Brunner/Mazel.

Choca, J. P., & Van Denburg, E. (1997). *Interpretative guide to the Millon Clinical Multiaxial Inventory* (2nd ed.). Washington, DC: American Psychological Association.

Ciarrochi, J., Chan, A., & Caputi, P. (2000). A critical evaluation of the emotional intelligence construct. *Personality and Individual Differences, 28,* 539–561.

Clark, M. E. (1993, March). *MMPI-2 Anger and Cynicism scales: Interpretive cautions.* Paper presented at the 28th Annual Symposium on Recent Developments in the Use of the MMPI/MMPI-2, St. Petersburg, FL.

Clarkin, J. F., & Hurt, S. W. (1988). Psychological assessment: Tests and rating scales. In J. A. Talbott, R. E. Hales, & S. C. Yodofsky (Eds.), *The American Psychiatric Press textbook of psychiatry* (pp. 225–246). Washington, DC: American Psychiatric Press.

Colligan, R. C., & Offord, K. P. (1986). [MMPI data research tape for Mayo Clinic patients referred for psychiatric evaluations.] Unpublished raw data.

Colligan R. C., Osborne, D., Swenson, W. M., & Offord, K. (1983). *The MMPI: Contemporary normative study.* New York: Praeger.

Collins, J. M., & Schmidt, F. L. (1993). Personality, integrity, and white collar crime: A construct validity study. *Personnel Psychology, 46,* 295–311.

Collis, J. M., & Messick, S. (Eds.). (2001). *Intelligence and personality: Bridging the gap in theory and measurement.* Mahwah, NJ: Erlbaum.

Consulting Psychologists Press. (1995). *CPI psychological inventory.* New York: Author.

Cort, D., Kappagoda, C. T., & Greene, R. L. (2001, March). *Prediction of compliance using the MMPI-2 in a multi-disciplinary preventative cardiology program.* Paper presented at the 36th Annual Symposium on Recent Developments in the Use of the MMPI-2/MMPI-A, Safety Harbor, FL.

Costa, P. T., Jr., & McCrae, R. R. (1992). *Revised NEO Personality Inventory (NOE-PI-PR) and NEO Five Factor Inventory (NEO-FFI) professional manual.* Odessa, FL: Psychological Assessment Resources.

Craig, R. J. (1993a). *Millon Clinical Multiaxial Inventory: A clinical research information synthesis.* Hillsdale, NJ: Erlbaum.

Craig, R. J. (1993b). *Psychological screening with the MCMI-II.* Odessa, FL: Psychological Assessment Resources.

Cramer, P. (1991). *The development of defense mechanisms: Theory, research, and assessment.* New York: Springer-Verlag.

Crits-Christoph, P., Luborsky, L., Dahl, L., Popp, C., Mellon, J., & Mark, D. (1988). Clinicians can agree in assessing relationship patterns in psychotherapy. *Archives of General Psychiatry, 45,* 1001–1004.

Cross, W. E. (1978). The Thomas and Cross model of psychological nigrescence: A review. *Journal of Black Psychology, 5*, 13–31.

Cross, W. E. (1991). *Shades of black: Diversity in African-American identity.* Philadelphia: Temple University Press.

Crowther, M. R., & Zeiss, A. M. (2002). Working with older adults: Relating interventions to aging. In N. D. Sundberg, A. A. Wineberger, & J. R. Taplin (Eds.), *Clinical psychology: Evolving theory, practice and research* (4th ed., pp. 302–329). Upper Saddle River, NJ: Prentice-Hall.

Cuellar, I., Arnold, B., & Maldonada, R. (1995). Acculturation Rating Scale for Mexican Americans–II: A revision of the original ARSMA scale. *Hispanic Journal of Behavioral Sciences, 17,* 275–304.

Cuellar, I., Harris, L., & Jasso, R. (1980). An acculturation scale for Mexican American normal and clinical populations. *Hispanic Journal of Behavioral Sciences, 2,* 199–217.

Cummings, N. (1991). The somatizing patient. In C. A. Austad & W. A. Berman (Eds.), *Psychotherapy in managed care: The optimal use of time and resources* (pp. 234–237). Washington, DC: American Psychological Association.

Cummings, N. (1999). Medical cost offset, meta-analysis, and implications for future research and practice. *Clinical Psychology: Science and Practice, 6,* 221–224.

Daldrup, R. J., Beutler, L. E., Engle, D., & Greenberg, L. S. (1988). *Focused expressive psychotherapy: Freeing the overcontrolled patient.* New York: Guilford Press.

Dana, R. H. (1993). *Multicultural assessment perspective in professional psychology.* Boston: Allyn & Bacon.

David, A. S. (1990). Insight and psychosis. *British Journal of Psychiatry, 156,* 798–808.

David, A. S. (1998). Schizophrenia and intellectual decline. *American Journal of Psychiatry, 155,* 1634–1635.

David, A. S. (1999). "To see oursels as others see us"—Aubrey Lewis's insight. *British Journal of Psychiatry, 175,* 210–216.

David, A.S., Malmberg, A., Brandt, L., Allebeck, P., & Lewis, G. (1997). IQ and risk for schizophrenia: A population-based cohort study. *Psychological Medicine, 27,* 1311–1323.

Davidson, M., Reichenberg, A., Rabinowitz, J., Weiser, M., Kaplan, Z., & Mark, M. (1999). Behavioral and intellectual markers for schizophrenia in apparently healthy male adolescents. *American Journal of Psychiatry, 156,* 1328–1335.

Davies, N., Russell, A., Jones, P., & Murray, R. M. (1998). Which characteristics of schizophrenia predate psychosis? *Journal of Psychiatric Research, 32,* 121–131.

Davies, M., Stankov, L., & Roberts, R. D. (1998). Emotional intelligence: In search of an elusive construct. *Journal of Personality and Social Psychology, 75,* 989–1015.

Davis, G. L., Hoffman, R. G., & Nelson, K. S. (1990). Differences between Native Americans and whites on the California Psychological Inventory. *Psychological Assessment, 2,* 238–242.

Dawda, D., & Hart, S. D. (2000). Assessing emotional intelligence: Reliability and validity of the Bar-On Emotional Quotient Inventory (EQ-i) in university students. *Personality and Individual Differences, 28,* 797–812.

Day, D. V., & Bedeian, A. G. (1991). Predicting job performance across organizations:

The interaction of work orientation and psychological climate. *Journal of Management, 17,* 589–600.

Deary, I. J. (2000). *Looking down on human intelligence.* Oxford, UK: Oxford University Press.

Deary, I. J., MacLennan, W. J., & Starr, J. M. (1999). Is age kinder to the initially more able? Differential ageing of verbal ability in the Healthy Old People in Edinburgh study. *Intelligence, 26,* 357–375.

Dempster, F. N., & Corkill, A. J. (1999). Individual differences in susceptibility to interference and general cognitive ability. *Acta Psychologica, 101,* 395–416.

DeNeve, K. M., & Cooper, H. (1998). The happy personality: A meta-analysis of 137 personality traits and subjective well being. *Psychological Bulletin, 124,* 197–229.

Derby, W. N. (2001). Writing the forensic neuropsychological report. In C. G. Armengol, E. Kaplan, & E. J. Moes (Eds.), *The consumer-oriented neuropsychological report* (pp. 203–224). Lutz, FL: Psychological Assessment Resources.

Derogatis, L. R. (1994). *SCL-90-R: Administration, scoring, and procedures manual.* Minneapolis, MN: National Computer Systems.

Derogatis, L. R., & Lynn, L. L. (1999). Psychological tests in screening for psychiatric disorder. In M. E. Maruish (Ed.), *The use of psychological testing for treatment planning and outcomes assessment* (pp. 41–79). Mahwah, NJ: Erlbaum.

Diener, E. (1984). Subjective well-being. *Psychological Bulletin, 95,* 542–575.

Digman, J. M. (1990). Personality structure: Emergence of the five-factor model. *Annual Review of Psychology, 41,* 417–440.

DiNardo, P. A., Brown, T. A., & Barlow, D. H. (1994). *Anxiety Disorders Interview Schedule for DSM-IV: Lifetime Version.* San Antonio, TX: Psychological Corporation.

Distler, L. S., May, P. R., & Tuma, A. H. (1964). Anxiety and ego strength as predictors of response to treatment in schizophrenic patients. *Journal of Consulting Psychology, 28,* 1970–1977.

Dowd, E. T., Milne, C. R., & Wise, S. L. (1991). The Therapeutic Reactance Scale: A measure of psychological reactance. *Journal of Counseling and Development, 69,* 541–545.

Dyer, E. D. (1987). Can university success and first-year job performance be predicted from academic achievement, vocational interest, personality, and biographical measures? *Psychological Reports, 61,* 655–671.

Eaton, W. W., Neufeld, K., Chen, L., & Cai, G. (2000). A comparison of self-report and clinical diagnostic interviews for depression. *Archives of General Psychiatry, 57,* 217–222.

Egan, G. (2002). *The skilled helper* (7th ed.). Brooks/Cole.

Egan, V. (1989). Links between personality, ability and attitudes in a low-IQ sample. *Personality and Individual Differences, 10,* 997–1001.

Egeland, B., Erickson, M., Butcher, J. N., & Ben-Porath, Y. S. (1991). MMPI-2 profiles of women at risk for child abuse. *Journal of Personality Assessment, 5,* 254–263.

Elliott, T. R., Anderson, W. P., & Adams, N. A. (1987). MMPI indicators of long-term therapy in a college counseling center. *Psychological Reports, 60,* 79–81.

Endler, N. S., & Summerfeldt, L. J. (1995). Intelligence, personality, psychopathology and adjustment. In D. H. Saklofske & M. Zeidner (Eds.), *International handbook of personality and intelligence* (pp. 249–284). New York: Plenum Press.

Entwisle, D. R., & Astone, N. M. (1994). Some practical guidelines for measuring youth's race/ethnicity and socioeconomic status. *Child Development, 65,* 1521–1540.

Essig, S., Mittenberg, W., Petersen, R., Strauman, S., & Cooper, J. (2001). Practices in forensic neuropsychology: Perspectives of neuropsychologists and trial attorneys. *Archives of Clinical Neuropsychology, 16*(3), 271–291.

Exner, J. E., Jr. (1974). *The Rorschach: A comprehensive system. Volume 1:* New York: Wiley.

Exner, J. E., Jr. (1986). *The Rorschach: A comprehensive system. Volume 1: Basic Foundations* (2nd ed.). New York: Wiley.

Exner, J. E., Jr. (1991). *The Rorschach: A comprehensive system. Volume 2: Interpretation* (2nd ed.). New York: Wiley.

Exner, J. E., Jr. (1993). *The Rorschach: A comprehensive system. Volume 1: Basic foundations* (3rd ed.). New York: Wiley.

Exner, J. E., Jr. (1995). *Alumni newsletter.* Asheville, NC: Rorschach Workshops.

Exner, J. E., Jr. (1996). *1996 Alumni newsletter.* Asheville, NC: Rorschach Workshops.

Exner, J. E., Jr. (1997). The future of Rorschach in personality assessment. *Journal of Personality Assessment, 68,* 37–46.

Exner, J. E., Jr. (2000a). *2000 Alumni newsletter.* Asheville, NC: Rorschach Workshops.

Exner, J. E., Jr. (2000b). *A primer for Rorschach interpretation.* Asheville, NC: Rorschach Workshops.

Exner, J. E., Jr. (2001a). A comment on "The misperception of psychopathology: Problems with the norms of the comprehensive system for the Rorschach." *Clinical Psychology: Science and Practice, 8,* 386–388.

Exner, J. E., Jr. (2001b). *A Rorschach workbook for the comprehensive system* (5th ed.). Asheville, NC: Rorschach Workshops.

Exner, J. E., Jr. (2002). *The Rorschach: A comprehensive system. Volume 1: Basic foundations* (4th ed.). New York: Wiley.

Exner, J. E., Jr., & Andronikof-Sanglade, A. (1992). Rorschach changes following brief and short-term therapy. *Journal of Personality Assessment, 59,* 59–71.

Exner, J. E., Jr., Colligan, S. C., Boll, T. J., Stischer, B., & Hillman, L. (1996). Rorschach findings concerning closed head injury patients. *Assessment, 3,* 317–326.

Exner, J. E., Jr., & Weiner, I. B. (1995). *The Rorschach: A comprehensive system. Volume 3. Assessment of children and adolescents* (2nd ed.). New York: Wiley.

Eysenck, H. J. (1944). General social attitudes. *Journal of Social Psychology, 19,* 207–227.

Eysenck, H. J. (1986). A critique of contemporary classification and diagnosis. In T. Millon & G. L. Klerman (Eds.), *Contemporary directions in psychopathology: Toward the DSM-IV* (pp. 73–98). New York: Guilford Press.

Eysenck, H. J. (1971). Relationship between intelligence and personality. *Perceptual and Motor Skills, 32,* 637–638.

Fabrigoule, C., Letenneur, L., Dartigues, J. F., Zarrouk, M., Commenges, D., & Barberger-Gateau, P. (1995). Social and leisure activities and risk of dementia: A prospective longitudinal study. *Journal of the American Geriatric Society, 43,* 485–490.

Faull, R., & Meyer, G. J. (1993, March). *Assessment of depression with the MMPI: Distinctions between Scale 2 and the DEP.* Paper presented at the midwinter meeting of the Society for Personality Assessment, San Francisco.

Faust, D., & Fogel, B. (1989). The development and initial validation of a sensitive bedsider cognitive screening test. *Journal of Nervous and Mental Disease, 177,* 25–31.

Felton, J. L., & Nelson, R. O. (1984). Inter-assessor agreement on hypothesized controlling variables and treatment proposals. *Behavioral Assessment, 6,* 199–208.

Fergusson, D. M., & Lynskey, M. T. (1996). Adolescent resiliency to family adversity. *Journal of Child Psychology and Psychiatry, 37,* 281–292.

Finn, S. E. (1990, October). *A model for providing test feedback with the MMPI-2.* Paper presented at the 25th Annual Symposium on Recent Developments in the Use of the MMPI/MMPI-2, Minneapolis, MN.

Finn, S. E. (1996a). Assessment feedback integrating MMPI-2 and Rorschach findings. *Journal of Personality Assessment, 67,* 543–557.

Finn, S. E. (1996b). *Manual for using the MMPI-2 as a therapeutic intervention.* Minneapolis: University of Minnesota Press.

Finn, S. E., & Butcher, J. N. (1991). Clinical objective personality assessment. In M. Hersen, A. E. Kazdin, & A. S. Bellack (Eds.), *The clinical psychology handbook* (2nd ed., pp. 362–373). New York: Pergamon Press.

Finn, S. E., & Martin, H. (1997). Therapeutic assessment with the MMPI-2 in managed care. In J. N. Butcher (Ed.), *Personality assessment in managed care: Using the MMPI-2 in treatment planning* (pp. 131–152). New York: Oxford University Press.

Finn, S. E., Moes, E. J., & Kaplan, E. (2001). The consumer's point of view. In C. G. Armengol, E. Kaplan, & E. J. Moes (Eds.), *The consumer-oriented neuropsychological report* (pp. 13–46). Lutz, FL: Psychological Assessment Resources.

Finn, S. E., & Tonsager, M. E. (1992). The effects of providing MMPI-2 test feedback to college students awaiting psychotherapy. *Psychological Assessment, 4,* 278–287.

First, M. B., Spitzer, R. L., Gibbon, M., & Williams, J. B. (1995). *Structured Clinical Interview for DSM-IV Axis I disorders—patient edition (SCID-I/P, Version 2.0).* New York: New York State Psychiatric Institute.

Fisher, C. T. (1994). *Individualizing psychological assessment.* Hillsdale, NJ: Erlbaum.

Fisher, D., Beutler, L. E., & Williams, O. B. (1999a). Making assessment relevant to treatment planning: The STS Clinician Rating Form. *Journal of Clinical Psychology, 55,* 825–842.

Fisher, D., Beutler, L. E., & Williams, O. B. (1999b). STS Clinician Rating Form: Patient assessment and treatment planning. *Journal of Clinical Psychology, 55,* 825–842.

Folstein, M. F., Folstein, S. E., & McHugh, P. R. (1975). A "mini-mental state": A practical method for grading the cognitive state of patients for the clinician. *Journal of Psychiatric Research, 12,* 189–198.

Fowler, R. D., & Matarazzo, J. D. (1988). Psychologists and psychiatrists as expert witnesses. *Science, 241,* 1143.

Frances, A., First, M. B., Widiger, T. A., Miele, G. M., Tilly, S. M., Davis, W. W., & Pincus, H. A. (1991). An A–Z guide to DSM-IV conundrums. *Journal of Abnormal Psychology, 100,* 407–412.

Frauenhoffer, D., Ross, M. J., Gfeller, J., Searight, H. R., & Piotrowski, C. (1998). Psychological test usage among licensed mental health practitioners: A multidisciplinary survey. *Journal of Psychological Practice, 4*(1), 28–33.

Freud, S. (1953). On psychotherapy. In J. Strachey (Ed. & Trans.), *The standard edition of the complete psychological works of Sigmund Freud* (Vol. 7, pp. 257–258). London: Hogarth Press. (Original work published 1905)

Friedman, A. F., Lewak, R. W., Nichols, D. S., & Webb, J. F. (2001). *Psychological assessment with the MMPI-2.* Mahway, NJ: Earlbaum.

Friesen, W., & Andrews, D. (1982). Self-management during counseling sessions: The behavioral assessment of process. *Criminal Justice and Behavior, 9,* 204–216.

Frueh, B. C., & Kinder, B. N. (1994). The susceptibility of the Rorschach inkblot test to malingering of combat-related PTSD. *Journal of Personality Assessment, 62,* 280–298.

Gallagher-Thompson, D., & Thompson, L. W. (1996). Applying cognitive-behavioral therapy to the problems of later life. In S. H. Zarit & B. G. Knight (Eds.), *A guide to psychotherapy and aging* (pp. 61–82). Washington, DC: American Psychological Association.

Ganellen, R. J. (1994). Attempting to conceal psychological disturbance: MMPI defensive response sets and the Rorschach. *Journal of Personality Assessment, 63,* 423–437.

Ganellen, R. J. (1996). *Integrating the Rorschach and the MMPI-2 in personality assessment.* Mahwah, NJ: Erlbaum.

Garb, H. N. (1984). The incremental validity of information used in personality assessment. *Clinical Psychology Review, 4,* 641–655.

Garb, H. N. (1998). *Studying the clinician: Judgment research and psychological assessment.* Washington, DC: American Psychological Association.

Garb, H. N. (1999). Call for a moratorium on the use of the Rorschach Inkblot Test in clinical and forensic settings. *Assessment, 6,* 313–315.

Garb, H. N., Florio, C. M., & Grove, W. M. (1998). The validity of the Rorschach and the Minnesota Multiphasic Personality Inventory: Results from meta-analyses. *Psychological Science, 9,* 402–404.

Garb, H. N., Wood, J. M., Nezworski, M. T., Grove, W. M., & Stejskal, W. J. (2001). Toward a resolution of the Rorschach controversy. *Psychological Assessment, 13*(4), 433–448.

Garfield, S. L., Heine, R. W., & Leventhal, M. (1954). An evaluation of psychological reports in a clinical setting. *Journal of Consulting Psychology, 18,* 281–286.

Garfield, S. L., & Kurtz, R. (1977). A study of eclectic views. *Journal of Consulting and Clinical Psychology, 45,* 75–83.

Gatchel, R. J., & Weisberg, J. N. (Eds.). (2000). *Personality characteristics of patients with pain.* Washington, DC: American Psychological Association.

Gaw, K. F., & Beutler, L. E. (1995). Integrating treatment recommendations. In L. E. Beutler & M. R. Berren (Eds.), *Integrative assessment of adult personality* (pp. 280–319). New York: Guilford Press.

Gelso, C. J., & Fretz, B. R. (1992). *Counseling psychology.* Orlando, FL: Harcourt Brace Jovanovich.

Gibertini, M., Brandenburg, N., & Retzlaff, P. (1986). The operating characteristics of the Millon Clinical Multiaxial Inventory. *Journal of Personality Assessment, 50,* 554–567.

Gibertini, M., & Retzlaff, P. (1988). Factor invariance of the Millon Clinical Multiaxial Inventory. *Journal of Psychopathology and Behavioral Assessment, 10,* 65–74.

Gibson, D. R. (1990). Personality correlates of logical and sociomoral judgment. *Journal of Personality and Social Psychology, 59,* 1296–1300.

Gilberstadt, H., & Duker, J. (l965). *A handbook for clinical and actuarial MMPI interpretation.* Philadelphia: W. B. Saunders.

Gillis, J. S., Lipkin, M. D., & Moran, T. J. (1981). Drug therapy decisions: A social judgement analysis. *The Journal of Nervous and Mental Disease, 169,* 439–447.

Gillis, J. S., & Moran, T. J. (1981). An analysis of drug decisions in a state psychiatric hospital. *Journal of Clinical Psychology, 37,* 32–42.

Goff, M., & Ackerman, P.L. (1992). Personality–intelligence relations: Assessment of typical intellectual engagement. *Journal of Educational Psychology, 84,* 537–552.

Gold, A., Deary, I. J., MacLeod, K. M., & Frier, B. M. (1995). The effect of IQ level on the degree of cognitive deterioration experienced during acute hypoglycaemia in normal humans. *Intelligence, 20,* 267–290.

Gold, J. (1998). Schizophrenia and intellectual decline. *American Journal of Psychiatry, 155,* 1633–1634.

Goldberg, D. (1972). *The detection of psychiatric disorders by questionnaire.* Oxford, UK: Oxford University Press.

Goldberg, L. R. (1990). An alternative description of personality: The Big Five factor structure. *Journal of Personality and Social Psychology, 59,* 1215–1229.

Goldberg, L. R., & Kilkowski, J. M. (1985). The prediction of semantic consistency in self-descriptions: Characteristics of persons and of terms that affect the consistency of responses to synonym and antonym pairs. *Journal of Personality and Social Psychology, 48,* 82–98.

Goleman, D. (1995). *Emotional intelligence.* New York: Bantam Books.

Good, B. J. (1992a). Culture and psychopathology: Directions for psychiatric anthropology. In T. Schwartz, G. M. White, & C. A. Lutz (Eds.), *New directions in psychological anthropology* (pp. 181–205). Cambridge, UK: Cambridge University Press.

Good, B. J. (1992b). Gender and counseling psychology: Current knowledge and directions for research and social action. In S. D. Brown & R. W. Lent (Eds.), *Handbook of counseling psychology* (2nd ed., pp. 383–416). New York: Wiley.

Goodman, R. (1995). The relationship between normal variation in IQ and common childhood pathology: A clinical study. *European Child and Adolescent Psychiatry, 4,* 187–196.

Gough, H. G. (1952). On making a good impression. *Journal of Educational Research, 46,* 33–42.

Gough, H. G. (1954). Some common misconceptions about neuroticism. *Journal of Consulting Psychology, 18,* 287–292.

Gough, H. G. (1957). *Manual for the California Psychological Inventory.* Palo Alto, CA: Consulting Psychologists Press.

Gough, H. G. (1964). Academic achievement in high school as predicted from the California Psychological Inventory. *Journal of Educational Psychology, 65,* 174–180.

Gough, H. G. (1966). Appraisal of social maturity by means of the CPI. *Journal of Abnormal Psychology, 71,* 189–195.

Gough, H. G. (1969). A leadership index on the California Psychological Inventory. *Journal of Counseling Psychology, 16,* 283–289.

Gough, H. G. (1984). A managerial potential scale for the California Psychological Inventory. *Journal of Applied Psychology, 69,* 233–240.

Gough, H. G. (1987). *The California Psychological Inventory administrator's guide.* Palo Alto, CA: Consulting Psychologists Press.

Gough, H. G. (1990). Testing for leadership with the California Psychological Inventory. In K. E. Clark & M. B. Clark (Eds.), *Measures of leadership* (pp. 355–379). West Orange, NJ: Leadership Library of America.

Gough, H. G. (1995a). Career assessment and the California Psychological Inventory. *Journal of Career Assessment, 3,* 101–122.

Gough, H. G. (1995b). *CPI narrative report.* Palo Alto, CA: Consulting Psychologists Press.

Gough, H. G. (1995c). *CPI profile report.* Palo Alto, CA: Consulting Psychologists Press.

Gough, H. G. (2000). The California Psychological Inventory. In C. E. Watkins, Jr., & V. L. Campbell (Eds.), *Testing and assessment in counseling practice.* Mahwah, NJ: Erlbaum.

Gough, H. G. (2002). *Comprehensive bibliography of the California Psychological Inventory, 1948–2002.* Palo Alto, CA: Consulting Psychologists Press.

Gough, H. G., & Bradley, P. (1992). Delinquent and criminal behavior as assessed by the revised California Psychological Inventory. *Journal of Clinical Psychology, 48,* 298–308.

Gough, H. G., & Bradley, P. (1996). *California Psychological Inventory Manual* (3rd ed.). Palo Alto, CA: Consulting Psychologists Press.

Gough, H. G., Bradley, P., & McDonald, J. S. (1991). Performance of residents in anesthesiology as related to measures of personality and interests. *Psychological Reports, 68,* 979–994.

Gough, H. G., & Lanning, K. (1986). Predicting grades in college from the California Psychological Inventory. *Educational and Psychological Measurement, 46,* 205–213.

Gough, H. G., & McAllister, L. W. (1995). *CPI configural analysis report: An interpretation of scale combinations.* Palo Alto, CA: Consulting Psychologists Press.

Gough, H. G., Wenk, E. A., & Rozynko, V. V. (1965). Parole outcome as predicted from the CPI, the MMPI, and a base expectancy table. *Journal of Abnormal Psychology, 70,* 432–441.

Graham, J. R. (1988, August). *Establishing validity of the revised form of the MMPI.* Symposium presented at the 96th Annual Convention of the Amercan Psychological Association, Atlanta, GA.

Graham, J. R. (1990). *MMPI-2: Assessing personality and psychopathology.* New York: Oxford University Press.

Graham, J. R., Ben-Porath, Y. S., & McNulty, J. (2000). *Using the MMPI-2 in outpatient mental health settings.* Minneapolis: University of Minnesota Press.

Graham, J. R., Watts, D., & Timbrook, R. (1991). Detecting fake-good and fake-bad MMPI-2 profiles. *Journal of Personality Assessment, 57,* 264–277.

Gray-Little, B. (1995). The assessment of psychopathology in racial and ethnic minorities. In J. N. Butcher (Ed.), *Clinical personality assessment: Practical approaches* (pp. 141–157). New York: Oxford University Press.

Greene, R. L. (2000). *The MMPI-2: An interpretive manual* (2nd ed.). Boston: Allyn & Bacon.

Grisso, T. (2001). *Evaluating competencies: Forensic assessments and instruments* (2nd ed.). New York: Kluwer/Plenum Press.

Groth-Marnat, G. (1999a). Financial efficacy of clinical assessment: Rational guidelines and issues for future research. *Journal of Clinical Psychology, 55,* 813–824.

Groth-Marnat, G. (1999b). *Handbook of psychological assessment* (3rd ed., rev.). New York: Wiley.

Groth-Marnat, G. (Ed.). (2000). *Neuropsychological assessment in clinical practice: A guide to test interpretation and integration.* New York: Wiley.

Groth-Marnat, G. (in press-a). The California Psychological Inventory. In G. Groth-Marnat (Ed.), *Handbook of psychological assessment* (4th ed.). New York: Wiley.

Groth-Marnat, G. (in press-b). The psychological report (general). In R. Fernandez-Ballesteros (Ed.), *Encyclopedia of psychological assessment.* Thousand Oaks, CA: Sage.

Groth-Marnat, G., & Edkins, G. (1996). Professional psychologists in general health care settings: A review of the financial efficacy of direct treatment interventions. *Professional Psychology: Research and Practice, 27,* 161–174.

Groth-Marnat, G., Roberts, R., & Beutler, L. E. (2001). Client characteristics and psychotherapy: Perspectives, support, interactions, and implications for training. *Australian Psychologist, 36,* 115–121.

Grundy, C. T., Lunnen, K. M., Lambert, M. J., Ashton, J. E., & Tovey, D. R. (1994). The Hamilton Rating Scale for Depression: One scale or many? *Clinical Psychology: Science and Practice, 1,* 197–205.

Haase, R. F., & Ivey, A. E. (1970). Influence of client pretesting on counseling outcome. *Journal of Consulting and Clinical Psychology, 34,* 128.

Hacker, D. (1999). *A writer's reference* (4th ed.). Boston: Bedford/St. Martin's.

Haddad, N. A. (1990). *Why nurses stay: The relationship of personality to job and career satisfaction.* Unpublished doctoral dissertation, Virginia Polytechnic Institute and State University, Falls Church.

Hamilton, M. (1959). The measurement of anxiety states by rating. *British Journal of Medical Psychology, 32,* 56–62.

Hamilton, M. (1960). A rating scale for depression. *Journal of Neurology, Neurosurgery, and Psychiatry, 23,* 56–62.

Handel, R. W., & Ben-Porath, Y. S. (2000). Multicultural assessment with the MMPI-2: Issues for research and practice. In R. H. Dana (Ed.), *Handbook of cross-cultural/multicultural personality assessment* (pp. 229–245). Mawah, NJ: Erlbaum.

Hansen, N. D., Pepitone-Arreola-Rockwell, F., & Greene, A. F. (2000). Multicultural competence: Criteria and case examples. *Professional Psychology: Research and Practice, 31*(6), 652–660.

Hargrave, G. E., & Hiatt, D. (1989). Use of the California Psychological Inventory in law enforcement selection. *Journal of Personality Assessment, 53,* 267–277.

Harvey, V. S. (1997). Improving readability of psychological reports. *Professional Psychology: Research and Practice, 28,* 271–274.

Hathaway, S. R. (1965). Personality inventories. In B. Wolman (Ed.), *Handbook of clinical psychology* (pp. 451–476). New York: McGraw-Hill.

Hathaway, S. R., & McKinley, J. C. (1940). A multiphasic personality schedule (Minnesota): I. Construction of the schedule. *Journal of Psychology, 10,* 249–254.

Hathaway, S. R., & McKinley, J. C. (1943a). *Manual for the Minnesota Multiphasic Personality Inventory.* New York: Psychological Corporation.

Hathaway, S. R., & McKinley, J. C. (1943b). *The Minnesota Multiphasic Personality Inventory.* New York: Psychological Corporation.

Haverkamp, B. E. (1993). Confirmatory bias in hypothesis testing for client identified and counselor self-generated hypotheses. *Journal of Counseling Psychology, 40,* 303–315.

Headland, T. N., Pike, K. L., & Harris, M. (Eds.). (1990). *Emics and etics: The insider/ outsider debate.* Newbury Park, CA: Sage.

Heilbrun, K. (1992). The role of psychological testing in forensic assessment. *Law and Human Behavior, 16,* 257–272.

Heilbrun, K. (2001). *Principles of forensic mental health assessment.* New York: Kluwer/Plenum Press.

Heller, S. S., Larrieu, J. A., D'Imperio, R., & Boris, N. W. (1999). Research on resilience to child maltreatment: Empirical considerations. *Child Abuse and Neglect, 23,* 321–338.

Helms, J. E. (1990). *Black and white racial identity: Theory, research, and practice.* New York: Greenwood Press.

Helms, J. E. (1992). Why is there no study of cultural equivalence in standardized cognitive ability testing? *American Psychologist, 47,* 1083–1101.

Helms, J. E. (1995). An update of Helm's White and People of Color Racial Identity models. In J. G. Ponterotto, J. M. Casas, L. A. Suzuki, & C. M. Alexander (Eds.), *Handbook of multicultural counseling* (pp. 181–188). Newbury Park, CA: Sage.

Helms, J. E., & Carter, R. (1990). Development of the white racial identity inventory. In J. Helms (Ed.), *Black and white racial identity: Theory, research, and practice* (pp. 1–26). New York: Greenwood Press.

Helson, R., & Pals, J. L. (2000). Creative potential, creative achievement, and personal growth. *Journal of Personality Assessment, 68,* 1–27.

Helson, R., & Picano, J. (1990). Is the traditional role bad for women? *Journal of Personality and Social Psychology, 59,* 311–320.

Helson, R., & Roberts, B. W. (1994). Ego development and personality change in adulthood. *Journal of Personality and Social Psychology, 66,* 911–920.

Helson, R., Roberts, B. W., & Agronick, G. (1995). Enduringness and change in creative personality and the prediction of occupational creativity. *Journal of Personality and Social Psychology, 69,* 1173–1183.

Helson, R., Stewart, A. J., & Ostrove, J. (1995). Identity in three cohorts of midlife women. *Journal of Personality and Social Psychology, 69,* 544–557.

Helson, R., & Wink, P. (1992). Personality change in women from the early 40s to the early 50s. *Psychology and Aging, 7,* 46–55.

Henry, W. P., Schacht, T. E., Strupp, H. H., Butler, S. F., & Binder, J. L. (1993). Effects of training in time-limited dynamic psychotherapy: Mediators of therapists' responses to training. *Journal of Consulting and Clinical Psychology, 61,* 441–447.

Herrnstein, R. J., & Murray, C. (1994). *The bell curve.* New York: Free Press.

Hilsenroth, M. J., & Handler, L. (1995). A survey of graduate students' experiences, interests, and attitudes about learning the Rorschach. *Journal of Personality Assessment, 64,* 243–257.

Hjemboe, S., & Butcher, J. N. (1991). Couples in marital distress: A study of demographic and personality factors as measured by the MMPI-2. *Journal of Personality Assessment, 57,* 216–237.

Hoffman, B. F. (1986). How to write a psychiatric report for litigation following a personal injury case. *American Journal of Psychiatry, 143,* 164–169.

Hoffman, C., Rice, D., & Sung, H. Y. (1996). Persons with chronic conditions: Their prevalence and costs. *Journal of the American Medical Association, 276,* 1473–1479.

Hogan, J. C. (1978). Personological dynamics of leadership. *Journal of Research in Personality, 12,* 390–395.

Holliman, N. B., & Montross, J. (1984). The effects of depression upon responses to the California Psychological Inventory. *Journal of Clinical Psychology, 40,* 1373–1378.

Hollon, S., & Mandell, M. (1979). Use of the MMPI to measure treatment effect In J. N. Butcher (Ed.), *New directions in MMPI research* (pp. 241–302). Minneapolis: University of Minnesota Press.

Holtzman, W. H., Thorpe, J. S., Swartz, J. D., & Herron, E. W. (1961). *Administration and scoring guide.* Cleveland, OH: Psychological Corporation.

Holub, R. J. (1992). *Forensic psychological testing: A survey of practices and beliefs.* Unpublished manuscript, Minnesota School of Professional Psychology, Bloomington.

Hooley, J. M., & Hiller, J. B. (2000). Personality and expressed emotion. *Journal of Abnormal Psychology, 109,* 40–44.

Hough, L. (1988). *Personality assessment for selection and placement decisions.* Minneapolis: Personnel Decisions Research Institute.

Houts, A. C. (2002). Discovery, invention, and the expansion of the diagnostic and statistical manual of mental disorders. In L. E. Beutler & M. Malik (Eds.), *Rethinking the DSM: Psychological perspectives.* Washington, DC: American Psychological Association.

Huesmann, L. R., Eron, D., & Yarmel, P. W. (1987). Intellectual functioning and aggression. *Journal of Personality and Social Psychology, 52,* 232–240.

Huffcutt, A. I., & Arthur, W., Jr. (1994). Hunger and Hunter (1984) revisited: Interview validity for entry-level jobs. *Journal of Applied Psychology, 79,* 184–190.

Hughes, D., Blazer, D., & Hybels, C. (1991). Duke social support index (DSSI): A working paper (rev.). Durham, NC: Duke University Medical Center, Center for the Study of Aging and Human Development.

Hunsley, J., & Bailey, J. M. (1999). The clinical utility of the Rorschach: Unfulfilled promises and an uncertain future. *Psychological Assessment, 11,* 266–177.

Hyer, L., & Associates. (1994). *Trauma victim: Theoretical issues and practical suggestions.* Muncie, IN: Accelerated Development.

Introduction. (1999). *American Journal of Managed Care, 5,* S764–S766.

Jacobs, J., Merhard, M., Delgado, A., & Strain, J. (1977). Screening for organic mental syndromes in the medically ill. *Annals of Internal Medicine, 86,* 40–46.

Jacobs, R. L. (1992). *Moving up the corporate ladder: A longitudinal study of motivation, personality, and managerial success in women and men.* Unpublished doctoral dissertation, Boston University.

James, W. (1907). *Pragmatism.* New York: Longmans, Green.

Jensen, A. (1980). *Bias in mental testing.* New York: Free Press.

Johnson, J. A. (2000). Predicting observers' ratings of the big five from the CPI, HPI, and NEO-PI-R: A comparative validity study. *European Journal of Personality, 14,* 1–19.

Kadden, R. M., Litt, M. D., Donovan, D., & Cooney, N. L. (1996). Psychometric properties of the California Psychological Inventory Socialization scale in treatment-seeking alcoholics. *Psychology of Addictive Behaviors, 10,* 131–146.

Karno, M., Beutler, L. E., & Harwood, T. M. (in press). Interactions between psychotherapy process and patient attributes that predict alcohol treatment effectiveness: A preliminary report. *Addictive Behaviors.*

Katon, W. J., & Walker, E. A. (1998). Medically unexplained symptoms in primary care. *Journal of Clinical Psychiatry, 59,* 15–21.

Katzman, R. (1993). Education and the prevalence of dementia and Alzheimer's disease. *Neurology, 43,* 13–20.

Kaufman, A. S., & Kaufman, J. C. (2001). Emotional intelligence as an aspect of general intelligence: What would David Wechsler say? *Emotion, 1,* 258–264.

Keilin, W. G., & Bloom, L. J. (1986). Child custody evaluation practices: A survey of experienced professionals. *Professional Psychology: Research and Practice, 17,* 338–346.

Keller, L. S., & Butcher, J. N. (1991). *Use of the MMPI-2 with chronic pain patients.* Minneapolis: University of Minnesota Press.

Kemp, B. J., & Vash, C. L. (1971). Productivity after injury in a sample of spinal cord injured persons: A pilot study. *Journal of Chronic Disease, 24,* 259–275.

Kendler, K. S. (1990). Toward a scientific psychiatric nosology: Strengths and limitations. *Archives of General Psychiatry, 47,* 969–973.

Kennedy, G. J. (2000). Personality, somatoform, and pain disorders. In G. J. Kennedy (Ed.), *Geriatric mental health care: A treatment guide for health professionals* (pp. 114–126). New York: Guilford Press.

Kessler, L., & Eaton, W. (Eds.). (1985). *Epidemiological methods in psychiatry: The NIMH Epidemiological Catchment Area Program.* New York: Academic Press.

Kihlstrom, J. F., & Cantor, N. (2000). Social intelligence. In R. J. Sternberg (Ed.), *Handbook of intelligence* (pp. 359–379). New York: Cambridge University Press.

Kleinmuntz, B. (1990). Why we still use our heads instead of formulas: Toward an integrative approach. *Psychological Bulletin, 107,* 296–310.

Knoff, H. M. (Ed.). (1986). *The assessment of child and adolescent personality.* New York: Guilford Press.

Kondo, K., Niino, M., & Shido, K. (1994). A case-control study of Alzheimer's disease in Japan—significance of life-styles. *Dementia, 5,* 314–326.

Konson, D. S., Steurwald, B. L., Newman, J. P., & Widom, C. S. (1994). The relation between socialization and antisocial behavior, substance abuse, and family conflict in students. *Journal of Personality Assessment, 63,* 473–488.

Kopta, S. M., Newman, F. L., McGovern, M. P., & Sandrock, D. (1986). Psychotherapeutic orientations: A comparison of conceptualizations, interventions, and treatment plan costs. *Journal of Consulting and Clinical Psychology, 54,* 369–374.

Krabbendam, L., Marcelis, M., Delespaul, P., Jolles, J., & van Os, J. (2001). Single or multiple familial cognitive risk factors in schizophrenia? *American Journal of Medical Genetics, 105,* 183–188.

Krishnamurthy, R., & Archer, R. P. (2001). An evaluation of the effects of Rorschach EB style on the diagnostic utility of the Depression Index. *Assessment, 8,* 105–109.

Kunce, J. T., & Anderson, W. P. (1976). Normalizing the MMPI. *Journal of Clinical Psychology, 32,* 776–780.

Kuperman, S. K., Golden, C.J., & Blume, H. G. (1979). Predicting pain treatment results by personality variables in organic and functional patients. *Journal of Clinical Psychology, 35,* 832–837.

Lambert, M. J., Hansen, N. B., Umpress, V., Lunnen, K., Okiishi, J., Burlingame, G. M., Huefner, J. C., & Reisinger, C. W. (1996). *Scoring and administration manual for the OQ-45.2.* Stevenson, MD: American Credentialing Services.

Landreville, P., Landry, J., Baillargeon, L., Guérette, A., & Matteau, E. (2001). Older adults' acceptance of psychological and pharmacological treatments for depression. *Journal of Gerontology: Psychological Sciences, 56B,* P285–P291.

Lane, R. D. (2000). Levels of emotional awareness: Neurological, psychological, and social perspectives. In R. Bar-On & J. D. A. Parker (Eds.), *The handbook of emotional intelligence: The theory and practice of development, evaluation, education, and application at home, school, and in the workplace* (pp. 171–191). San Francisco: Jossey-Bass.

Lanning, K. (1989). Detection of invalid response patterns on the California Psychological Inventory. *Applied Psychological Measurement, 13,* 45–56.

Larsen, R. J. (1992). Neuroticism and selective encoding and recall of symptoms: Evidence from a combined concurrent-retrospective study. *Journal of Personality and Social Psychology, 62,* 480–488.

Laurent, A., Moreaud, O., Bosson, J. L., Naegele, B., Boucharlat, J., Saoud, M., Dalery, J., & d'Amato, T. (1999). Neuropsychological functioning among nonpsychotic siblings and parents of schizophrenic patients. *Psychiatry Research, 87,* 147–157.

Lawton, M. P. (1988). Scales to measure competence in everyday activities. *Psychopharmacology Bulletin, 24,* 609–614.

Lawton, M. P., & Brody, E. M. (1969). Assessment of older people: Self-maintaining and instrumental activities of daily living. *Gerontologist, 9,* 179–185.

Lazarus, R. S. (1991a). *Emotion and adaptation.* New York: Oxford University Press.

Lazarus, R. S. (1991b). Psychological stress in the workplace. In P. L. Parrewé (Ed.), *Handbook on job stress* (pp. 1–13). Corte Madera, CA: Select Press.

Leary, T. (1957). *Interpersonal diagnosis of personality.* New York: Ronald Press.

Lees-Haley, P. R. (1992). Psychodiagnostic test usage by forensic psychologists. *American Journal of Forensic Psychology, 10,* 25–30.

Lees-Haley, P. R. (1997). MMPI-2 base rates for 492 personal injury plaintiffs: inplications and challenges for forensic assessment. *Journal of Clinical Psychology, 53,* 745–755.

Lees-Haley, P. R., Smith, H. W., Williams, C. W., & Dunn, J. T. (1996). Forensic neuropsychological test usage: An empirical survey. *Archives of Clinical Neuropsychology, 11*, 45–51.

Leserman, J., Petitto, J. M., Perkins, D. O., Folds, J. D., Golden, R. N., & Evans, D. L. (1997). Severe stress, depressive symptoms, and changes in lymphocyte subsets in human immunodeficiency virus—infected men: A 2–year follow-up study. *Archives of General Psychiatry, 54*, 279–285.

Leventhal, A. M. (1966). An anxiety scale for the CPI. *Journal of Clinical Psychology, 22*, 459–461.

Lewak, R. W., & Hogan, R. S. (2001). Deceptions in psychological testing. *American Journal of Forensic Psychiatry, 22*, 57–81.

Lewak, R. W., Marks, P. A., & Nelson, G. E. (1991). *Therapist guide to the MMPI and MMPI-2: Providing feedback and treatment.* Muncie, IN: Accelerated Development.

Lewandowski, D., & Graham, J. R. (1972). Empirical correlates of frequently occurring two-point MMPI code types: A replicated study. *Journal of Consulting and Clinical Psychology, 39*, 467–472.

Lezak, M. D. (1995). *Neuropsychological assessment* (3rd ed.). New York: Oxford University Press.

Lichtenberg, P. A. (1999). *Handbook of assessment in clinical gerontology.* New York: Wiley.

Lilienfeld, S. O. (1996). The MMPI-2 Antisocial Practices Content Scale: Consruct validity and comparison with the Psychopathic Deviate Scale. *Psychological Assessment, 8*, 281–293.

Litz,, B. T., Gray, M. J., Bryant, R. A., & Adler, A. B. (2002). Early interventions for trauma: Current status and future directions. *Clinical Psychology: Science and Practice, 9*, 112–134.

Loehlin, J. C. (1997). A test of J. R. Harris's theory of peer influences on personality. *Journal of Personality and Social Psychology, 72*, 1197–1201.

Lovitt, R. (1988). Current practice of psychological assessment: Response to Sweeney, Clarkin, and Fitzgibbon. *Professional Psychology: Research and Practice, 19*, 516–521.

Lowman, R. L. (1991). *The clinical practice of career assessment: Interests, abilities, and personality.* Washington, DC: American Psychological Association.

Lowman, R. L., & Carson, A. D. (2000). Integrating assessment data into career counseling. In D. A. Luzzo (Ed.), *Career counseling of college students: An empirical guide to strategies that work* (pp. 121–136). Washington, DC: American Psychological Association.

Lubin, B., Larsen, R. M., & Matarazzo, J. D. (1984). Patterns of psychological test usage in the United States: 1935–1982. *American Psychologist, 39*, 451–454.

Lubin, B., Larsen, R. M., Matarazzo, J., & Seever, M. (1985). Psychological assessment services and psychological test usage in private practice and military settings. *Psychotherapy in Private Practice, 4*, 19–29.

Lubin, B., Wallis, R. R., & Paine, C. (1971). Patterns of psychological test usage in the United States. *Professional Psychology, 2*, 70–74.

Luborsky, L. (1984). *Principles of psychoanalytic psychotherapy: A manual for supportive–expressive treatment.* New York: Basic Books.

Luborsky, L., & Crits-Christoph, P. (1990). *Understanding transference: The core conflictual relationship method*. New York: Basic Books.

Lynam, D., Moffitt, T.E., & Stouthamer-Loeber, M. (1993). Explaining the relation between IQ and delinquency: Class, race, test motivation, school failure, or self-control? *Journal of Abnormal Psychology, 102,* 187–196.

Macklin, M. L., Metzger, L. J., Litz, B. T., McNally, R. J., Lasko, N. B., Orr, S. P., & R. K. Pitman (1998). Lower precombat intelligence is a risk factor for posttraumatic stress disorder. *Journal of Consulting and Clinical Psychology, 66,* 323–326.

Maddux, J. E. (2002). Stopping the "madness": Positive psychology and the deconstruction of the illness ideology and the DSM. In C. R. Snyder & S. Lopez (Eds.), *The handbook of positive psychology* (pp. 13–25). New York: Oxford University Press.

Maloney, M. P. (1985). *A clinician's guide to forensic psychological assessment*. New York: Free Press.

Manos, N. (1985). Adaptation of the MMPI in Greece: Translation, standardization, and coss-cultural comparison. In J. N. Butcher & C. D. Spielberger (Eds.), *Advances in personality assessment* (Vol. 4, pp. 159–208). Hillsdale, NJ: Erlbaum.

Marks, P. A., Seeman, W., & Haller, D. L. (1974). *The actuarial use of the MMPI with adolescents and adults*. Baltimore: Williams & Wilkins.

Maruish, M. E. (Ed.). (1999). *The use of psychological testing and treatment planning* (2nd ed.). Mahwah, NJ: Erlbaum.

Maruish, M. E. (Ed.). (2000). *Handbook of psychological testing in primary care settings*. Mahwah, NJ: Erlbaum.

Matarazzo, J. D. (1972). *Wechsler's measurement and appraisal of adult intelligence* (5th ed.). New York: Oxford University Press.

Matarazzo, J. D. (1990). Psychological assessment versus psychological testing: Validation from the Binet to the school, clinic, and courtroom. *American Psychologist, 45,* 999–1017.

Matthews, G. (1997a). Extraversion, emotion and performance: A cognitive-adaptive model. In G. Matthews (Ed.), *Cognitive science perspectives on personality and emotion.* (pp. 339–442). Amsterdam: Elsevier.

Matthews, G. (1997b). Intelligence, personality and information-processing: An adaptive perspective. In J. Kingma & W. Tomic (Eds.), *Advances in cognition and educational practice: Reflections on the concept of intelligence* (Vol. 4, pp. 175–200). Stamford, CT: JAI Press.

Matthews, G. (1997c). An introduction to the cognitive science of personality and emotion. In G. Matthews (Ed.), *Cognitive science perspectives on personality and emotion* (pp. 3–30). Amsterdam: Elsevier.

Matthews, G. (1999). Personality and skill: A cognitive-adaptive framework. In P. L. Ackerman, P. C. Kyllonen, & R. D. Roberts (Eds.), *Learning and individual differences: Process, trait, and content determinants* (pp. 251–273). Washington, DC: American Psychological Association.

Matthews, G., Saklofske, D. H., Costa, P. T., Jr., Deary, I. J., & Zeidner, M. (1998). Dimensional models of personality: A framework for systematic clinical assessment. *European Journal of Personality Assessment, 14,* 36–49.

Matthews, G., Zeidner, M., & Roberts, R. D. (2002). *Emotional intelligence: Science and myth*. Cambridge, MA: MIT Press.

Matthews, G., & Zeidner, M. (2000). Emotional intelligence, adaptation to stressful encounters, and health outcomes. In R. Bar-On & J. D. A. Parker (Eds.), *Handbook of emotional intelligence: The theory and practice of development, evaluation, education, and application at home, school, and in the workplace* (pp. 459–489). New York: Jossey-Bass.

May, R. R. (1980). *Sex and fantasy: Patterns of male and female development.* New York: Horton.

Mayer, J. D., Salovey, P. R., & Caruso, D. R. (2000a). Competing models of emotional intelligence. In R. J. Sternberg (Ed.), *Handbook of human intelligence* (2nd ed.). New York: Cambridge University Press.

Mayer, J. D., Salovey, P. R., & Caruso, D. R. (2000b). Emotional intelligence as Zeitgeist, as personality, and as a mental ability. In R. Bar-On & J. D. A. Parker (Eds.), *Handbook of emotional intelligence: The theory and practice of development, evaluation, education, and application at home, school, and in the workplace.* San Francisco: Jossey-Bass.

Mayer, J. D., Salovey, P., Caruso, D. R., & Sitarenios, G.(2001). Emotional intelligence as a standard intelligence. *Emotion, 1,* 232–242.

Mazure, C., Nelson, C., & Price, L. H. (1986). Reliability and validity of the symptoms of major depressive illness. *Archives of General Psychiatry, 43,* 451–456.

McAllister, L. W. (1996). *A practical guide to CPI interpretation* (3rd ed.). Palo Alto, CA: Consulting Psychologists Press.

McCann, J. T. (1998). Defending the Rorschach in court: An analysis of admissibility using legal and professional standards. *Journal of Personality Assessment, 70,* 125–144.

McCrae, R. R. (2000). Emotional intelligence from the perspective of the five-factor model of personality. In R. Bar-On & J. D. A. Parker (Eds.), *Handbook of emotional intelligence: The theory and practice of development, evaluation, education, and application at home, school, and in the workplace* (pp. 263–276). San Francisco: Jossey-Bass.

McCrae, R. R., & Costa, P. T. (1997). Conceptions and correlates of openness to experience. In R. Hogan, J. Johnson, & S. Briggs (Eds.), *Handbook of personality psychology* (pp. 826–847). San Diego, CA: Academic Press.

McCrae, R. R., Costa, P. T., & Piedmont, R. L. (1993). Folk concepts, natural language, and psychological constructs: The California Psychological Inventory and the five-factor model. *Journal of Personality, 61,* 1–26.

McDaniel, M., Whetzel, D. L., Schmidt, F. L., & Maurer, S. D. (1994). The validity of employment interviews: A comprehensive review and meta-analysis. *Journal of Applied Psychology, 79,* 599–616.

McFarland, S. G., & Sparks, C. M. (1985). Age, education, and the internal consistency of personality scales. *Journal of Personality and Social Psychology, 49,* 1692–1702.

McGorry, P. D., & McConville, S. B. (1999). Insight in psychosis: An elusive target. *Comprehensive Psychiatry, 40,* 131–142.

McLemore, C., & Benjamin, L. S. (1979). Whatever happened to interpersonal diagnosis?: A psychosocial alternative to DSM-III. *American Psychologist, 34,* 17–34.

McLeod, C. C., Budd, M. A., & McClelland, D. C. (1997). Treatment of somatization in primary care. *General Hospital Psychiatry, 19,* 251–258.

McNulty, J., Graham, J. R., Ben-Porath, Y. S., & Stein, L. A. R. (1997). Comparative validity of MMPI-2 scores of African American and Caucasian health center clients. *Psychological Assessment, 9*(4), 464–470.

Megargee, E. I. (1972). *The California Psychological Inventory handbook.* San Francisco: Jossey-Bass.

Megargee, E. I. (1995). Assessment research in correctional settings: Methodological issues and practical problems. *Psychological Assessment, 7,*(3), 359–366.

Melton, G. B., Petrila, J., Poythress, N. G., & Slobogin, C. (1997). *Psychological evaluations for the courts: A handbook for mental health professionals and lawyers* (2nd ed.). New York: Guilford Press.

Meyer, G. J. (1993). The impact of response frequency on the Rorschach constellation indices and on their validity with diagnostic and MMPI-2 criteria. *Journal of Personality Assessment, 60,* 153–180.

Meyer, G. J. (1997). On the integration of personality assessment methods: The Rorschach and MMPI. *Journal of Personality Assessment, 68,* 297–330.

Meyer, G. J. (2001). Evidence to correct misperceptions about Rorschach norms. *Clinical Psychology: Science and Practice, 8,* 389–396.

Meyer, G. J., & Archer, R. P. (2001). The hard science of Rorschach research: What do we know and where do we go? *Psychological Assessment, 13,* 486–502.

Meyer, G. J., Finn, S. E., Eyde, L. D., Kay, G. G., Moreland, K. L., Dies, R. R., Eisman, E. J., Kubiszyn, T. W., & Reed, G. M. (2001). Psychological testing and psychological assessment: A review of evidence and issues. *American Psychologist, 56,* 128–165.

Millon, T. (1969). *Modern psychopathology.* Philadelphia: W. B. Saunders.

Millon, T. (1977). *Millon Clinical Multiaxial Inventory.* Minneapolis, MN: National Computer Systems.

Millon, T. (1981). *Disorders of personality.* New York: Wiley.

Millon, T. (1986a). Personality prototypes and their diagnostic criteria. In T. Millon & G. Klerman (Eds.), *Contemporary directions in psychopathology: Toward DSM-IV* (pp. 639–669). New York: Guilford Press.

Millon, T. (1986b). A theoretical derivation of pathological personalities. In T. Millon & G. L. Klerman (Eds.), *Contemporary directions in psychopathology: Toward DSM-IV* (pp. 671–712). New York: Guilford Press.

Millon, T. (1987). *Millon Clinical Multiaxial Inventory–II: Manual for the MCMI-II.* Minneapolis, MN: National Computer systems.

Millon, T. (1990). *Toward a new personology: An evolutionary model.* New York: Wiley.

Millon, T. (1994). *The Millon Clinical Multiaxial Inventory–III manual.* Minneapolis, MN: National Computer Systems.

Millon, T. (1997). *The Millon Clinical Multiaxial Inventory–III manual* (2nd ed.). Minneapolis, MN: National Computer Systems.

Millon, T., Davis, R., & Millon, C. (1997). *MCMI-III manual.* Minneapolis, MN: National Computer Systems.

Millon, T., Green, C., & Meagher, R. (1982). *Millon Behavioral Health Inventory manual* (3rd ed). Minneapolis, MN: National Computer Systems.

Moffitt, T. E., Gabrielli, W. F., Mednick, S. A., & Schulsinger, F. (1981). Socioeconomic status, IQ, and delinquency. *Journal of Abnormal Psychology 90,* 152–156.

Mohr, D. C., Geedkin, D. E., Likosky, W., Beutler, L., Gatto, N., & Langan, M. K.

(1997). Identification of Beck Depression Inventory items related to multiple sclerosis. *Journal of Behavioral Medicine, 20*, 407–414.

Mollinare, V., Aames, A., & Essa, M. (1994). Prevalence of personality disorders in two geropsychiatric inpatient units. *Journal of Geriatric Psychiatry and Neurology, 7*, 209–215.

Monroe, S. M. (1982). Life events assessment: Current practices, emerging trends. *Clinical Psychology Review, 2*, 435–453.

Monte, C. F. (1995). *Beneath the mask: An introduction to theories of personality.* Fort Worth, TX: Harcourt Brace.

Moore, J. E., Armentraut, D. P., Parker, J. C., & Kivlahan, D. R. (1986). Empirically derived pain-patient MMPI subgroups: Prediction of treatment outcomes. *Journal of Behavioral Medicine, 9*, 51–63.

Moore, O., Cassidy, E., Carr, A., & O'Callaghan, E. (1999). Unawareness of illness and its relationship with depression and self-deception in schizophrenia. *European Psychiatry, 14*, 264–269.

Moos, R. H. (1974). *Family Environment Scale, Form R.* Palo Alto, CA: Consulting Psychologists Press.

Morgan, C. D., & Murray, H. A. (1935). A method for investigating fantasies: The Thematic Apperception Test. *Archives of Neurological Psychiatry, 34*, 289–306.

Mostofsky, D., & Barlow, D. H. (2000). *The management of stress and anxiety in medical disorders.* Needham Heights, MA: Allyn & Bacon.

Mughal, S., Walsh, J., & Wilding, J. (1996). Stress and work performance: The role of trait anxiety. *Personality and Individual Differences, 20*, 685–691.

Munley, P. H., Bains, D. S., Bloem, W. D., & Busby, R. M. (1997). Posttraumatic stress disorder and the MMPI-2. *Journal of Traumatic Stress, 8*(1), 171–178.

Munley, P. H., Busby, R. M., & Jaynes, G. (1997). MMPI-2 findings in schizophrenia and depression. *Psychological Assessment, 9*(4), 508–511.

Murphy, J. W., & Longino, C. F., Jr. (1992). What is the justification for a qualitative approach to aging studies? *Aging and Society, 12*, 143–156.

Murray, S. G. (1980). Personality and other characteristics of adult women with low and high profiles on the SCII or SVIB occupational scales. *Journal of Applied Psychology, 66*, 422–430.

Mussman, M. (1964). Teachers' evaluations of psychological reports. *Journal of School Psychology, 3*, 35–37.

Myers, I. B., & McCaulley, M. H. (1985). *A guide to the development and use of the Myers-Briggs Type Indicator.* Palo Alto, CA: Consulting Psychologists Press.

National Advisory Commission on Criminal Justice Standards and Goals. (1973). *Report on corrections.* Washington, DC: Author.

Newman, K. (2001). Family values. In A. J. Cherlin (Ed.), *Public and private families* (2nd ed., pp. 113–126). New York: McGraw-Hill.

Newton, N. A., Brauer, D. Gutmann, D. L., & Grunes, J. (1986). Psychodynamic therapy with the aged: A review. In T. L. Brink (Ed.), *Clinical gerontology: A guide to assessment and intervention* (pp. 205–230). New York: Haworth Press.

Newton, N. A., & Lazarus, L. W. (1992). Behavioral and psychotherapeutic interventions. In J. E. Birren, B. R. Sloane, & G. D. Cohen (Eds.), *Handbook of mental health and aging* (pp. 699–719). San Diego, CA: Academic Press.

Norcross, J. C. (Ed). (2002). *Psychotherapy relationships that work: Therapist contributions and responsiveness to patient needs.* New York: Oxford University Press.

Norcross, J. C., & Prochaska, J. O. (1988). A study of eclectic (and integrative) views revisited. *Professional Psychology: Research and Practice, 19*, 170–174.

Nunnally, J. C. (1978). *Psychometric theory.* New York: McGraw-Hill.

Okazaki, S., & Sue, S. (1995). Cultural considerations in psychological assessment of Asian-Americans. In J. N. Butcher (Ed.), *Clinical personality assessment: Practical approaches* (pp. 107– 115). New York: Oxford University Press.

Ones, D. S., Viswesvaran, C., & Reiss, A. D. (1996). Role of social desirability in personality testing for personnel selection: The red herring. *Journal of Applied Psychology, 81*, 660–679.

Ott, A., Breteler, M. M. B., van Harskamp, F., Claus, J. J., van der Cammen, T. J. M., Grobbee, D. E., & Hofman, A. (1995). Prevalence of Alzheimer's disease and vascular dementia: Association with education. *British Medical Journal, 310*, 970–973.

Otto, R. K., & Heilbrun, K. (2002). The practice of forensic psychology. *American Psychologist, 57*, 5–18.

Ownby, R. L. (1997). *Psychological reports* (3rd ed.). New York: Wiley.

Paniagua, F. A. (1994). *Assessing and treating culturally diverse clients: A practical guide.* Thousand Oaks, CA: Sage.

Parker, C. H., Hanson, R. K., & Hunsley, J. (1988). MMPI, Rorschach, and WAIS: A meta-analytic comparison of reliability, stability, and validity. *Psychological Bulletin, 103*, 367–373.

Parker, J. D. A. (2000). Emotional intelligence: Clinical and therapeutic implications. In R. Bar-On & J. D. A. Parker (Eds.) *Handbook of emotional intelligence* (pp. 490–504). San Francisco: Jossey-Bass.

Parkison, S., & Fishburne, J. (1984). MMPI normative data for a male active duty Army population. In *Proceedings of the Psychology in the Department of Defense, Ninth Symposium* (USAFA No. TR-84–2). Colorado Springs, CO: U.S. Air Force Academy.

Paulhus, D. L., Bruce, M. N., & Trapnell, P. D. (1995). Effects of self-presentation strategies on personality profiles and their structures. *Personality and Social Psychology Bulletin, 21*, 100–108.

Pearlin, L., Mullan, J., Semple, S., & Skaff, M. (1990). Caregiving and the stress process: An overview of concepts and their measures. *The Gerontologist, 30(5)*, 583–591.

Pedersen, N. L., Reynolds, C. A., & Gatz, M. (1996). Sources of covariation among Mini-Mental State Examination scores, education and cognitive abilities. *Journal of Gerontology, 51B*, P55–P63.

Pereda, M., Ayuso-Mateos, J. L., Gomez del Barro, A., Echevarria, S., Farinas, M. C., Garcia Palomo, D., Gonzalez Macias, J., & Vazquez-Barquero, J. L. (2000). Factors associated with neuropsychological performance in HIV-seropositive subjects without AIDS. *Psychological Medicine, 30*, 205–217.

Perry, W., Potterat, E., Auslander, L., Kaplan, E., & Jeste, D. (1996). A neuropsychological approach to the Rorschach in patients with dementia of the Alzheimer type. *Assessment, 3*, 351–363.

Persons, J. B., Mooney, K. A., & Padesky, C. A. (1995). Interrater reliability of cognitive-behavioral case formulations. *Cognitive Therapy and Research, 19*, 21–34.

Petrides, K. V., & Furnham, A. (2000). On the dimensional structure of emotional intelligence. *Personality and Individual Differences, 29*, 313–320.

Phinney, J. S. (1992). The multigroup ethnic identity measure: A new scale for use with diverse groups. *Journal of Adolescent Research, 7,* 156–176.

Phinney, J. S. (1996). When we talk about American ethnic groups, what do we mean? *American Psychologist, 51,* 918–927.

Pieniadz, J., & Kelland, D. Z. (2001). Reporting scores in neuropsychological assessment: Ethicality, validity, practicality, and more. In C. G. Armengol, E. Kaplan, & E. J. Moss (Eds.), *The consumer-oriented neuropsychological report* (pp. 123–140). Lutz, FL: Psychological Assessment Resources.

Piotrowski, C. (1998). Assessment of pain: A survey of practicing clinicians. *Perceptual and Motor Skills, 86,* 181–182.

Piotrowski, C. (1999). Assessment practices in the era of managed care: Current status and future directions. *Journal of Clinical Psychology, 55,* 787–796.

Piotrowski, C., & Belter, R. W. (1999). Internship training in psychological assessment: Has managed care had an impact? *Assessment, 6,* 381–385.

Piotrowski, C., & Keller, J. W. (1989). Psychological testing in outpatient mental health facilities: A national study. *Professional Psychology: Research and Practice, 20,* 423–425.

Piotrowski, C., & Lubin, B. (1990). Assessment practices of health psychologists: Survey of APA Division 38 clinicians. *Professional Psychology: Research and Practice, 21,* 99–l06.

Piotrowski, C., & Zalewski, C. (1993). Training in psychodiagnostic testing in APA-approved PsyD and PhD clinical psychology programs. *Journal of Personality Assessment, 61,* 394–405.

Podboy, J. W., & Kastl, A. J. (1993). The international misuse of standardized psychological tests in complex trials. *American Journal of Forensic Psychology, 11,* 47–54.

Pope, K. S., Butcher, J. N., & Seelen, J. (1993). *The MMPI, MMPI-2, and MMPI-A in court: A practical guide for expert witnesses and attorneys.* Washington, DC: American Psychological Association.

Pope, K. S., Butcher, J. N., & Seelen, J. (1999). *The MMPI/MMPI-2/MMPI-A in court: Assessment, testimony, and cross-examination* (2nd ed.) Washington, DC: American Psychological Association.

Presley, G., Smith, C., Hilsenroth, M., & Exner, J. E., Jr. (2001). Clinical utility of the Rorschach with African Americans. *Journal of Personality Assessment, 77,* 491–507.

Pruit, S. D., Klapow, J. C., Epping-Jordan, J. E., & Dresselhaus, T. R. (1999). Moving behavioral medicine to the front line: A model for the integration of behavioral and medical science in primary care. *Professional Psychology: Research and Practice, 29,* 230–236.

Pustell, H. B. (1958). A note on use of the MMPI in college counseling. *Journal of Counseling Psychology, 5,* 69–70.

Quereshi, M. Y., & Kleman, R. (1996). Validation of selected MMPI-2 basic and content scales. *Current Psychology: Developmental, Learning, Personality, Social-Psychology, 15*(3), 249–253.

Quill, T. E. (1985). Somatization disorder: One of medicine's blind spots. *Journal of the American Medical Association., 254,* 3075–3079.

Raab, E., Rickels, K., & Moore, E. (1964). A double blind evaluation of tybamate in anxious neurotic medical clinic patients. *American Journal of Psychiatry, 120,* 1005–1007.

Rapaport, D., Gill, M., & Schafer, R. (1946). *Diagnostic psychological testing* (Vol. 1). Chicago: Year Book Medical.

Rawls, D. J., & Rawls, J. R. (1986). Personality characteristics and personal history data of successful and less successful executives. *Psychological Reports, 23,* 1032–1034.

Reckase, M. D. (1996). Test construction in the 1990's: Recent approaches every psychologist should know. *Psychological Assessment, 8,* 354–359.

Reich, J., Steward, M. S., Tupin, J. P., & Rosenblatt, R. M. (1985). Prediction of response to treatment in chronic pain patients. *Journal of Clinical Psychology, 46,* 425–427.

Retzlaff, P. (1992). Professional training in psychological testing: New teachers and new tests. *Journal of Training and Practice in Professional Psychology, 6*(1), 45–50.

Retzlaff, P. (Ed.). (1995). *Tactical psychotherapy of the personality disorders: An MCMI-III based approach.* Needham Heights, MA: Allyn & Bacon.

Retzlaff, P. (1996). MCMI-III diagnostic validity: Bad test or bad validity study? *Journal of Personality Assessment, 66,* 431–437.

Retzlaff, P. (1999). Comment on the validity of the MCMI-III. *Law and Human Behavior, 24,* 499–500.

Retzlaff, P., & Gibertini, M. (1987). Factor structure of the MCMI basic personality scales and common item artifact. *Journal of Personality Assessment, 51,* 588–594.

Retzlaff, P., & Gibertini, M. (1994). Neuropsychometric issues and problems. In R. Vanderploeg (Ed.), *Clinician's guide to neuropsychological assessment* (pp. 277–300). Hillsdale, NJ: Erlbaum.

Retzlaff, P., Ofman, P., Hyer, L., & Matheson, S. (1994). MCMI-II high-point codes: Severe personality disorder and clinical syndrome extensions. *Journal of Clinical Psychology, 50,* 228–234.

Retzlaff, P., Sheehan, E., & Fiel, A. (1991). MCMI-II report style and bias: Profile and validity scales analysis. *Journal of Personality Assessment, 56,* 466–477.

Retzlaff, P., Sheehan, E., & Lorr, M. (1990). MCMI-II scoring: Weighted and unweighted algorithms. *Journal of Personality Assessment, 55,* 219–223.

Retzlaff, P., Stoner, J., & Kleinsasser, D. (2002). Validity of the MCMI-III in corrections. *International Journal of Offender Therapy and Comparative Criminology, 46,* 319–332.

Reynolds, J. F., Mair, D. C., & Fischer, P. C. (1995). *Writing and reading mental health records* (2nd ed.). Mahwah, NJ: Erlbaum.

Robbins, E., Waters, J., & Herbert, P. (1997). Competency to stand trial evaluations: A study of actual practice in two states. *Journal of the American Academy of Psychiatry and Law, 25,* 469–483.

Roberts, R. D., Goff, G. N., Anjoul, F., Kyllonen, P. C., Pallier, G., & Stankov, L. (2001). The Armed Services Vocational Aptitude Battery: Not much more than acculturated learning (Gc)!? *Learning and Individual Differences, 12,* 81–103.

Roberts, R. D., Zeidner, M., & Matthews, G. (2001). Does emotional intelligence meet traditional standards for an intelligence? Some new data and conclusions. *Emotion, 1,* 196–231.

Robins, L. N., Helzer, J. E., Croughan, J., & Ratcliff, K. S. (l98l). National Institute of Mental Health Diagnostic Interview Schedule: Its history, characteristics, and validity. *Archives of General Psychiatry, 38,* 38l–389.

Robins, L. N., Wing, J., Wittchen, H. U., Babor, T. F., Burke, J., Farmer, A., Jablenski, A., Pickens, R., Regier, D. A., Sartorius, N., & Towle, L. H. (1988). The Composite International Diagnostic Interview: An epidemiological instrument suitable for use in conjunction with different diagnostic systems and in different cultures. *Archives of General Psychiatry, 45,* 1069–1077.

Robinson, D. L. (1985). How personality relates to intelligence test performance: Implications for a theory of intelligence, aging research, and personality assessment. *Personality and Individual Differences, 6,* 203–216.

Robinson, D. L. (1986). The Wechsler Adult Intelligence Scale and personality assessment: Towards a biologically based theory of intelligence and cognition. *Personality and Individual Differences, 7,* 153–159.

Rodgers, B., & Mann, S. A. (1986). The reliability and validity of PSE assessments by lay interviewers: A national population survey. *Psychological Medicine, 16,* 689–700.

Rogers, R., & Cavanaugh, J. L. (1983). Usefulness of the Rorschach: A survey of forensic psychologists. *Journal of Psychiatry and Law, 11,* 55–67.

Rogers, R., Bagby, R. M., & Chakraborty, D. (1993). Feigning schizophrenic disorders on the MMPI-2: Detection of coached simulators. *Journal of Personality Assessment, 60,* 215–226.

Rogers, R., Salekin, R. T., & Sewell, K. W. (1999). Validation of the Millon Clinical Multiaxial Inventory for Axis II disorders: Does it meet the *Daubert* standard? *Law and Human Behavior, 23,* 425–443.

Rogler, L. H., Malgady, R., & Rodriguez, O. (1989). *Hispanics and mental health: A framework for research.* Bronx, NY: Fordham University, Hispanic Research Center.

Rokke, P. D., & Scogin, F. (1995). Depression treatment preferences in younger and older adults. *Journal of Clinical Geropsychology, 1,* 243–257.

Rolls, E.T. (1999). *The brain and emotion.* New York: Oxford University Press.

Root, M. P. P. (Ed.). (1992). *Racially mixed people in America.* Newbury Park, CA: Sage.

Rorer, L. G., & Widiger, T. (1983). Personality structure and assessment. *Annual Review of Psychology, 34,* 431–463.

Rorschach, H. (1921). *Psychodiagnostik.* Bern: Bircher.

Rucker, C. (1967). Technical language in the school psychologist's report. *Psychology in the Schools, 4,* 146–150.

Rushton, J. P. (1995). *Race, evolution, and behavior: A life history perspective.* New Brunswick, NJ: Transaction.

Russell, A. J., Munro, J. C., Jones, P. B., & Hemsley, D. R., & Murray, R. M. (1997). Schizophrenia and the myth of intellectual decline. *American Journal of Psychiatry, 154,* 635–639.

Rutter, M. (1994). Beyond longitudinal data: Causes, consequences, changes, and continuity. *Journal of Consulting and Clinical Psychology, 62,* 928–940.

Saklofske, D. H., Austin, E. J., & Minski, P. S. (in press). Factor structure and validity of a trait emotional intelligence measure. *Personality and Individual Differences.*

Saklofske, D. H., Kelly, I. W., & Janzen, B. L. (1995). Neuroticism, depression, and depression proneness. *Personality and Individual Differences, 18*, 27–31.

Saklofske, D. H., & Kostura, D. D. (1990). Extraversion–introversion and intelligence. *Personality and Individual Differences, 6*, 547–551.

Saklofske, D. H., & Zeidner M. (Eds.). (1995). *International handbook of personality and intelligence.* New York: Plenum Press.

Salovey, P., Bedell, B. T., Detweiler, J. B., & Mayer, J. D. (2000). Current directions in emotional intelligence research. In M. Lewis & J. M. Haviland-Jones (Eds.), *Handbook of emotions* (2nd ed., pp. 504–520). New York: Guilford Press.

Salthouse, T. A. (1996). The processing-speed theory of adult age differences in cognition. *Psychological Review, 103*, 403–428.

Sandler, J. Z., Hulgus, Y. F., & Agich, G. J. (1994). On values in recent American psychiatric classification. *Journal of Medicine and Philosophy, 19*, 261–277.

Santy, P. A., Endicott, J., Jones, D. R., Rose, R. M., Patterson, J., Holland, A. W., Faulk, D. M., & Marsh, R. (1993). Results of a structured psychiatric interview to evaluate NASA astronaut candidates. *Military Medicine, 158*, 5–9.

Sarason, I. G., Levine, H. M., Basham, R. B., & Sarason, B. R. (1983). Assessing social support: The Social Support Questionnaire. *Journal of Personality and Social Psychology, 44*, 127–139.

Sarchione, C. D., Cuttler, M. J., Muchinsky, P., & Nelson-Gray, R. O. (1998). Prediction of dysfunctional job behaviors among law enforcement officers. *Journal of Applied Psychology, 83*, 904–912.

Satz, P. (1993). Brain reserve capacity on symptom onset after brain injury: A formulation and review of the evidence for threshold theory. *Neuropsychology, 7*, 273–295.

Satz, P., Morgenstern, H., Miller, E. N., Selnes, O. A., McArthur, J. C., Cohen, B. A., Wesch, J., Becker, J. T., Jacobson, L., D'Elia, L. F., van Gorp, W., & Visscher, B. (1993). Low education as a possible risk factor for cognitive abnormalities in HIV-1: Findings from the Multicenter AIDS Cohort Study (MACS). *Journal of Acquired Immune Deficiency Syndromes, 6*, 503–511.

Savasir, I., & Erol, N. (1990). The Turkish MMPI: Translation, standardization, and validation. In J. N. Butcher & C. D. Spielberger (Eds.), *Advances in personality assessment* (Vol. 8, pp. 49–62). Hillsdale, NJ: Erlbaum.

Scandell, D. J., & Wlazelek, B. G. (1996). Self-presentation strategies on the NEO-Five Factor Inventory: Implications for detecting faking. *Psychological Reports, 79*, 1115–1121.

Schill, T., & Wang, T. (1990). Correlates of the MMPI-2 Anger content scale. *Psychological Reports, 67*, 800–804.

Schmand, B., Smit, J. H., Geerlings, M. I., & Lindeboom, J. (1997). The effects of intelligence and education on the development of dementia. A test of the brain reserve hypothesis. *Psychological Medicine, 27*, 1337–1344.

Schofield, P. W., Mosesson, R. E., Stern, Y., & Mayeux, R. (1995). The age at onset of Alzheimer's disease and an intracranial area measurement: A relationship. *Archives of Neurology, 52*, 95–98.

Schofield, W. (1950). Changes in responses to the MMPI following certain therapies. *Psychological Monographs, 64*(5, Whole No. 311).

Schofield, W. (1953). A further study of the effects of therapies on MMPI responses. *Journal of Abnormal and Social Psychology, 48*, 67–77.

Schretlen, D. J. (1988). The use of psychological tests to identify malingered symptoms of mental disorder. *Clinical Psychology Review, 8,* 451–476.

Schroer, A. C. P., & Dorn, F. J. (1986). Enhancing the career and personal development of gifted college students. *Journal of Counseling and Development, 64,* 567–571.

Schulz, R., & Tompkins, C. A. (1990). Life events and changes in social relationships: Examples, mechanisms, and measurement. *Journal of Social and Clinical Psychology, 9,* 69–77.

Schutte, N. S., Malouff, J. M., Hall, L. E., Haggerty, D. J., Cooper, J. T., Golden, C. J., & Dornheim, L. (1998). Development and validation of a measure of emotional intelligence. *Personality and Individual Differences, 25,* 167–177.

Schwartz, C. E., Kozora, E., & Zeng, Q. (1996). Towards patient collaboration in cognitive assessment: Specificity, sensitivity, and incremental validity of self-report. *Annals of Behavioral Medicine, 18,* 177–184.

Schwean, V. L., & Saklofske, D. H. (1998). WISC-III assessment of children with attention-deficit/hyperactivity disorder. In A. Pripitera & D. H. Saklofske (Eds.), *WISC-III clinical use and interpretation* (pp. 91–118). San Diego, CA: Academic Press.

Scogin, F. (2000). *The first session with seniors.* San Francisco: Jossey-Bass.

Scogin, F., Rohen, N., & Bailey, E. (2000). Geriatric Depression Scale. In M. Maruish (Ed.), *Handbook of psychological assessment in primary care settings* (pp. 491–508). Mahwah, NJ: Erlbaum.

Scogin, F., Schumacher, J., Gardner, J., & Chaplin, W. (1995). Predictive validity of psychological testing in law enforcement settings. *Professional Psychology: Research and Practice, 26*(1), 68–71.

Seligman, M. E. P., & Csikszentmihalyi, M. (2000). Positive psychology: An introduction. *American Psychologist, 55,* 5–14.

Shaffer, T. W., Erdberg, P., & Haroian, J. (1999). Current nonpatient data for the Rorschach, WAIS-R, and MMPI-2. *Journal of Personality Assessment, 73,* 305–316.

Shapiro, D. (1976). *Neurotic styles.* New York: Basic Books.

Shealy, R. C., Lowe, J. D., & Ritzier, B. A. (1980). Sleep onset insomnia: Personality outcomes. *Journal of Consulting and Clinical Psychology, 48,* 659–661.

Shefler, G., & Tishby, O. (1998). Interjudge reliability and agreement about the patient's central issue in time-limited psychotherapy (TLP) and its relation to TLP outcome. *Psychotherapy Research, 8,* 426–438.

Sheikh, J. I., & Yesavage, J. A. (1986). Geriatric Depression Scale: Recent evidence and development of a shorter version. *Clinical Gerontology, 5,* 165–172.

Sheldon, K. M., & King, L. (2001). Why positive psychology is necessary. *American Psychologist, 56,* 216–217.

Shiang, J., Kjellander, C., Huang, K., & Bogumill, S. (1998). Developing cultural competency in clinical practice: Treatment considerations for Chinese cultural groups in the United States. *Clinical Psychology: Science and Practice, 5,* 182–210.

Shondrick D. D., Ben-Porath, Y. S., & Stafford, K. (1992, May). *Forensic assessment with the MMPI-2: Characteristics of individuals undergoing court-ordered evaluations.* Paper presented at the 27th Annual Symposium on Recent Developments in the Use of the MMPI/MMPI-2, Minneapolis, MN.

Shure, G.H., & Rogers, M.S. (1963). Personality factor stability for three ability levels. *Journal of Psychology, 55,* 445–456.

Siegel, C., & Fischer, S. K. (1981). *Psychiatric records in mental health care.* New York: Brunner/Mazel.

Sipps, G. J., Berry, G. W., & Lynch E. M. (1987). WAIS-R and social intelligence: A test of established assumptions that uses the CPI. *Journal of Clinical Psychology, 43,* 499–504.

Skre, I., Onstad, S., Torgersen, S., & Kringlen, E. (1991). High interrater reliability for the Structured Clinical Interview for the DSM-III-R Axis I (SCID-I). *Acta Psychiatrica Scandanavica, 84,* 167–173.

Smith, D., & Dumont, F. (1997). Eliminating overconfidence in psychodiagnosis: Strategies for training and practice. *Clinical Psychology—Science and Practice, 4,* 335–345.

Snowdon, D. A., Kemper, S. J., Mortimer, J. A., Greiner, L. H., Wekstein, D. R., & Markesbery, W. R. (1996). Linguistic ability in early life and cognitive function and Alzheimer's disease in later life: Findings from the Nun Study. *Journal of the American Medical Association, 275,* 528–532.

Sobel, D. S. (2000). Mind matters, money matters: The cost effectiveness of mind–body medicine. *Journal of the American Medical Association, 284,* 1705.

Soskin, W. F. (1959). Influence of four types of data on diagnostic conceptualization in psychological testing. *Journal of Abnormal and Social Psychology, 58,* 69–78.

Spickard, P. R. (1992). The illogic of American racial categories. In P. P. M. Root (Ed.), *Racially mixed people in America* (pp. 12–23). Newbury Park, CA: Sage.

Spielberger, C. D., Gorsuch, R. L., Lushene, R., Vagg, P. R., & Jacobs, G. A. (1983a). *Manual for the State–Trait Anxiety Inventory.* Palo Alto, CA: Consulting Psychologists Press.

Spielberger, C. D., Gorsuch, R. L., Lushene, R., Vagg, P. R., & Jacobs, G. A. (1983b). *State–Trait Anxiety Inventory.* Palo Alto, CA: Consulting Psychologists Press.

Spitzer, R. L., Williams, J. B. W., & Gibbon, M. (1986). *The Structured Clinical Interview for DSM-III-R—patient version.* New York: New York State Psychiatric Institute.

Spitzer, R. L., Williams, J. B. W., Gibbon, M., & First, M. B. (1990). *User's guide for the structured clinical interview for DSM-III-R: SCID.* Washington, DC: American Psychiatric Press.

Spitzer, R. L., Williams, J. B. W., Gibbon, M., & First, M. B. (1992). The Structured Clinical Interview for DSM-III-R (SCID-I): History, rationale, and description. *Archives of General Psychiatry, 49,* 624–629.

Spitzer, R. L., Williams, J. B. W., Kroenke, K., Linzer, M., deGruy, F. V., III, Hahn, S. R., Brody, D., & Johnson, J. G. (1994). Utility of a new procedure for diagnosing mental disorders in primary care: The PRIME-MD 1000 Study. *Journal of the American Medical Association, 272,* 1749–1756.

Staal, W. G., Hijman, R., Pol, H. E. H., & Kahn, R. S. (2000). Neuropsychological dysfunctions in siblings discordant for schizophrenia. *Psychiatry Research, 95,* 227–235.

Standage, K. (1990). A classification of respondents to the CPI Socialization scale: Associations with diagnosis and other clinical variables. *Personality and Individual Differences, 11,* 335–341.

Standage, K., Smith, D., & Norman, R. (1988). A classification of respondents to the

CPI Socialization scale: Associations with psychiatric diagnosis and implications for research. *Personality and Individual Differences, 9*, 231–236.

Stern, R. A., Silva, S. G., Chaisson, N., & Evans, D. L. (1996). Influence of cognitive reserve on neuropsychological functioning in asymptomatic Human Immunodeficiency Virus-1 infection. *Archives of Neurology, 53*, 148–153.

Stern, Y., Gurland, B., Tatemichi, T. K., Tang, M. X., Wilder, D., & Mayeux, R. (1994). Influence of education and occupation on the incidence of Alzheimer's disease. *Journal of the American Medical Association, 271*, 1004–1010.

Sternberg, R. J., & Grigorenko, E. L. (2001). Unified psychology. *American Psychologist, 56*, 1069–1079.

Sternberg, R. J., Wagner, R. K., Williams, W. M., & Horvath, J. A. (1995). Testing common sense. *American Psychologist, 50*, 912–927.

Strupp, H. H., & Binder, J. L. (1984). *Psychotherapy in a new key.* New York: Basic Books.

Strupp, H. H., Horowitz, L. M., & Lambert, M. J. (1997). *Measuring patient changes in mood, anxiety, and personality disorders: Toward a core battery.* Washington, DC: American Psychological Association.

Sue, S. W., Fujino, D. C., Hu, L. T., Takeuchi, D. T., & Zane, N. W. S. (1991). Community mental health services for racial and ethnic minority groups: A test of the cultural responsiveness hypothesis. *Journal of Counseling Psychology, 59*, 533–540.

Sue, S. W., & Sue, D. (1990). *Counseling the culturally different: Theory and practice* (2nd ed.). New York: Wiley.

Suen, H. K. (1990). *Principles of test theories.* Hillsdale, NJ: Erlbaum.

Suinn, R., Rickard-Figueroa, K., Lew, S., & Vigil, P. (1987). The Suinn–Lew Asian Self-Identity Acculturation Scale: An initial report. *Educational and Psychological Measurement, 47*, 401–407.

Summerfeldt, L. J., & Antony, M. M. (2002). Structured and semistructured diagnostic interviews. In M. M. Antony & D. H. Barlow (Eds.), *Handbook of assessment and treatment planning for psychological disorders* (pp. 3–37). New York: Guilford Press.

Sundberg, N. D. (1961). The practice of psychological testing in clinical services in the United States. *American Psychologist, 16*, 79–83.

Swaab, D. F. (1991). Brain aging and Alzheimer's disease: "Wear and tear" versus "use it or lose it." *Neurobiology of Aging, 12*, 317–324.

Sweeney, J. A., Clarkin, J. F., & Fitzgibbon, M. L. (1987). Current practice of psychological assessment. *Professional Psychology: Research and Practice, 18*, 377–380.

Tallent N. (1993). *Psychological report writing* (4th ed.). Englewood Cliffs, NJ: Prentice-Hall.

Tallent, N., & Reiss, W. J. (1959a). Multidisciplinary views on the preparation of written clinical psychological reports: I. Spontaneous suggestions for content. *Journal of Clinical Psychology, 15*, 218–221.

Tallent, N., & Reiss, W. J. (1959b). Multidisciplinary views on the preparation of written clinical psychological reports: II. Acceptability of certain common content variables and styles of expression. *Journal of Clinical Psychology, 15*, 218–221.

Tellegen A., & Ben-Porath, Y. S. (1992). The new uniform T scores for the MMPI: Rationale, derivation, and appraisal. *Psychological Assessment, 4,* 145–155.

Thorndike, E. L. (1920). Intelligence and its use. *Harper Magazine, 140,* 227–235.

Thorndike, E. L. (1940). *Human nature and social order.* New York: Macmillan.

Topping, G. D., & O'Gorman, J. G. (1997). Effects of faking set on validity of the NEO-FFI. *Personality and Individual Differences, 23,* 117–124.

Turner, S. M., DeMers, S. T., Fox, H. R., & Reed, G. M. (2001). APA's guidelines of test user qualifications: An executive summary. *American Psychologist, 56*(12), 1099–1113.

Vaillant, G. E. (2000). Adaptive mental mechanisms: Their role in a positive psychology. *American Psychologist, 55,* 89–98.

Vandiver, B. J., Cross, W. E., Worrell, F. C., & Fhagen-Smith, P. E. (2002). Validating the Cross Racial Identity Scale. *Journal of Counseling Psychology, 49,* 71–85.

Vassend, O., Watten, R., Myhrer, T., & Syvertsen, J. L. (1994). Negative affectivity and intellectual ability: A study of their relation to self-reported physical symptoms, perceived daily stress and mood, and disciplinary problems in military recruits. *Social Science and Medicine, 39,* 583–590.

Vernon, P. E. (1953). *Personality tests and assessments.* London: Methuen.

Viglione, D. J. (1999). A review of recent research addressing the utility of the Rorschach. *Psychological Assessment, 11,* 251–265.

Viglione, D. J., Brager, R. C., & Haller, N. (1988). Usefulness of structural Rorschach data in identifying inpatients with depressive symptoms: A preliminary study. *Journal of Personality Assessment, 52,* 524–529.

Wagner, E. E., & Dobbins, R. D. (1967). MMPI profiles of parishioners seeking pastoral counseling. *Journal of Consulting Psychology, 31,* 83–84.

Wakefield, H., & Underwager, R. (1993). Misuse of psychological tests in forensic settings: Some horrible examples. *American Journal of Forensic Psychology, 11,* 55–75.

Walters, G. D., White, T. W., & Greene, R. L. (1988). Use of the MMPI to identify malingering and exaggeration of psychiatric symptomology in male prison inmates. *Journal of Consulting and Clinical Psychology, 56,* 111–117.

Watkins, C. E., Jr., Campbell, V. L., Nieberding, R., & Hallmark, R. (1995). Contemporary practice of psychological assessment by clinical psychologists. *Professional Psychology: Research and Practice, 26,* 54–60.

Watson, D., & Pennebaker, J. W. (1989). Health complaints, stress, and distress: Exploring the central role of negative affectivity. *Psychological Review, 96,* 234–254.

Wechsler, D. (1987). *Wechsler Memory Scale—Revised manual.* New York: Psychological Corporation.

Wechsler, D. A. (1997). *WAIS-III administration and scoring manual.* San Antonio, TX: Psychological Corporation.

Weed, N. C., Butcher, J. N., Ben-Porath, Y. S., & McKenna, T. (1992). New measures for assessing alcohol and drug abuse: The APS and AAS. *Journal of Personality Assessment, 58,* 389–404.

Weiner, I. B. (1993). Clinical considerations in the conjoint use of the Rorschach and the MMPI. *Journal of Personality Assessment, 60,* 148–152.

Weiner, I. B. (1997). Current status of the Rorschach inkblot method. *Journal of Personality Assessment, 68,* 5–19.

Weiner, I. B. (1999). What the Rorschach can do for you: Incremental validity in clinical applications. *Assessment, 6,* 327–338.

Weiner, I. B. (2001). Advancing the science of psychological assessment: The Rorschach inkblot method as exemplar. *Psychological Assessment, 13,* 423–432.

Weiner, I. B., & Exner, J. E., Jr. (1991). Rorschach changes in long-term and short-term psychotherapy. *Journal of Personality Assessment, 56,* 453–465.

Weiner, I. B., Exner, J. E., Jr., & Sciara, A. (1996). Is the Rorschach welcome in the courtroom? *Journal of Personality Assessment, 67,* 422–424.

Weiner, J. (1985). Teachers' comprehension of psychological reports. *Psychology in the Schools, 22,* 60–64.

Weiss, D. S. (1981). A multigroup study of personality patterns in creativity. *Perceptual and Motor Skills, 52,* 735–746.

Wells, A., & Matthews, G. (1994). Attention and emotion: A clinical perspective. Hove, UK: Erlbaum.

Westen, D. (1991). Social cognition and object relations. *Psychological Bulletin, 109,* 429–455.

Wetter, M. W., Baer, R. A., Berry, D. T., Robison, L. H., & Sumpter, J. (1993). MMPI-2 profiles of motivated fakers given specific symptom information. *Psychological Assessment, 5,* 317–323.

Wetter, M. W., Baer, R. A., Berry, D. T., Smith, G. T., & Larsen, L. (1992). Sensitivity of the MMPI-2 validity scales to random responding and malingering. *Psychological Assessment, 4,* 369–374.

Whalley, L. J., Starr, J. M., Athawes, M. B., Hunter, M. A., Pattie, A., & Deary, I. J. (2000). Childhood mental ability and dementia. *Neurology, 55,* 1455–1459.

Whisman, M. A., Strosahl, K., Fruzzetti, A. E., Schmaling, K. B., Jacobson, N. S., & Miller, D. M. (1989). A structured interview version of the Hamilton Rating Scale for Depression: Reliability and Validity. *Psychological Assessment, 1,* 238–241.

Widiger, T. A., & Spitzer, R. L. (1991). Sex bias in the diagnosis of personality disorders: Conceptual and methodological issues. *Clinical Psychology Review, 11,* 1–22.

Wills, T. A. (1978). Perceptions of clients by professional helpers. *Psychological Bulletin, 85,* 968–1000.

Wing, J. K., Nixon, J. M., Mann, S. A., & Leff, J. P. (1977). Reliability of the PSE (ninth edition) used in a population study. *Psychological Medicine, 7,* 505–516.

Wink, P., & Helson, R. (1993). Personality change in women and their partners. *Journal of Personality and Social Psychology, 65,* 597–605.

Witteman, C., & Koele, P. (1999). Explaining treatment decisions. *Psychotherapy Research, 9,* 100–114.

Wohlwill, J., & Carson, D. (Eds.). (1972). *Environment and the social sciences.* Washington, DC: American Psychological Association.

Wolber, G. J., & Carne, W. F. (1993). *Writing psychological reports, a guide for clinicians.* Sarasota, FL: Professional Resource Press.

Wood, J. M., Nezworski, M. T., Garb, H. N., & Lilienfeld, S. O. (2001). The misperception of psychopathology: Problems with the norms of the comprehensive system for the Rorschach. *Clinical Psychology: Science and Practice, 8,* 350–373.

Wood, J. M., Nezworski, M. T., & Stejskal, W. J. (1996). The comprehensive system for the Rorschach: A critical examination. *Psychological Science, 7,* 3–10.

Woody, R. H. (1980). Critical discussion. In R. H. Woody (Ed.), *Encyclopedia of clinical assessment* (Vol. 2). San Francisco: Jossey-Bass.

Wright, B. A., & Fletcher, B. (1982). Uncovering hidden resources: A challenge in assessment. *Professional Psychology, 13,* 229–235.

Yang, J., McCrae, R. R., Costa, P. T., Dai, X., Yao, S., Cai, T., & Gao, B. (1999). Cross-cultural personality assessment in psychiatric populations: The NEO-PI-R in the People's Republic of China. *Psychological Assessment, 11,* 359–368.

Yee, A. H. (1983). Ethnicity and race: Psychological perspectives. *Educational Psychologist, 18,* 14–24.

Yee, A. H., Fairchild, H. H., Weizmann, F., & Wyatt, G. E. (1993). Addressing psychology's problem with race. *American Psychologist, 48,* 1132–1140.

Yesavage, J. A., Brink, T. L., Rose, T. L., Lum, O., Huang, V., Adey, M., & Leirer, V. O. (1983). Development and validation of a geriatric depression screening scale: A preliminary report. *Journal of Psychiatric Research, 17,* 37–49.

Yokley, J. M., & Reuter, J. M. (1989). The computer-assisted Child Diagnostic System: A research and development project. *Computers in Human Development, 5,* 277–295.

Yzaguirre, R., & Perez, S. M. (1995, January). Racial/ethnic categories: A symposium. *Bulletin of the Institute for Children, Youth, and Family, 13,* 2–10.

Zarit, S. H., & Zarit, J. M. (1998). *Mental disorders in older adults: Fundamentals of assessment and treatment* (pp. 83–85). New York: Guilford Press.

Zeidner, M. (1995). Personality trait correlates of intelligence. In D. H. Saklofske & M. Zeidner (Eds.), *International handbook of personality and intelligence* (pp. 299–347). New York: Plenum Press.

Zeidner, M. (1998). *Test anxiety.* New York: Plenum Press.

Zeidner, M., & Matthews, G. (2000). Personality and intelligence. In R. J. Sternberg (Ed.), *Handbook of human intelligence* (2nd ed.). New York: Cambridge University Press.

Zeidner, M., Matthews, G., & Saklofske, D. H. (1998). Intelligence and mental health. In N. Adler, R. Parke, C. Peterson, R. Roskoski, R. Schwarzer, R. Silver, D. Spiegel, & H. Friedman (Eds.), *Encyclopedia of mental health* (Vol. 2, pp. 521–534). San Diego, CA: Academic Press.

Zeidner, M., & Saklofske, D. H. (1996). Adaptive and maladaptive coping. In M. Zeidner & N. S. Endler (Eds.), *Handbook of coping: Theory, research, applications* (pp. 505–531). New York: Wiley.

Zimmerman, M. (1983). Methodological issues in the assessment of life events: A review of issues and research. *Clinical Psychology Review, 3,* 339–370.

Ziskin, J. (1995) *Coping with psychiatric and psychological testimony.* Los Angeles, CA: Law and Psychology Press.

Zuckerman, E. L. (2000). *Clinician's thesaurus: The guidebook for writing psychological reports* (5th ed.). New York: Guilford Press.

Zuckerman, M. (1990). Some dubious premises in research and theory on racial differences: Scientific, social, and ethical issues. *American Psychologist, 45,* 1297–1303.

Zuckerman, M. (1999). *Vulnerability to psychopathology.* Washington, DC: American Psychological Association.

Index

Page numbers followed by an *f* indicate figure, *t* indicate table.